ESSENTIALS OF PHYSIOLOGY
for Paramedical Students

ESSENTIALS OF PHYSIOLOGY
for Paramedical Students

K Sembulingam PhD
Formerly at
MR Medical College, Kalaburagi, Karnataka, India
Sri Ramachandra Medical College and Research Institute Chennai, Tamil Nadu, India
School of Health Sciences, Universiti Sains Malaysia, Kelantan, Malaysia
Sri Lakshmi Narayana Institute of Medical Sciences, Puducherry, India
Sri Manakula Vinayagar Medical College and Hospital, Puducherry, India
Shri Sathya Sai Medical College and Research Institute, Nellikuppam, Tamil Nadu, India
Madha Medical College & Research Institute, Chennai, Tamil Nadu, India

Prema Sembulingam PhD
Formerly at
MR Medical College, Kalaburagi, Karnataka, India
Sri Ramachandra Medical College and Research Institute, Chennai, Tamil Nadu, India
School of Health Sciences, Universiti Sains Malaysia, Kelantan, Malaysia
Sri Lakshmi Narayana Institute of Medical Sciences, Puducherry, India
Sathyabama University Dental College and Hospital, Chennai, Tamil Nadu, India
Sri Manakula Vinayagar Medical College and Hospital, Puducherry, India
Shri Sathya Sai Medical College and Research Institute, Nellikuppam, Tamil Nadu, India
Madha Medical College & Research Institute, Chennai, Tamil Nadu, India

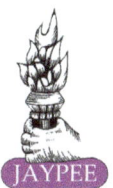

JAYPEE BROTHERS MEDICAL PUBLISHERS
The Health Sciences Publisher
New Delhi | London

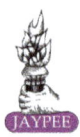 **Jaypee Brothers Medical Publishers (P) Ltd**

Headquarters
Jaypee Brothers Medical Publishers (P) Ltd
EMCA House, 23/23-B
Ansari Road, Daryaganj
New Delhi - 110 002, India
Landline: +91-11-23272143,+91-11-23272703, +91-11-23282021,+91-11-23245672
Head Office : 011-43574357
Email: jaypee@jaypeebrothers.com

Corporate Office
Jaypee Brothers Medical Publishers (P) Ltd
4838/24, Ansari Road, Daryaganj
New Delhi 110 002, India
Phone: +91-11-43574357
Fax: +91-11-43574314
Email: jaypee@jaypeebrothers.com

Overseas Office
J.P. Medical Ltd
83 Victoria Street, London
SW1H 0HW (UK)
Phone: +44 20 3170 8910
Fax: +44 (0)20 3008 6180
Email: info@jpmedpub.com

Website: www.jaypeebrothers.com
Website: www.jaypeedigital.com

© 2021, Jaypee Brothers Medical Publishers

The views and opinions expressed in this book are solely those of the original contributor (s)/author (s) and do not necessarily represent those of editor (s) of the book.

All rights reserved. No part of this publication may be reproduced, stored or transmitted in any form or by any means, electronic, mechanical, photocopying, recording or otherwise, without the prior permission in writing of the publishers/editors.

All brand names and product names used in this book are trade names, service marks, trademarks or registered trademarks of their respective owners. The publisher is not associated with any product or vendor mentioned in this book.

Medical knowledge and practice change constantly. This book is designed to provide accurate, authoritative information about the subject matter in question. However, readers are advised to check the most current information available on procedures included and check information from the manufacturer of each product to be administered, to verify the recommended dose, formula, method and duration of administration, adverse effects and contraindications. It is the responsibility of the practitioner to take all appropriate safety precautions. Neither the publisher nor the author (s)/editor (s) assume any liability for any injury and/or damage to persons or property arising from or related to use of material in this book.

This book is sold on the understanding that the publisher is not engaged in providing professional medical services. If such advice or services are required, the services of a competent medical professional should be sought.

Every effort has been made where necessary to contact holders of copyright to obtain permission to reproduce copyright material. If any have been inadvertently overlooked, the publisher will be pleased to make the necessary arrangements at the first opportunity. The **CD/ DVD-ROM** (if any) provided in the sealed envelope with this book is complimentary and free of cost. **Not meant for sale**.

Inquiries for bulk sales may be solicited at: jaypee@jaypeebrothers.com

Essentials of Physiology for Paramedical Students

First Edition: **2021**

ISBN: 978-93-5025-116-4

In Loving Memory of

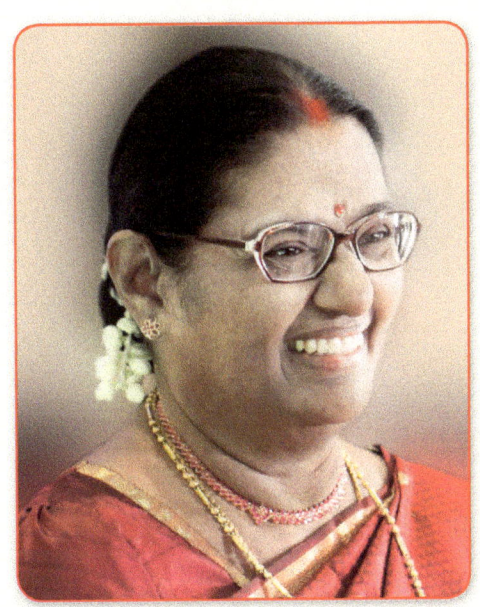

Dr Prema Sembulingam

Preface

We, the authors of "*Essentials of Medical Physiology*" and "*Essentials of Physiology for Dental Students*" are proud to bring out another textbook in Physiology, titled "*Essentials of Physiology for Paramedical Students*". This is the outcome of the requests, wishes and friendly orders from different category of people including students of health sciences and staff.

The primary aim of this book is to meet the needs of all students of health sciences specifically, in getting knowledge of recent developments in the field of physiology, in knowing the important applied aspects of various topics and also from examination point of view.

This book will be very much beneficial to students of Nursing, Pharmacy, Allied Health Science, Biotechnology, all other paramedical courses and health-related courses.

Though we have planned to publish such book for health sciences students long back, it was possible to execute it now only due to various reasons.

It could not have been possible to bring this book out but for the efforts and hard work from my life partner and the co-author of all our books Dr Prema Sembulingam. Her encouragements, emotional support, and her expectations and dreams of publishing this book will be evergreen in memory for years to come.

Though we miss her now, the efforts and work rendered by her for this book also could not be forgotten. That made me to mention "We" in this preface.

We wish to continue our services to the students' community through this book. We are confident that the opinions, comments, and valuable suggestions from one and all coming across for this book will help us to improve it further to meet the needs of everyone who have Physiology as a subject in their career.

We thank all our friends who had helped us in processing the script of this book.

We are grateful to **Shri Jitendar P Vij** (Group Chairman), **Mr Ankit Vij** (Managing Director), **Mr MS Mani** (Group President) and **Ms Chetna Malhotra Vohra** (Associate Director–Content Strategy) of M/s Jaypee Brothers Medical Publishers (P) Ltd, New Delhi, India for publishing the book in the same format as we wanted.

We are also grateful to **Dr Madhu Choudhary** (Publishing Head–Education), **Ms Pooja Bhandari** (Production Head) and **Ms Sunita Katla** (Executive Assistant to Group Chairman and Publishing Manager) for coordinating the processing of this edition. We thank **Dr Sneha Kashyap** (Development Editor), **Ms Seema Dogra** (Cover Visualizer), **Ms Geeta Srivastava** (Proofreader), **Ms Neelam Kakriya** (Proofreader), **Mr Dinesh Bhardwaj** (Typesetter), **Mr Varun Rajoria** (Graphic Designer) and all other staff of M/s Jaypee Brothers Medical Publishers (P) Ltd, New Delhi, India for their wholehearted contribution while formatting the book.

K Sembulingam
DrSembu@gmail.com

Contents

Section 1: General Physiology

1. Cell 1
2. Cell Junctions 11
3. Transport Through Cell Membrane 14
4. Homeostasis 20

Section 2: Blood and Body Fluids

5. Body Fluids 23
6. Blood 28
7. Red Blood Cells 33
8. Erythropoiesis 37
9. Hemoglobin and Iron Metabolism 41
10. Erythrocyte Sedimentation Rate, Packed Cell Volume, Blood Indices and Anemia 44
11. White Blood Cells 49
12. Immunity 54
13. Platelets 60
14. Hemostasis 62
15. Coagulation of Blood 64
16. Blood Groups and Blood Transfusion 69
17. Reticuloendothelial System, Tissue Macrophage and Spleen 74
18. Lymphatic System, Lymph, Tissue Fluid and Edema 77

Section 3: Muscle Physiology

19. Classification of Muscles 83
20. Structure of Skeletal Muscle 85
21. Properties of Skeletal Muscle 89
22. Changes During Muscular Contraction 94
23. Neuromuscular Junction 100
24. Smooth Muscle 103

Section 4: Digestive System

25. Overview of Digestive System 109
26. Mouth and Salivary Secretion 112
27. Stomach and Gastric Secretion 117
28. Pancreas and Pancreatic Secretion 125
29. Liver and Biliary System 130
30. Small Intestine, Large Intestine and their Secretions 137
31. Movements of Gastrointestinal Tract 142

Section 5: Renal Physiology and Skin

32. Overview of Renal System 149
33. Nephron 151
34. Juxtaglomerular Apparatus 155
35. Renal Circulation 158
36. Urine Formation 160
37. Concentration of Urine 166
38. Acidification of Urine and Role of Kidney in Acid-base Balance 170
39. Renal Function Tests, Renal Failure, Dialysis and Diuretics 173
40. Micturition 177
41. Skin 182
42. Body Temperature 186

Section 6: Endocrinology

43. Overview of Endocrine System 191
44. Pituitary Gland 196
45. Thyroid Gland 205
46. Parathyroid Glands and Physiology of Bone 212
47. Endocrine Functions of Pancreas 218
48. Adrenal Cortex 224
49. Adrenal Medulla 231
50. Endocrine Functions of Other Organs and Local Hormones 234

Section 7: Reproductive System

51. Male Reproductive System 239
52. Female Reproductive System 248
53. Menstrual Cycle 253
54. Pregnancy, Parturition, Mammary Glands and Lactation 262
55. Fertility Control 268

Section 8: Cardiovascular System

56. Overview of Cardiovascular System 275
57. Properties of Cardiac Muscle 280
58. Cardiac Cycle 284
59. Heart Sounds and Cardiac Murmur 289
60. Electrocardiogram and Arrhythmia 292
61. Cardiac Output 298
62. Heart Rate 301
63. Blood Pressure 305
64. Arterial Pulse and Venous Pulse 313
65. Regional Circulation and Fetal Circulation 317
66. Hemorrhage, Circulatory Shock and Heart Failure 324
67. Cardiovascular Adjustments during Exercise 328

Section 9: Respiratory System and Environmental Physiology

68. Respiratory Tract and Pulmonary Circulation 333
69. Mechanics of Respiration 338
70. Pulmonary Function Tests 342
71. Ventilation and Dead Space 347
72. Exchange and Transport of Respiratory Gases 350
73. Regulation of Respiration 356
74. Diseases and Disorders of Respiration 360
75. High Altitude, Deep Sea Physiology and Exposure to Cold and Heat 366
76. Artificial Respiration 371
77. Effects of Exercise on Respiration 374

Section 10: NERVOUS SYSTEM

78. Overview of Nervous System, Neuron and Neuroglia 377
79. Receptors, Synapse and Neurotransmitters 387
80. Reflex Activity 395
81. Spinal Cord 400
82. Somatosensory System and Somatomotor System 412
83. Physiology of Pain 419
84. Thalamus and Hypothalamus 423
85. Cerebellum 430
86. Basal Ganglia 434
87. Cerebral Cortex, Limbic System and Reticular Formation 437
88. Proprioceptors, Posture, Equilibrium and Vestibular Apparatus 447
89. Electroencephalogram, Epilepsy and Sleep 454
90. Higher Intellectual Functions 460
91. Cerebrospinal Fluid 464
92. Autonomic Nervous System 468

Section 11: Special Senses

93. Eye 475
94. Visual Process and Field of Vision 482
95. Visual Pathway 487
96. Pupillary Reflexes, Refractive Errors and Color Vision 491
97. Ear 498
98. Auditory Pathway 502
99. Mechanism of Hearing and Auditory Defects 504
100. Sensations of Taste and Smell 508

Index 515

SECTION 1 GENERAL PHYSIOLOGY

CHAPTER 1

Cell

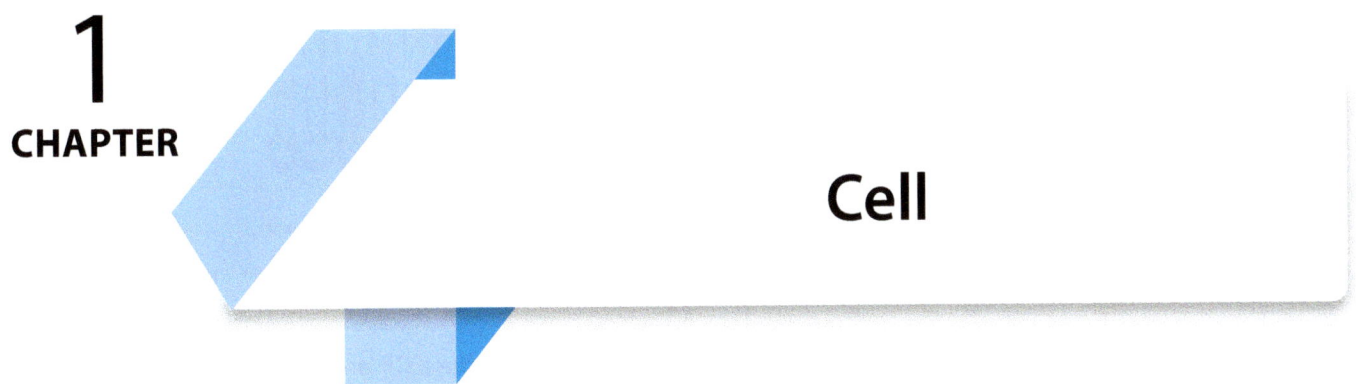

CHAPTER OUTLINE

- CELL, TISSUE, ORGAN AND SYSTEM
- STRUCTURE OF THE CELL
- CELL MEMBRANE
- CYTOPLASM
- ORGANELLES IN CYTOPLASM
- ORGANELLES WITH LIMITING MEMBRANE
- ORGANELLES WITHOUT LIMITING MEMBRANE
- NUCLEUS
- DEOXYRIBONUCLEIC ACID: DNA
- GENE
- RIBONUCLEIC ACID: RNA
- GENE EXPRESSION
- CELL DEATH

CELL, TISSUE, ORGAN AND SYSTEM

CELL

All living organisms are composed of many blocks of cells. Each single has all the characteristics of life.

Cell is **defined** as the structural and functional unit of the living body.

TISSUE

Tissue is defined as the group of cells having similar function. Tissues are classified into four primary tissues.

Primary tissues are:

1. *Epithelial tissue:* Squamous, columnar and cuboidal epithelial cells.
2. *Connective tissue:* Connective tissue proper, cartilage, bone and blood.
3. *Muscle tissue:* Skeletal muscle, smooth muscle and cardiac muscle.
4. *Nervous tissue:* Neurons and supporting cells.

ORGAN

An organ is the structure that is formed by two or more primary types of tissues. Some organs are composed of all the four types of primary tissues. Organs may be **tubular** like intestine or **hollow** like stomach.

SYSTEM

System is the group of organs which work together to carry out specific functions of the body. Each system performs a specific function.

For example, digestive system is concerned with digestion of food particles. Cardiovascular system is responsible for transport of substances between the organs. Respiratory system is concerned with the supply of oxygen and removal of carbon dioxide. Endocrine system is concerned with growth of the body and regulation and maintenance of normal life. Nervous system controls the locomotion and other activities including the intellectual functions.

STRUCTURE OF THE CELL

Each cell is formed by a cell body and a cell membrane or plasma membrane that covers the cell body.

Important parts of a cell are:

I. Cell membrane.
II. Cytoplasm with organelles.
III. Nucleus.

CELL MEMBRANE

Cell membrane is a protective sheath that envelops the cell body **(Fig. 1.1)**. It separates the fluid outside the cell called extracellular fluid (ECF) and the fluid inside the cell called intracellular fluid (ICF). It is a **semipermeable membrane** and allows free exchange of certain substances between ECF and ICF. Thickness of the cell membrane varies from 75 to 111Å.

COMPOSITION OF CELL MEMBRANE

Cell membrane is composed of three types of substances:

Section 1: General Physiology

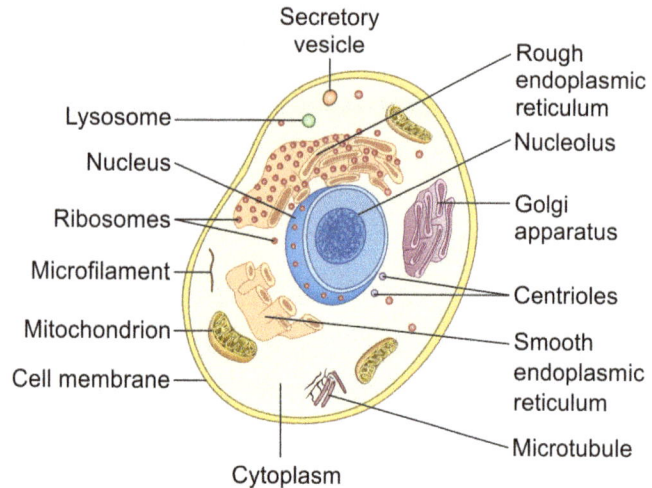

FIGURE 1.1: Structure of the cell.

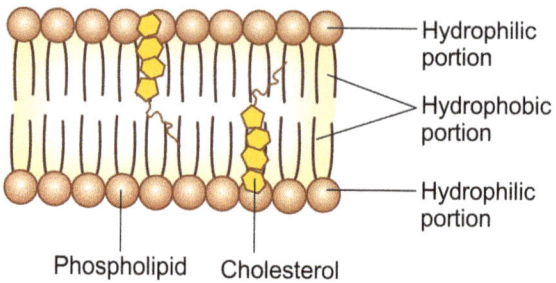

FIGURE 1.3: Lipids of the cell membrane.

1. Proteins (55%).
2. Lipids (40%).
3. Carbohydrates (5%).

■ STRUCTURE OF CELL MEMBRANE

Cell membrane is called a **unit membrane** or a three-layered membrane. Three layers of cell membrane are, one **electron-lucent lipid layer** in the center and two **electron-dense protein layers**. The two electron-dense protein layers are placed on either side of the central lipid layer. Carbohydrate molecules are found on the surface of the cell membrane.

Lipid Layer of Cell Membrane

It is a bilayered structure formed by a thin film of lipids (Fig. 1.2). It is fluid in nature and the portions of the membrane along with the dissolved substances move to all areas of the cell membrane. Major lipids are phospholipids and cholesterol.

1. Phospholipids

Phospholipid molecules are formed by phosphorus and fatty acids. Each phospholipid molecule resembles the headed pin in shape (Fig. 1.3). Outer part of phospholipid molecule is the head portion which is water soluble (hydrophilic). The inner part is the tail portion that is not soluble in water (hydrophobic). The hydrophobic tail portions meet in the center of the membrane. The hydrophilic head portions of outer layer face the ECF and those of the inner layer face the cytoplasm.

2. Cholesterol

Cholesterol molecules are arranged in between the phospholipid molecules.

Functions of lipid layer

Lipid layer is semipermeable in nature and allows only the fat-soluble substances like oxygen, carbon dioxide and alcohol to pass through it. It does not allow the water-soluble materials like glucose, urea and electrolytes to pass through it.

Protein Layers of the Cell Membrane

Protein layers of the cell membrane are electron-dense layers situated on either side of the central lipid layer. The protein molecules present in these layers are mostly glycoproteins. Protein molecules are classified into two categories:

1. Integral proteins

Integral proteins or **transmembrane proteins** or intrinsic proteins, are tightly bound with the cell membrane. These protein molecules pass through the entire thickness of the cell membrane from one side to the other side.

2. Peripheral proteins

Peripheral proteins also known as **peripheral membrane proteins** do not penetrate the cell membrane but are embedded partially in the outer and inner surfaces of the cell membrane. These protein molecules are loosely bound with the cell membrane and so dissociate readily from the cell membrane.

Functions of protein layers

1. Integral proteins provide the structural integrity of the cell membrane.
2. Channel proteins help in the diffusion of water-soluble substances such as glucose and electrolytes (Chapter 3).
3. Carrier or transport proteins help in the transport of substances across the cell membrane by means of active or passive transport (Chapter 3).
4. Some carrier proteins act as pumps, by which ions are transported actively across the cell membrane.

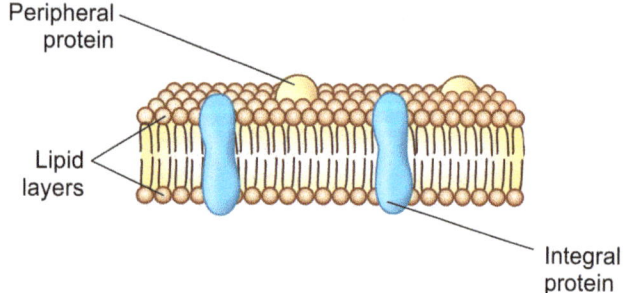

FIGURE 1.2: Diagram of the cell membrane.

5. Receptor proteins serve as the receptor sites for hormones and neurotransmitters.
6. Some of the protein molecules form the enzymes and control chemical (metabolic) reactions within the cell membrane.
7. Some proteins act as antigens and induce the process of antibody formation (Chapter 15).
8. Some proteins called cell adhesion molecules are responsible for attachment of cells to their neighbors or to basal lamina.

Carbohydrates of the Cell Membrane

Carbohydrate molecules form a thin loose covering over the entire surface of the cell membrane called **glycocalyx**. Some carbohydrate molecules are attached with proteins and form **glycoproteins** and some are attached with lipids and form **glycolipids**.

Functions of carbohydrates

1. Carbohydrate molecules are negatively charged and do not permit the negatively charged substances to move in and out of the cell.
2. Glycocalyx from neighboring cells helps in the tight fixation of cells with one another.
3. Some of the carbohydrate molecules form receptors for some hormones.

■ FUNCTIONS OF CELL MEMBRANE

Functions of proteins in cell membrane are listed in **Box 1.1**.

■ CYTOPLASM

Cytoplasm present inside cell contains a clear liquid portion called **cytosol** which contains many substances such as

BOX 1.1: Functions of cell membrane.

1. Protective function
Cell membrane protects the cytoplasm and the organelles present in the cytoplasm
2. Selective permeability
Cell membrane acts as a semipermeable membrane, which allows only some substances to pass through it and acts as a barrier for other substances
3. Absorptive function
Nutrients are absorbed into the cell through the cell membrane
4. Excretory function
Metabolites and other waste products from the cell are excreted out through the cell membrane
5. Exchange of gases
Oxygen enters the cell from blood and carbon dioxide leaves the cell and enters blood through the cell membrane
6. Maintenance of shape and size of cell
Cell membrane is responsible for the maintenance of shape and size of the cell

BOX 1.2: Cytoplasmic organelles.

Organelles with limiting membrane
1. Endoplasmic reticulum
2. Golgi apparatus
3. Lysosome
4. Peroxisome
5. Secretory vesicles
6. Mitochondria
7. Nucleus
Organelles without limiting membrane
1. Ribosomes
2. Centrosome
3. Cytoskeleton

proteins, carbohydrates, lipids and electrolytes. In addition to these substances, many organelles are also present in cytoplasm.

■ ORGANELLES IN CYTOPLASM

All the cells in the body contain some common structures called organelles in the cytoplasm. Some organelles are bound by limiting membrane and others do not have limiting membrane **(Box 1.2)**. The organelles carry out the various functions of the cell **(Table 1.1)**.

■ ORGANELLES WITH LIMITING MEMBRANE
■ 1. ENDOPLASMIC RETICULUM

Endoplasmic reticulum is made up of tubules and microsomal vesicles. It is of two types namely, rough endoplasmic reticulum and smooth endoplasmic reticulum.

Rough Endoplasmic Reticulum

It is the endoplasmic reticulum with rough, bumpy or bead-like appearance. Rough appearance is due to the attachment of granular ribosomes to its outer surface. Hence, it is also called the **granular endoplasmic reticulum (Fig. 1.4)**. Rough endoplasmic reticulum is vesicular or tubular in structure.

Functions of rough endoplasmic reticulum

i. Rough endoplasmic reticulum is concerned with the **synthesis of proteins** in the cell. Examples are synthesis of insulin from β-cells of islets of Langerhans in pancreas and antibodies from B lymphocytes.
ii. It also plays an important role in degradation of worn out cytoplasmic organelles. It wraps itself around the worn-out organelles and forms a vacuole which is called the **autophagosome**. Autophagosome is digested by lysosomal enzymes.

Smooth Endoplasmic Reticulum

Smooth endoplasmic reticulum is also called as **agranular endoplasmic reticulum** because of its smooth appearance without the attachment of ribosome. It is formed by many interconnected tubules. So, it is also called tubular endoplasmic reticulum.

Section 1: General Physiology

TABLE 1.1: Functions of cytoplasmic organelles.

Organelles	Functions
Rough endoplasmic reticulum	1. Synthesis of proteins 2. Degradation of worn-out organelles
Smooth endoplasmic reticulum	1. Synthesis of lipids and steroids 2. Role in cellular metabolism 3. Storage and metabolism of calcium 4. Catabolism and detoxification of toxic substances
Golgi apparatus	1. Processing, packaging, labelling and delivery of proteins and lipids
Lysosomes	1. Degradation of macromolecules 2. Degradation of worn-out organelles in cytoplasm 3. Removal of excess of secretory products 4. Secretion of perforin, granzymes, melanin and serotonin 5. Degradation of own cell
Peroxisomes	1. Breakdown of excess fatty acids 2. Detoxification of hydrogen peroxide and other metabolic products 3. Oxygen utilization 4. Acceleration of gluconeogenesis 5. Degradation of purine to uric acid 6. Role in the formation of myelin 7. Role in the formation of bile acids
Mitochondria	1. Production of energy 2. Synthesis of ATP 3. Initiation of apoptosis
Ribosomes	1. Synthesis of proteins
Centrosome	1. Movement of chromosomes during cell division
Cytoskeleton	1. Determination of shape of the cell 2. Provide support and stability of the cell 3. Movement of substances within the cell 4. Role in mitosis
Nucleus	1. Control of all activities of the cell 2. Synthesis of RNA 3. Sending genetic instruction to cytoplasm for protein synthesis 4. Formation of subunits of ribosomes 5. Control of cell division 6. Storage of hereditary information in genes (DNA)

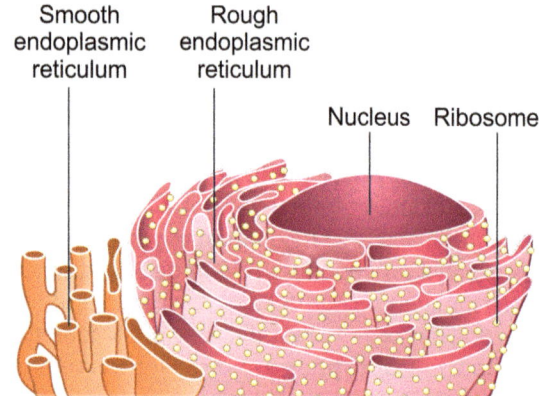

FIGURE 1.4: Endoplasmic reticulum.

Functions of smooth endoplasmic reticulum

i. It is responsible for synthesis of cholesterol and steroid.
ii. It is concerned with various metabolic processes of the cell because of the presence of many enzymes on its outer surface.
iii. It is concerned with the storage and metabolism of calcium.
iv. It is also concerned catabolism and **detoxification** of toxic substances like some drugs and **carcinogens** (cancer producing substances) in liver.

Rough endoplasmic reticulum and smooth endoplasmic reticulum are interconnected and continuous with one another.

■ 2. GOLGI APPARATUS

Golgi apparatus or Golgi body or Golgi complex is present in all the cells except red blood cells. It consists of 5 to 8 flattened membranous sacs called **cisternae (Fig. 1.5)**.

Golgi apparatus is situated near the nucleus. It has two ends or faces namely, **cis face** and **trans face**. The cis face is positioned near the endoplasmic reticulum.

Reticular vesicles from endoplasmic reticulum enter the Golgi apparatus through cis face. The trans face is situated near the cell membrane. The processed substances make their exit from Golgi apparatus through trans face.

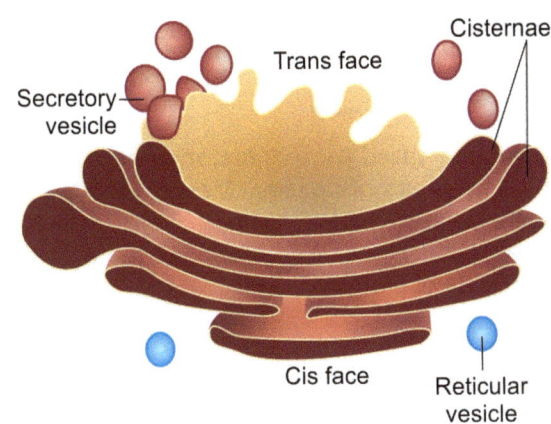

FIGURE 1.5: Golgi apparatus.

Functions of Golgi Apparatus

i. It is concerned with the processing and delivery of substances such as proteins and lipids to different parts of the cell.
ii. It functions like a **post office** because, it packs the processed materials into the secretory granules, secretory vesicles, and lysosomes and dispatch them either out of the cell or to another part of the cell.
iii. It also functions like a **shipping department** of the cell because it sorts out and labels the materials for distribution to their proper destinations.

■ 3. LYSOSOMES

Lysosomes are small globular structures having small granules which contain lysosomal enzymes. Lysosomal enzymes are synthesized in rough endoplasmic reticulum and transported to the Golgi apparatus. Here, these enzymes are processed and packed in the form of small vesicles. These vesicles are pinched off from Golgi apparatus and become the lysosomes.

Types of Lysosomes
Lysosomes are of two types
  i. Primary lysosome which is pinched off from Golgi apparatus. It is inactive in spite of having the hydrolytic enzymes.
  ii. Secondary lysosome which is active lysosome formed by the fusion of a primary lysosome with phagosome or endosome.

Functions of Lysosomes
Lysosomes contain about 50 different **hydrolytic enzymes**, known as **acid hydroxylases** through which the functions of lysosomes are executed. Important lysosomal enzymes are proteases, lipases, amylases and nucleases.

i. Degradation of macromolecules
Macromolecules such as bacteria are engulfed by the cell by means of endocytosis (Chapter 3). Macromolecules engulfed by the cell via endocytosis are called **endosomes**. Other macromolecules engulfed by the cell via phagocytosis are called **phagosomes** or **vacuoles**.

Primary lysosome fuses with the endosome or phagosome to form **secondary lysosome.** Secondary lysosome becomes acidic and the lysosomal enzymes are activated. Macromolecules are digested and degraded by these enzymes. Secondary lysosome containing these **degraded waste products** moves through cytoplasm and fuses with cell membrane. Now the waste products are eliminated by **exocytosis**.

Because of their degradation activity, lysosomes are often called **garbage disposal system** or **waste disposal system** of the cell.

ii. Degradation of worn-out organelles
The rough endoplasmic reticulum wraps itself around the worn-out organelles and form **autophagosomes.** One **primary lysosome** fuse with one autophagosome and form the **secondary lysosome**. Enzymes in the secondary lysosome are activated. Now, these enzymes digest the contents of autophagosome.

iii. Removal of excess secretory products in the cells
Lysosomes in the cells of the secretory glands remove the excess secretory products by degrading the secretory granules.

iv. Secretory function: Secretory lysosomes
Lysosomes having secretory function called secretory lysosomes are found in some of the cells. The conventional lysosomes are modified into secretory lysosomes by combining with secretory granules. Examples are secretory lysosomes of melanocytes which secrete melanin.

v. Degradation of own cells
When a cell is damaged and about to die, lysosomes are burst and release the enzymes. These enzymes digest and degrade their own cell. Hence, the lysosomes are also called "**suicidal bags**" of the cell.

■ 4. PEROXISOMES

Peroxisomes or **microbodies** are pinched off from endoplasmic reticulum. Peroxisomes contain some **oxidative enzymes** such as catalase, urate oxidase and D-amino acid oxidase.

Functions of Peroxisomes
Peroxisomes:
  i. Breakdown the excess fatty acids.
  ii. Degrade the toxic substances like hydrogen peroxide and other metabolic products by means of detoxification.
  iii. Form the major site of oxygen utilization in the cells.
  iv. Accelerate gluconeogenesis from fats.
  v. Degrade purine to uric acid.
  vi. Participate in the formation of myelin.
  vii. Play a role in the formation of bile acids.

■ 5. SECRETORY VESICLES

Secretory vesicles are globular structures, formed in the endoplasmic reticulum, and processed and packed in Golgi

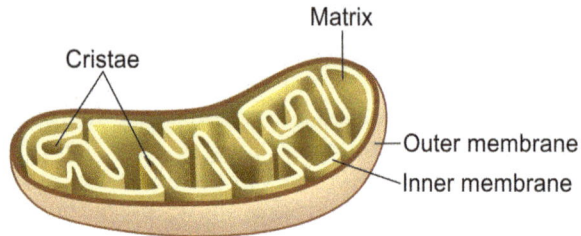

FIGURE 1.6: Structure of mitochondrion.

apparatus. When necessary, the secretory vesicles rupture and release the secretory substances into the cytoplasm.

■ 6. MITOCHONDRION

Mitochondrion (plural 'mitochondria') is a rod or oval-shaped structure covered by a double layered membrane **(Fig. 1.6)**. The outer membrane is smooth and encloses the contents of mitochondrion. It contains various enzymes such as acetyl-CoA synthetase and glycerophosphate acetyltransferase.

Inner membrane contains enzymes and other protein molecules which are involved in respiration and ATP synthesis. Because of these functions, the enzymes and other protein molecules of inner membrane are collectively known as **respiratory chain** or electron transport system. Mitochondria contain their own DNA which is responsible for many enzymatic actions.

Functions of Mitochondrion

i. Production of energy

Mitochondrion is called the '**power house of the cell**' because it produces the energy required for the cellular activities. The energy is produced by oxidation of the food substances like proteins, carbohydrates and lipids by the oxidative enzymes in cristae. During oxidation, water and carbon dioxide are produced with release of energy. The released energy is stored in mitochondria and used later for synthesis of ATP.

ii. Synthesis of ATP

Components of respiratory chain in the mitochondrion are responsible for the synthesis of ATP by utilizing the energy through oxidative phosphorylation. The ATP molecules defuse throughout the cell from mitochondrion. Whenever energy is needed for cellular activity, the ATP molecules are broken down.

iii. Apoptosis

Mitochondria are involved in initiation of apoptosis (see below) also.

■ ORGANELLES WITHOUT LIMITING MEMBRANE

■ 1. RIBOSOMES

Ribosomes are small granular structures. Some ribosomes are attached to rough endoplasmic reticulum while others are present as free ribosomes in the cytoplasm. The ribosomes are made up of proteins (35%) and RNA (65%). The RNA present in ribosomes is called **ribosomal RNA (rRNA)**.

Functions of Ribosomes

Ribosomes are called **protein factories** because of their role in the synthesis of proteins. Messenger RNA passes the genetic code for protein synthesis from nucleus to the ribosomes. Ribosomes, in turn arrange the amino acids into small units of proteins.

■ 2. CENTROSOME

Centrosome is situated near the center of the cell close to the nucleus. It consists of two cylindrical structures called **centrioles** which are responsible for the movement of chromosomes during cell division.

■ 3. CYTOSKELETON

Cytoskeleton of the cell is a complex network that gives shape, support and stability to the cell. It is also essential for the cellular movements and the response of the cell to external stimuli. The cytoskeleton consists of three major protein components, viz.: microtubules, intermediate filaments and microfilaments.

Microtubules

Microtubules are straight and hollow tubular structures formed by bundles of globular protein called α- and β-tubulins **(Fig. 1.7)**.

Intermediate Filaments

Intermediate filaments form a network around the nucleus and extend to the periphery of the cell **(Fig. 1.8)**.

Microfilaments

Microfilaments are long and fine thread-like structures, which are made up of nontubular contractile proteins called actin and myosin **(Fig. 1.9)**.

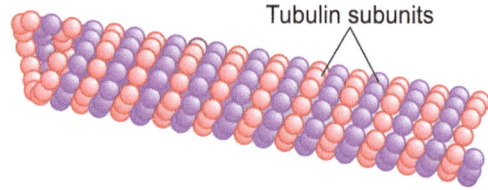

FIGURE 1.7: Microtubules.

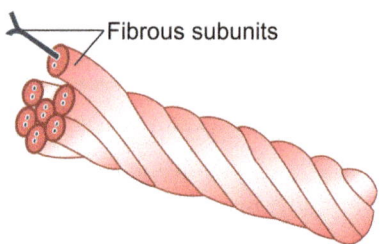

FIGURE 1.8: Intermediate filament.

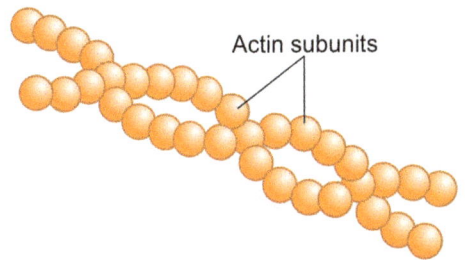

FIGURE 1.9: Microfilament of ectoplasm.

Functions of Cytoskeleton

Cytoskeleton:
i. Determine the shape of the cell.
ii. Give structural strength to the cell.
iii. Act like **conveyor belts** which allow the movement of granules, vesicles, protein molecules and some organelles like mitochondria to different parts of the cell.
vi. Form the spindle fibers, which separate the chromosomes during mitosis.

NUCLEUS

Nucleus is the largest organelle of the cell. It is present in all the cells in the body except the red blood cells. The cells with nucleus are called **eukaryotes** and those without nucleus are known as **prokaryotes**. Presence of nucleus is necessary for cell division.

Most of the cells have only one nucleus (**uninucleated**). Few types of cells like skeletal muscle cells have many nuclei (**multinucleated**). Generally, the nucleus is located near the center of the cell. It is mostly spherical in shape. However, the shape and situation of nucleus vary in different cells.

STRUCTURE OF NUCLEUS

Nuclear Membrane

Nucleus is covered by a double layered membrane called nuclear membrane. It encloses the fluid called nucleoplasm. Nuclear membrane is porous and permeable in nature and it allows nucleoplasm to communicate with the cytoplasm.

Nucleoplasm

Nucleoplasm is a highly viscous fluid that forms the ground substance of nucleus. It is similar to cytoplasm present outside the nucleus. It surrounds chromatin and nucleolus.

Chromatin

Chromatin is a thread-like material made up of large molecules of **deoxyribonucleic acid (DNA)**. The DNA molecules are compactly packed with the help of a specialized basic protein called **histone**. It forms the major bulk of nuclear material. Just before cell division, the chromatin condenses to form chromosome.

Chromosomes

Chromosome is the rod-shaped nuclear structure that carries a complete blueprint of all the hereditary characteristics of that species. A chromosome is formed by a single DNA and each DNA contains many genes.

Diploid cells and haploid cells

All the dividing cells of the body except reproductive cells contain 23 pairs of chromosomes. Each pair consists of one chromosome inherited from mother and one from father. The cells with 23 pairs of chromosomes are called diploid cells. Reproductive cells or gametes or sex cells which contain only 23 single chromosomes are called haploid cells.

Sex chromosomes and autosomes

Among the 23 pairs of chromosomes, one pair is concerned with determination of sex of the person. These chromosomes are called sex chromosomes. Remaining 22 pair of chromosomes that are not concerned with sex determination are named as autosomes.

Among the sex chromosomes, one is called x chromosome and another one is called y chromosomes. The cells of females have two X chromosomes and cells of males have one X chromosome and one Y chromosome.

Nucleolus

Nucleolus is a small, round granular structure of the nucleus. Each nucleus contains one or more nucleoli. The nucleolus contains **ribonucleic acid (RNA)** and some proteins, which are similar to those found in ribosomes. The RNA is synthesized by five different pairs of chromosomes and stored in the nucleolus.

FUNCTIONS OF NUCLEUS

Nucleus is considered as brain of the cells. Major functions of nucleus are the control of cellular activities and storage of hereditary material. So, it is also called **control center**. Functions of nucleus are listed in **Box 1.3**.

BOX 1.3: Functions of nucleus.

1. Control of all the cellular activities that include metabolism, protein synthesis, growth and reproduction (cell division)
2. Synthesis of ribonucleic acid (RNA)
3. Formation of subunits of ribosomes
4. Sending genetic instruction to the cytoplasm for protein synthesis through messenger RNA (mRNA)
5. Control of the cell division through genes
6. Storage of hereditary information (in genes) and transformation of this information from one generation of the species to the next.

DEOXYRIBONUCLEIC ACID: DNA

Deoxyribonucleic acid (DNA) is a nucleic acid that carries the genetic information to the offspring of an organism. DNA forms the chemical basis of hereditary characters. It contains the instruction for the synthesis of proteins in the ribosomes. Gene is a part of a DNA molecule.

DNA is present in mitochondria and the nucleus (chromosome) of the cell. DNA in mitochondria is called **non-chromosomal DNA**. DNA present in the nucleus forms the component of chromosomes, which carries the hereditary information. The hereditary information that is encoded in DNA is called **genome.** Each DNA molecule is divided into discrete units called genes.

STRUCTURE OF DNA

DNA is a double-stranded complex nucleic acid. It is formed by deoxyribose, phosphoric acid and four types of bases. Each DNA molecule consists of two polynucleotide chains, which are twisted around one another in the form of a double helix. The two chains are formed by the sugar deoxyribose and phosphate. These two substances form the backbone of DNA molecule. Both chains of DNA are connected with each other by some organic bases **(Fig. 1.10)**.

Each chain of DNA molecule consists of many nucleotides.

Each nucleotide is formed by:

1. Deoxyribose: Sugar.
2. Phosphate.
3. One of the following organic (nitrogenous) bases:
   Purines:
      i. Adenine (A)
      ii. Guanine (G).
   Pyrimidines:
      i. Thymine (T)
      ii. Cytosine (C).

Strands of DNA are arranged in such a way that both are bound by specific pairs of bases. The adenine of one strand binds specifically with thymine of opposite strand. Similarly, the cytosine of one strand binds with guanine of the other strand.

GENE

Gene is the basic **hereditary unit** of the cell. It is a portion of DNA molecule that contains the message or code for the synthesis of a specific protein from amino acids. It is like a book that contains the information necessary for protein synthesis.

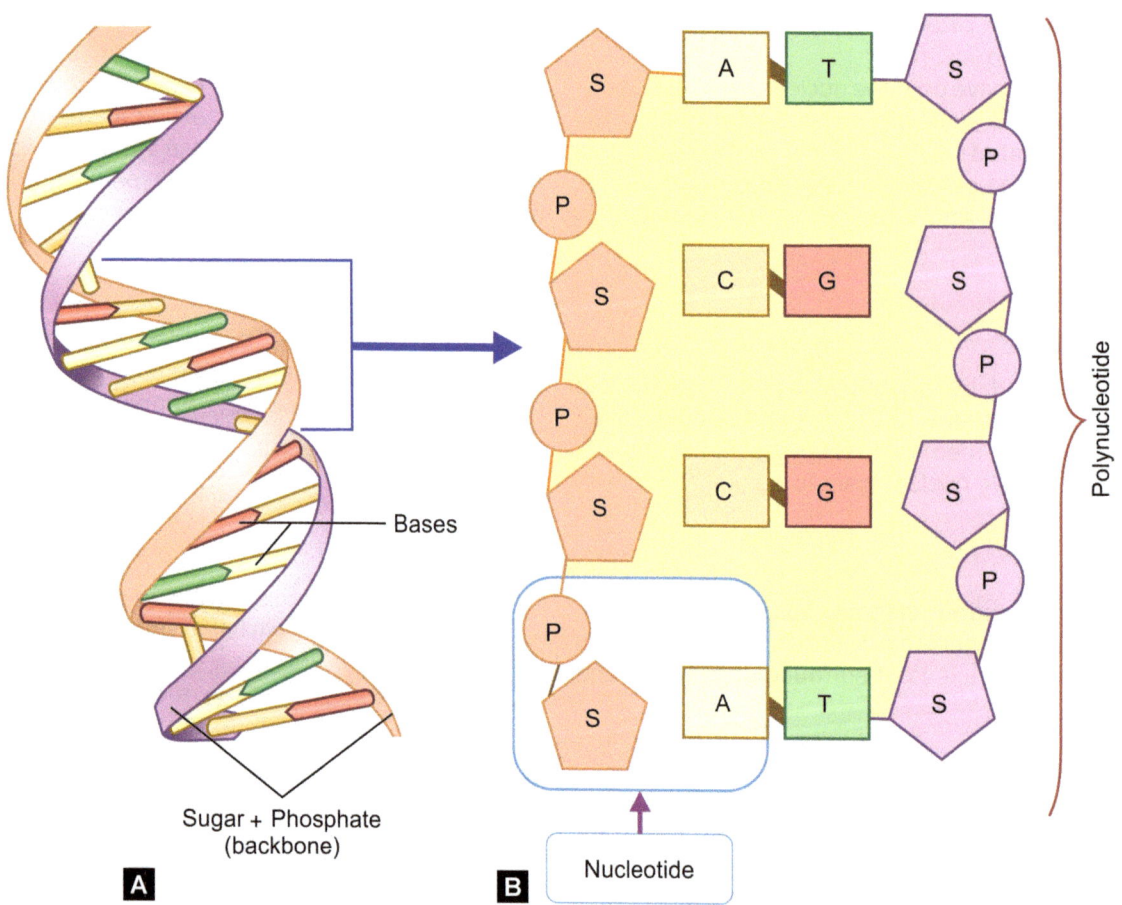

FIGURE 1.10: Structure of DNA. **A.** Double helical structure of DNA. **B.** Magnified view of the components of DNA. A = Adenine, C = Cytosine, G = Guanine, P = Phosphate, S = Sugar, T = Thymine.

BOX 1.4: Common chromosomal disorders.

1. Turner's syndrome
• Genetic disorder that affects females
• It is due to partial or complete missing of one of the two sex (X) chromosomes
• This disorder is characterized by short stature, infertility, heart abnormalities, renal problems and learning difficulties

2. Down syndrome
• Genetic disorder that occurs due to the presence of an extra copy of chromosome 21
• The person has 47 chromosomes instead of usual 46
• It is characterized by physical disabilities and mental retardation

GENETIC DISORDERS

Genetic disorder is a disease or condition that occurs due to absence of a gene or a defective gene or by a chromosomal abnormality. Examples are sickle cell anemia, Alzheimer's diseases and diabetes.

CHROMOSOMAL DISORDERS

Chromosomal disorder is a genetic disorder caused by abnormalities in chromosome. It may be due to any change in structure (structural abnormality) or number (numerical abnormality) of chromosomes. Refer **Box 1.4** for common chromosomal disorders.

RIBONUCLEIC ACID: RNA

Ribonucleic acid (RNA) is a nucleic acid that contains a long chain of nucleotide units. Various functions coded in the genes are carried out in the cytoplasm of the cell by RNA. RNAs is formed from DNA.

TYPES OF RNA

RNA is of three types. Each type of RNA plays a specific role in protein synthesis. Three types of RNA are given below.

1. Messenger RNA (mRNA)

Messenger RNA carries the **genetic code** of amino acid sequence for synthesis of protein from DNA to the cytoplasm.

2. Transfer RNA (tRNA)

Transfer RNA is responsible for decoding the genetic message present in mRNA.

3. Ribosomal RNA (rRNA)

Ribosomal RNA is present within the ribosome and forms a part of the structure of ribosome. It is responsible for the assembly of protein from amino acids in the ribosome.

STRUCTURE OF RNA

Each RNA molecule consists of a single strand of polynucleotide unlike the double-stranded DNA.

Each nucleotide in RNA is formed by:

1. Ribose: Sugar.
2. Phosphate.
3. One of the following organic bases:
   Purines:
   i. Adenine (A)
   ii. Guanine (G).
   Pyrimidines:
   i. Uracil (U)
   ii. Cytosine (C).

Uracil replaces the thymine of DNA and it has similar structure of thymine.

GENE EXPRESSION

Gene expression is the process by which the information (code word) encoded in the gene is converted into functional gene product or document of instruction (RNA) that is used for protein synthesis.

Gene expression involves two steps namely, transcription and translation.

TRANSCRIPTION OF GENETIC CODE

Transcription means copying. It indicates the copying of genetic code from DNA to RNA. Proteins are synthesized in the ribosomes which are present in the cytoplasm. However, the synthesis of different proteins depends upon information (**sequence of codon**) encoded in the genes of the DNA which is present in the nucleus. Since DNA is a macromolecule, it cannot pass through the pores of the nuclear membrane and enter the cytoplasm. But, the information from DNA must be sent to ribosome. So, the gene has to be transcribed (copied) into mRNA which is developed from DNA.

Thus, the first stage in the protein synthesis is transcription of genetic code. It involves the formation of mRNA and simultaneous copying or transfer of information from DNA to mRNA. The mRNA enters the cytoplasm from the nucleus and activates the ribosome resulting in protein synthesis.

TRANSLATION OF GENETIC CODE

Translation is the process by which protein synthesis occurs in the ribosome of the cell under the direction of genetic instruction carried by mRNA from DNA. Or, it is the process by which the mRNA is read by ribosome to produce a protein. This involves the role of other two types of RNA, namely tRNA and rRNA.

The mRNA moves out of nucleus into the cytoplasm. Now, a group of ribosomes called **polysome** gets attached to mRNA. The sequence of **codons** in mRNA are exposed and recognized by the complementary sequence of base in tRNA. The complementary sequence of base is called **anticodon**. According to the sequence of bases in anticodon, different amino acids are transported from the cytoplasm into the ribosome by tRNA that acts as a carrier. With the help of rRNA, the protein molecules are assembled from amino acids. The protein synthesis occurs in the ribosomes which are attached to rough endoplasmic reticulum.

CELL DEATH

Cell death occurs by two distinct processes:
1. Apoptosis.
2. Necrosis.

APOPTOSIS

Apoptosis is defined as the **programmed cell death** under genetic control. It is also called **cell suicide**. This type of programmed cell death is a normal phenomenon and it is essential for normal development of the body.

Main function of apoptosis is to remove unwanted cells without causing any stress or damage to the neighboring cells.

NECROSIS

Necrosis (means 'dead' in Greek) is the uncontrolled and **unprogrammed cell death** due to unexpected and accidental damage. It is also called '**cell murder**' because the cell is killed by extracellular or external events. After necrosis, the harmful chemical substances released from the dead cells cause damage and inflammation of neighboring tissues.

Common causes of necrosis are injury, infection, inflammation, infarction and cancer. Necrosis is induced by both physical and chemical events such as heat, radiation, trauma, hypoxia due to lack of blood flow, and exposure to toxins.

CHAPTER 2

Cell Junctions

CHAPTER OUTLINE

- **DEFINITION AND CLASSIFICATION**
- **OCCLUDING JUNCTIONS**
  - TIGHT JUNCTION
- **COMMUNICATING JUNCTIONS**
  - GAP JUNCTION
  - CHEMICAL SYNAPSE
- **ANCHORING JUNCTIONS**
  - ADHERENS JUNCTIONS
  - FOCAL ADHESIONS
  - DESMOSOME
  - HEMIDESMOSOME

DEFINITION AND CLASSIFICATION

Cell junction is defined as the connection between neighboring cells or the contact between the cell and extracellular matrix. It is also called **membrane junction**.

Connection between two cells is called **intercellular junctions**. Tight junction, gap junction, adherence junction and desmosome are intercellular junctions. Contact between the cell and extracellular matrix are focal adherence and hemidesmosome. Cells junctions are mostly formed by cell junction proteins.

Cell junctions are classified into three types:

I. Occluding junction.
II. Communicating junction.
III. Anchoring junction.

OCCLUDING JUNCTIONS

Cell junctions which prevent the movement of ions and molecules from one cell to another cell are called the occluding junctions. Tight junctions belong to this category.

TIGHT JUNCTION

Tight junction is formed by the tight fusion of the cell membranes from the adjacent cells. The area of the fusion is very tight and forms a ridge. This type of junction is present in the apical margins of epithelial cells in intestinal mucosa, wall of renal tubule, capillary wall and choroid plexus **(Fig. 2.1)**.

Proteins involved in tight junction are occludin, claudin, JAMs, cingulin, symplekin and ZO–1, 2, 3.

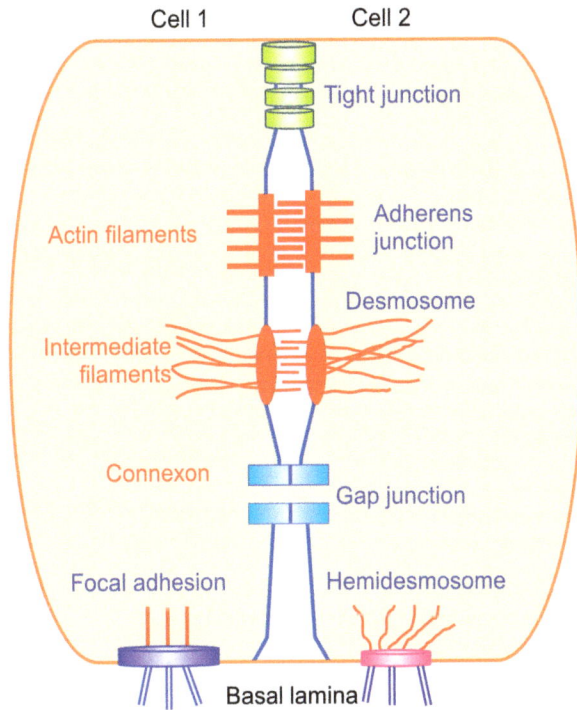

FIGURE 2.1: Different types of cell junctions.

Functions of Tight Junction

1. The tight junction holds the neighboring cells of the tissues firmly and thus provide strength and stability to the tissues **(Table 2.1)**

TABLE 2.1: Cell junctions.

Junction types	Proteins involved	Functions	Examples
Tight junction	1. Occludin 2. Claudin 3. JAMs 4. Cingulin 5. Symplekin 6. ZO–1, 2, 3	1. Strength and stability to tissues 2. Selective permeability 3. Fencing function 4. Maintenance of cell polarity 5. Formation of blood-brain barrier	1. Epithelial lining of intestinal mucosa and renal tubule 2. Endothelium in capillary wall and choroid plexus
Gap junction	1. Connexins	1. Allows passage of small molecules, ions and chemical messengers 2. Propagation of action potential	1. Epithelial lining 2. In syncytium of heart 3. Epithelium of intestine
Adherens junction	1. Cadherins	1. Cell to cell attachment	1. Epithelial lining 2. In intercalated disks of cardiac muscle 3. Epidermis
Focal adhesions	1. Integrins	Cell attachment to: 1. Basal lamina 2. Extracellular matrix	1. Epithelial lining
Desmosome	1. Cadherins	1. Cell to cell attachment	1. Epithelial lining 2. Skin
Hemidesmosome	1. Integrins	Cell attachment to: 1. Basal lamina 2. Extracellular matrix	1. Epithelial lining

2. It provides the barrier or **gate function** by which the interchange of ions, water and macromolecules between the cells is regulated.
3. It acts like a fence by preventing the lateral movement of integral membrane proteins and lipids from cell membrane.
4. By the **fencing function**, the tight junctions maintain the cell polarity by keeping the proteins in the apical region of the cell membrane.
5. Tight junctions in the brain capillaries form the **blood-brain barrier** (BBB) which prevents the entrance of many harmful substances from the blood into the brain tissues.

COMMUNICATING JUNCTIONS

Cell junctions, which permit the movement of ions and molecules from one cell to another cell, are called communicating junctions.

Communication junctions are of two types:

1. Gap junction.
2. Chemical synapse.

GAP JUNCTION OR NEXUS

Gap junction is also called **nexus**. It is present in heart, basal part of epithelial cells of intestinal mucosa, etc.

Structure of Gap Junction

Membranes of the two adjacent cells lie very close to each other and the **intercellular space** becomes a narrow channel. Cytoplasm of both the cells is interconnected and molecules move from one cell to another cell through these channels without having contact with extracellular fluid (ECF). The channel is surrounded by 6 subunits of proteins which are called **connexins** or **connexons**.

Functions of Gap Junction

1. Diameter of the channel in the gap junction is about 1.5 to 3 nm. So, the substances having molecular weight less than 1,000 such as glucose can pass through this junction easily.
2. It helps in the exchange of chemical messengers between the cells.
3. It helps in rapid propagation of action potential from one cell to another cell.

CHEMICAL SYNAPSE

Chemical synapse is the junction between a nerve fiber and a muscle fiber or between two nerve fibers, through which the signals are transmitted by the release of chemical transmitter. Refer Chapter 79 for details.

ANCHORING JUNCTIONS

Anchoring junctions are the junctions, which provide firm structural attachment between two cells or between a cell and the extracellular matrix. Anchoring junctions are divided into four types.

1. ADHERENS JUNCTIONS: CELL TO CELL JUNCTION

Adherens junction is a **cell to cell junction** that is the junction found between the cells. The connection occurs through the actin filaments. Adherens junctions are present in the intercalated disk of cardiac muscles (Chapter 56) and epidermis of the skin. Proteins involved in this junction are cadherins.

2. FOCAL ADHESIONS: CELL TO MATRIX JUNCTION

Focal adhesion is a **cell to matrix junction** that is junction between the cell and the extracellular matrix. The connection occurs through the actin filaments. This type of junction is seen in epithelia of various organs. Proteins involved in this junction are integrins.

3. DESMOSOME: CELL TO CELL JUNCTION

Desmosome is also **cell to cell junction**, but here the membranes of the cells are thickened and connected by intermediate filaments. So, desmosome functions like tight junction. This type of junction is found in areas subjected for stretching such as the skin. Proteins involved in this junction are cadherins.

4. HEMIDESMOSOME: CELL TO MATRIX JUNCTION

Hemidesmosome is also **cell to matrix junction** and the connection is through intermediate filaments. It is like half desmosome because here, the membrane of only one cell thickens. So, this is known as hemidesmosome or half desmosome. Mostly, the hemidesmosome connects the cells with their basal lamina. Proteins involved in this junction are integrins **(Table 2.1)**.

Chapter 3

Transport Through Cell Membrane

CHAPTER OUTLINE

- **IMPORTANCE OF TRANSPORT MECHANISM**
- **BASIC MECHANISM OF TRANSPORT**
- **PASSIVE TRANSPORT**
  - SIMPLE DIFFUSION
  - FACILITATED OR CARRIER MEDIATED DIFFUSION
  - SPECIAL TYPES OF PASSIVE DIFFUSION
- **ACTIVE TRANSPORT**
  - MECHANISM OF ACTIVE TRANSPORT
  - CARRIER PROTEINS
- **SUBSTANCES TRANSPORTED BY ACTIVE TRANSPORT**
- **TYPES OF ACTIVE TRANSPORT**
- **PRIMARY ACTIVE TRANSPORT**
- **SECONDARY ACTIVE TRANSPORT**
- **SPECIAL CATEGORIES OF ACTIVE TRANSPORT OR VESICULAR TRANSPORT**

■ IMPORTANCE OF TRANSPORT MECHANISM

Transport mechanism in the body is necessary for the supply of essential substances such as nutrients, water, electrolytes, etc. and to remove unwanted substances like waste materials, carbon dioxide, etc. from tissues.

■ BASIC MECHANISM OF TRANSPORT

Mechanism of transport of substances across the cell membrane is of two types:

 I. Passive transport.
 II. Active transport.

■ PASSIVE TRANSPORT

Passive transport is the transport of substances along the concentration gradient or electrical gradient or both (electrochemical gradient). During this, the substances move from the region of higher concentration to the region of lower concentration. It is also known as **diffusion** or **downhill movement**. It does not need energy.

Passive transport or diffusion is of two types:

 A. Simple diffusion.
 B. Facilitated diffusion.

■ SIMPLE DIFFUSION

Simple diffusion is of two types:

1. Simple diffusion through lipid layer.
2. Simple diffusion through protein layer.

Simple Diffusion Through Lipid Layer

Lipid soluble substances such as oxygen, carbon dioxide and alcohol are transported by simple diffusion through the lipid layer of the cell membrane **(Fig. 3.1A)**.

Simple Diffusion Through Protein Layer

There are specific protein channels that extend from cell membrane through which the simple diffusion takes place. Water-soluble substances like electrolytes are transported through these channels. The protein channels are selectively permeable to only one type of ion. Accordingly, the channels are named after the ions diffusing through these channels like sodium channels, potassium channels, etc.

Protein Channels

Protein channels are of two types:

1. Ungated channels which are opened continuously.
2. Gated channels which are closed all the time and are opened only when required **(Fig. 3.1B)**.

Gated channels

Gated channels are divided into three categories **(Fig. 3.1C)**:

1. **Voltage-gated channels** which open by change in the electrical potential.
   Examples: Calcium channels present in neuromuscular junction (Chapter 23).

Chapter 3: Transport Through Cell Membrane

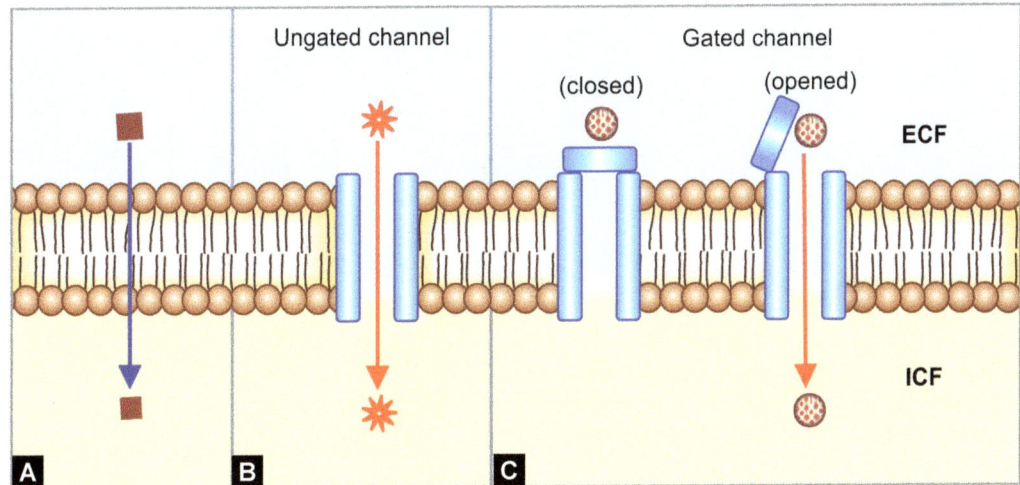

FIGURE 3.1: Hypothetical diagram of simple diffusion through the cell membrane.
A. Diffusion through lipid layer. B. Diffusion through ungated channel. C. Diffusion through gated channel.

2. **Ligand-gated channels** that open in the presence of hormonal substances (ligand).
   Examples: Sodium channels which are opened by acetylcholine in neuromuscular junction.
3. **Mechanically gated channels** which are opened by some mechanical factors such pressure and force.
   Examples: Sodium channels in pressure receptors called Pacinian corpuscles (Chapter 79).

■ FACILITATED OR CARRIER MEDIATED DIFFUSION

In this type of diffusion, some carrier proteins help the transport of substances. The water-soluble substances with larger molecules cannot pass through the protein channels by simple diffusion. Such substances are transported with the help of carrier proteins. This type of diffusion is faster than the simple diffusion. Glucose and amino acids are transported by this method **(Fig. 3.2)**.

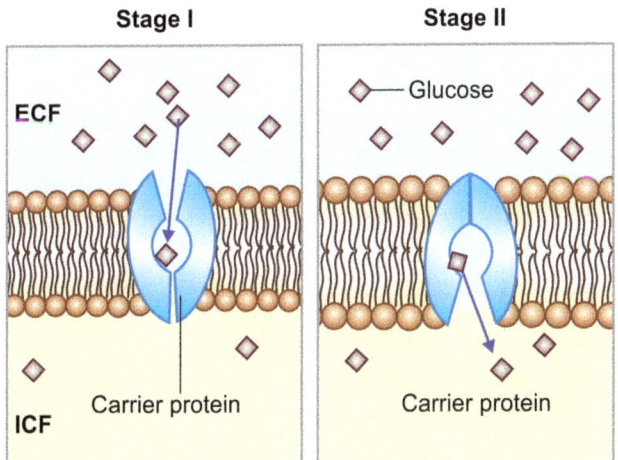

FIGURE 3.2: Hypothetical diagram of facilitated diffusion from higher concentration to lower concentration. Stage I: Glucose binds with carrier protein. Stage II: Conformational change occurs in the carrier protein and glucose is released into ICF.
ECF = Extracellular fluid. ICF = Intracellular fluid.

■ SPECIAL TYPES OF PASSIVE TRANSPORT

In additions to diffusion, there are some special types of passive transport, viz.:

1. Bulk flow.
2. Filtration.
3. Osmosis.

1. Bulk Flow

Bulk flow is the movement of large quantity of substances from a region of high pressure to the region of low pressure. Example is the exchange of gases across the respiratory membrane in lungs (Chapter 72).

2. Filtration

Filtration is the process by which water and solutes move from an area of high hydrostatic pressure to an area of low hydrostatic pressure. Filtration process is seen at the arterial end of the capillaries where movement of fluid occurs along with dissolved substances from blood into the interstitial fluid (Chapter 18). It also occurs in glomeruli of kidneys (Chapter 36).

3. Osmosis

Osmosis is defined as movement of water or any other solvent from an area of lower concentration to an area of higher concentration through a semipermeable membrane **(Fig. 3.3)**.

Osmosis is of two types:

i. **Endosmosis** by which water moves into the cell.
ii. **Exosmosis** by which water moves out of the cell.

Osmotic Pressure, Colloidal Osmotic Pressure and Oncotic Pressure

Osmotic pressure is the pressure created by the solutes in a fluid. Colloidal osmotic pressure is the osmotic pressure exerted by **colloidal substances** in the body.

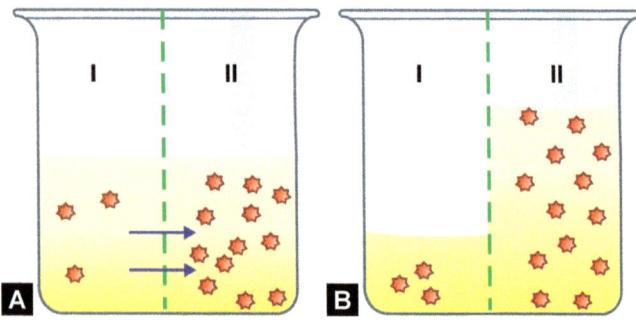

FIGURE 3.3: Osmosis. Red objects = Solute. Yellow shade = Water. Green dotted line = Semipermeable membrane. **A.** Concentration of solute is high in compartment II and low in compartment I. So, water moves from I to II through semipermeable membrane. **B.** Entrance of water into II exerts osmotic pressure.

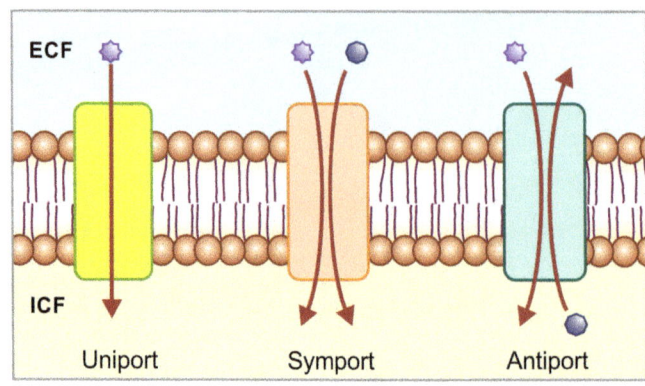

FIGURE 3.4: Carrier proteins of active transport. ECF = Extracellular fluid, ICF = Intracellular fluid.

Oncotic pressure is the osmotic pressure exerted by the colloidal substances (proteins) of the plasma. It is about 25 mm Hg.

■ ACTIVE TRANSPORT

Active transport is the transport of substances against the chemical or electrical or electrochemical gradient. It is also called **uphill transport (Table 3.1)**. Active transport requires energy, which is obtained mainly by breakdown of ATP. It also needs a carrier protein.

■ MECHANISM OF ACTIVE TRANSPORT

When a substance that has to be transported across the cell membrane comes near the cell, it combines with the carrier protein of the cell membrane and forms substance-protein complex. This complex moves towards the inner surface of the cell membrane. Now, the substance is released from the carrier proteins. The same carrier protein moves back to the outer surface of the cell membrane to transport another molecule of the substance.

■ CARRIER PROTEINS

Carrier proteins involved in active transport are of two types:

1. Uniport.
2. Symport or antiport.

Uniport

Uniport is the carrier protein that can carry only one substance in a single direction. It is also known as uniport pump.

Symport or Antiport

Symport is the carrier protein that transports two different substances in the same direction. Antiport is the carrier protein that transports two different substances in opposite directions **(Fig. 3.4)**

■ SUBSTANCES TRANSPORTED BY ACTIVE TRANSPORT

Substances transported by active transport are in ionic form and non-ionic form. The substances in ionic form are sodium, potassium, calcium, hydrogen, chloride and iodide. The substances in non-ionic form are glucose, amino acids and urea.

■ TYPES OF ACTIVE TRANSPORT

Active transport is of two types:

A. Primary active transport.
B. Secondary active transport.

■ PRIMARY ACTIVE TRANSPORT

Primary active transport is the type of transport mechanism in which the energy is liberated directly from breakdown of ATP. By this method, the substances like sodium, potassium, calcium, hydrogen and chloride are transported across the cell membrane.

TABLE 3.1: Passive transport vs active transport.

Description	Passive transport	Active transport
Definition	Transport along concentration or electrical or electrochemical gradient	Transport against concentration or electrical or electrochemical gradient
Another name	Downhill movement	Uphill movement
Energy	Does not require energy	Requires energy
Substances transported	Oxygen Carbon dioxide Alcohol Water Electrolytes	Ionic substances: Sodium Potassium Calcium Hydrogen Chloride Iodide Non-ionic substances: Glucose Amino acids Urea Macromolecules

Primary Active Transport of Sodium and Potassium: Sodium-Potassium Pump

Sodium (Na^+) and potassium (K^+) ions are transported across the cell membrane by sodium-potassium (Na^+-K^+) pump which is also called Na^+-K^+ ATPase pump. This pump is formed by a carrier protein and it is present in all cells of the body.

Mechanism of action of Na^+-K^+ pump

Three sodium ions from the cell get attached to the receptor sites of sodium ions on the inner surface of the carrier protein. Two potassium ions outside the cell bind to the receptor sites of potassium ions located on the outer surface of the carrier protein.

This pump obtains energy by breakdown of ATP into adenosine diphosphate (ADP) with the release of one high-energy phosphate. Refer **Figure 3.5** for details.

Electrogenic activity of Na^+-K^+ pump

The Na^+-K^+ pump moves three sodium ions outside the cell and two potassium ions inside cell. Thus, when the pump works once, there is a net loss of one positively charged ion from the cell. Continuous activity of the Na^+-K^+ pumps causes reduction in the number of positively charged ions inside the cell, leading to increase in the negativity inside the cell. This activity is called the electrogenic activity of Na^+-K^+ pump.

Transport of Calcium Ions

Calcium ions are actively transported from inside to outside the cell by **calcium pump** with the help of a separate carrier protein. The energy is obtained from ATP.

Transport of Hydrogen Ions

Hydrogen ions are actively transported across the cell membrane by **hydrogen pump** with the help of another carrier protein. It also obtains energy from ATP.

■ SECONDARY ACTIVE TRANSPORT

Secondary active transport is the transport of a substance along with sodium ions by a common carrier protein.

Secondary active transport if of two types:

1. *Cotransport*: Transport of the substance in the same direction along with sodium.
2. *Countertransport*: Transport of the substance in the opposite direction to that of sodium.

Sodium Cotransport

In this, along with sodium, another substance is carried with the help of a carrier protein called symport (the protein that transports two different molecules in the same direction across the cell membrane).

Examples: Transport of glucose, amino acids, chloride, iodine, iron and urate ions **(Fig. 3.6)**.

Sodium Countertransport

In this process, the substances are transported across the cell membrane in exchange for sodium ions by the carrier protein called antiport (the carrier protein that transports two different ions or molecules in opposite direction across the cell membrane).

Examples: Sodium-calcium countertransport and sodium-hydrogen countertransport in the tubular cells **(Fig. 3.7)**.

■ SPECIAL CATEGORIES OF ACTIVE TRANSPORT OR VESICULAR TRANSPORT

In addition to primary and secondary active transport systems, some special categories of active transport systems also exist in the body.

Special categories of active transport are:

1. Endocytosis.
2. Exocytosis.
3. Transcytosis.

■ ENDOCYTOSIS

Endocytosis is the transport mechanism by which the **macromolecules** enter the cell.

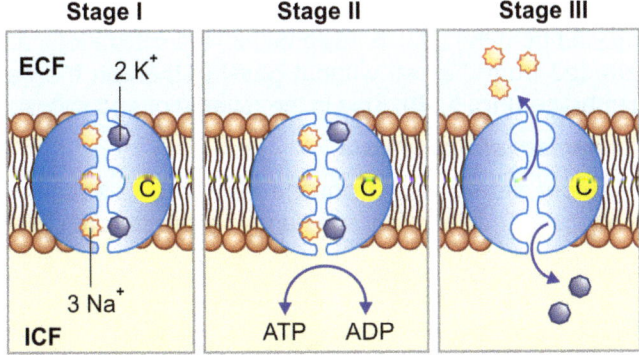

FIGURE 3.5: Hypothetical diagram of sodium-potassium (Na^+-K^+) pump. C = Carrier protein. Stage I: Three Na^+ from intracellular fluid (ICF) and two K^+ from extracellular fluid (ECF) bind with 'C'. Stage II: Binding of Na^+ and K^+ to 'C' activates the enzyme ATPase. ATPase causes breakdown of ATP into adenosine diphosphate (ADP) with the release of one high-energy phosphate. Stage III: Conformational change occurs in 'C' followed by release of Na^+ into ECF and K^+ into ICF.

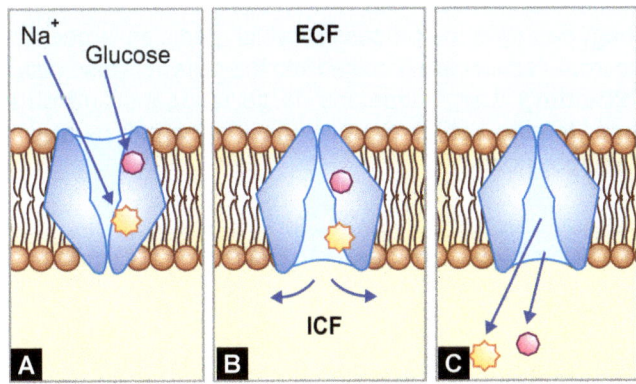

FIGURE 3.6: Sodium (Na^+) cotransport. **A.** Na^+ and glucose from extracellular fluid (ECF) bind with carrier protein. **B.** Conformational change occurs in the carrier protein. **C.** Na^+ and glucose are released into intracellular fluid (ICF).

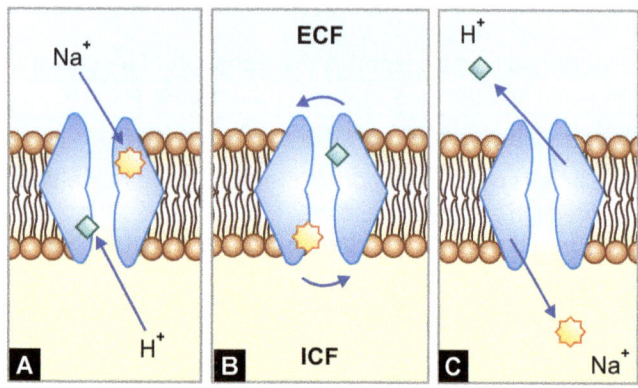

FIGURE 3.7: Sodium (Na⁺) countertransport. **A.** Na⁺ from extracellular fluid (ECF) and hydrogen (H⁺) from intracellular fluid (ICF) bind with carrier protein. **B.** Conformational change occurs in the carrier protein. **C.** Na⁺ enters ICF and H⁺ enters ECF.

Endocytosis is of three types:
a. Pinocytosis.
b. Phagocytosis.
c. Receptor-mediated endocytosis.

a. *Pinocytosis*

Pinocytosis is the process by which macromolecules such as bacteria and antigens are taken into the cells. It is otherwise called **cell drinking**.

Mechanism of pinocytosis

  i. Macromolecules (in the form of droplets of fluid) bind to the outer surface of the cell membrane.
 ii. Now, the cell membrane evaginates and engulfs the droplets.
iii. Engulfed droplets are converted into vesicles and vacuoles, which are called **endosomes (Fig. 3.8)**.
 iv. Endosome travels into the interior of the cell.
  v. **Primary lysosome** in the cytoplasm fuses with the endosome and forms the **secondary lysosome**.
 vi. Now, hydrolytic enzymes present in the secondary lysosome are activated resulting in digestion and degradation of the **endosomal contents**.

b. *Phagocytosis*

Phagocytosis is the process by which particles larger than macromolecules are engulfed into the cells. It is also called **cell eating**. Larger bacteria, larger antigens and other larger foreign bodies are taken inside the cell by means of phagocytosis.

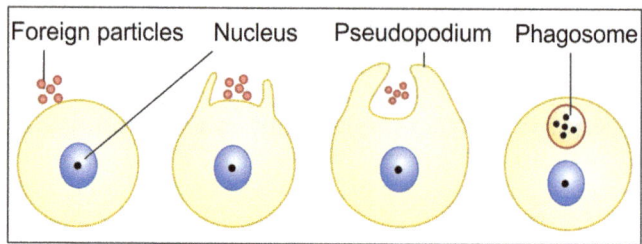

FIGURE 3.9: Process of phagocytosis.

Only few cells in the body such as neutrophils, monocytes and the tissue macrophages show phagocytosis. Among these cells, the macrophages are the largest phagocytic cells.

Mechanism of phagocytosis

  i. When the bacteria or the foreign body enters the body, first the phagocytic cell sends pseudopodium (cytoplasmic extension) around the bacteria or the foreign substance.
 ii. Then, these particles are engulfed and are converted into endosome-like vacuole. The vacuole is very large and it is usually called the **phagosome**.
iii. Phagosome travels into the interior of the cell.
 iv. **Primary lysosome** fuses with this phagosome and forms **secondary lysosome**.
  v. Hydrolytic enzymes present in the secondary lysosome are activated resulting in digestion and degradation of the **phagosomal contents (Fig. 3.9)**.

c. *Receptor-mediated Endocytosis*

Receptor-mediated endocytosis is the transport of macromolecules with the help of a receptor protein called **clathrin**. Receptor-mediated endocytosis plays an important role in the transport of various types of macromolecules such as hormones, antibodies, lipids, growth factors, toxins, bacteria and viruses.

■ EXOCYTOSIS

Exocytosis is the process by which the substances are expelled from the cell. In this process, the substances are extruded from the cell without passing through the cell membrane **(Fig. 3.10)**. This is the reverse of endocytosis.

Mechanism of exocytosis

Secretory substances from the cells are released by exocytosis. The secretory substances of the cell are stored

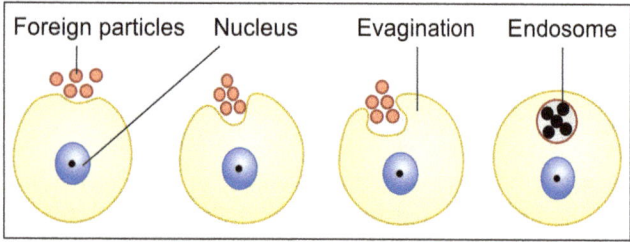

FIGURE 3.8: Process of pinocytosis.

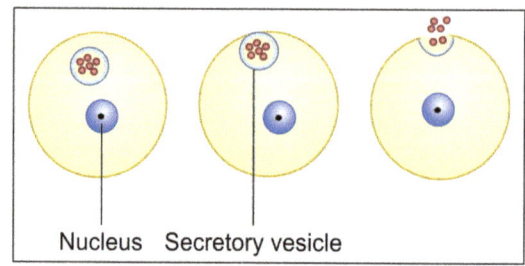

FIGURE 3.10: Process of exocytosis.

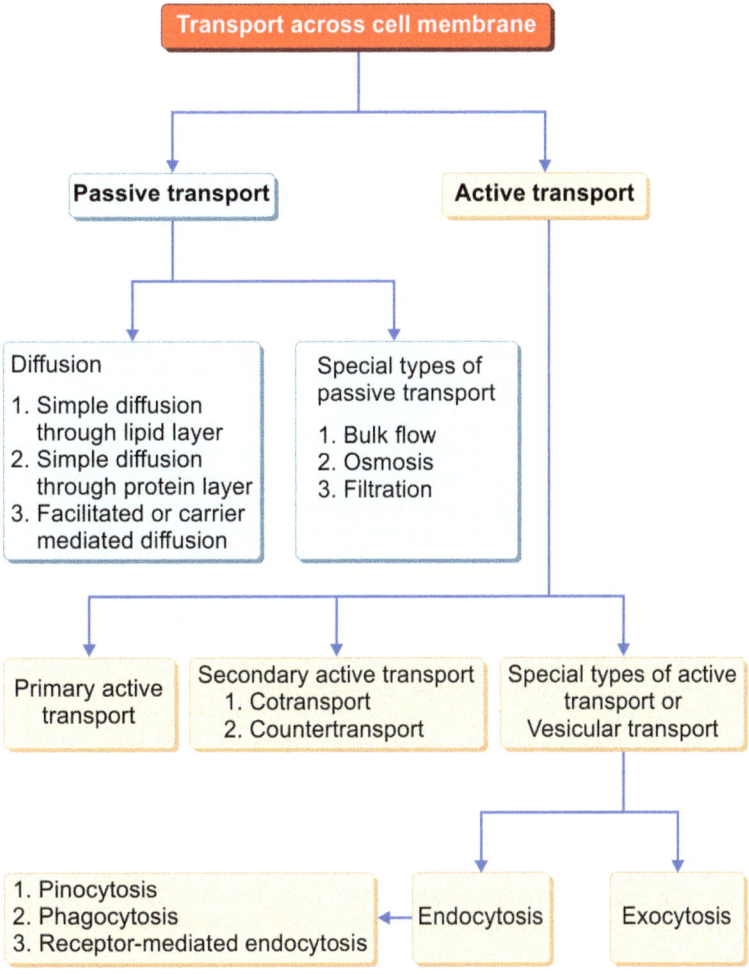

FIGURE 3.11: Types of transport mechanisms across cell membrane.

in the form of **secretory vesicles** in the cytoplasm. When required, the vesicles move towards the cell membrane and get fused with it. Later, the contents of the vesicles are released out of the cell **(Fig. 3.11)**.

■ TRANSCYTOSIS

Transcytosis is a transport mechanism in which an extracellular macromolecule enters through one side of a cell, migrates across cytoplasm of the cell and exits through the other side by means of exocytosis.

Examples are movement of proteins and pathogens like HIV from capillary blood into interstitial fluid through endothelial cells of the capillary.

Chapter 4: Homeostasis

CHAPTER OUTLINE

- DEFINITION
- INTERNAL ENVIRONMENT
- COMPONENTS OF HOMEOSTATIC SYSTEM
- MECHANISM OF ACTION OF HOMEOSTATIC SYSTEM
- NEGATIVE FEEDBACK
- POSITIVE FEEDBACK
- FEED-FORWARD CONTROL

DEFINITION

'**Homeostasis**' means the maintenance of constant **internal environment** of the body (**homeo** means same; stasis means standing). The controlled internal environment is also called '**Milieu interieur**'.

INTERNAL ENVIRONMENT

Internal environment in the body is the **extracellular fluid (ECF)** in which the cells live. It is the fluid outside the cell and it constantly moves throughout the body. ECF includes blood, which circulates in the vascular system and **interstitial fluid** which is present in between the cells. ECF contains nutrients, ions and all other substances necessary for the survival of the cells.

Normal healthy living of large organisms including human beings depends upon constant maintenance of internal environment within the physiological limits. If the internal environment deviates beyond the **set limits**, body suffers from malfunction or dysfunction. Therefore, the ultimate goal of an organism is to have a normal healthy living, which is achieved by the maintenance of internal environment within set limits.

COMPONENTS OF HOMEOSTATIC SYSTEM

Homeostatic system in the body includes three components:

1. Sensors or Detectors or Receptors

Sensors recognize the deviation in any activity in internal environment and transmit the message to control center (Fig. 4.1).

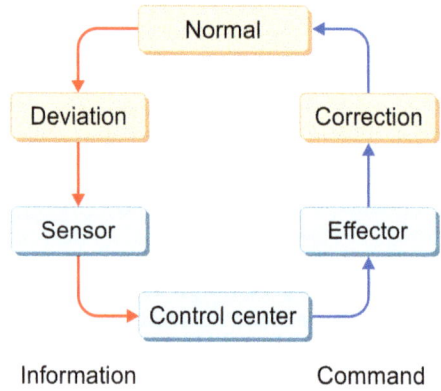

FIGURE 4.1: Components of homeostatic system.

2. Control Center or Integrator Center

Control center receives the message from sensors and immediately sends commands to concerned effectors.

3. Effectors

Effectors receive the commands from the center and either accelerate or inhibit the activity so that normalcy is restored.

MECHANISM OF ACTION OF HOMEOSTATIC SYSTEM

Homeostatic mechanism in the body maintains the normalcy of various systems. Whenever there is any change in behavioral pattern of any system, the effectors bring back the normalcy either by inhibiting and reversing the change or by supporting and accelerating the change.

Chapter 4: Homeostasis

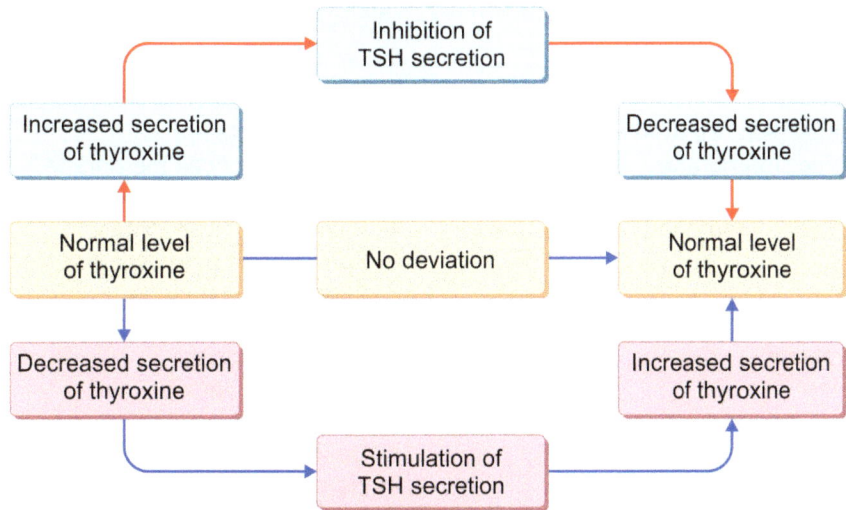

FIGURE 4.2: Negative feedback mechanism: Secretion of thyroxine. TSH = Thyroid-stimulating hormone.

Homeostatic mechanism functions by three types of feedback control systems:

1. Negative feedback.
2. Positive feedback.
3. Feed-forward control.

■ NEGATIVE FEEDBACK

Negative feedback mechanism is the one by which a particular system reacts in such a way as to stop the change or reverse the direction of change. After receiving a message, the effectors send the inhibitory signals back to the system. Now, the system stabilizes its own function either by stopping the signals or by reversing the signals.

Example is the regulation of thyroxin secretion by thyroid gland. Thyroid-stimulating hormone (TSH) released from pituitary gland stimulates thyroid gland, which in turn secretes thyroxin. When thyroxin level increases in blood, it inhibits the secretion of TSH from pituitary so that, the secretion of thyroxine from thyroid gland decreases **(Fig. 4.2)**. On the other hand, if thyroxin secretion is less, it induces pituitary gland to release TSH. Now, TSH stimulates thyroid gland to secrete thyroxin (Chapter 45).

■ POSITIVE FEEDBACK

Positive feedback mechanism is the one in which the system reacts in such a way as to amplify (increase the intensity of) the change in the same direction. Positive feedback is less common than the negative feedback. However, it has its own significance, particularly during emergency conditions.

One of the positive feedbacks occurs during the blood clotting. Blood clotting is necessary to arrest bleeding during injury and it occurs in three stages:

1. Formation of prothrombin activator.
2. Conversion of prothrombin into thrombin.
3. Conversion of fibrinogen into fibrin by thrombin.

Thrombin formed in the second stage stimulates the formation of more prothrombin activator in addition to converting fibrinogen into fibrin **(Fig. 4.3)**. It causes formation of more and more amount of prothrombin activator so that the blood clotting process is accelerated and blood loss is prevented quickly (Chapter 15). Other processes where positive feedback occurs are milk ejection reflex (Chapter 44) and parturition and both the processes involve oxytocin secretion.

■ FEED-FORWARD CONTROL

In addition to positive and negative feedback, homeostasis mechanism has feed-forward control system also.

Feed-forward control system is the control system in homeostasis that anticipates the change or deviation that may occur in a later stage and takes appropriate control action to avoid the disturbance. Whereas the feedback control systems detect the deviation only when it happens.

Examples is secretion of gastric juice (along with salivary secretion) even before entrance of food in mouth (Chapter 27).

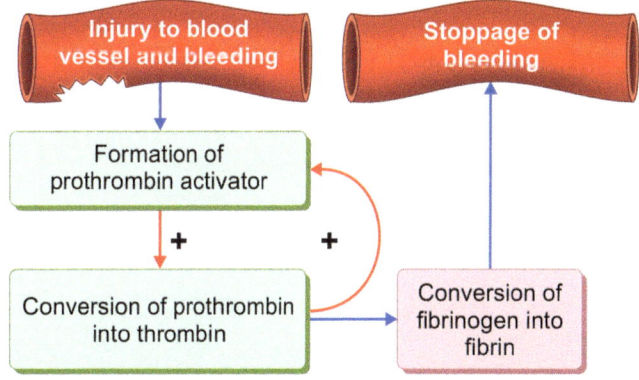

FIGURE 4.3: Positive feedback mechanism: Coagulation of blood. Once formed, thrombin induces the formation of more prothrombin activator.

MODEL QUESTIONS IN GENERAL PHYSIOLOGY

■ LONG QUESTIONS

1. Describe the mechanism of active transport of substances through cell membrane.
2. Describe the mechanism of passive transport of substances through cell membrane.

■ SHORT QUESTIONS

1. Cell membrane.
2. Proteins of cell membrane.
3. Endoplasmic reticulum.
4. Ribosomes.
5. Mitochondria.
6. Golgi apparatus.
7. Cytoskeleton.
8. Tight junctions.
9. Gap junctions.
10. Endocytosis.
11. Negative feedback.
12. Positive feedback.

■ VERY SHORT ANSWER QUESTIONS

1. Integral proteins.
2. Lipid layer of cell membrane.
3. List the organelles present in cytoplasm.
4. Functions of lysosomes.
5. Functions of peroxisomes.
6. Functions of nucleus.
7. Apoptosis.
8. Cellular necrosis.
9. Adherence junction.
10. Focal adhesion.
11. Desmosome.
12. Hemidesmosome.
13. Protein channels.
14. Phagocytosis.
15. Exocytosis.

SECTION 2 BLOOD AND BODY FLUIDS

Chapter 5: Body Fluids

CHAPTER OUTLINE

- **TOTAL BODY WATER**
- **COMPARTMENTS OF BODY FLUIDS**
- **COMPOSITION OF BODY FLUIDS**
- **MEASUREMENT OF BODY FLUID VOLUME**
  - INDICATOR DILUTION METHOD
  - MEASUREMENT OF TOTAL BODY WATER
  - MEASUREMENT OF EXTRACELLULAR FLUID VOLUME
  - MEASUREMENT OF PLASMA VOLUME
  - MEASUREMENT OF BLOOD VOLUME
- MEASUREMENT OF INTRACELLULAR FLUID VOLUME
- MEASUREMENT OF INTERSTITIAL FLUID VOLUME
- **CONCENTRATION OF BODY FLUIDS**
- **MAINTENANCE OF WATER BALANCE**
- **APPLIED PHYSIOLOGY**
  - DEHYDRATION
  - OVERHYDRATION OR WATER INTOXICATION

■ TOTAL BODY WATER

Body is formed by solids and fluids. Fluid part is more than two third of the whole body. Water forms most of the fluid part of the body.

In human beings, the total body water varies from 45% to 75% of body weight. In a normal young adult male, body contains 60 to 65% of water and 35 to 40% of solids. In a normal young adult female, the water is 50 to 55% and solids are 45 to 50%.

Total quantity of body water in an average human being weighing about 70 kg is about 40 L.

■ COMPARTMENTS OF BODY FLUIDS: DISTRIBUTION OF BODY FLUIDS

Compartments and distribution of body fluids with the quantity is given in **Table 5.1**. Water moves between different compartments **(Fig. 5.1)**. Total body water (40 L) is distributed into two major fluid compartments:

1. **Intracellular fluid** (ICF) forming 55% of the total body water (22 L).
2. **Extracellular fluid** (ECF) forming 45% of the total body water (18 L). ECF is divided into five subunits. Refer **Table 5.1** for details.

■ COMPOSITION OF BODY FLUIDS

Body fluids contain water and solids. Solids are organic and inorganic substances.

■ ORGANIC SUBSTANCES

Organic substances present in body fluids are glucose, amino acids and other proteins, fatty acids and other lipids, hormones and enzymes.

■ INORGANIC SUBSTANCES

Inorganic substances present in body fluids are sodium, potassium, calcium, magnesium, chloride, bicarbonate, phosphate and sulfate. Differences between ECF and ICF are given in **Table 5.2**.

■ MEASUREMENT OF BODY FLUID VOLUME

Volume of different compartments of the body fluid is measured by indicator dilution method or dye dilution method.

■ INDICATOR DILUTION METHOD

Principle

A known quantity of a substance such as a dye is administered into a specific body fluid compartment. This substance is called the **marker substance** or **indicator**. After administration into the body fluid, the marker substance is allowed to mix thoroughly with the fluid compartment. Then, a sample of fluid is drawn and the concentration of the marker substance is determined.

TABLE 5.1: Subunits of extracellular fluid.

Subunit of ECF	%	L
I. Interstitial fluid and lymph	20.0	12.0
II. Plasma	7.5	2.75
III. Fluids in bones	7.5	
IV. Fluid in dense connective tissues such as cartilage	7.5	3.25

V. Transcellular fluid
  1. Cerebrospinal fluid
  2. Intraocular fluid
  3. Digestive juices
  4. Serous fluid
    a. Intrapleural fluid
    b. Pericardial fluid
    c. Peritoneal fluid
  5. Synovial fluid in joints
  6. Fluid in urinary tract
	2.5	

ECF 45% of body fluid. Total quantity of ECF is 18L.

TABLE 5.2: Differences between extracellular fluid (ECF) and intracellular fluid (ICF).

Substance	ECF	ICF
Sodium	142 mEq/L	10 mEq/L
Calcium	5 mEq/L	1 mEq/L
Potassium	4 mEq/L	140 mEq/L
Magnesium	3 mEq/L	28 mEq/L
Chloride	103 mEq/L	4 mEq/L
Bicarbonate	28 mEq/L	10 mEq/L
Phosphate	4 mEq/L	75 mEq/L
Sulfate	1 mEq/L	2 mEq/L
Proteins	2 g/dL	16 g/dL
Amino acids	30 mg/dL	200 mg/dL
Glucose	90 mg/dL	0 to 20 mg/dL
Lipids	0.5 g/dL	2 to 95 g/dL
Partial pressure of oxygen	35 mm Hg	20 mm Hg
Partial pressure of carbon dioxide	46 mm Hg	50 mm Hg
Water	15 to 20 L (18)	20 to 25 L (22)
pH	7.4	7.0

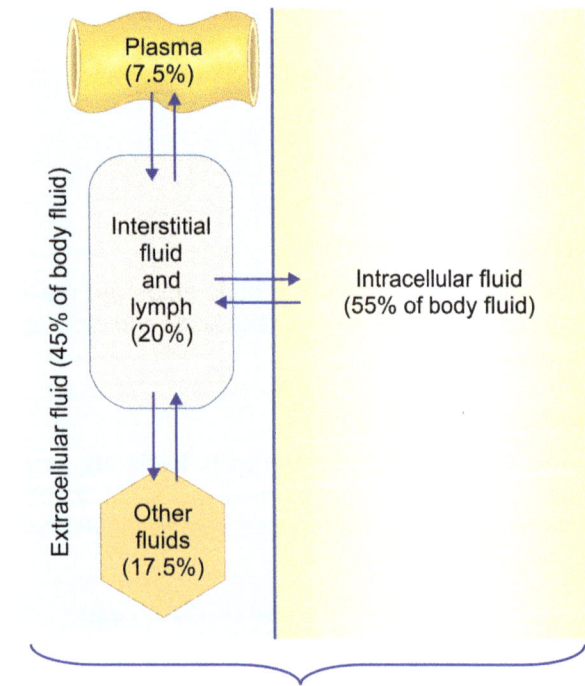

FIGURE 5.1: Body fluid compartments and movement of fluid between different compartments. Other fluids = Transcellular fluid, fluid in bones and fluid in connective tissue.

Formula to Measure the Body Fluid Volume by Indicator Dilution Method

Quantity of fluid in the compartment is measured by using the formula:

$$V = \frac{M}{C}$$

Where,
- V = The volume of fluid in the compartment
- M = Mass or total quantity of marker substance injected
- C = Concentration of the marker substance in the sample fluid

Correction factor

Some amount of marker substance is lost through urine during distribution. So, the formula is corrected as follows:

$$\text{Volume} = \frac{M - \text{Amount of substance excreted}}{C}$$

Uses of Indicator Dilution Method

Indicator dilution or dye dilution method is used to measure ECF volume, plasma volume and the volume of total body water.

■ MEASUREMENT OF TOTAL BODY WATER

Marker substance for measuring TBW should be distributed through all the compartments of body fluid. Such marker substances are deuterium oxide, tritium oxide and antipyrine.

Deuterium oxide and tritium oxide mix with fluids of all the compartments within few hours after injection. Since plasma is part of total body fluid, the concentration of marker substances can be obtained from sample of plasma. And, the formula for indicator dilution method is applied to calculate total body water.

MEASUREMENT OF EXTRACELLULAR FLUID VOLUME

ECF volume is measured by using the substances, which can pass through the capillary membrane freely and remain only in the ECF but not enter into the cell.

Such marker substances are:
1. Radioactive sodium, chloride, bromide, sulfate and thiosulfate.
2. Non-metabolizable saccharides like inulin, mannitol, raffinose and sucrose.

When any of the above substances is injected into blood, it mixes with the fluid of all sub-compartments of ECF within 30 minutes to 1 hour. The indicator dilution method is applied to calculate ECF volume. Since ECF includes plasma, the concentration of the marker substance can be obtained in the sample of plasma.

Example for Measurement of ECF Volume

Quantity of sucrose injected (M) : 150 mg
Urinary excretion of sucrose : 10 mg
Concentration of sucrose in plasma (C): 0.01 mg/mL

$$\text{Sucrose space} = \frac{\text{Mass} - \text{Amount lost in urine}}{\text{Concentration of sucrose in plasma}}$$

$$= \frac{150 - 10 \text{ mg}}{0.01 \text{ mg/mL}}$$

$$= 14,000 \text{ mL}$$

Therefore, the ECF volume = 14 L

MEASUREMENT OF PLASMA VOLUME

The substance, which binds with plasma proteins strongly and diffuses into interstitium only in small quantities or does not diffuse at all, is used to as marker substance to measure plasma volume.

Measurement of Plasma Volume by Indicator or Dye Dilution Technique

Principles and other details of this technique are same as that of ECF volume. The dye which is used to measure plasma volume is **Evans blue** or **T-1824**.

Procedure

A small quantity of blood (3 to 4 mL) is drawn from the subject and a known quantity of the dye is added. This is used as control sample in the procedure. Then, a known volume of dye is injected intravenously. After 10 minutes, a sample of blood is drawn. Then, another 4 samples of blood are collected at the interval of 10 minutes. All the 5 samples are centrifuged and plasma is separated from the samples. In each sample of plasma, the concentration of the dye is measured by colorimetric method and the average concentration is found. The subject's urine is collected and the amount of dye excreted in the urine is measured.

Calculation

Plasma volume is determined by using the formula:

$$\text{Volume} = \frac{\text{Amount of dye injected} - \text{Amount excreted}}{\text{Average concentration of dye in plasma}}$$

MEASUREMENT OF BLOOD VOLUME

Measurement of total blood volume involves two steps:
1. Determination of plasma volume.
2. Determination of blood cell volume.

Plasma volume is determined by indicator dilution technique as mentioned above. Blood cell volume is determined by hematocrit value.

It is usually done by centrifuging the blood and measuring the packed cell volume (Chapter 10). PCV is expressed in percentage. If this is deducted from 100, the percentage of plasma is known. From this, and from the volume of plasma, the amount of total blood is calculated by using the formula:

$$\text{Blood volume} = \frac{100 \times \text{Amount of plasma}}{100 - \text{PCV}}$$

MEASUREMENT OF INTRACELLULAR FLUID VOLUME

Intracellular fluid volume cannot be measured directly. It is calculated from the values of volume of total body water and ECF volume:

ICF volume = Total fluid volume − ECF volume

MEASUREMENT OF INTERSTITIAL FLUID VOLUME

Interstitial fluid volume also cannot be measured directly. It is calculated from the values of ICF volume and plasma volume as given below:

Interstitial fluid volume = ICF volume − Plasma volume

CONCENTRATION OF BODY FLUIDS

Concentration of body fluids is expressed in three ways:
1. Osmolality.
2. Osmolarity.
3. Tonicity.

OSMOLALITY

Osmolality is the concentration of osmotically active substance in a solution. It is expressed as the number of particles (osmoles) per kilogram of solvent (osmoles/kg H_2O).

OSMOLARITY

Osmolarity is another term to express the osmotic concentration. It is the number of particles (osmoles) per liter of solution (osmoles/L).

Osmotic pressure in solutions depends upon osmolality. However, in practice, the osmolarity and not osmolality is considered to determine the osmotic pressure.

Mole and Osmole

A mole (mol) is the molecular weight of a substance in gram. Millimole (mMol) is 1/1,000 of a mole. One osmole (Osm) is the expression of amount of osmotically active particles. It is the molecular weight of a substance in grams divided by number of freely moving particles liberated in solution of each molecule. One milliosmole (mOsm) is 1/1,000 of an osmole.

■ TONICITY

Tonicity is the measure of effective osmolality. In terms of tonicity, the solutions are classified into three categories:

1. Isotonic fluid
2. Hypertonic fluid
3. Hypotonic fluid

1. Isotonic Fluid

Fluid which has the same effective osmolality (tonicity) as body fluids is called isotonic fluid. Examples are 0.9% sodium chloride solution (normal saline) and 5% glucose solution.

2. Hypertonic Fluid

Fluid which has greater effective osmolality than the body fluids is called hypertonic fluid. Example is 2% sodium chloride solution.

3. Hypotonic Fluid

Fluid which has less effective osmolality than the body fluids is called hypotonic fluid. Example is 0.3% sodium chloride solution.

■ MAINTENANCE OF WATER BALANCE

Body has several mechanisms which work together to maintain the water balance. The important mechanisms involve hypothalamus (Chapters 84) and kidneys (Chapter 36).

■ APPLIED PHYSIOLOGY

Fluid balance exists in the body because of equal intake and removal of fluid. Abnormal level of fluids in the body is called fluid imbalance.

Fluid imbalance results in:
1. Dehydration or
2. Water intoxication.

■ DEHYDRATION

Definition

Dehydration is defined as excessive loss of water from the body. Body requires certain amount of fluid intake daily for normal functions. Minimum daily requirement of water intake is about 1 L. This varies with the age and activity of the individual. The most active individuals need 2 to 3 L of water intake daily. Dehydration occurs when fluid loss is more than what is consumed.

Classification of Dehydration

Dehydration is of three types:

1. *Mild dehydration*: It occurs when fluid loss is about 5% of total body fluids. Dehydration is not very serious and can be treated easily by rehydration.
2. *Moderate dehydration*: Moderate dehydration occurs when fluid loss is about 10%. Dehydration becomes little serious and immediate treatment should be given by rehydration.
3. *Severe dehydration*: It occurs when fluid loss is about 15%. Dehydration becomes severe and requires hospitalization and emergency treatment. When fluid loss is more than 15%, dehydration becomes very severe and life threatening.

Causes of Dehydration

Common causes of dehydration are severe diarrhea, vomiting, excess loss of water through urine, insufficient intake of water, prolonged exposure to heat.

Signs and Symptoms of Dehydration

Mild and moderate dehydration

1. Dryness of the mouth and excess thirst.
2. Decrease in sweating and decrease in urine formation.
3. Headache and dizziness.
4. Weakness and cramps in legs and arms.

Severe dehydration

1. Decrease in blood volume, cardiac output and blood pressure.
2. Hypovolemic cardiac shock and fainting.

Very severe dehydration

1. Damage of organs such as brain, liver and kidneys.
2. Mental depression and confusion.
3. Renal failure.
4. Convulsions and coma.

Treatment of Dehydration

Treatment depends upon the severity of dehydration. In mild dehydration, the best treatment is drinking of water and stopping fluid loss. However, in severe dehydration drinking water alone is ineffective because it cannot compensate the salt loss. So, the effective treatment for severe dehydration is oral rehydration therapy.

Oral Rehydration Therapy

Oral rehydration therapy (ORT) is the treatment for dehydration in which an **oral rehydration solution (ORS)** is administered orally. ORS was formulated by World Health Organization (WHO). This solution contains anhydrous glucose, sodium chloride, potassium chloride and trisodium citrate.

In case of very severe dehydration, proper treatment is intravenous administration of necessary fluid and electrolytes.

■ OVERHYDRATION OR WATER INTOXICATION

Definition

Overhydration, hyperhydration, water excess or water intoxication is defined as the condition in which body has too much water.

Causes for Water Intoxication

Overhydration occurs when more fluid is taken than that can be excreted. It also develops in some conditions such as heart failure, renal disorders and hypersecretion of antidiuretic hormone.

Signs and Symptoms

1. Behavioral changes occur first. Person becomes drowsy and inattentive.
2. Nausea and vomiting occur.
3. There is sudden loss of weight, followed by weakness and blurred vision.
4. Muscular symptoms such as cramps, twitching, poor coordination and paralysis develop.
5. Severe conditions of water intoxication result in:
    i. **Delirium** (extreme mental condition characterized by confused state and illusion).
    ii. **Seizures** (sudden uncontrolled involuntary muscular contractions).
    iii. **Coma** (profound state of unconsciousness, in which the person fails to respond to external stimuli and cannot perform voluntary actions).

Treatment of Water Intoxication

Mild water intoxication requires only fluid restriction. In very severe cases, the treatment includes administration of drugs such as diuretics to increase water loss through urine or and intravenous administration of saline to restore sodium.

CHAPTER 6

Blood

CHAPTER OUTLINE

- DEFINITION
- PROPERTIES OF BLOOD
- COMPOSITION OF BLOOD
- PLASMA PROTEINS
- BLOOD VOLUME
- FUNCTIONS OF BLOOD

DEFINITION

Blood is defined as a red color fluid that circulates through vascular system in humans and other vertebrates, carrying nutrients and oxygen to all parts of the body and waste products including carbon dioxide from all parts of the body.

PROPERTIES OF BLOOD

1. Color

Blood is red in color. Arterial blood is scarlet red because of more O_2 and venous blood is purple red because of more CO_2.

2. Volume

See below for details of blood volume.

3. Reaction and pH

Blood is slightly alkaline and its pH in normal conditions is 7.4.

4. Specific gravity

Specific gravity of total blood : 1.052 to 1.061
Specific gravity of blood cells : 1.092 to 1.101
Specific gravity of plasma : 1.022 to 1.026

5. Viscosity

Blood is five times more viscous than water. It is mainly due to red blood cells and plasma proteins.

COMPOSITION OF BLOOD

Blood contains the blood cells which are called **formed elements** and the liquid portion known as plasma.

BLOOD CELLS

Three types of cells are present in the blood:

1. Red blood cells (RBCs) or erythrocytes.
2. White blood cells (WBCs) or leukocytes.
3. Platelets or thrombocytes.

Hematocrit Value

Hematocrit is the volume of RBCs in blood expressed in percentage. It is also called **packed cell volume** (PCV). Its normal value is 45%.

If blood is collected in a hematocrit tube along with a suitable anticoagulant and centrifuged for 30 minutes at a speed of 3,000 revolutions per minute (rpm), the red blood cells settle down at the bottom leaving clear plasma at the top. Plasma forms 55% and red blood cells form 45% of the total blood. In between the plasma and the red blood cells, there is a thin layer of white buffy coat (Fig. 10.2). This white buffy coat is formed by the aggregation of white blood cells and platelets.

PLASMA

Plasma is a straw-colored clear liquid part of blood. It contains 91 to 92% of water and 8 to 9% of solids. The solids are the organic substances (**Box 6.1**) and inorganic substances (**Box 6.2**). Plasma also has some gases (**Box 6.2**)

Table 6.1 gives the normal values of some important substances in blood.

SERUM

Serum is the clear fluid that oozes out from blood clot. When the blood is shed or collected in a container, it clots

BOX 6.1: Organic substances present in plasma.

I. Plasma proteins
1. Albumin
2. Globulin
3. Fibrinogen

II. Amino acids
1. Essential amino acids
2. Non-essential amino acids

III. Carbohydrates
1. Glucose

IV. Fats
1. Triglycerides
2. Cholesterol
3. Phospholipids

V. Internal secretions
1. Hormones

VI. Enzymes
1. Amylase
2. Carbonic anhydrase
3. Acid phosphatase
4. Alkaline Phosphatase
5. Lipase
6. Esterase
7. Protease
8. Transaminase

VII. Non-protein nitrogenous substances
1. Ammonia
2. Creatine
3. Creatinine
4. Xanthi
5. Hypoxanthine
6. Urea
7. Uric acid

VIII. Antibodies

BOX 6.2: Inorganic substances and gases present in plasma.

Inorganic substances
1. Sodium
2. Calcium
3. Potassium
4. Magnesium
5. Bicarbonate
6. Chloride
7. Phosphate
8. Iodide
9. Iron
10. Copper

Gases
1. Oxygen
2. Carbon dioxide
3. Nitrogen

TABLE 6.1: Normal values of some important substances in blood.

Substance	Normal value
1. Fasting glucose	70 to 100 mg/dL
2. Creatinine	0.5 to 1.5 mg/dL
3. Urea	15 to 40 mg/dL
4. Cholesterol	Up to 200 mg/dL
5. Plasma proteins	6.4 to 8.3 g/dL
6. Bilirubin	0.5 to 1.5 mg/dL
7. Iron	50 to 150 µg/dL
8. Copper	100 to 200 mg/dL
9. Calcium	9 to 11 mg/dL 4.5 to 5.5 mEq/L
10. Sodium	135 to 145 mEq/L
11. Potassium	3.5 to 5.0 mEq/L
12. Magnesium	1.5 to 2.0 mEq/L
13. Chloride	100 to 110 mEq/L
14. Bicarbonate	22 to 26 mEq/L

because of the conversion of fibrinogen into fibrin. After about 45 minutes, serum oozes out of the clot. For clinical investigations, serum is separated from blood cells by centrifuging. Volume of the serum is almost the same as that of plasma (55%). It is different from plasma only by the absence of fibrinogen, i.e. serum contains all the other constituents of plasma except fibrinogen. Fibrinogen is absent in serum because it is converted into fibrin during blood clotting. Thus,

Serum = Plasma – Fibrinogen

■ PLASMA PROTEINS

Plasma proteins are:
1. Serum albumin.
2. Serum globulin.
3. Fibrinogen.

Serum contains only albumin and globulin. Fibrinogen is absent in serum because, it is converted into fibrin during blood clotting. Because of this, the albumin and globulin are usually called **serum albumin** and **serum globulin**.

Globulin is of three types namely, α-globulin, β-globulin and γ-globulin.

■ NORMAL VALUES

Normal values of the plasma proteins are given in **Table 6.2**.

Albumin/Globulin Ratio

The ratio between plasma level of albumin and globulin is called albumin/globulin (A/G) ratio. It is an important indicator of some liver and kidney diseases. Normal A/G ratio is 2:1.

■ ORIGIN OF PLASMA PROTEINS

In embryonic stage, the plasma proteins are synthesized by the **mesenchyme cells**. In adults, the plasma proteins are synthesized mainly from reticuloendothelial cells of liver and also from spleen, bone marrow, disintegrating blood cells and general tissue cells. Gamma globulin is synthesized from B lymphocytes.

TABLE 6.2: Normal value and molecular weight of plasma proteins.

Plasma protein	Normal value	Molecular weight
Serum albumin	4.7 g/dL	69,000
Serum globulin	2.3 g/dL	1,56,000
Fibrinogen	0.3 g/dL	4,00,000
Total proteins	7.3 g/dL (6.4 to 8.3 g/dL)	—

■ PROPERTIES OF PLASMA PROTEINS

1. Molecular Weight

Molecular weight of plasma proteins is given in **Table 6.2**.

2. Oncotic Pressure

Plasma proteins exert oncotic or osmotic pressure in the blood (Chapter 3). Normally, it is about 25 mm Hg. Albumin plays a major role in exerting oncotic pressure.

3. Specific Gravity

Specific gravity of the plasma proteins is 1.022 to 1.026.

4. Buffer Action

Acceptance of hydrogen ions is called buffer action. Plasma proteins have 1/6 of total buffering action of the blood.

■ FUNCTIONS OF PLASMA PROTEINS

1. Role in Coagulation of Blood

Fibrinogen is essential for the coagulation of blood (Chapter 15).

2. Role in Defense Mechanism of Body

Gamma globulins play an important role in the defense mechanism of the body by acting as antibodies. These proteins are also called **immunoglobulins** (Chapter 12).

3. Role in Transport Mechanism

Plasma proteins are essential for the transport of various substances in the blood.

4. Role in Maintenance of Oncotic Pressure in Blood

At the capillary level, most of the substances are exchanged between blood and tissues. However, because of their large size, the plasma proteins cannot pass through the capillary membrane easily and remain in the blood. In the blood, these proteins exert the oncotic pressure or colloidal osmotic pressure. Albumin generates about 70% of oncotic pressure. Oncotic pressure exerted by the plasma proteins is about 25 mm Hg. Refer Chapter 3 for definition of osmotic pressure and oncotic pressure.

5. Role in Regulation of Acid-base Balance

Plasma proteins, particularly the albumin, play an important role in regulating the acid-base balance in the blood. This is because of the virtue of their buffering action.

6. Role in Viscosity of Blood

Plasma proteins provide viscosity to the blood, which is important to maintain the blood pressure. Albumin provides maximum viscosity than the other plasma proteins.

7. Role in Erythrocyte Sedimentation Rate (ESR)

Globulin and fibrinogen accelerate the tendency of **rouleaux formation** (Chapter 7) by the red blood cells. Rouleaux formation is responsible for ESR, which is an important diagnostic and prognostic tool (Chapter 10).

8. Role in Suspension Stability of Red Blood Cells

During circulation, the red blood cells remain suspended uniformly in the blood. This property of the red blood cells is called the suspension stability. Globulin and fibrinogen help in the suspension stability of the red blood cells.

9. Role in Production of Trephone Substances

Trephone substances are necessary for nourishment of tissue cells in culture. These substances are produced by leukocytes from the plasma proteins.

10. Role as Reserve Proteins

During fasting, inadequate food intake or inadequate protein intake, the plasma proteins are utilized by the body tissues as the last source of energy. Because of this, the plasma proteins are called reserve proteins.

■ PLASMAPHERESIS AND THERAPEUTIC PLASMA EXCHANGE

Plasmapheresis

Plasmapheresis is an experimental procedure done in animals to demonstrate the importance of plasma proteins.

Procedure

Plasmapheresis is usually demonstrated in dogs. Blood is removed completely from the body of the dog. Red blood cells are separated from plasma and are washed in saline and reinfused into the body of the same dog along with a physiological solution called **Locke's solution.**

Due to sudden lack of proteins, the animal undergoes a state of shock. If the animal is fed with diet containing sufficiently high quantity of proteins, the normal level of plasma proteins is restored within 7 days and the animal survives. The new plasma proteins are also synthesized by the liver of the dog.

If the experiment is done in animals after removal of liver, even if the diet contains adequate quantity of proteins, the plasma proteins are not produced. The shock persists in the animal and leads to death.

Thus, this experiment 'plasmapheresis' is used to demonstrate importance of plasma proteins for survival and synthesis of plasma proteins by the liver.

Therapeutic Plasma Exchange

Therapeutic plasma exchange is a blood purification procedure by which plasma is replaced by blood substitutes. Patient's blood is passed through a machine which removes the plasma and returns the blood cells to patient's blood stream along with blood substitutes. This procedure for an effective temporary treatment of many autoimmune diseases.

In an **autoimmune disease**, the immune system attacks body's own tissues through antibodies (Chapter 12). The antibodies that are proteins in nature circulate in the bloodstream before attacking the target tissues. This procedure is used to remove these antibodies from the blood.

Though purification producer is used to remove antibodies from the blood, it cannot prevent the production of antibodies by the immune system of the body. So, it can provide only a temporary benefit of protecting the tissues from the antibodies. The patients must go for repeated sessions of this treatment.

■ APPLIED PHYSIOLOGY: VARIATIONS IN PLASMA PROTEIN LEVEL

Level of plasma proteins vary independently of one another. However, in several conditions, the quantity of albumin and globulin change in opposite direction. Elevation of all fractions of plasma proteins is called **hyperproteinemia** and decrease in all fractions of plasma proteins is called **hypoproteinemia**.

■ BLOOD VOLUME

■ NORMAL BLOOD VOLUME

Average volume of blood in a normal adult is 5 L. Total amount of blood present in the circulatory system, blood reservoirs, organs and tissues together constitute blood volume. It is about 8% of the body weight in a normal young healthy adult weighing about 70 kg.

In newborn baby it is 450 mL. It increases during growth and reaches 5 L at the time of puberty. In females it is slightly less and is about 4.5 L.

■ VARIATIONS IN BLOOD VOLUME

Physiological Variations

1. *Age*: Blood volume is less at birth and it increases as the age advances. At birth and at 24 hours after birth, the blood volume is about 80 mL/kg body weight. At the age of 15 years, the blood volume is about 70 mL/kg body weight, which is almost the adult volume.
2. *Sex*: In males, blood volume is slightly more than in females because of increase in erythropoietic activity, body weight and surface area of the body. In females, it is slightly less because of loss of blood through menstruation, more fats and less body surface area.
3. *Surface are of the body*: Blood volume is directly proportional to the surface area of the body.
4. *Body weight*: Blood volume is directly proportional to body weight.
5. *Atmospheric temperature*: Exposure to cold environment reduces the blood volume and exposure to warm environment increases the blood volume.
6. *Pregnancy*: During early stage of pregnancy, blood volume increases by 20 to 30%.
7. *Exercise*: Exercise increases the blood volume by increasing the release of erythropoietin and production of more RBCs.
8. *Posture*: Standing (erect posture) for a long time, reduces the blood volume by about 15%.
9. *High altitude*: Blood volume increases in high altitude.
10. *Emotion*: Excitement increases blood volume.

Pathological Variations

Hypervolemia

Increase in blood volume is called hypervolemia. It occurs in the following pathological conditions.

1. Hyperthyroidism
2. Hyperaldosteronism
3. Cirrhosis of the liver
4. Congestive cardiac failure

Hypovolemia

Decrease in blood volume is called hypovolemia. It occurs in the following pathological conditions.

1. Hemorrhage or blood loss.
2. Fluid loss.
3. Hemolysis.
4. Anemia.
5. Hypothyroidism.

■ REGULATION OF BLOOD VOLUME

Various mechanisms are involved in the regulation of blood volume. Important ones are the renal and hormonal mechanisms. Hypothalamus plays a vital role in the activation of these two mechanisms during the regulation of blood volume.

When blood volume increases, hypothalamus causes loss of fluid from the body. When the blood volume reduces, hypothalamus induces retention of water. Hypothalamus regulates the extracellular fluid (ECF) volume and blood volume by acting mainly through kidneys and sweat glands and by inducing thirst. This function of hypothalamus is described in Chapter 84.

Hormones also are involved in the regulation of blood volume through the regulation of ECF volume.

Hormones regulating blood volume through ECF volume are:

1. Antidiuretic hormone (Chapter 44).
2. Aldosterone (Chapter 48).
3. Cortisol (Chapter 48).
4. Atrial natriuretic peptide (Chapter 50).

■ MEASUREMENT OF BLOOD VOLUME

Refer Chapter 5 for measurement of blood volume.

FUNCTIONS OF BLOOD

1. NUTRITIVE FUNCTION

Nutritive substances such as glucose, amino acids, lipids and vitamins derived from digested food are absorbed from gastrointestinal tract and carried by blood to different parts of the body for growth and production of energy.

2. RESPIRATORY FUNCTION

Transport of respiratory gases is done by the blood. It carries oxygen from alveoli of lungs to different tissues and carbon dioxide from tissues to alveoli.

3. EXCRETORY FUNCTION

Waste products formed in the tissues during various metabolic activities are removed by blood and carried to the excretory organs like kidney, skin, liver, etc. for excretion.

4. TRANSPORT OF HORMONES AND ENZYMES

Hormones which are secreted by ductless (endocrine) glands are released directly into the blood. The blood transports these hormones to their target organs/tissues. Blood also transports enzymes.

5. REGULATION OF WATER BALANCE

This helps in the regulation of water content of the body.

6. REGULATION OF ACID-BASE BALANCE

Plasma proteins and hemoglobin act as buffers and help in the regulation of acid-base balance.

7. REGULATION OF BODY TEMPERATURE

Because of the high specific heat of blood, it is responsible for maintaining the thermoregulatory mechanism in the body, i.e. the balance between heat loss and heat gain in the body.

8. STORAGE FUNCTION

Water and some important substances like proteins, glucose, sodium and potassium are constantly required by the tissues. Blood serves as a readymade source for these substances. And, these substances are taken from blood during the conditions like starvation, fluid loss, electrolyte loss, etc.

9. DEFENSIVE FUNCTION

Blood plays an important role in the defense of the body. The white blood cells are responsible for this function. Neutrophils and monocytes engulf the bacteria by phagocytosis. Lymphocytes are involved in development of immunity. Eosinophils are responsible for detoxification; disintegration and removal of foreign proteins (Chapters 11 and 12).

Chapter 7

Red Blood Cells

CHAPTER OUTLINE

- DEFINITION
- NORMAL COUNT
- MORPHOLOGY
- PROPERTIES
- LIFESPAN
- FATE
- FUNCTIONS
- VARIATIONS IN NUMBER
- HEMOLYSIS AND FRAGILITY

■ DEFINITION

Red blood cells (RBCs) or **erythrocytes** are the **non-nucleated** formed elements in the blood. Red color of the RBC is due to the presence of hemoglobin.

■ NORMAL RBC COUNT

RBC count ranges between 4 and 5.5 million/cu mm of blood. In adult males, it is 5 million/cu mm and in adult females it is 4.5 million/cu mm.

■ MORPHOLOGY OF RED BLOOD CELLS

NORMAL SHAPE

Normally, RBCs are disk shaped and biconcave. The central portion is thinner and periphery is thicker. Biconcave contour of RBCs has some mechanical and functional advantages.

Advantages of Biconcave Shape of RBCs

Biconcave shape of RBCs has some functional advantages which are given in **Box 7.1**.

> **BOX 7.1:** Advantages of biconcave shape of RBCs.
>
> 1. Biconcave shape helps in equal and rapid diffusion of oxygen and other substances into the interior of the cell.
> 2. Large surface area is provided for absorption or removal of different substances from the cell.
> 3. Minimal tension is offered on the membrane when the volume of cell alters.
> 4. Because of biconcave shape, while passing through minute capillaries, RBCs squeeze through the capillaries very easily without getting damaged.

NORMAL SIZE

Diameter : 7.2 µ (6.9 to 7.4 µ)
Thickness : At the periphery it is thicker with 2.2 µ and at the center it is thinner with 1 µ **(Fig. 7.1)**.
This difference in thickness is because of the biconcave shape
Surface area : 120 sq µ
Volume : 85 to 90 cu µ

NORMAL STRUCTURE

RBC is a non-nucleated cell. Because of the absence of nucleus, the DNA is also absent. Other organelles such as mitochondria and Golgi apparatus also are absent in RBC. Since, mitochondria are absent, the energy is produced from glycolytic process.

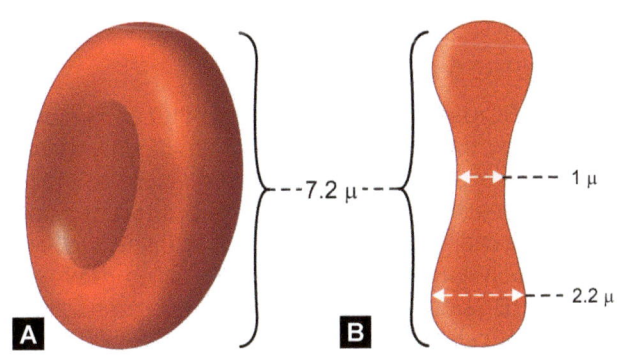

FIGURE 7.1: Dimensions of RBC.
A. Surface view. **B.** Sectioned view.

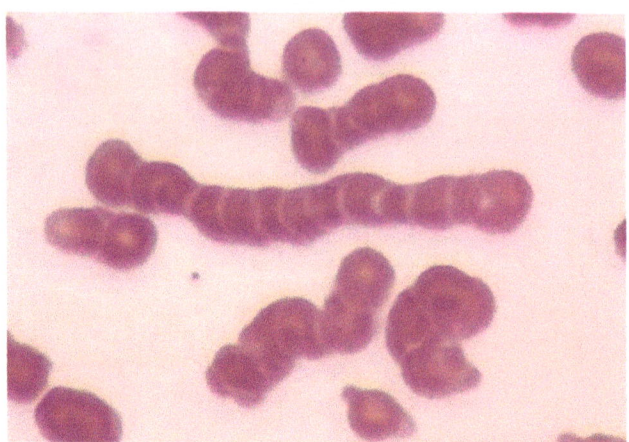

FIGURE 7.2: Rouleaux formation (*Courtesy:* Dr Nivaldo Medeiros).

■ PROPERTIES OF RED BLOOD CELLS

■ 1. ROULEAUX FORMATION

When blood is taken out of the blood vessel, the RBCs pile up one above another like the pile of coins. This property of the RBCs is called rouleaux (pleural = rouleau) formation **(Fig. 7.2)**. It is accelerated by plasma proteins namely globulin and fibrinogen.

■ 2. SPECIFIC GRAVITY

Specific gravity of RBC is 1.092 to 1.101.

■ 3. PACKED CELL VOLUME

Packed cell volume (PCV) is the volume of the RBCs expressed in percentage. It is also called **hematocrit** value. It is 45% of the blood and the plasma volume is 55% (Chapter 10).

■ 4. SUSPENSION STABILITY

During circulation, the RBCs remain suspended or dispersed uniformly in the blood. This property of the RBCs is called the suspension stability (Chapter 10).

■ LIFESPAN OF RED BLOOD CELLS

Average lifespan of RBC is about 120 days. After the lifetime, the senile (old) RBCs are destroyed in reticuloendothelial system.

■ FATE OF RED BLOOD CELLS

When the RBCs become older (120 days), the cell membrane becomes very fragile. So, these cells are destroyed while trying to squeeze through the capillaries which have lesser or equal diameter as that of RBC. The destruction occurs mainly in the capillaries of spleen because these capillaries are very much narrow. So, the spleen is called **graveyard of RBCs**. RBCs are also destroyed by reticuloendothelial cells (Kupffer cells) of liver.

Destroyed RBCs are fragmented and hemoglobin is released from the fragmented parts.

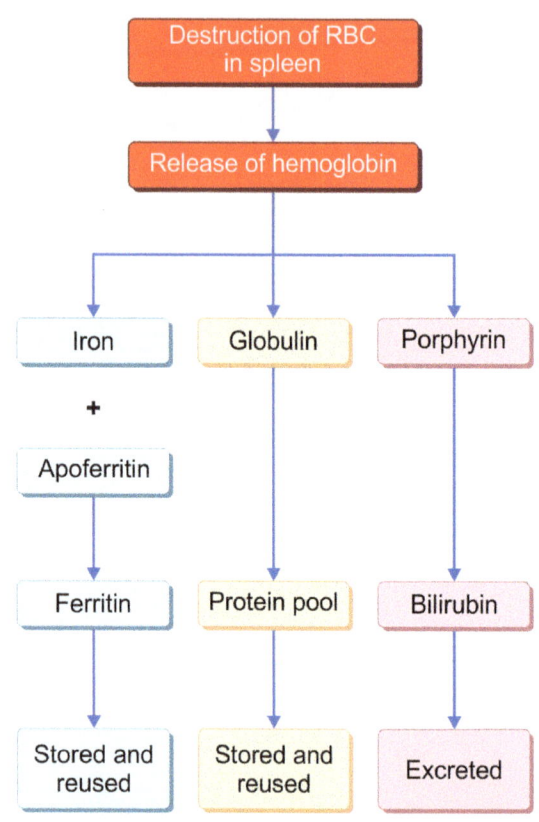

FIGURE 7.3: Fate of RBC.

Hemoglobin is degraded into iron, **globin** and **porphyrin**. Iron combines with the protein called **apoferritin** to form **ferritin** which is stored in the body and reused later. Globin enters the protein depot for later use **(Fig. 7.3)**. The porphyrin is degraded into **bilirubin**, which is excreted by liver through bile (Chapter 29).

Daily 10% of senile RBCs are destroyed in normal young healthy adults. It causes release of about 0.6 g/dL of hemoglobin into the plasma. From this 0.9 to 1.5 mg/dL bilirubin is formed.

■ FUNCTIONS OF RED BLOOD CELLS

1. *Transport of O_2 from the Lungs to the Tissues*

Hemoglobin combines with oxygen to form **oxyhemoglobin** which is transported by blood. In blood, about 97% of oxygen is transported in the form of oxyhemoglobin (Chapter 72).

2. *Transport CO_2 from the Tissues to the Lungs*

Hemoglobin combines with carbon dioxide and form **carbhemoglobin**.

3. *Buffering Action in Blood*

Hemoglobin functions as a good buffer. By this action, it regulates the hydrogen ion concentration and thereby plays a role in the maintenance of acid-base balance.

4. *In Blood Group Determination*

RBCs carry the blood group antigens like A antigen, B antigen and Rh factor. This helps in determination of blood group and enables to prevent the reactions due to incompatible blood transfusion (Chapter 16).

VARIATIONS IN NUMBER OF RED BLOOD CELLS

PHYSIOLOGICAL VARIATIONS

A. Increase in RBC Count: Polycythemia

Increase in the RBC count is known as polycythemia. It occurs in both physiological and pathological conditions. When it occurs in physiological conditions it is called **physiological polycythemia**. The increase in number during this condition is marginal and temporary. It occurs in the following conditions.

1. Age

At birth, the RBC count is 8 to 10 million/cu mm of blood. The count decreases within 10 days after birth due to destruction of RBCs. Because of excess destruction of RBCs and liberation of bilirubin, **physiological jaundice** develops in some newborn babies between 2 to 3 days after birth. Such type of jaundice lasts only for few days.

However, in infants and growing children, the cell count is more than the value in adults.

2. Sex

Before puberty and after menopause, in females the RBC count is similar to that in males. During reproductive period of females, the count is less than of males (4.5 million/cu mm).

3. High altitude

In people living in mountains (above 10,000 feet from mean sea level), the RBC count is more than 7 million/cu mm. It is due to hypoxia (decreased oxygen supply to tissues) in high altitude. Hypoxia stimulates kidney to secrete a hormone called erythropoietin which stimulates the bone marrow to produce more RBCs.

4. Muscular exercise

RBC count increases after muscular exercise. It is because of mild hypoxia which increases the sympathetic activity secretion of adrenaline from adrenal medulla. Adrenaline contracts spleen and RBCs are released into blood. Hypoxia also causes secretion of erythropoietin which stimulates the bone marrow to produce more RBCs.

5. Emotional conditions

The RBC count increases during the emotional conditions such as anxiety. It is because of increase in the sympathetic activity and contraction of spleen.

6. Increased environmental temperature

Generally increased temperature increases all the activities in the body including production of RBCs.

7. After meals

There is a slight increase in the RBC count after taking meals. It is because of need for more oxygen for metabolic activities.

B. Decrease in RBC Count

Decrease in RBC count occurs in the following physiological conditions.

1. High barometric pressures

At high barometric pressures as in deep sea, where the oxygen tension of blood is higher, the RBC count decreases.

2. During sleep

Generally, all the activities of the body are decreased during sleep including production of RBCs.

3. Pregnancy

In pregnancy, the RBC count decreases. It is because of increase in ECF volume. Increase in ECF volume, increases the plasma volume also resulting in **hemodilution**. So, there is a relative reduction in the RBC count.

PATHOLOGICAL VARIATIONS

A. Increase in RBC Count: Pathological Polycythemia

Pathological polycythemia is the abnormal increase in the RBC count. The count increases above 7 million/cu mm of the blood. Polycythemia is of two types, the primary polycythemia and secondary polycythemia.

Primary polycythemia: Polycythemia vera

Primary polycythemia is otherwise known as polycythemia vera. It is a disease characterized by persistent increase in RBC count above 14 million/cu mm of blood. This is always associated with increased WBC count above 24,000/cu mm of blood. Polycythemia vera occurs because of red bone marrow malignancy.

Secondary polycythemia

It is the pathological condition in which polycythemia occurs because of diseases in some other system such as respiratory disorders, congenital heart disease and chemical poisons.

All these conditions lead to hypoxia which stimulates release of erythropoietin. Erythropoietin stimulates the bone marrow resulting in increased RBC count.

B. Decrease in RBC Count: Anemia

Anemia is the abnormal decrease in RBC count. It is described in Chapter 10.

HEMOLYSIS AND FRAGILITY OF RBC

DEFINITION

Hemolysis

Hemolysis is the destruction of blood cells. To define more specifically, it is the process, which involves rupture of RBC and liberation of hemoglobin.

Fragility

Susceptibility of RBC to hemolysis or tendency to break easily is called fragility (fragile = easily broken).

Fragility is of two types:

1. **Osmotic fragility** which occurs due to exposure to hypotonic saline.
2. **Mechanical fragility** which occurs due to **mechanical trauma** (wound or injury).

Normally, old RBCs are destroyed in the reticuloendothelial system. Abnormal hemolysis is the process by which even younger RBCs are destroyed in large number by the presence of hemolytic agents or hemolysins.

■ PROCESS OF HEMOLYSIS

Normally, plasma and RBCs are in **osmotic equilibrium**. When the osmotic equilibrium is disturbed, the cells are affected. For example, when the RBCs are immersed in hypotonic saline the cells swell and rupture by bursting because of endosmosis. Hemoglobin is released from the ruptured RBCs.

■ CONDITIONS WHEN HEMOLYSIS OCCURS

1. Hemolytic jaundice.
2. Antigen antibody reactions.
3. Poisoning by chemicals or toxins.

■ HEMOLYSINS

Hemolysins or hemolytic agents are the substances, which cause destruction of RBCs.

Hemolysins are of two types:

1. Chemical substances.
2. Substances of bacterial origin or substances found in body.

Chemical Substances

Chemical substances such as alcohol, benzene, chloroform, ether, acids, alkalis and poisons like carbolic acid, nitrobenzene and resin cause hemolysis. Venom of poisonous snakes like cobra also cause hemolysis.

Substances of Bacterial Origin

Hemolysis is caused by toxic substances or toxins from bacteria such as *Streptococcus, Staphylococcus, Tetanus bacillus,* etc.

Chapter 8

Erythropoiesis

CHAPTER OUTLINE

- **DEFINITION**
- **SITE OF ERYTHROPOIESIS**
  - IN FETAL LIFE
  - IN NEWBORN BABIES, CHILDREN AND ADULTS
- **PROCESS OF ERYTHROPOIESIS**
  - STEM CELLS
  - CHANGES DURING ERYTHROPOIESIS
  - STAGES OF ERYTHROPOIESIS
- **FACTORS NECESSARY FOR ERYTHROPOIESIS**
  - STIMULATING FACTORS
  - MATURATION FACTORS
  - FACTORS NECESSARY FOR HEMOGLOBIN FORMATION

■ DEFINITION

Erythropoiesis is the process of origin, development and maturation of erythrocytes. **Hemopoiesis** is the process of origin, development and maturation of all the blood cells.

■ SITE OF ERYTHROPOIESIS

■ IN FETAL LIFE

In fetal life, the erythropoiesis occurs in three different stages.

1. *Mesoblastic Stage*

During first 2 or 3 months of intrauterine life, the RBCs are produced from mesenchymal cells of **yolk sac**.

2. *Hepatic Stage*

During the next 3 months of intrauterine life, RBCs are produced mainly from the liver. Some cells are produced from the spleen and other lymphoid organs are also.

3. *Myeloid Stage*

During the last 3 months of intrauterine life, the RBCs are produced from red bone marrow and liver.

■ IN NEWBORN BABIES, CHILDREN AND ADULTS

1. Up to the age of 20 years: RBCs are produced from red bone marrow of all bones.
2. After the age of 20 years: RBCs are produced from all the membranous bones and ends of long bones.

■ PROCESS OF ERYTHROPOIESIS

■ STEM CELLS

In bone marrow, RBCs develop from the **hematopoietic stem cells** which are called uncommitted **pluripotent hematopoietic stem cells** (PHSC). PHSC are not designed to form a particular type of blood cell; hence the name **uncommitted PHSC (Fig. 8.1)**. When the cells are designed to form a particular type of blood cell, these cells are called **committed PHSC**.

Committed PHSCs are of two types:

1. **Lymphoid stem cells** (LSC) which give rise to lymphocytes and natural killer (NK) cells.
2. **Colony-forming blastocytes**, which give rise to all the other blood cells except lymphocytes. When grown in cultures, these cells form colonies hence, name colony-forming blastocytes.

   Different units of colony-forming cells are:
   i. Colony-forming unit-erythrocytes (CFU-E) from which RBCs develop.
   ii. Colony-forming unit-granulocytes/monocytes (CFU-GM) from which granulocytes (neutrophils, basophils and eosinophils) and monocytes develop.

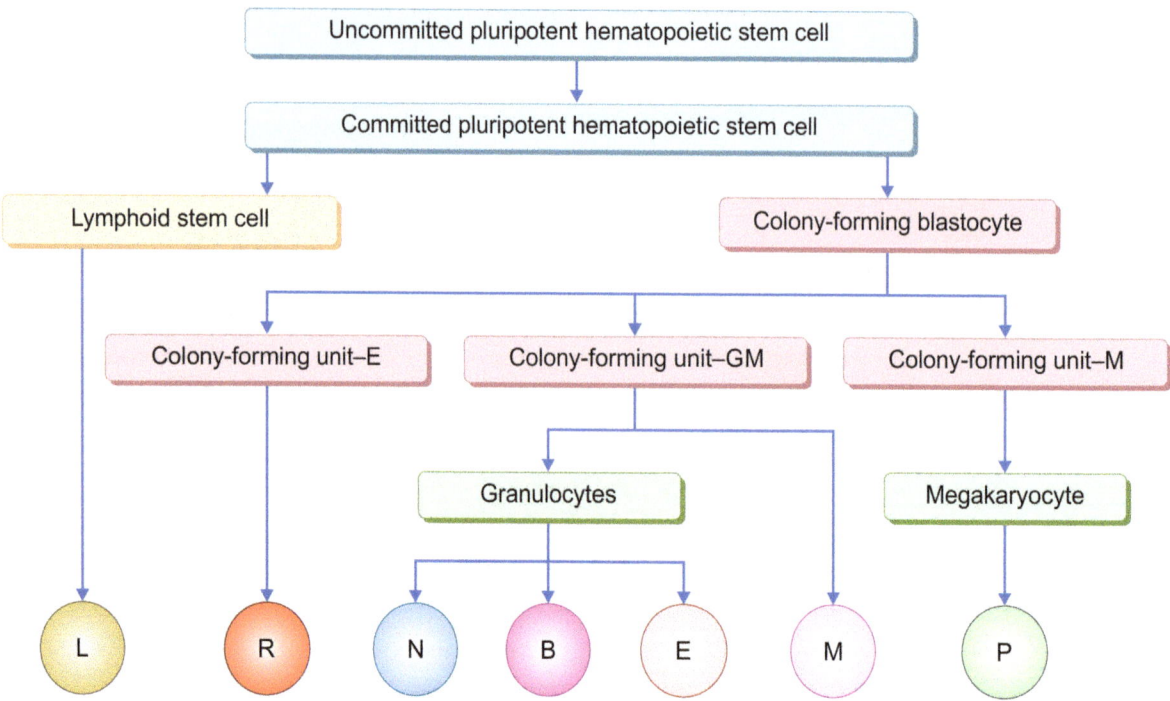

FIGURE 8.1: Stem cells.
L = Lymphocyte, R = Red blood cell, N = Neutrophil, B = Basophil, E = Eosinophil, M = Monocyte, P = Platelet.

iii. Colony-forming unit-megakaryocytes (CFU-M) from which platelets develop.

CHANGES DURING ERYTHROPOIESIS

When the cells of CFU-E pass through different stages and finally become the matured RBCs, four important changes are noticed:

1. Size of the cell is reduced from the diameter of 25 to 7.2 μ.
2. Nucleoli and nucleus disappear.
3. Hemoglobin appears.
4. Staining properties of the cytoplasm are changed.

STAGES OF ERYTHROPOIESIS

1. Proerythroblast (Megaloblast)

Proerythroblast or megaloblast is very large with a diameter of about 20 μ. Nucleus is large with two or more nucleoli and a **chromatin network**. Hemoglobin is absent. The cytoplasm is basophilic in nature. Proerythroblast multiplies several times and finally forms early normoblast **(Fig. 8.2)**.

2. Early Normoblast

It is smaller than proerythroblast with a diameter of about 15 μ. The nucleoli disappear from the nucleus and condensation of chromatin network occurs. The cytoplasm is basophilic in nature. So, this cell is also called **basophilic erythroblast**. This cell develops into intermediate normoblast.

3. Intermediate Normoblast

It is smaller than the early normoblast with a diameter of 10 to 12 μ. Chromatin network in nucleus shows further condensation. **Hemoglobin** starts appearing. Because of small quantity of acidic hemoglobin, the cytoplasm becomes polychromatic. So, this cell is called polychromophilic or **polychromatic erythroblast**. This cell develops into late normoblast.

4. Late Normoblast

Diameter of the cell decreases further to about 8 to 10 μ. Quantity of hemoglobin increases making the cytoplasm almost acidophilic. So, the cell is now called **orthochromatic erythroblast**. Nucleus becomes very small with very much condensed chromatin network and is called **ink spot nucleus**. At the end of this stage, nucleus disappears by the process called **pyknosis**. Late normoblast develops into reticulocyte.

5. Reticulocyte

Reticulocyte or **immature RBC** is slightly larger than matured RBC. The **reticular network** or reticulum that is formed from the disintegrated organelles are present in the cytoplasm.

In newborn babies, the reticulocyte count is 2 to 6% of RBCs, i.e. 2 to 6 reticulocytes are present for every 100 RBCs. Number of reticulocytes decreases during the 1st week after birth. Later, the reticulocyte count remains constant at or below 1%.

6. Matured Erythrocyte

Matured erythrocyte is small with a diameter of 7.2 μ. It has hemoglobin but no nucleus. Reticular network disappears and the cell becomes biconcave in shape.

Important events during erythropoiesis are given in **Table 8.1**.

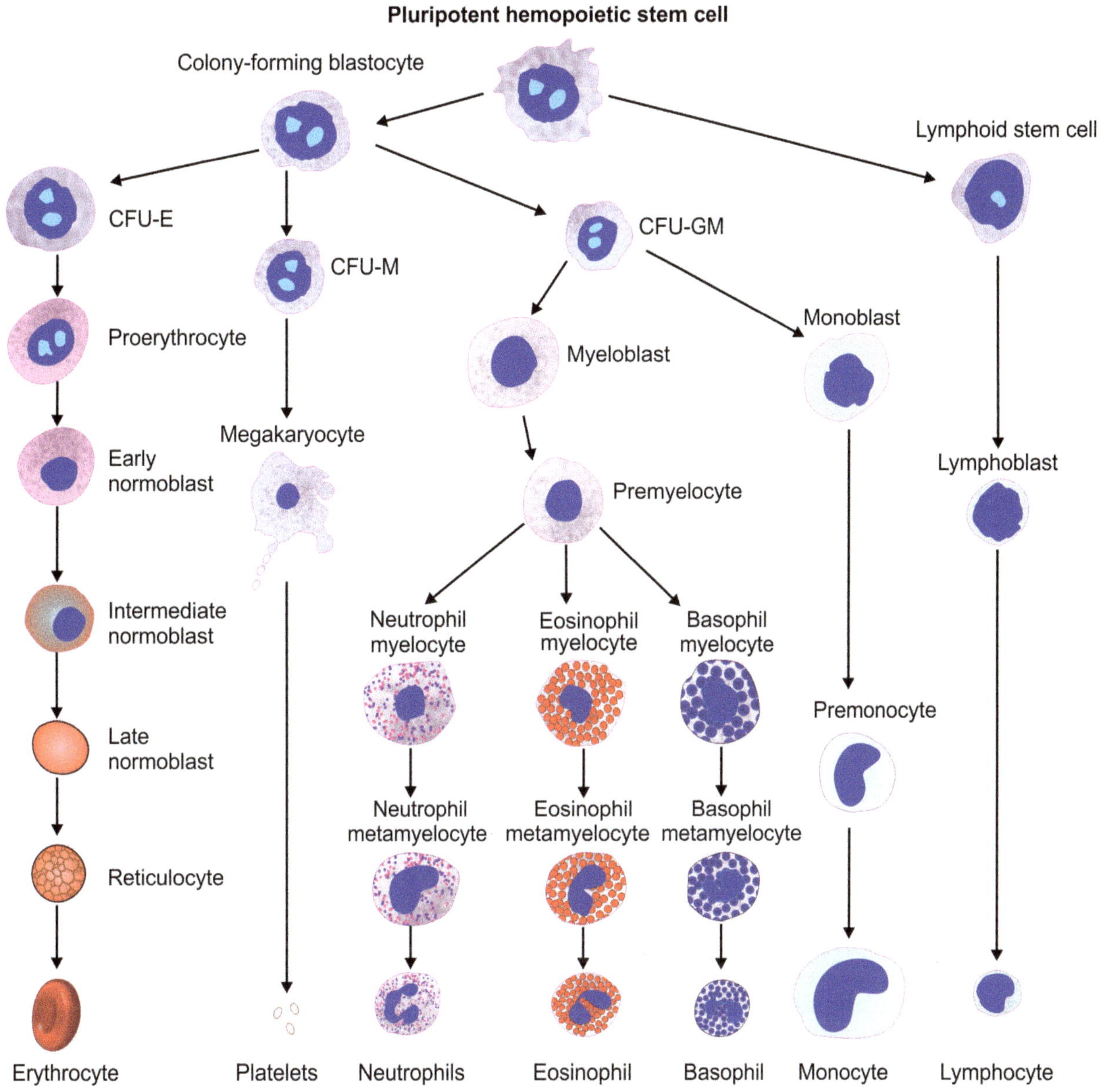

FIGURE 8.2: Stages of hemopoiesis. CFU-E = Colony-forming unit-erythrocyte. CFU-M = Colony-forming unit-megakaryocyte, CFU-GM = Colony-forming unit-granulocyte/monocyte.

■ FACTORS NECESSARY FOR ERYTHROPOIESIS

Development and maturation of erythrocytes require many factors which are classified into three categories:

■ STIMULATING FACTORS

1. *Hypoxia*

Hypoxia (reduced availability of oxygen to the tissues) is the most important stimulating factor for erythropoiesis. It stimulates erythropoiesis by inducing secretion of erythropoietin from kidney.

2. *Erythropoietin*

Erythropoietin is a hormone secreted by peritubular capillaries in the kidney. Hypoxia is the stimulant for erythropoietin secretion.

Erythropoietin promotes erythropoiesis by stimulating production of proerythroblasts, development of proerythroblasts into matured RBCs and release of matured erythrocytes into blood.

3. *Thyroxine*

Being a general metabolic hormone, thyroxine accelerates the process of erythropoiesis at many levels.

4. *Role of Sex Hormones*

Testosterone has mild erythropoietic action after puberty.

5. *Hematopoietic Growth Factors*

Hematopoietic growth factors or growth inducers are the interleukins 3, 6 and 11 and **stem cell factor** (steel

TABLE 8.1: Changes during erythropoiesis.

Stage of erythropoiesis	Diameter (μ)	Nucleus	Staining property	Important event
1. Proerythroblast	20	Has two or more nucleoli and chromatin network	Basophilic	Synthesis of hemoglobin starts
2. Early normoblast	15	No nucleoli Dense chromatin network	Basophilic	Nucleoli disappear
3. Intermediate normoblast	10 to 12	Further condensation of chromatin network	Polychromophilic or Polychromatic	Hemoglobin starts appearing
4. Late normoblast	8 to 10	Small with very much condensed chromatin Ink-spot nucleus	Acidophilic	Nucleus disappears by pyknosis
5. Reticulocyte	7 to 7.5	Absent	Basophilic	Reticulum is formed Cell enters capillary from site of production
6. Matured RBC	7.2	Absent	Acidophilic	Reticulum disappears Cell attains biconcavity

factor). Generally, these factors stimulate the proliferation of PHSCs.

6. Vitamins

Vitamins B_3, B_6, C, D and E are necessary for erythropoiesis **(Table 8.2)**. Deficiency of these vitamins causes anemia.

■ MATURATION FACTORS

Vitamin B_{12}, intrinsic factor and folic acid are necessary for the maturation of RBCs.

1. Vitamin B_{12} (Cyanocobalamin)

Vitamin B_{12} is essential for synthesis of DNA, cell division and maturation in RBCs. It is also called **extrinsic factor** since it is obtained mostly from diet. It is also produced in the large intestine by the intestinal flora. It is absorbed from the small intestine in the presence of intrinsic factor of Castle. Deficiency of vitamin B_{12} causes **pernicious anemia** (macrocytic anemia).

2. Intrinsic Factor of Castle

Intrinsic factor is produced in gastric mucosa by the parietal cells of the gastric glands. It is essential for the absorption of vitamin B_{12} from intestine. Absence of intrinsic factor also leads to pernicious anemia because of failure of vitamin B_{12} absorption.

3. Folic Acid

Folic acid is also essential for the synthesis of DNA. Deficiency of folic acid decreases the DNA synthesis causing maturation failure. Here the cells are larger and remain in megaloblastic (proerythroblastic) stage which leads to **megaloblastic anemia**.

■ FACTORS NECESSARY FOR HEMOGLOBIN FORMATION

Various materials are essential for the formation of hemoglobin in the RBCs such as:

1. First class proteins and amino acids are required for formation of globin.
2. Iron is necessary for formation of heme part of the hemoglobin.
3. Copper helps absorption of iron from GI tract.
4. Cobalt and nickel help utilization of iron during hemoglobin synthesis.
5. Vitamins C, B_2, B_3, and B_6 are essential for hemoglobin synthesis.

TABLE 8.2: Factors necessary for erythropoiesis.

Stimulating factors	Maturation factors	Factors necessary for hemoglobin formation
1. Hypoxia 2. Erythropoietin 3. Thyroxine 4. Hematopoietic growth factors 5. Vitamins: B_3, B_6, C, D and E	1. Vitamin B_{12} 2. Intrinsic factor 3. Folic acid	1. First class proteins and amino acids 2. Iron 3. Copper 4. Cobalt and nickel 5. Vitamins: C, B_2, B_3 and B_6

Chapter 9: Hemoglobin and Iron Metabolism

CHAPTER OUTLINE

- DEFINITION
- NORMAL HEMOGLOBIN CONTENT
- FUNCTIONS
- STRUCTURE
- TYPES OF NORMAL HEMOGLOBIN
- ABNORMAL HEMOGLOBIN
- ABNORMAL HEMOGLOBIN DERIVATIVES
- SYNTHESIS
- DESTRUCTION
- IRON METABOLISM

DEFINITION

Hemoglobin (Hb) is the iron-containing coloring pigment of red blood cell (RBC). It forms 95% of dry weight of RBC and 30 to 34% of wet weight. Molecular weight of hemoglobin is 68,000.

NORMAL HEMOGLOBIN CONTENT

Average hemoglobin content in blood is 14 to 16 g/dL. At the time of birth, infants and growing children, hemoglobin content is high because of increased number of RBCs.

Hemoglobin content in a normal adult male is 15 g/dL and in normal adult female is 14.5 g/dL.

FUNCTIONS OF HEMOGLOBIN

TRANSPORT OF RESPIRATORY GASES

Major function of hemoglobin is the transport of respiratory gases. It transports:

1. Oxygen from the lungs to tissues.
2. Carbon dioxide from tissues to lungs (Chapter 72).

BUFFER ACTION

Hemoglobin acts as a buffer and plays an important role in acid-base balance.

STRUCTURE OF HEMOGLOBIN

Hemoglobin is a conjugated protein. It consists of a protein called **globin** and an iron-containing pigment called **heme**.

Iron is present in an unstable ferrous (Fe^{2+}) form. Heme part is called **porphyrin**. It is formed by four **pyrrole rings** (tetrapyrrole). The iron is attached to each pyrrole ring and globin molecule.

Globin is made up of four polypeptide chains. Among the four polypeptide chains, two are α-chains with 141 amino acids and other two chains are β-chains with 146 amino acids.

TYPES OF NORMAL HEMOGLOBIN

Hemoglobin is of two types. Both the types of hemoglobin differ from each other structurally and functionally.

1. Adult Hemoglobin (HbA)

In adult hemoglobin, the globin contains two α-chains and two β-chains.

2. Fetal Hemoglobin (HbF)

In fetal hemoglobin, globin has two α-chains and two γ-chains instead of β-chains.

Functionally, fetal hemoglobin has **more affinity** for oxygen than adult hemoglobin. And, the oxygen-hemoglobin dissociation curve of fetal blood is shifted to left (Chapter 72).

ABNORMAL HEMOGLOBIN

Abnormal types of hemoglobin are produced because of structural changes in the polypeptide chains caused by mutation in the genes of the globin chains. Abnormal hemoglobin is of two categories:

1. Abnormal Hemoglobin in Hemoglobinopathies

Hemoglobinopathy is a genetic disorder caused by abnormal polypeptide chains of hemoglobin. Some of the hemoglobinopathies are HbS, HbC, HbE, HbH and HbM.

TABLE 9.1: Formation of abnormal hemoglobin derivatives.

Derivative	Formation
Carboxyhemoglobin	By combination of hemoglobin with carbon monoxide
Methemoglobin	By oxidation of hemoglobin from ferrous state to ferric state
Sulfhemoglobin	By combination of hemoglobin with hydrogen sulfide

2. Abnormal Hemoglobin in Thalassemia and Related Disorders

In thalassemia, abnormal hemoglobin is present with decreased polypeptide chains (Chapter 10).

ABNORMAL HEMOGLOBIN DERIVATIVES

Abnormal hemoglobin which is formed by the combination of hemoglobin with substances other than oxygen and carbon dioxide is called **hemoglobin derivative**.

High levels of hemoglobin derivatives in blood produce serious effects by preventing the transport of oxygen. It results in oxygen lack in tissues, which may be fatal. Abnormal hemoglobin derivatives are of three types:

1. CARBOXYHEMOGLOBIN

Carboxyhemoglobin or **carbon monoxyhemoglobin** is the abnormal hemoglobin derivative formed by the combination of carbon monoxide with hemoglobin **(Table 9.1)**. Since hemoglobin has 200 times more affinity for **carbon monoxide** than oxygen, it hinders the transport of oxygen resulting in hypoxia (Chapter 74). Normal carboxyhemoglobin level is 1 to 3% of total hemoglobin.

Signs and Symptoms of Carbon Monoxide Poisoning

1. While breathing air with less than 1% of carbon monoxide, the hemoglobin saturation is 15 to 20% and mild symptoms such as headache and nausea appear.
2. While breathing air with more than 1% carbon monoxide, the hemoglobin saturation is 30 to 40%. It causes severe symptoms like convulsions, cardiorespiratory arrest, unconsciousness and coma.
3. When hemoglobin saturation increases above 50%, death occurs.

2. METHEMOGLOBIN

Methemoglobin is the abnormal hemoglobin derivative formed when iron molecule of hemoglobin is oxidized from normal ferrous state to ferric state. Methemoglobin is also called **ferrihemoglobin**. Normal methemoglobin level is less than 3% of total hemoglobin.

Common sources of methemoglobin are contaminated well waters with nitrates and nitrites, explosives, naphthalene balls and nitrous oxide.

3. SULFHEMOGLOBIN

Sulfhemoglobin is the abnormal hemoglobin derivative formed by the combination of hemoglobin with hydrogen sulfide. It is caused by drugs such as sulfonamides. Normal sulfhemoglobin level is less than 1% of total hemoglobin.

SYNTHESIS OF HEMOGLOBIN

Synthesis of hemoglobin actually starts in proerythroblastic stage. However, hemoglobin appears only in intermediate normoblastic stage. Synthesis of the hemoglobin is continued until the stage of reticulocyte. Heme is synthesized from **succinyl-CoA** and glycine in the mitochondria. Polypeptide chains of globin are produced in the ribosomes.

SUBSTANCES NECESSARY FOR HEMOGLOBIN SYNTHESIS

Various factors are essential for the formation of hemoglobin in the RBC. Refer Chapter 8 for details.

DESTRUCTION OF HEMOGLOBIN

After the lifespan of 120 days, the RBC is destroyed in the reticuloendothelial system, particularly in spleen and the hemoglobin is released into plasma. Soon, the hemoglobin is degraded in the reticuloendothelial cells and split into globin, iron and porphyrin.

Globin is utilized for the resynthesis of hemoglobin. Iron is stored in the body. Porphyrin is converted into **biliverdin**. Most of the biliverdin is converted into **bilirubin**. Bilirubin and biliverdin are together called the **bile pigments**. Refer Chapter 29 for details of bile pigments.

IRON METABOLISM

Iron is an essential mineral. It is the important component of proteins which are involved in oxygen transport. Iron is important for the formation of hemoglobin and myoglobin. Iron is also necessary for the formation of other substances like **cytochrome, cytochrome oxidase, peroxidase** and **catalase.**

Total quantity of iron in the body is about 4 g. Normal blood level of iron is 50 to 150 µg/dL.

DIETARY IRON

Dietary iron is available in two forms called heme and nonheme.

Heme iron is present in fish, meat and chicken. Iron in these sources is found in the form of heme. Heme iron is absorbed easily from intestine.

Iron in the form of nonheme is available in vegetables, grains and cereals. Nonheme iron is not absorbed easily as heme iron. Cereals, flours and products of grains which are enriched or fortified (strengthened) with iron, become good dietary sources of nonheme iron, particularly for children and women.

ABSORPTION OF IRON

Iron is absorbed from small intestine through enterocytes by pinocytosis and transported into the blood. Iron is present mostly in ferric (Fe^{3+}) form. It is converted into ferrous form (Fe^{2+}) which is absorbed into the blood.

■ TRANSPORT OF IRON

Immediately after absorption into blood, iron combines with a **β-globulin** called **apotransferrin** and forms **transferrin**. And iron is transported in blood in the form of transferrin. Iron combines loosely with globin and can be released easily at any region of the body.

■ STORAGE OF IRON

Iron is stored in large quantities in reticuloendothelial cells and hepatocytes in liver. It is stored in other cells also but in small quantities. In the cytoplasm of the cell, iron is stored as **ferritin** in large amount. Small quantity of iron is also stored as **hemosiderin**.

■ DAILY LOSS OF IRON

In males, about 1 mg of iron is excreted everyday through feces. In females, the amount of iron loss is very much high. This is because of the menstruation. During every menstrual cycle, about 50 mL of blood is lost by which 25 mg of iron is lost. This is why the iron content is always less in females than in males.

■ REGULATION OF TOTAL IRON IN THE BODY

Absorption and excretion of iron are maintained almost equally under normal physiological conditions. When the iron storage is saturated in the body, it automatically decreases further absorption of iron from the gastrointestinal tract by feedback mechanism.

■ APPLIED PHYSIOLOGY: IRON DEFICIENCY ANEMIA

Deficiency of iron causes decrease in hemoglobin synthesis resulting in iron deficiency anemia. Refer Chapter 10 for details.

Chapter 10: Erythrocyte Sedimentation Rate, Packed Cell Volume, Blood Indices and Anemia

CHAPTER OUTLINE

- **ERYTHROCYTE SEDIMENTATION RATE**
  - DEFINITION
  - DETERMINATION
  - NORMAL VALUES
  - SIGNIFICANCE OF DETERMINING ESR
  - APPLIED PHYSIOLOGY: VARIATIONS
- **PACKED CELL VOLUME**
  - DEFINITION
  - METHOD OF DETERMINATION
- **SIGNIFICANCE OF DETERMINING PCV**
  - NORMAL VALUES
  - APPLIED PHYSIOLOGY: VARIATIONS
- **BLOOD INDICES**
  - DIFFERENT BLOOD INDICES
- **ANEMIA**
  - DEFINITION
  - CLASSIFICATION
  - SIGNS AND SYMPTOMS

ERYTHROCYTE SEDIMENTATION RATE

DEFINITION

Erythrocyte sedimentation rate (ESR) is the rate at which the erythrocytes settle down. Normally, when the blood is in circulation, the red blood cells (RBCs) remain suspended uniformly. This property is called **suspension stability** of RBCs. If blood is mixed with an anticoagulant and allowed to stand undisturbed on a vertical tube, the red cells settle down due to gravity with a supernatant layer of clear plasma.

DETERMINATION OF ESR

ESR is determined by two methods:

1. Westergren Method

In this method, **Westergren tube** is used to determine ESR. This tube is 300 mm long and opened on both ends **(Fig. 10.1A)**. It is marked 0 to 200 mm from above downwards. 1.6 mL of blood is mixed with 0.4 mL of 3.8% **sodium citrate** (anticoagulant). The ratio of blood and anticoagulant is 4:1. This blood is loaded in the Westergren tube up to '0' mark above. Tube is placed vertically in the Westergren stand and left undisturbed and reading is taken after 1 hour.

2. Wintrobe Method

In this method, **Wintrobe tube** is used to determine ESR. This tube is a short and opened on one end and closed on the other end **(Fig. 10.1B)**. It is 110 mm long with 3 mm bore. It is used for determining ESR and PCV. It is marked on both sides. On one side, the marking is 0 to 100 (for ESR) and on other side, 100 to 0 (for PCV) from above downwards.

About 1 mL of blood is mixed with an anticoagulant called **ethylenediaminetetra acetic acid** (**EDTA**). Blood is loaded in the tube up to '0' mark above. Tube is placed on the Wintrobe stand and left undisturbed and reading is taken after 1 hour.

NORMAL VALUES OF ESR

Normal values of ESR in both Westergren method and Wintrobe method are given in **Table 10.1**.

SIGNIFICANCE OF DETERMINING ESR

ESR is an easy, inexpensive test which helps in diagnosis as well as prognosis. **Prognosis** means monitoring the course of disease and response of the patient to therapy. Determination of ESR is especially helpful in assessing the progress of patients treated for certain chronic disorders such as pulmonary tuberculosis and rheumatoid arthritis.

APPLIED PHYSIOLOGY: VARIATIONS OF ESR

Physiological Variation

1. *Age:* ESR is less in children and infants because of large number of RBCs.

Chapter 10: Erythrocyte Sedimentation Rate, Packed Cell Volume, Blood Indices and Anemia

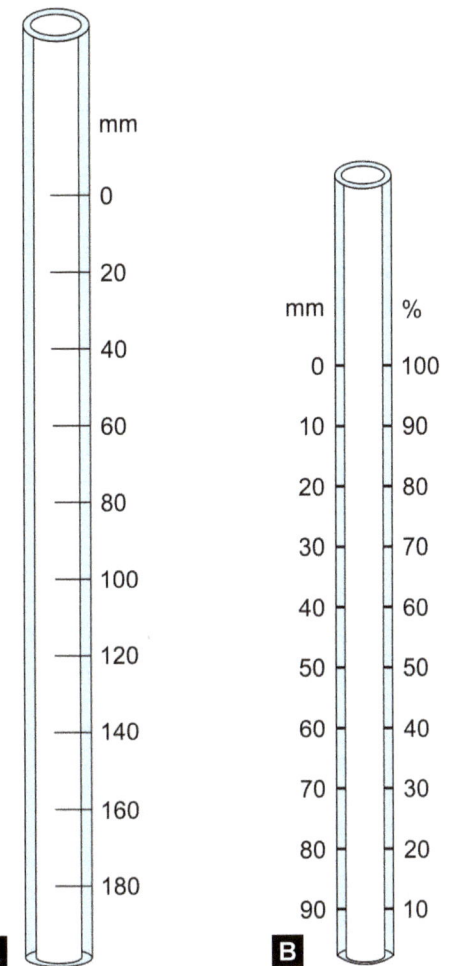

FIGURE 10.1: ESR tubes.
A. Westergren tube: Used to determine ESR.
B. Wintrobe tube: Used to determine ESR and PCV.

2. *Sex*: ESR is more in females than in males because of decreased number of RBCs.
3. *Menstruation*: ESR increases during menstruation because of loss of blood and RBCs.
4. *Pregnancy*: From 3rd month to parturition, ESR increases up to 35 mm in 1 hour because of hemodilution.

Pathological Variation

ESR increases in tuberculosis, all types of anemia except sickle cell anemia, rheumatoid arthritis, rheumatic fever and liver diseases.

TABLE 10.1: Normal values of erythrocyte sedimentation rate (ESR).

ESR	Westergren method (mm in 1 hour)	Wintrobe method (mm in 1 hour)
Males	3 to 7	0 to 9
Females	5 to 9	0 to 15
Infants	0 to 2	0 to 5

ESR decreases in allergic conditions, sickle cell anemia, peptone shock and polycythemia.

■ PACKED CELL VOLUME

■ DEFINITION

Packed cell volume (PCV) is the volume of the RBCs in the blood that is expressed in percentage. It is also called hematocrit value.

■ METHOD OF DETERMINATION

Blood is mixed with the anticoagulant EDTA or **heparin** and filled in Wintrobe tube up to the 100 or 0 mark above. The tube with the blood is centrifuged at a speed of 3,000 revolutions per minute (rpm) for 30 minutes.

At the end of 30 minutes, the tube is taken out and the reading is taken. RBCs are packed at the bottom and this is the backed cell volume. The plasma remains above this. In between the RBCs and the plasma, there is a **white buffy coat**, which is formed by white blood cells (WBCs) and the platelets **(Fig. 10.2)**.

■ SIGNIFICANCE OF DETERMINING PCV

Determination of PCV helps in:

1. Diagnosis and treatment of anemia.
2. Diagnosis and treatment of polycythemia.
3. Determination of severity of dehydration and recovery from dehydration after treatment.
4. Decision of blood transfusion.

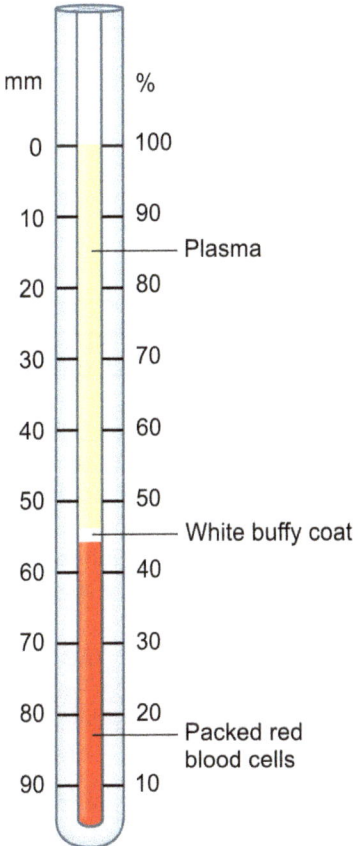

FIGURE 10.2: Packed cell volume.

NORMAL VALUES OF PCV

Normal PCV:

In males   : 40 to 45%
In females   : 38 to 42%

APPLIED PHYSIOLOGY: VARIATIONS IN PCV

PCV increases in polycythemia, dehydration and **dengue shock syndrome** (dengue fever of grade III or IV severity). **Dengue fever** is a tropical disease caused by flavivirus, transmitted by mosquito *Aedes aegypti*.

PCV decreases in anemia, cirrhosis of liver and pregnancy.

BLOOD INDICES

Blood indices are the calculations derived from RBC count, hemoglobin content of blood and PCV. Blood indices help in diagnosis of the type of anemia.

DIFFERENT BLOOD INDICES

Blood indices are four in number:

1. Mean Corpuscular Volume

Mean corpuscular volume (MCV) is the average volume of a single RBC and it is expressed in cubic microns (cu μ).

Normal MCV is 90 cu μ (78 to 90 cu μ). When MCV is normal, the RBC is called **normocyte**. When MCV increases, the cell is known as a **macrocyte** and when it decreases, the cell is called **microcyte**.

2. Mean Corpuscular Hemoglobin

Mean corpuscular hemoglobin (MCH) is the quantity or amount of hemoglobin present in one RBC. It is expressed in picogram (pg).

Normal MCH is 30 pg (27 to 32 pg).

3. Mean Corpuscular Hemoglobin Concentration

Mean corpuscular hemoglobin concentration (MCHC) is the concentration of hemoglobin in one RBC. It is the amount of hemoglobin expressed in relation to the volume of one RBC. So, the unit of expression is percentage. This is the most important absolute value in the diagnosis of anemia.

Normal MCHC is 30% (30 to 38%). When MCHC is normal, the RBC is **normochromic**. When MCHC decreases, the RBC is known as **hypochromic**. In pernicious anemia and megaloblastic anemia, RBCs are macrocytic and normochromic or hypochromic. In iron deficiency anemia, RBCs are microcytic and hypochromic.

A single RBC cannot be hyperchromic because, the amount of hemoglobin cannot increase beyond normal level.

4. Color Index

Color index (CI) is the ratio between the percentage of hemoglobin and the percentage of RBCs in the blood. Actually, it is the average hemoglobin content in one cell of a patient compared to the average hemoglobin content in one cell of a normal person.

Normal color index is 1.0 (0.8 to 1.2). Color index is useful in determining the type of anemia.

ANEMIA

DEFINITION

Anemia is a blood disorder characterized by the reduction in red blood cell count, hemoglobin content and packed cell volume.

CLASSIFICATION OF ANEMIA

Anemia is classified by two methods namely, morphological classification and etiological classification.

Morphological Classification

By this method, anemia is classified by the morphology (size and color) of RBC. Size of RBC is expressed as mean corpuscular volume (MCV). Color of RBC depends upon hemoglobin concentration in RBC and it is expressed as mean corpuscular hemoglobin concentration (MCHC).

By this method, anemia is classified into four types:

1. Normocytic normochromic anemia.
2. Macrocytic normochromic anemia.
3. Macrocytic hypochromic anemia.
4. Microcytic hypochromic anemia **(Table 10.2)**.

Etiological Classification

In this method, anemia is classified by the cause. Etiology means the study of cause or origin of any disease.

By method, anemia is classified into five types:

1. Hemorrhagic anemia.
2. Hemolytic anemia.
3. Nutrition deficiency anemia.
4. Aplastic anemia.
5. Anemia of chronic diseases.

1. Hemorrhagic anemia

Hemorrhage means excess loss of blood (Chapter 66). Anemia due to hemorrhage is known as hemorrhagic

TABLE 10.2: Morphological classification of anemia.

Type of anemia	Size of RBC	MCV (cu μ)	Color of RBC	MCHC (%)
Normocytic normochromic	Normal	90	Normal	30
Macrocytic normochromic	Large	More than 90	Normal	30
Macrocytic hypochromic	Large	More than 90	Less	Less than 30
Microcytic hypochromic	Small	Less than 78	Less	Less than 30

anemia or **blood loss anemia**. It occurs both in acute and chronic hemorrhagic conditions.

RBCs are **normocytic** and **normochromic** in acute hemorrhage and **microcytic** and **hypochromic** in chronic hemorrhage.

2. *Hemolytic anemia*

Hemolysis means destruction of RBCs. Anemia due to excess destruction of RBCs is called hemolytic anemia.

It is classified into two types, extrinsic hemolytic anemia and intrinsic hemolytic anemia.

Extrinsic hemolytic anemia

This type of anemia caused by destruction of RBCs by external factors. Healthy RBCs are hemolyzed by factors outside the blood cells such as antibodies, chemicals and drugs. Refer **Table 10.3** for various causes of extrinsic hemolytic anemia.

Intrinsic hemolytic anemia

This type of anemia is caused by destruction of RBCs due to defective RBCs. There is production of unhealthy RBCs, which are short lived and are destroyed soon. Intrinsic hemolytic anemia is often inherited and it includes sickle cell anemia and thalassemia.

Sickle cell anemia

Sickle cell anemia is an inherited blood disorder characterized by sickle-shaped RBCs. It occurs when a person inherits two abnormal genes (one from each parent). In sickle cell anemia, hemoglobin becomes abnormal with normal α-chains and abnormal β-chains. Because of this, RBCs attain sickle (crescent) shape and become more fragile leading to hemolysis.

Thalassemia

Thalassemia is an inherited disorder characterized by abnormal hemoglobin. In normal hemoglobin, the number of α- and β-polypeptide chains is equal. In thalassemia, the number of these chains is not equal. This causes defective formation of RBCs or hemolysis of the matured RBCs. Thalassemia is of two types, α-thalassemia and β-thalassemia.

3. *Nutrition deficiency anemia*

Nutrition deficiency anemia is the type of anemia that occurs due to deficiency of a nutritive substance necessary for erythropoiesis.

Nutrition deficiency anemia are of four types:

i. Iron deficiency anemia

Iron deficiency anemia is the most common type of anemia. It develops due to inadequate availability of iron for hemoglobin synthesis. RBCs are **microcytic and hypochromic**.

ii. Protein deficiency anemia

Protein deficiency decreases the hemoglobin synthesis resulting in anemia. **RBCs are** macrocytic and hypochromic.

TABLE 10.3: Etiological classification of anemia.

Type of anemia	Causes		Morphology of RBC
Hemorrhagic anemia	Excess loss of blood by internal or external bleeding		Acute loss: Normocytic and normochromic
			Chronic loss: Microcytic and hypochromic
Hemolytic anemia	Extrinsic hemolytic anemia: i. Liver failure ii. Renal disorder iii. Hypersplenism iv. Burns v. Infections such as hepatitis and malaria vi. Drugs such as penicillin vii. Poisoning by lead, coal and tar viii. Presence of isoagglutinins like anti-Rh ix. Autoimmune diseases		Normocytic, normochromic
	Intrinsic hemolytic anemia Hereditary disorders	Sickle cell anemia	Sickle shape
		Thalassemia	Irregular, microcytic and hypochromic
Nutrition deficiency anemia	Iron deficiency		Microcytic, hypochromic
	Protein deficiency		Macrocytic, hypochromic
	Vitamin B_{12} deficiency		Macrocytic, normochromic/hypochromic
	Folic acid deficiency		Megaloblastic, hypochromic
Aplastic anemia	Bone marrow disorder		Normocytic, normochromic
Anemia of chronic diseases	i. Non-infectious inflammatory diseases such as rheumatoid arthritis ii. Chronic infections like tuberculosis iii. Chronic renal failure		Normocytic, normochromic

iii. Vitamin B_{12} deficiency: Pernicious anemia

Vitamin B_{12} is a maturation factor for RBC and deficiency of this causes pernicious anemia, which is also called **Addison's anemia**. It occurs because of less intake of vitamin B_{12} or poor absorption of vitamin B_{12}. Vitamin B_{12} is absorbed from the stomach with the help of intrinsic factor of Castle, which is secreted in the gastric mucosa. Decrease in the production of intrinsic factor causes poor absorption of vitamin B_{12}. RBCs are **macrocytic and normochromic/hypochromic**.

iv. Folic acid deficiency: Megaloblastic anemia

Folic acid is necessary for the maturation of RBC. Deficiency of this leads to defective DNA synthesis making the nucleus to remain immature. RBCs are **megaloblastic and hypochromic**.

4. Aplastic anemia

Aplastic anemia is due to the bone marrow disorder. The red bone marrow is reduced and replaced by fatty tissues. RBCs are **normocytic and normochromic**.

5. Anemia due to chronic diseases

Anemia occurs due to some chronic diseases such as rheumatoid arthritis, tuberculosis and chronic renal failure **(Table 10.3)**. RBCs are **normocytic and normochromic**.

■ SIGNS AND SYMPTOMS OF ANEMIA

1. Skin, Hair and Nails

In anemic patients, the color of the skin becomes pale. Skin also loses the elasticity and becomes thin and dry. Loss of hair is common with thinning and early graying. The nails become brittle and easily breakable.

2. Cardiovascular System

There is increase in heart rate and cardiac output. Heart is dilated and cardiac murmurs are produced.

3. Respiratory System

Rate and force of respiration increases. Sometimes, it leads to breathlessness and **dyspnea** (difficulty in breathing). Oxygen-hemoglobin dissociation curve is shifted to right.

4. Digestive System and Metabolism

Anorexia (loss of appetite), nausea, vomiting, abdominal discomfort and constipation are common. In pernicious anemia, there is atrophy of papillae in tongue. In aplastic anemia, necrotic lesions appear in mouth and pharynx. Basal metabolic rate increases in severe anemia.

5. Kidney

Kidney function is disturbed. Albuminuria is common.

6. Reproduction System

In females, the menstrual cycle is disturbed. There may be menorrhagia, oligomenorrhea or amenorrhea (Chapter 53).

7. Neuromuscular System

Common neuromuscular symptoms are headache, lack of concentration, restlessness, drowsiness, dizziness or vertigo, and fainting. Muscles become weak and the patient feels lack of energy and fatigued often and easily.

Chapter 11

White Blood Cells

CHAPTER OUTLINE

- WBC VS RBC
- CLASSIFICATION
- MORPHOLOGY
- NORMAL COUNT
- APPLIED PHYSIOLOGY: VARIATIONS
- LIFESPAN
- PROPERTIES
- FUNCTIONS
- LEUKOPOIESIS

WBC VS RBC

White blood cells (WBCs) or **leukocytes** are the colorless and nucleated formed elements of blood (leuko means white or colorless).

Compared to RBCs, the WBCs are larger in size and lesser in number. Yet functionally, these cells are as important as RBCs. WBCs play important role in defense mechanism of body. WBCs differ from RBCs in many aspects. Differences between these two types of blood cells are given in **Table 11.1**.

CLASSIFICATION OF WHITE BLOOD CELLS

White blood cells are classified into two groups depending upon the presence or absence of granules in the cytoplasm, viz. granulocytes with granules and agranulocytes without granules.

GRANULOCYTES

Depending upon staining property of granules, the granulocytes are classified into three types:

1. Neutrophils : Granules take both acidic and basic stains.
2. Eosinophils : Granules take acidic stain.
3. Basophils : Granules take basic stain.

AGRANULOCYTES

Agranulocytes have plain cytoplasm without granules. Agranulocytes are of two types:

1. Monocytes.
2. Lymphocytes.

TABLE 11.1: Differences between white blood cell and red blood cell.

Feature	WBC	RBC
1. Color	Colorless	Red
2. Number	Less: 4,000 to 11,000/cu mm	More: 4.5 to 5.5 million/cu mm
3. Size	Larger with maximum diameter of 18 μ	Smaller with maximum diameter of 7.4 μ
4. Shape	Irregular	Disk shaped and Biconcave
5. Hemoglobin	Absent	Present
6. Nucleus	Present	Absent
7. Granules	Present in some types	Absent
8. Types	Many types	Only one type
9. Lifespan	Shorter Ranges from ½ to 15 days	Longer 120 days
10. Functions	Defense and immunity	Transport of oxygen and carbon dioxide Buffering action

MORPHOLOGY OF WHITE BLOOD CELLS

NEUTROPHILS

Neutrophils are called **polymorphonuclear leukocytes** because the nucleus is multilobed. Number of lobes in

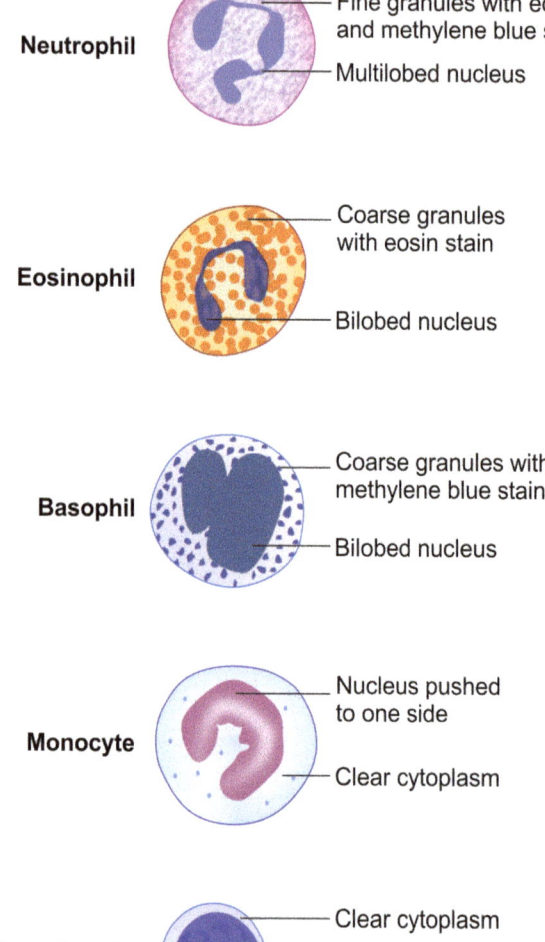

FIGURE 11.1: Different white blood cells.

the nuclei varies from 1 to 6 **(Fig. 11.1)**. Granules are fine or small in size. When stained with **Leishman's stain** which contains acidic eosin and basic methylene blue, the granules take both the stains equally. So, the granules appear violet in color. Diameter of cell is 10 to 12 μ. Neutrophils are ameboid and phagocytic in nature.

■ EOSINOPHILS

Eosinophils have coarse (larger) granules in the cytoplasm, which stain pink or reddish orange with eosin. Normally, nucleus is bilobed and spectacle shaped. Diameter of this cell varies between 10 and 14 μ.

■ BASOPHILS

Basophils also have coarse granules in the cytoplasm and the granules stain purple blue with methylene blue. Nucleus is bilobed. Diameter of this cell is 8 to 10 μ.

■ MONOCYTES

Monocytes are the largest leukocytes with diameter of 14 to 18 μ. The cytoplasm is clear without granules. The nucleus is round, oval, horseshoe shaped, bean shaped or kidney shaped. Nucleus is placed either in the center of the cell or pushed to one side and a large amount of cytoplasm is seen.

■ LYMPHOCYTES

Lymphocytes also do not have granules in the cytoplasm. Nucleus is oval, bean shaped or kidney shaped and occupies the whole of the cytoplasm. A rim of cytoplasm may or may not be seen.

Depending upon the size, the lymphocytes are divided into two types:

1. *Large lymphocytes*: Younger cells with a diameter of 10 to 12 μ.
2. *Small lymphocytes*: Older cells with a diameter of 7 to 10 μ.

■ NORMAL LEUKOCYTE COUNT

1. **Total leukocyte count** *(TC)*: 4,000 to 11,000/cu mm of blood.
2. **Differential WBC count** *(DC)*: Given in **Table 11.2**.

■ APPLIED PHYSIOLOGY: VARIATIONS IN LEUKOCYTE COUNT

Leukocytosis

Leukocytosis is the increase in total WBC count. Leukocytosis occurs in both physiological and pathological conditions.

Leukopenia

Leukopenia is the decrease in total WBC count. Generally, the term leukopenia is used for pathological conditions only.

■ PHYSIOLOGICAL VARIATIONS

1. *Age:* In infants and children, total WBC count is more; it is about 20,000/cu mm in infants and about 10,000 to 15,000/cu mm of blood in children.
2. *Sex:* WBC count is slightly more in males than in females.

TABLE 11.2: Normal count, diameter and lifespan of white blood cells.

WBC	Percentage	Absolute value (per cu mm)	Diameter (μ)	Lifespan (days)
1. Neutrophils	50 to 70	3,000 to 6,000	10 to 12	2 to 5
2. Eosinophils	2 to 4	150 to 300	10 to 14	7 to 12
3. Basophils	0 to 1	0 to 100	8 to 10	12 to 15
4. Monocytes	2 to 6	200 to 600	14 to 15	2 to 5
5. Lymphocytes	20 to 30	1,500 to 3000	7 to 12	½ to 1

3. *Diurnal variation:* WBC count is minimum in early morning and maximum in the afternoon.
4. *Exercise:* Count increases slightly.
5. *Sleep:* Count decreases slightly.
6. *Emotional conditions like anxiety:* WBC count increases slightly.
7. *Pregnancy:* WBC count increases.
8. *Menstruation:* Count increases.
9. *Parturition:* Count increases.

PATHOLOGICAL VARIATIONS

Leukocytosis

WBC count increases in the following pathological conditions:

1. Infections.
2. Allergy.
3. Common cold.
4. Tuberculosis.
5. Glandular fever.

Leukopenia

WBC count decreases in the following pathological conditions:

1. Anaphylactic shock.
2. Cirrhosis of liver.
3. Disorders of spleen.
4. Pernicious anemia.
5. Typhoid and paratyphoid.
6. Viral infections.

Leukemia

Leukemia is a type of **blood cancer** characterized by production of large number of leukocytes including immature and abnormal leukocytes. Leukocyte count increases more than 10,00,000/ cu mm.

Leukemia is caused by genetic mutation in DNA of bone morrow cells.

LIFESPAN OF WHITE BLOOD CELLS

Lifespan of WBCs is not constant. It depends upon the demand in the body and their function. Lifespan of these cells may be as short as half a day or it may be long. Lifespan of different WBCs is given in **Table 11.2**.

PROPERTIES OF WHITE BLOOD CELLS

1. Diapedesis

Diapedesis is the process by which the leukocytes squeeze through the narrow blood vessels.

2. Ameboid Movement

Neutrophils, monocytes and lymphocytes show amebic movement characterized by protrusion of the cytoplasm and change in the shape.

3. Chemotaxis

Chemotaxis is the attraction of WBCs towards the injured tissues by the chemical substances released at the site of injury.

4. Phagocytosis

Neutrophils and monocytes engulf the foreign bodies by means of phagocytosis. Refer Chapter 3 for phagocytosis.

FUNCTIONS OF WHITE BLOOD CELLS

WBCs play an important role in defense mechanism. These cells protect the body from invading organisms or foreign bodies either by destroying or inactivating them. However, in defense mechanism, each type of WBCs acts in a different way.

FUNCTIONS OF NEUTROPHILS

Along with monocytes, the neutrophils provide the **first line of defense** against the invading microorganisms. Neutrophils wander freely all over the body through the tissues.

Neutrophils move by diapedesis towards the site of infection by means of **chemotaxis**. Chemotaxis occurs due to the attraction by some chemical substances called **chemoattractants**, which are released from the infected area. After reaching the area, the neutrophils engulf the bacteria and then destroy them by means of **phagocytosis** (Chapter 3).

Pus and Pus Cells

Pus cells are the dead WBCs killed by toxins released from bacteria during the battle between WBCs and bacteria.

Pus is the whitish yellow fluid formed in the area of infected tissue. It consists of dead WBCs, bacteria or foreign bodies, serum and cellular debris.

FUNCTIONS OF EOSINOPHILS

Eosinophils are responsible for defense mechanism of the body against the parasites and parasitic worms. During parasitic infections, there is a production of a large number of eosinophils which move towards the tissues affected by parasites. Eosinophil count increases also during allergic diseases, like asthma.

Eosinophils are responsible for detoxification, disintegration and removal of foreign proteins.

FUNCTIONS OF BASOPHILS

Basophils help in healing processes. So, their number increases during healing process.

Basophils also play an important role in allergy or acute hypersensitivity reactions (allergy). This is because of the presence of receptors for IgE in basophil membrane. Basophils also secrete heparin.

Section 2: Blood and Body Fluids

■ FUNCTIONS OF MONOCYTES

Monocytes are the largest cells among the leukocytes. Like neutrophils, monocytes also are motile and phagocytic in nature. These cells wander freely through all tissues of the body and provide the first line of defense along with neutrophils. Basophils also secrete heparin.

Monocytes are the precursors of the **tissue macrophages**. The matured monocytes stay in the blood only for few hours. Afterwards these cells enter the tissues from the blood and become tissue macrophages.

Examples of tissue macrophages are **Kupffer cells** in liver, **alveolar macrophages** in lungs and macrophages in spleen. Functions of macrophages are discussed in Chapter 17.

■ FUNCTIONS OF LYMPHOCYTES

Lymphocytes are responsible in development of immunity. Depending upon the function, the lymphocytes are divided into two types:

1. T lymphocytes which are concerned with cellular immunity.
2. B lymphocytes which are concerned with humoral immunity.

Functions of these two types of lymphocytes are explained in detail in Chapter 12.

■ LEUKOPOIESIS

Leukopoiesis is the development and maturation of leukocytes (Figs. 8.2 and 11.2).

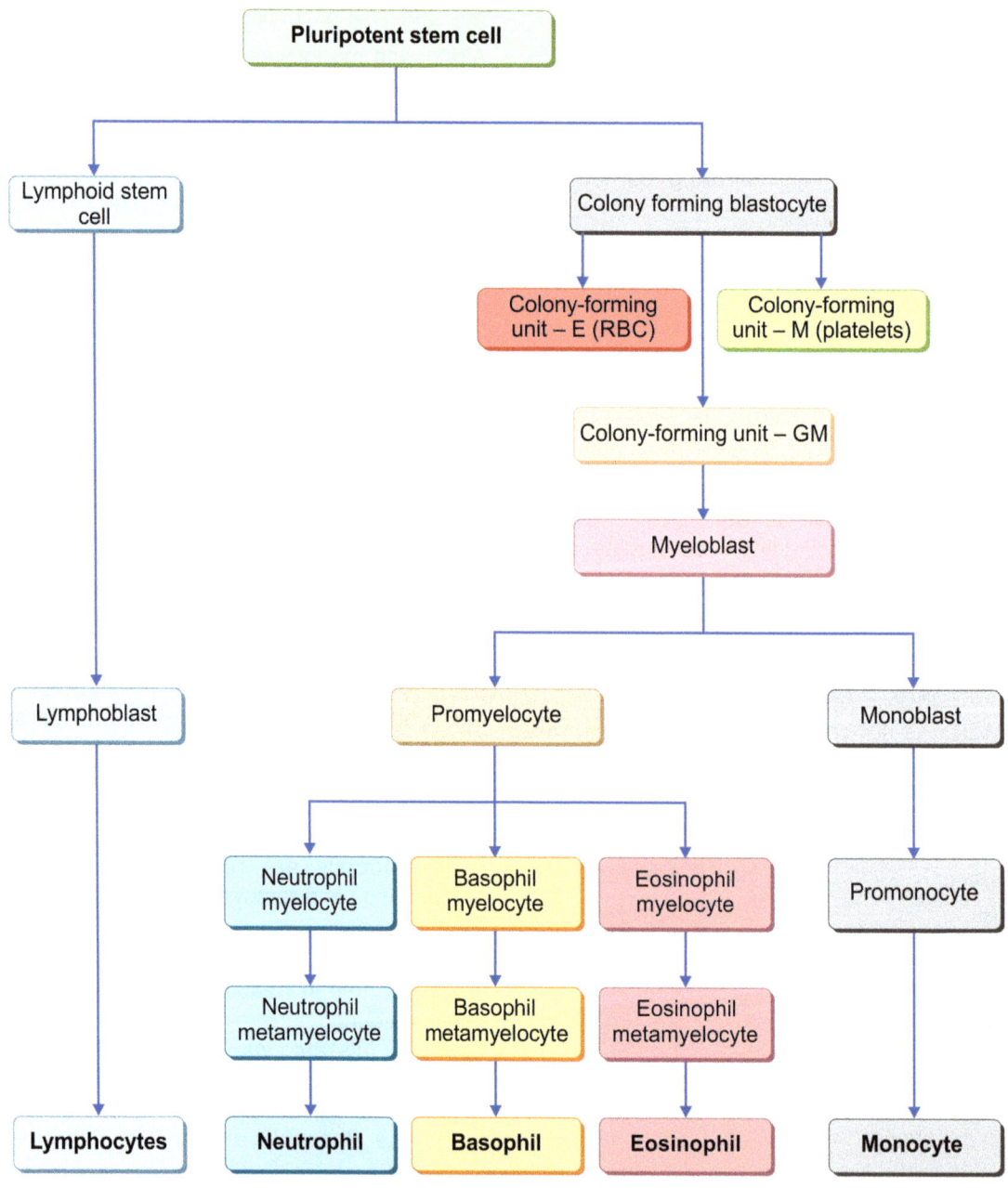

FIGURE 11.2: Leukopoiesis.
E = Erythrocytes, M = Magakaryocyte, GM = Granulocyte/Monocyte, RBC = Red blood cell.

■ STEM CELLS

Committed pluripotent stem cell gives rise to leukocytes through various stages. Details of stem cells are given in Chapter 8.

■ FACTORS NECESSARY FOR LEUKOPOIESIS

Leukopoiesis is influenced by **hematopoietic growth factors** and colony-stimulating factors (CSFs). Hematopoietic growth factors are discussed in Chapter 8.

Colony-stimulating Factors

Colony-stimulating factors are proteins which cause the formation of **colony-forming blastocytes**.

Colony-stimulating factors are of three types:

1. **Granulocyte-CSF** (G-CSF) secreted by monocytes and endothelial cells.
2. **Granulocyte-monocyte-CSF** (GM-CSF) secreted by monocytes, endothelial cells and T lymphocytes.
3. **Monocyte-CSF** (M-CSF) secreted by monocytes and endothelial cells.

Chapter 12

Immunity

CHAPTER OUTLINE

- **DEFINITION AND TYPES OF IMMUNITY**
- **DEVELOPMENT AND PROCESSING OF LYMPHOCYTES**
- **ANTIGENS**
- **DEVELOPMENT OF CELL-MEDIATED IMMUNITY**
- **DEVELOPMENT OF HUMORAL IMMUNITY**
- **NATURAL KILLER CELL**
- **CYTOKINES**
- **IMMUNIZATION**
- **IMMUNE DEFICIENCY DISEASES**
- **AUTOIMMUNE DISEASES**

■ DEFINITION AND TYPES OF IMMUNITY

Immunity is defined as the capacity of the body to resist the **pathogenic agents**. It is the ability of the body to resist the entry of different types of foreign bodies such as bacteria, virus, toxic substances, etc.

Immunity is of two types, innate immunity and acquired immunity.

■ INNATE IMMUNITY OR NON-SPECIFIC IMMUNITY

Innate immunity is the inborn capacity of the body to resist the pathogens. If any organism enters the body, innate immunity eliminates it before the development of any disease. This type of immunity represents the first line of defense against any type of pathogens. Therefore, it is also called **non-specific immunity**.

Examples of innate immunity are destruction of bacteria by salivary lysozyme and destruction of bacteria by acidity in urine and vaginal fluid.

■ ACQUIRED IMMUNITY OR SPECIFIC IMMUNITY

Acquired immunity is the resistance developed in the body against any specific foreign body such as bacteria, viruses, toxins, vaccines or transplanted tissues. So, this type of immunity is also called **specific immunity**.

Lymphocytes are responsible for acquired immunity **(Fig. 12.1)**.

Types of Acquired Immunity

Two types of acquired immunity develop in the body:

I. Cell-mediated immunity or cellular immunity.
II. Humoral immunity.

■ DEVELOPMENT AND PROCESSING OF LYMPHOCYTES

In fetus, lymphocytes develop from bone marrow. All the lymphocytes are released in the circulation and are differentiated into two categories, T lymphocytes and B lymphocytes.

■ T LYMPHOCYTES

T lymphocytes are processed in **thymus**. The processing occurs during the period between just before birth and few months after birth. **Thymosin** secreted by thymus accelerates proliferation and activation of lymphocytes in thymus.

Types of T Lymphocytes

During the processing, T lymphocytes are transformed into four types:

1. Helper T cells or inducer T cells.
2. Cytotoxic T cells or killer T cells.
3. Suppressor T cells.
4. Memory T cells.

Storage of T Lymphocytes

After the transformation, all the types of T lymphocytes leave the thymus and are stored in lymphoid tissues of lymph nodes, spleen, bone marrow and the gastrointestinal (GI) tract.

■ B LYMPHOCYTES

B lymphocytes were first discovered in the **bursa of Fabricius** in birds, hence the name B lymphocytes. The

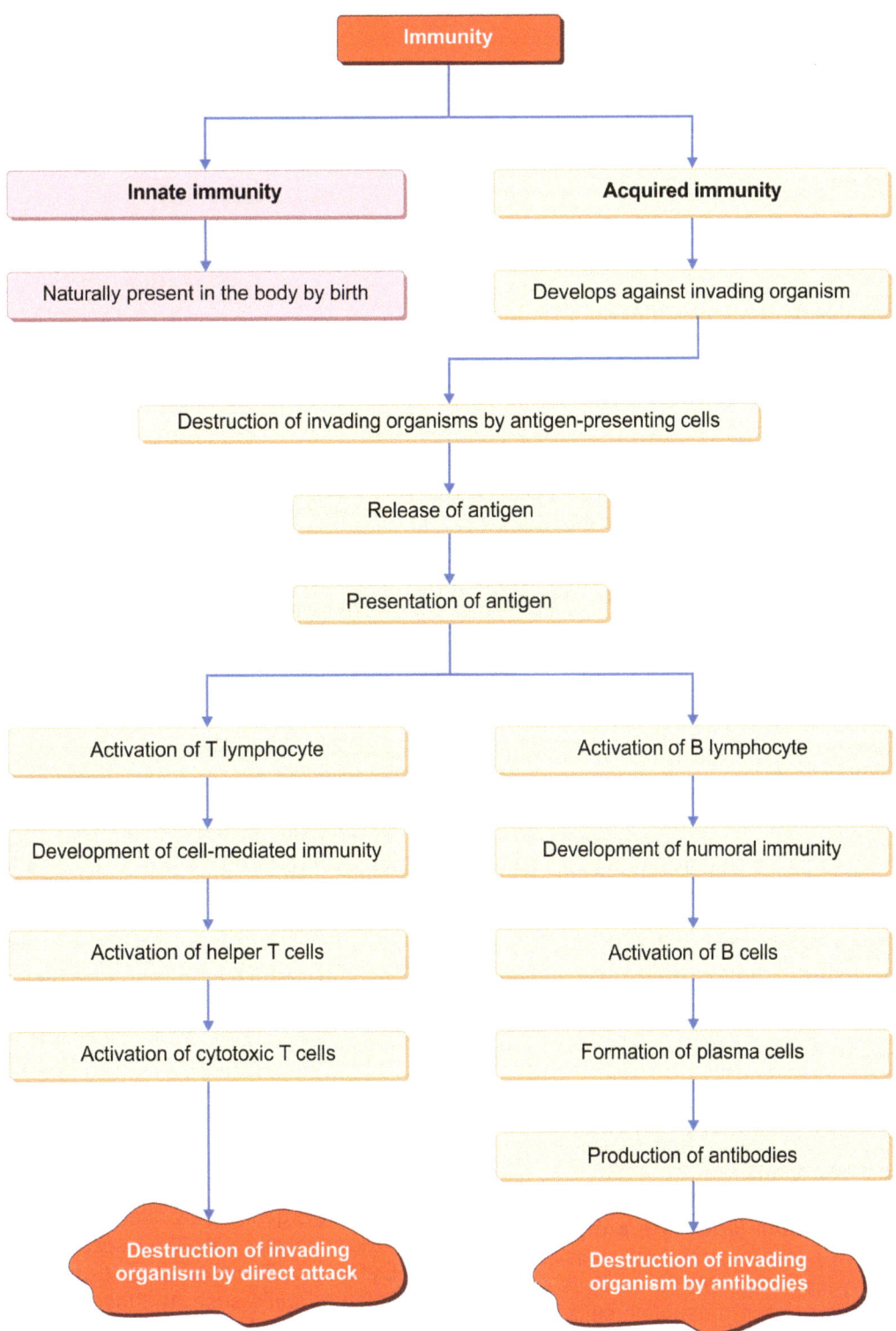

FIGURE 12.1: Schematic figure showing development of immunity.

bursa of Fabricius is a lymphoid organ situated near the cloaca of birds. Bursa is absent in mammals, and the processing of B lymphocytes takes place in bone marrow and liver.

Types of B Lymphocytes

After processing, the B lymphocytes are transformed into two types:

1. Plasma cells.
2. Memory cells.

Storage of B Lymphocytes

After the transformation, B lymphocytes are stored in the lymphoid tissues of lymph nodes, spleen, bone marrow and the GI tract.

ANTIGENS

DEFINITION AND TYPES

Antigens are the substances, which induce specific immune reactions in the body. The antigens are conjugated proteins such as lipoproteins, glycoproteins and nucleoproteins.

Antigens are of two types:

1. **Autoantigens** or **self-antigens** which are present on the body's own cells like 'A' antigen and 'B' antigen on the RBCs.
2. **Foreign antigens** or **non-self-antigens** which enter the body from outside.

DEVELOPMENT OF CELL-MEDIATED IMMUNITY

INTRODUCTION

Cell-mediated immunity or **cellular immunity** or **T cell immunity** is offered by T lymphocytes. Cellular immunity is the major defense mechanism against infections by viruses, fungi and few bacteria. It is also responsible for **delayed allergic reactions** and **rejection of transplanted tissues**.

Cell-mediated immunity starts developing when T cells come in contact with the antigens. Usually, the invading microbial or non-microbial organisms carry the **antigenic materials**. These antigenic materials are released from invading organisms and are presented to the helper T cells by antigen-presenting cells.

ANTIGEN-PRESENTING CELLS

Antigen-presenting cells are the special type of cells in the body which induce the release of antigenic materials from invading organisms and later present these materials to the helper T cells. Major antigen-presenting cells are **macrophages**. **Dendritic cells** in spleen, lymph nodes and skin also function like antigen-presenting cells.

Role of Antigen-presenting Cells

Invading foreign organisms are either engulfed by macrophages through phagocytosis or trapped by dendritic cells. Later, the antigen from these organisms is digested into small peptides. The antigenic peptide products move towards the surface of antigen-presenting cells and bind with **human leukocyte antigen** (HLA). The HLA is present in the molecule of class II **major histocompatibility complex** (MHC) which is situated on the surface of the antigen-presenting cells.

Presentation of Antigen

Antigen-presenting cells present their class II MHC molecules together with antigen bound HLA to the helper T cells. This activates the helper T cells through series of events **(Fig. 12.2)**.

Sequence of Events During Activation of Helper T Cells

1. Helper T cell recognizes the antigen bound to class II MHC molecule which is situated on the surface of

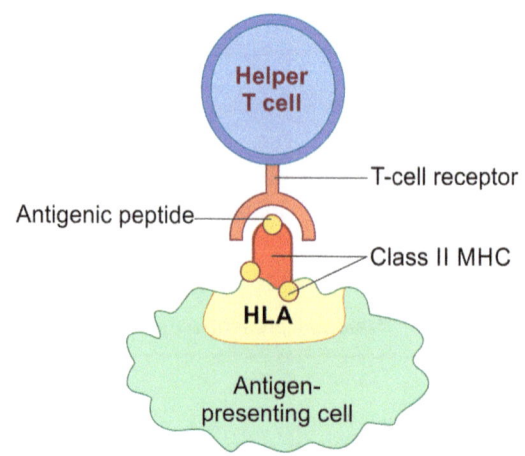

FIGURE 12.2: Antigen presentation. Antigen-presenting cells present their class II MHC molecules together with antigen bound HLA to the helper T cells.

MHC = Major histocompatibility complex. HLA = Human leukocyte antigen.

antigen-presenting cell. Helper T cell recognizes the antigen with the help of its own surface receptor protein called **T cell receptor**.

2. At the same time, macrophages (antigen presenting cells) release interleukin-1 which facilitates the activation and proliferation of helper T cells.
3. Proliferated helper T cells enter the circulation for further actions.
4. Simultaneously the antigen bound to class II MHC molecules activate the B cells also resulting in development of humoral immunity (see below).

ROLE OF HELPER T CELLS

Helper T cells which enter the circulation, activate all the other T cells and B cells. Helper T cells are of two types namely Helper-1 (TH1) cells and Helper-2 (TH2) cells.

TH1 cells are concerned with cellular immunity and TH2 cells are concerned with humoral immunity.

ROLE OF CYTOTOXIC T CELLS

Cytotoxic T cells that are activated by helper T cells destroy the invading organisms by attacking them directly by their cytotoxic substances like the lysosomal enzymes.

Cytotoxic T cells also destroy cancer cells, transplanted cells such as those of transplanted heart or kidney. Cytotoxic T cells destroy even the body's **own tissues** which are affected by the foreign bodies such as viruses. Many viruses are entrapped in the membrane of affected cells. Antigen of the viruses attracts the cytotoxic T cells which now kill the affected cells also along with viruses. Because of this, cytotoxic T cell is called **killer T cell**.

ROLE OF SUPPRESSOR T CELLS

Suppressor T cells or **regulatory T cells** suppress the activities of the killer T cells. Thus, suppressor T cells prevent the killer T cells from destroying the body's own tissues along with invaded organisms. Suppressor cells suppress the activities of helper T cells also.

ROLE OF MEMORY T CELLS

Some of the T cells activated by an antigen do not enter the circulation, but remain in lymphoid tissue. These T cells are called memory T cells.

In later periods, the memory cells migrate to various lymphoid tissues throughout the body. When the body is exposed to the same organism for the second time, the memory cells identify the organism and immediately activate the other T cells. So, the invading organism is destroyed very quickly. The response of the T cells is also more powerful this time.

SPECIFICITY OF T CELLS

Each T cell is designed to be activated only by one type of antigen. It is capable of developing immunity against that antigen only. This property is called the specificity of T cells.

DEVELOPMENT OF HUMORAL IMMUNITY
INTRODUCTION

Humoral immunity or **B cell immunity** is the immunity mediated by antibodies. **Antibodies** are secreted by B lymphocytes and released into the blood and lymph. The blood and lymph are the body fluids (humours or humors in Latin). Since the B lymphocytes provide immunity through humors, this type of immunity is called humoral immunity.

The antibodies produced by B lymphocytes are gamma globulins. These anti-bodies fight against the invading organisms. The humoral immunity is the major defense mechanism against the bacterial infection.

As in the case of cell-mediated immunity, the macrophages and other antigen-presenting cells play an important role in the development of humoral immunity also.

ROLE OF ANTIGEN-PRESENTING CELLS

Ingestion of foreign organisms and digestion of their antigen by the antigen-presenting cells are already explained.

Presentation of Antigen

The antigen-presenting cells present their class II MHC molecules together with antigen bound HLA to B lymphocytes. This activates the B cells through series of events.

Sequence of Events During Activation of B Cells

1. B cell recognizes the antigen bound to class II MHC molecule which is situated on the surface of antigen-presenting cell. B lymphocytes recognizes the antigen with the help of its own surface receptor protein called **B cell receptor**.
2. At the same time, macrophages (antigen-presenting cells) release interleukin-1 which facilitates the activation and proliferation of B cells.
3. Proliferated B cells carry out further actions.
4. Simultaneously the antigen bound to class II MHC molecules activates the helper T cells also resulting in development of cell-mediated immunity (already explained).

Transformation B Cells

Proliferated B cells are transformed into two types of cells:
1. Plasma cells.
2. Memory cells.

ROLE OF PLASMA CELLS

Plasma cells destroy the foreign organisms by producing the antibodies. Antibodies are released into lymph and then transported into the circulation. Antibodies are produced until the end of lifespan of each plasma cell which may be from several days to several weeks.

ROLE OF MEMORY B CELLS

Memory B cells occupy the lymphoid tissues throughout the body. Memory cells are in inactive form until the body is exposed to the same organism for the second time.

During the second exposure, memory cells are activated by the antigen and produce more quantity of antibodies at a faster rate, than in the first exposure. The antibodies produced during the second exposure to foreign antigen are also more potent than those produced during first exposure. This phenomenon forms the basic principle of vaccination against the infections.

ROLE OF HELPER T CELLS

Helper T cells are simultaneously activated by antigen. Activated helper T cells secrete two substances called interleukin-2 and B cell growth factor, which promote:

1. Activation of a greater number of B lymphocytes.
2. Proliferation of plasma cells.
3. Production of antibodies.

ANTIBODIES

An antibody is defined as a protein that is produced by B lymphocytes in response to the presence of an antigen. Antibody is γ-globulin in nature and so it is also called **immunoglobulin** (Ig).

Structure of Antibodies

Antibodies are formed by two pairs of chains, namely one pair of heavy or long chains and one pair of light or short chains. Each heavy chain consists of about 400 amino acids and each light chain consists of about 200 amino acids.

Actually, each antibody has two halves, which are identical. The two halves are held together by **disulfide bonds** (S–S). Each half of the antibody consists of one heavy chain (H) and one light chain (L). The two chains in each half are also joined by disulfide bonds (S–S). The disulfide bonds allow the movement of amino acid chains. In each antibody, the light chain is parallel to one end of the heavy chain. The light chain and the part of heavy chain parallel to it form one arm. The remaining part of the heavy chain forms another arm. A hinge joins both the arms **(Fig. 12.3)**.

Each chain of the antibody includes two regions:
1. Constant region.
2. Variable region.

Types of Antibodies and their Functions

Five types of antibodies are identified:
1. *IgA (Ig alpha):* Plays a role in localized defense mechanism in external secretions like tear.
2. *IgD (Ig delta):* Involved in recognition of the antigen by B lymphocytes.
3. *IgE (Ig epsilon):* Involved in allergic reactions
4. *IgG (Ig gamma):* Responsible for complement fixation.
5. *IgM (Ig mu):* Also responsible for complement fixation.

Among these antibodies, IgG forms 75% of the antibodies in the body.

Actions of Antibodies

Antibodies protect the body from the invading organisms in two ways, by direct actions and through complement system.

1. Direct actions of antibodies

Antibodies directly inactivate the invading organism by any one of the following methods:

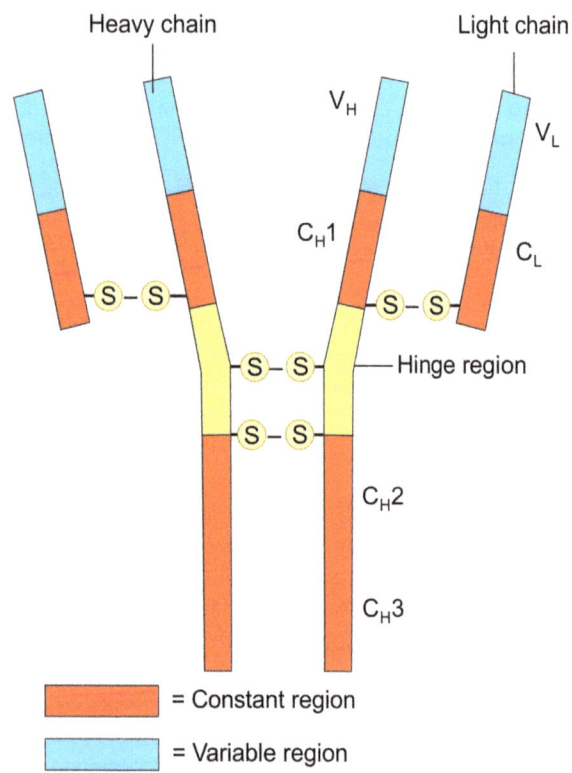

FIGURE 12.3: Structure of antibody (IgG) molecule. VL = Variable region of light chain, VH = Variable region of heavy chain, CL = Constant region of light chain, C_H1, C_H2 and C_H3 = Constant regions of heavy chains.

i. *Agglutination:* In this, the foreign bodies such as RBCs or bacteria, with antigens on their surfaces, are held together in a clump by the antibodies.
ii. *Precipitation:* In this, the soluble antigens like tetanus toxin are converted into insoluble forms and then precipitated.
iii. *Neutralization:* During this, the antibodies cover the toxic sites of antigenic products.
iv. *Lysis:* In this, the antibodies rupture the cell membrane of organisms and then destroy them.

2. Actions of antibodies through complement system

Complement system is the one that enhances or accelerates various activities during the fight against the invading organisms. It contains plasma enzymes, which are identified by numbers from C1 to C9.

Specificity of B Lymphocytes

Each B lymphocyte is designed to be activated only by one type of antigen. It is also capable of producing antibodies against that antigen only. This property is called **B lymphocyte specificity**.

■ NATURAL KILLER CELL

Natural killer (NK) cell is a large granular cell with indented nucleus. It is considered as the third type of lymphocyte. It is not a phagocytic cell, but its granules contain hydrolytic enzymes which causes lysis of cells of invading organisms.

Natural killer cell destroys the viruses, viral infected or damaged cells, which might form tumors, malignant cells and prevents development of cancerous tumors. It secretes cytokines such as interleukin-2, interferons, colony-stimulating factor (GM-CSF) and tumor necrosis factor-α.

■ CYTOKINES

Cytokines are the hormone-like small proteins acting as intercellular messengers (cell signaling molecules) by binding to specific receptors of target cells. These **non-antibody proteins** are secreted by WBCs and some other types of cells. Their major function is the activation and regulation of general immune system of the body.

Common cytokines are interleukins, interferons, tumor necrosis factors, chemokines, defensins, cathelicidins and platelet-activating factor.

■ IMMUNIZATION

Immunization is a procedure by which the body is prepared to fight against a specific disease. It is used to induce immune resistance of the body to a specific disease. Immunization is of two types namely passive immunization and active immunization.

■ PASSIVE IMMUNIZATION

Passive immunization immunity is produced without challenging the immune system of the body. It is done by administration of serum or gamma globulins from a person who is already immunized (affected by the disease) to a non-immune person. Passive immunization is acquired either naturally or artificially.

1. Passive Natural Immunization

Passive natural immunization is acquired from the mother before and after birth. Before birth, maternal antibodies (mainly IgG) are transported to fetus through placenta. After birth, the antibodies (IgA) are transported through breast milk.

2. Passive Artificial Immunization

Passive artificial immunization is developed by injecting previously prepared antibodies using serum from humans or animals.

ACTIVE IMMUNIZATION

Active immunization or immunity is acquired by activating the immune system of body. Body develops resistance against disease by producing antibodies following the exposure to antigens.

Active immunity is acquired either naturally or artificially.

1. Active Natural Immunization

Naturally acquired active immunity involves activation of immune system in the body to produce antibodies. It is achieved during infections.

2. Active Artificial Immunization

Active artificial immunization is a type of immunization achieved by the administration of vaccines or toxoids.

Vaccines

Vaccine is a substance that is administered into the body in order to develop or increase immunity against a particular disease. Vaccine is prepared from dead pathogens or live but attenuated (artificially weakened) organisms. Vaccine induces immunity against the pathogen, either by production of antibodies or by activation of T lymphocytes.

Vaccines are used to prevent many diseases such as smallpox, measles, mumps, poliomyelitis, tuberculosis, rubella, yellow fever, rabies, typhoid, influenza, hepatitis B, etc.

Toxoids

Toxoid is a substance which is processed to destroy its toxicity, but retains its capacity to induce antibody production by immune system. Toxoid consists of weakened components or toxins secreted by the pathogens. Toxoids are used to develop immunity against diseases like diphtheria, tetanus, cholera, etc.

Active artificial immunity may be effective life-long or for short period. It is effective lifelong against the diseases such as mumps, measles, smallpox, tuberculosis and yellow fever. It is effective only for short period against some diseases like cholera (about 6 months) and tetanus (about 1 year).

IMMUNE DEFICIENCY DISEASES

Immune deficiency diseases are group of diseases in which some components of immune system are missing or defective. Normally, defense mechanism protects the body from invading pathogenic organism. When the defense mechanism fails or becomes faulty (defective), the organisms of even low virulence produce severe disease. Such organisms, which take advantage of defective defense mechanism, are called **opportunists**.

Common immune deficiency disease is acquired immune deficiency syndrome (AIDS).

ACQUIRED IMMUNE DEFICIENCY SYNDROME

AIDS is an infectious disease caused by **human immune deficiency virus** (HIV). AIDS is the most common problem throughout the world because of rapid increase in the number of victims. Infection occurs when a glycoprotein from HIV binds to surface receptors of T lymphocytes, monocytes, macrophages and dendritic cells leading to destruction of these cells. It causes slow progressive decrease in immune function resulting in opportunistic infections of various types. The common **opportunistic infections** which kill the AIDS patient are pneumonia and skin cancer.

AUTOIMMUNE DISEASES

Autoimmune disease is defined as condition in which the immune system mistakenly attacks body's own cells and tissues. Normally, an antigen induces the immune response in the body. The condition in which the immune system fails to give response to an antigen is called tolerance. This is true with respect to body's own antigens that are called **self-antigens** or **autoantigens**.

Normally, body has the tolerance against self-antigen. However, in some occasions, the tolerance fails or becomes incomplete against self-antigen. This state is called **autoimmunity** and it leads to the activation of T lymphocytes or production of **autoantibodies** from B lymphocytes. T lymphocytes (cytotoxic T cells) or autoantibodies attack the body's normal cells whose surface contains the self-antigen or autoantigen.

COMMON AUTOIMMUNE DISEASES

1. Diabetes mellitus.
2. Myasthenia gravis.
3. Hashimoto's thyroiditis.
4. Graves' disease.
5. Rheumatoid arthritis.

Chapter 13

Platelets

CHAPTER OUTLINE

- MORPHOLOGY
- STRUCTURE AND COMPOSITION
- NORMAL COUNT AND VARIATIONS
- PROPERTIES
- FUNCTIONS
- DEVELOPMENT
- LIFESPAN AND FATE
- APPLIED PHYSIOLOGY: PLATELET DISORDERS

■ MORPHOLOGY

Platelets or **thrombocytes** are the formed elements of blood. Platelets are small, colorless, nonnucleated and moderately refractive bodies.

■ SIZE OF PLATELETS

Diameter : 2.5 µ (2 to 4 µ)
Volume   : 7.5 cu µ (7 to 8 cu µ)

Shape of Platelets

Normally, platelets are of several shapes, viz. spherical or rod shaped and become oval or disk shaped when inactivated. Sometimes, the platelets have dumbbell shape, comma shape, cigar shape or any other unusual shape.

■ STRUCTURE AND COMPOSITION

Platelets are constituted by cell membrane, microtubules and cytoplasm.

■ CELL MEMBRANE

Cell membrane is 6 nm thick and contains lipids in the form of phospholipids, cholesterol and glycolipids, carbohydrates as glycocalyx, and glycoproteins and proteins.

■ MICROTUBULES

Microtubules form a ring around cytoplasm below cell membrane. These tubules are made up of proteins called **tubulin**. Microtubules provide structural support for inactivated platelets to maintain the disk-like shape (Fig. 13.1).

■ CYTOPLASM

Cytoplasm of the platelets contains the cellular organelles, Golgi apparatus, endoplasmic reticulum, mitochondria, microtubule, microvessels, filaments and granules. Platelet granules are of two types namely alpha granules and dense granules. Granules of each type contain different substances.

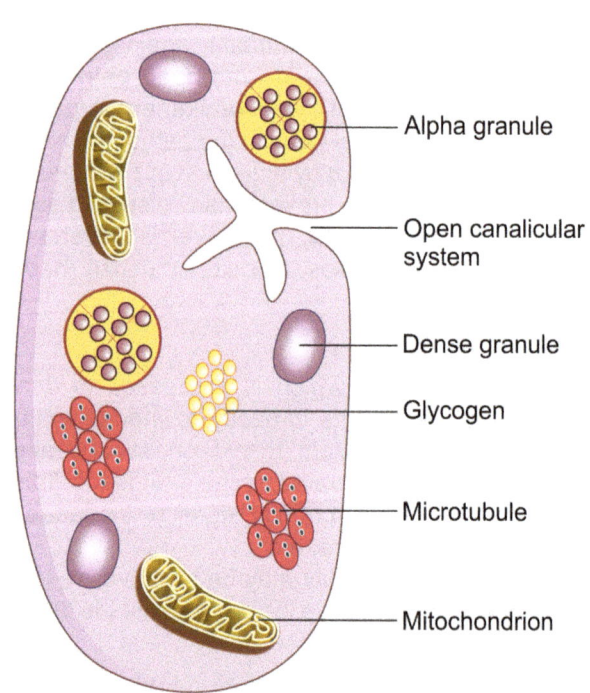

FIGURE 13.1: Platelet under electron microscope.

NORMAL COUNT AND VARIATIONS

Normal platelet count is 2,50,000. It ranges between 2,00,000 and 4,00,000/cu mm of blood.

PHYSIOLOGICAL VARIATIONS

1. *Age:* Platelets are less in infants (1,50,000 to 2,00,000/cu mm) and reaches normal level at 3rd month after birth.
2. *Sex:* There is no difference in the platelet count between males and females. In females, it is reduced during menstruation.
3. *High altitude:* Platelet count increases.
4. *After meals:* After taking food, the platelet count increases.

PATHOLOGICAL VARIATIONS

Refer applied physiology of this chapter.

PROPERTIES OF PLATELETS

1. ADHESIVENESS

Adhesiveness is the property of sticking to a rough surface. While coming in contact with any rough surface the platelets are activated and stick to the surface.

2. AGGREGATION (GROUPING OF PLATELETS)

Aggregation is the grouping of platelets. Activated platelets group together and become sticky.

3. AGGLUTINATION

Agglutination is the clumping together of platelets.

FUNCTIONS OF PLATELETS

1. ROLE IN BLOOD CLOTTING

Platelets are responsible for the formation of intrinsic **prothrombin activator**. This substance is responsible for the onset of blood clotting (Chapter 15).

2. ROLE IN CLOT RETRACTION

In the blood clot, the blood cells including platelets are entrapped in between the fibrin threads. The cytoplasm of platelets contains the contractile proteins namely actin, myosin and thrombosthenin which are responsible for clot retraction (Chapter 15).

3. ROLE IN PREVENTION OF BLOOD LOSS (HEMOSTASIS)

Platelets accelerate hemostasis by three ways:
  i. Platelets secrete 5-HT, which causes the constriction of blood vessels.
  ii. Due to the adhesive property, the platelets seal the damage in blood vessels like capillaries.
  iii. By formation of temporary plug also platelets seal the damage in blood vessels (Chapter 14).

4. ROLE IN REPAIR OF RUPTURED BLOOD VESSEL

Platelet-derived growth factor (PDGF) formed in cytoplasm of platelets is useful for the repair of the endothelium and other structures of the ruptured blood vessels.

5. ROLE IN DEFENSE MECHANISM

By the property of agglutination, platelets encircle the foreign bodies and destroy them by phagocytosis.

DEVELOPMENT OF PLATELETS

Platelets are formed from bone marrow. The pluripotent stem cell gives rise to the CFU-M. This develops into **megakaryocyte**. The cytoplasm of megakaryocyte form pseudopodium. A portion of pseudopodium is detached to form platelet, which enters the circulation **(Figs. 8.1 and 8.2)**.

Production of platelets is influenced by **thrombopoietin**. Thrombopoietin is a glycoprotein like erythropoietin, which is secreted by liver and kidneys.

LIFESPAN AND FATE OF PLATELETS

Average lifespan of platelets is about 10 days. Older platelets are destroyed by tissue macrophage system in spleen.

APPLIED PHYSIOLOGY: PLATELET DISORDERS

Platelet disorders are given in **Box 13.1**.

BOX 13.1: Platelet disorders.

Thrombocytopenia
Decrease in platelet count
Occurs in
1. Acute infections
2. Chickenpox
3. Smallpox
4. Splenomegaly
5. Typhoid
6. Tuberculosis
7. Purpura
Leads to thrombocytopenic purpura (Chapter 15)

Thrombocytosis
Increase in platelet count
Occurs in
1. Allergic conditions
2. Asphyxia
3. Hemorrhage
4. Bone fractures
5. Surgical operations
6. Splenectomy
7. Rheumatic fever
8. Trauma (wound or injury or damage caused by external force)

Thrombocythemia
Persistent and abnormal increase in platelet count
Occurs in
1. Carcinoma
2. Chronic leukemia
3. Hodgkin's disease

Chapter 14

Hemostasis

CHAPTER OUTLINE

- DEFINITION
- STAGES OF HEMOSTASIS

DEFINITION

Hemostasis is defined as arrest or stoppage of bleeding.

STAGES OF HEMOSTASIS

When a blood vessel is injured, the injury initiates a series of reactions resulting in hemostasis.

Hemostasis occurs in three stages:
1. Vasoconstriction.
2. Platelet plug formation.
3. Coagulation of blood.

1. VASOCONSTRICTION

Immediately after injury, the blood vessel constricts and decreases the loss of blood from damaged portion. Usually, arterioles and small arteries constrict. The vasoconstriction is purely a local phenomenon.

When the blood vessels are cut, the endothelium is damaged and the collagen is exposed. Platelets adhere to this collagen, and get activated. Activated platelets secrete **serotonin** and other vasoconstrictor substances which cause constriction of the blood vessels **(Fig. 14.1)**. Adherence of platelets to the collagen is accelerated by **von Willebrand factor**. This factor acts as a bridge between a specific glycoprotein present on the surface of platelet and collagen fibrils.

2. FORMATION OF PLATELET PLUG

The platelets get adhered to the collagen of ruptured blood vessel and secrete **ADP** and **thromboxane A$_2$**.

These two substances attract more and more platelets and activate them. All these platelets aggregate together and form a loose temporary platelet plug or temporary hemostatic plug, which closes the vessel and prevents further blood loss. The platelet aggregation is accelerated by platelet-activating factor (PAF).

3. COAGULATION OF BLOOD

During this process, the fibrinogen is converted into fibrin. The fibrin threads get attached to the loose platelet plug, which blocks the ruptured part of blood vessels and prevents further blood loss completely. The mechanism of blood coagulation is explained in the next chapter.

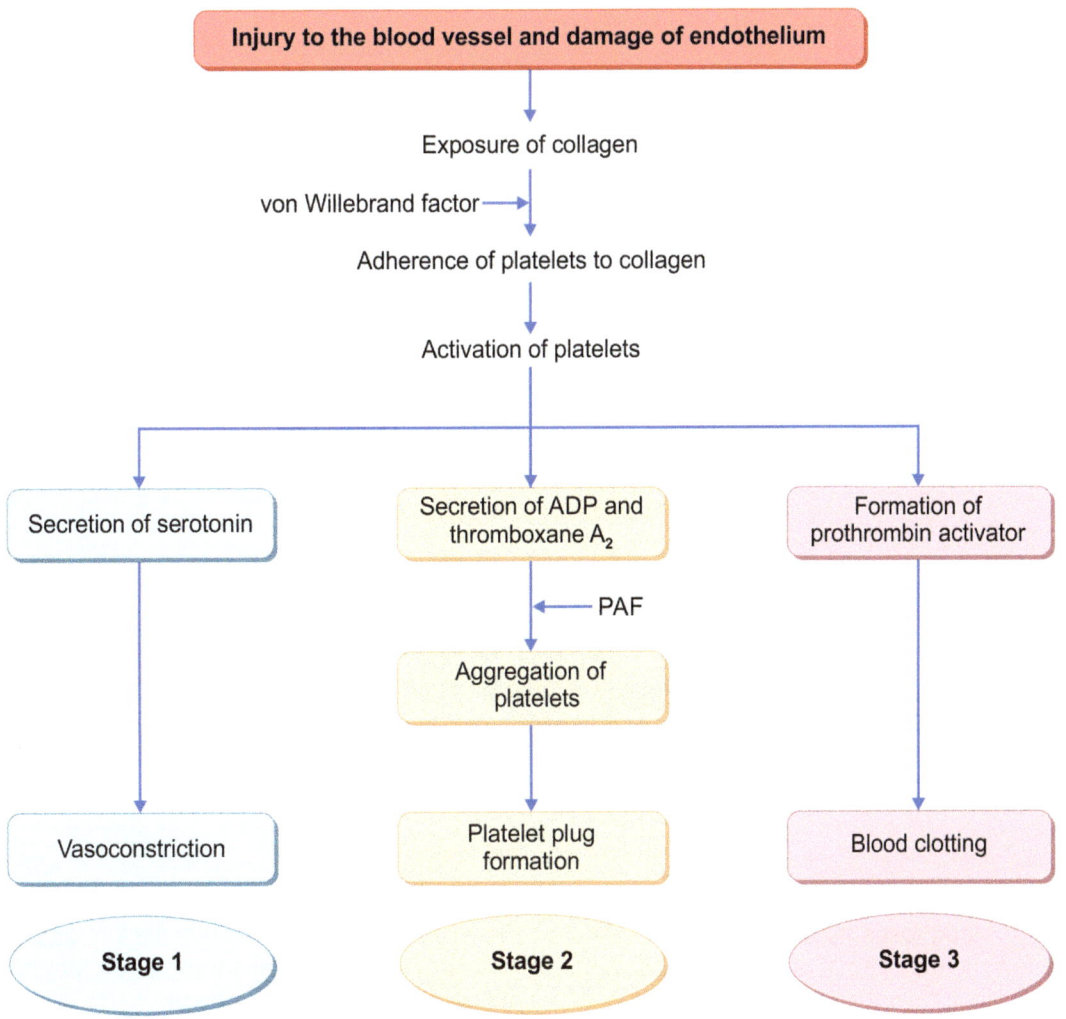

FIGURE 14.1: States of hemostasis.
ADP = Adenosine diphosphate, PAF = Platelet-activating factor.

15 CHAPTER

Coagulation of Blood

CHAPTER OUTLINE

- DEFINITION
- FACTORS INVOLVED IN BLOOD CLOTTING
- SEQUENCE OF CLOTTING MECHANISM
- BLOOD CLOT
- ANTICLOTTING MECHANISM IN THE BODY
- ANTICOAGULANTS
- PHYSICAL METHODS TO PREVENT BLOOD CLOTTING
- PROCOAGULANTS
- TESTS FOR CLOTTING
- APPLIED PHYSIOLOGY

DEFINITION

Blood coagulation or **blood clotting** is defined as the process in which blood loses its fluidity and becomes a jelly-like mass few minutes after it is shed out or collected in a container.

FACTORS INVOLVED IN BLOOD CLOTTING

Coagulation of blood occurs through a series of reactions due to the activation of a group of substances. The substances necessary for clotting are called **clotting factors**. Thirteen clotting factors are identified and listed in **Table 15.1**.

SEQUENCE OF CLOTTING MECHANISM

ENZYME CASCADE THEORY

Normally, all the factors are present in the form of inactive proenzymes. These proenzymes must be activated into enzymes to enforce blood clotting. Enzyme cascade theory explains how various reactions involved in the conversion of proenzymes to active enzymes take place in the form of a cascade. **Cascade** refers to a process that occurs through a series of steps, each step initiating the next, until the final step is reached.

Stages of Blood Clotting

Blood clotting occurs in three stages:
1. Formation of prothrombin activator.
2. Conversion of prothrombin into thrombin.
3. Conversion of fibrinogen into fibrin.

STAGE 1: FORMATION OF PROTHROMBIN ACTIVATOR

Blood clotting commences with the formation of prothrombin activator. This occurs through two pathways, intrinsic pathway and extrinsic pathway.

Intrinsic Pathway for the Formation of Prothrombin Activator

In this, the formation of prothrombin activator is initiated by platelets, which are within the blood itself **(Fig. 15.1)**.

TABLE 15.1: Clotting factors.

Factors	Name
I	Fibrinogen
II	Prothrombin
III	Thromboplastin (tissue factor)
IV	Calcium
V	Labile factor (proaccelerin or accelerator globulin)
VI	Presence has not been proved
VII	Stable factor
VIII	Antihemophilic factor (antihemophilic globulin)
IX	Christmas factor
X	Stuart-Prower factor
XI	Plasma thromboplastin antecedent
XII	Hageman factor (contact factor)
XIII	Fibrin-stabilizing factor (fibrinase)

Sequence of events in intrinsic pathway

i. During injury, the blood vessel is ruptured, endothelium is damaged and the collagen beneath endothelium is exposed.
ii. When factor XII (Hageman factor) comes in contact with collagen, it is converted into activated factor XII in the presence of **kallikrein** and **HMW kinogen** (high molecular weight kinogen).
iii. Activated factor XII converts factor XI into activated factor XI in the presence of HMW kininogen.
iv. Activated factor XI activates factor IX in the presence of factor IV (calcium).
v. Activated factor IX activates factor X in the presence of factor VIII and calcium.
vi. When platelet comes in contact with collagen of damaged blood vessel, it gets activated and releases phospholipids.
vii. Now, the activated factor X reacts with platelet phospholipid and factor V to form prothrombin activator. This needs presence of calcium ions.
viii. Factor V is also activated by positive feedback effect of thrombin (see below).

Extrinsic Pathway for the Formation of Prothrombin Activator

In this, the formation of prothrombin activator is initiated by the tissue thromboplastin which is formed from the injured tissues.

Sequence of events in extrinsic pathway

i. Damaged tissues release factor III (tissue thromboplastin).
ii. Glycoprotein and phospholipid components of thromboplastin convert factor X into activated factor X, in the presence of factor VII.
iii. Activated factor X reacts with factor V and phospholipid component of tissue thromboplastin to form prothrombin activator. This reaction requires the presence of calcium ions.

■ STAGE 2: CONVERSION OF PROTHROMBIN INTO THROMBIN

Sequence of Events in Stage 2

i. Prothrombin activator that is formed in intrinsic and extrinsic pathways converts prothrombin into thrombin in the presence of calcium ions (factor IV).
ii. Once formed thrombin initiates the formation of more thrombin molecules. Initially formed thrombin activates factor V. Factor V in turn accelerates formation of both extrinsic and intrinsic prothrombin activator which converts prothrombin into thrombin. This effect of thrombin is called **positive feedback effect (Fig. 15.1)**.

■ STAGE 3: CONVERSION OF FIBRINOGEN INTO FIBRIN

Sequence of Events in Stage 3

i. Thrombin converts fibrinogen into **activated fibrinogen** which is called **fibrin monomer**.
ii. Fibrin monomer polymerizes with other monomer molecules and form loosely arranged strands of fibrin.
iii. Later these loose strands are modified into dense and tight fibrin threads by fibrin-stabilizing factor (factor XIII) in the presence of calcium ions **(Fig. 15.1)**. All the tight fibrin threads are aggregated to form a meshwork of stable clot.

■ BLOOD CLOT

■ DEFINITION

Blood clot is defined as the mass of coagulated blood which contains RBCs, WBCs and platelets entrapped in fibrin meshwork. **External blood clot** is also called **scab**. It adheres to the opening of damaged blood vessel and prevents blood loss.

■ CLOT RETRACTION

Clot retraction is the process which involves contraction of blood clot 30 to 45 minutes after formation and oozing of **serum** out of clot. The contractile proteins namely, actin, myosin and **thrombosthenin** in the cytoplasm of platelets are responsible for clot retraction.

■ FIBRINOLYSIS

Fibrinolysis is the process that involves breakdown and dissolution of blood clot inside the blood vessel. It helps to remove the clot from lumen of the blood vessel.

Fibrinolysis requires **plasmin** or **fibrinolysin** which is derived from inactive **plasminogen.** Plasminogen is synthesized in liver and it is incorporated with other proteins in the blood clot. Plasminogen is converted into plasmin by **tissue plasminogen activator** (t-PA), lysosomal enzymes and thrombin. Plasmin causes lysis of clot by dissolving and digesting the fibrin threads.

■ ANTICLOTTING MECHANISM IN THE BODY

Under physiological conditions, intravascular clotting does not occur. It is because of following factors:

1. Continuous circulation of blood.
2. Smooth endothelial lining of the blood vessels.
3. Presence of natural anticoagulant called heparin that is produced by mast cells and basophils.
4. All the clotting factors are in inactive state.

■ ANTICOAGULANTS

Anticoagulants are the substances, which prevent or postpone coagulation of blood.

Anticoagulants are of three types:

I. Anticoagulants used to prevent blood clotting inside the body, i.e. in vivo.
II. Anticoagulants used to prevent clotting of blood that is collected from the body, i.e. in vitro.
III. Anticoagulants used to prevent blood clotting both in vivo and in vitro.

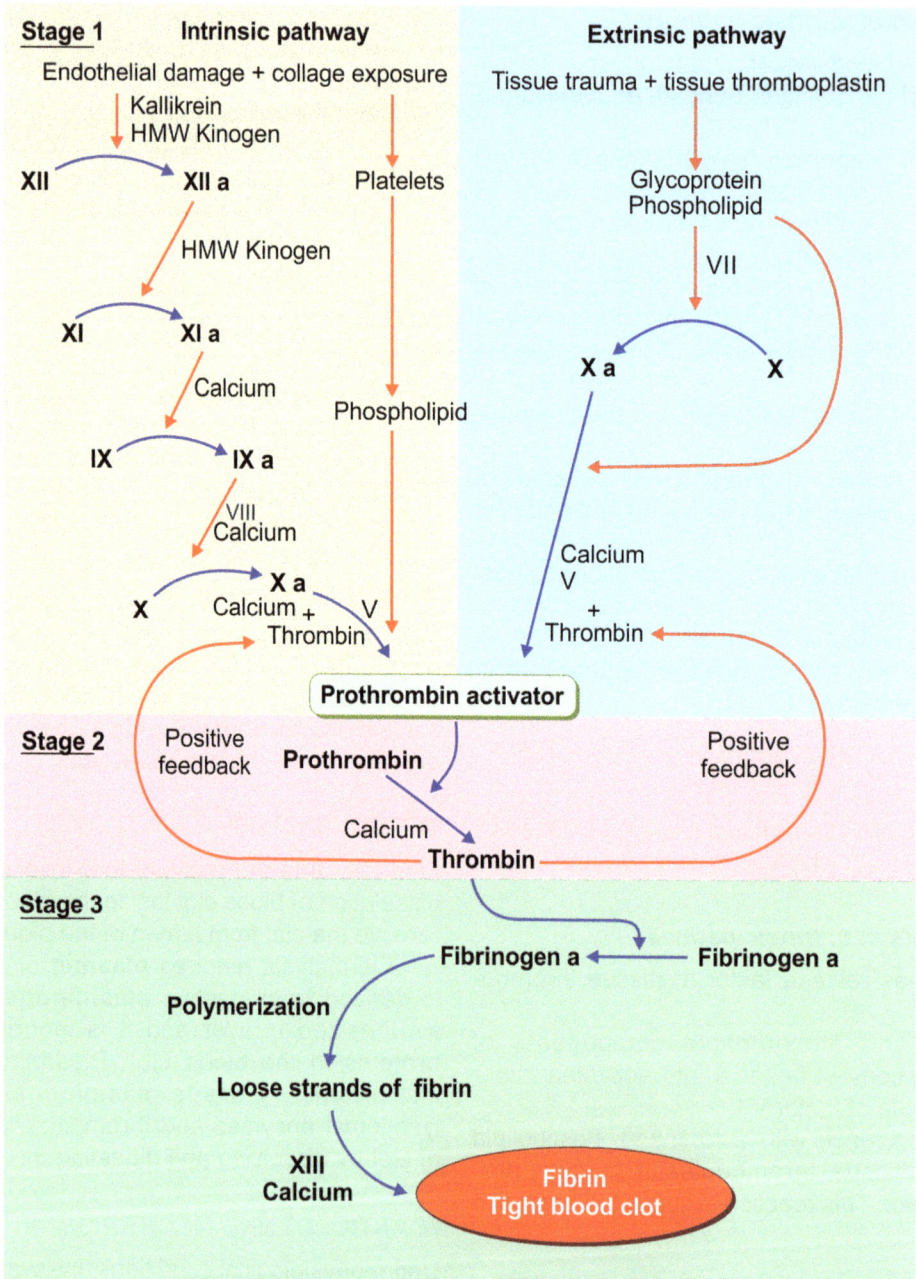

FIGURE 15.1: Stages of blood coagulation.
+ = Thrombin induces formation of more thrombin (positive feedback), a = Activated, HMW = High molecular weight.

1. HEPARIN

Heparin is a naturally produced anticoagulant in the body. It is produced by **mast cells** which are present in large numbers in liver and lungs. Heparin is also produced by basophils.

Mechanism of Action of Heparin

Heparin
  i. Prevents blood clotting by directly suppressing the activity of thrombin.
  ii. Combines with antithrombin III present in circulation and removes thrombin from circulation.
  iii. Activates antithrombin III.
  iv. Inactivates the active form of other clotting factors like IX, X, XI and XII.

Uses of Heparin

Heparin is used as an anticoagulant both in vivo and in vitro. Heparin is widely used as an anticoagulant during surgery and dialysis. It is also used to preserve the blood before transfusion.

In laboratory also heparin is also used as anticoagulant in vitro while collecting blood for various investigations.

2. COUMARIN DERIVATIVES

Dicoumoral and warfarin are the derivatives of coumarin. Coumarin derivatives prevent blood clotting by inhibiting the action of vitamin K. Vitamin K is essential for the formation of various clotting factors namely, II, VII, IX and X.

Uses

Dicoumoral and warfarin are the commonly used **oral anticoagulants** (in vivo).

3. EDTA

Ethylenediaminetetra acetic acid (EDTA) is a strong anticoagulant. It prevents blood clotting by removing calcium from blood.

Uses

EDTA is used as an anticoagulant both in vivo and in vitro. It is administered intravenously in cases of lead poisoning (in vivo). It is also used as an anticoagulant in the laboratory (in vitro).

4. OXALATE COMPOUNDS

Oxalate compounds prevent coagulation by forming calcium oxalate, which is precipitated later. Thus, these compounds reduce the blood calcium level and lack of calcium prevents coagulation.

Uses

Oxalate compounds are used as in vitro anticoagulants. Oxalate is poisonous so it cannot be used in vivo.

5. CITRATES

Sodium, ammonium and potassium citrates are used as anticoagulants. Citrate combines with calcium in blood to form insoluble calcium citrate. Like oxalate, citrate also removes calcium from blood and prevents coagulation.

Uses

Citrates are used as an anticoagulant both in vivo and in vitro. Citrates are used to store blood in the blood bank and in laboratory.

6. OTHER SUBSTANCES, WHICH PREVENT BLOOD CLOTTING

Peptone, proteins from venom of copper-head snake and hirudin (from leech) are the known anticoagulants.

PHYSICAL METHODS TO PREVENT BLOOD CLOTTING

Blood clotting is prevented by collecting the blood in a container with smooth surface like a **silicon-coated container**. The smooth surface inhibits the activation of factor XII and platelets. So, the formation of prothrombin activator is prevented.

Blood clotting is also postponed by storing blood at 5°C.

PROCOAGULANTS

Procoagulants or **hemostatic agents** are the substances, which accelerate the process of blood coagulation. Examples are thrombin, extracts of lungs and thymus, sodium or calcium alginate and oxidized cellulose

TESTS FOR CLOTTING

1. BLEEDING TIME

Bleeding time is the time interval from oozing of blood after a cut or injury till arrest of bleeding. Usually, it is determined by **Duke method** using blotting paper or filter paper method. Its normal duration is 3 to 6 minutes. It is prolonged in **purpura**.

2. CLOTTING TIME

Clotting time is the time interval from oozing of blood after a cut or injury till the formation of clot. It is usually determined by capillary tube method. Its normal duration is 3 to 8 minutes. And it is prolonged in **hemophilia**.

3. PROTHROMBIN TIME

It is the time taken by blood to clot after adding tissue thromboplastin to it. Blood is collected and oxalated so that, the calcium is precipitated and prothrombin is not converted into thrombin. Thus, the blood clotting is prevented. Then a large quantity of tissue thromboplastin with calcium is added to this blood. Calcium nullifies the effect of oxalate. The tissue thromboplastin activates prothrombin and blood clotting occurs.

During this procedure, the time taken by blood to clot after adding tissue thromboplastin is determined. Prothrombin time indicates the total quantity of prothrombin present in the blood.

Normal duration of prothrombin time is about 12 seconds. It is prolonged in deficiency of prothrombin and other factors like factors I, V, VII and X. However, it is normal in hemophilia.

APPLIED PHYSIOLOGY

1. BLEEDING DISORDERS

Bleeding disorders are the diseases characterized by prolonged bleeding time or clotting time. The bleeding disorders are of three types.

i. Hemophilia

Hemophilia is a group of sex-linked inherited blood disorders characterized by prolonged clotting time. In this disorder males are affected and the females are the carriers. Because of prolonged clotting time, even a mild trauma causes excess bleeding which can lead to death. Damage of skin while falling or extraction of a tooth may cause excess bleeding for few weeks.

Cause for hemophilia

Hemophilia is caused by lack of prothrombin activator which is due to the deficiency of factor VIII, IX or XI.

Types of hemophilia

Depending upon the deficiency of the factor involved, hemophilia is classified into three types:

a. *Hemophilia A or classic hemophilia*: Due to the deficiency of factor VIII.
b. *Hemophilia B or* **Christmas disease**: Due to the deficiency of factor IX.
c. *Hemophilia C*: Due to the deficiency of factor XI.

ii. Purpura

It is a disorder characterized by prolonged bleeding time. However, the clotting time is normal. Characteristic feature of this disease is spontaneous bleeding under the skin from ruptured capillaries. It causes small tiny hemorrhagic spots under the skin which are called **purpuric spots** (purple colored patch-like appearance). That is why this disease is called purpura.

Types and causes of purpura

Purpura is classified into different types depending upon the causes.

i. *Thrombocytopenic purpura*: Due to the deficiency of platelets (thrombocytopenia).
ii. *Idiopathic thrombocytopenic purpura*: Due to unknown cause.
iii. *Thrombasthenic purpura*: Due to structural or functional abnormality of platelets.

iii. von Willebrand Disease

von Willebrand disease is a bleeding disorder characterized by excess bleeding even with a mild injury. It is due to inherited deficiency of **von Willebrand factor** which is a protein secreted by endothelium of damaged blood vessels and platelets. Deficiency of von Willebrand factor suppresses platelet adhesion. It also causes deficiency of factor VIII. This results in excess bleeding.

■ 2. THROMBOSIS

Thrombosis or **intravascular blood clotting** refers to coagulation of blood inside the blood vessels. Normally, blood does not clot in the blood vessel because of some factors which are already explained. But some abnormal conditions can cause thrombosis.

Common causes for thrombosis are injury to blood vessels, sluggishness of blood flow, agglutination of RBCs. Poisoning by snake venom, mercury, and arsenic compounds.

Complications of Thrombosis

1. Thrombus

Thrombus is the solid mass of platelets, red cells and/or clot, which is formed during thrombosis. It occludes the blood vessel.

2. Embolism and embolus

Embolism is the process in which the thrombus or part of it is detached and carried in bloodstream and occludes the small blood vessels resulting in arrests of blood flow to any organ or region of the body. Embolus is the thrombus or part of it, which arrests the blood flow. Obstruction of blood flow by embolism is common in lungs (**pulmonary embolism**), brain (**cerebral embolism**) and heart (**coronary embolism**).

3. Ischemia

Insufficient blood supply to an organ or area of body by the obstruction of blood vessels is called ischemia. Ischemia results in tissue damage because of hypoxia (lack of oxygen). Ischemia also causes discomfort, pain and tissue death.

4. Necrosis and infarction

Necrosis is a general term that refers to tissue death caused by loss of blood supply, injury, infection, inflammation, physical agents or chemical substances. Infarction means the tissue death due to loss of blood supply. The area of tissue that undergoes infarction is called infarct.

Chapter 16: Blood Groups and Blood Transfusion

CHAPTER OUTLINE

- BLOOD GROUPS
- ABO BLOOD GROUPS
  - LANDSTEINER'S LAW
  - ABO SYSTEM
  - DETERMINATION OF ABO GROUP
  - IMPORTANCE OF ABO GROUPS IN BLOOD TRANSFUSION
  - MATCHING AND CROSSMATCHING
- RH FACTOR
- APPLIED PHYSIOLOGY
  - TRANSFUSION REACTIONS DUE TO ABO INCOMPATIBILITY
- TRANSFUSION REACTIONS DUE TO Rh INCOMPATIBILITY
- IMPORTANCE OF KNOWING BLOOD GROUP
- BLOOD TRANSFUSION
  - DEFINITION AND TYPES
  - CONDITIONS WHEN BLOOD TRANSFUSION IS NECESSARY
  - PRECAUTIONS TO BE TAKEN
  - BLOOD SUBSTITUTES
  - EXCHANGE TRANSFUSION
  - AUTOLOGOUS BLOOD TRANSFUSION

■ BLOOD GROUPS

Blood groups were discovered by Austrian Scientist **Karl Landsteiner** in 1901. He was honored with Nobel Prize in 1930 for this discovery.

More than 20 genetically determined blood group systems are known today. But Landsteiner discovered two blood group systems called ABO system and Rh system. These two blood group systems are the most important ones that are determined before blood transfusions.

■ ABO BLOOD GROUPS

Determination of ABO blood groups depends upon the immunological reaction between **antigen** and **antibody**. Landsteiner found two antigens on the surface of RBCs and named them as A antigen and B antigen. He noticed the **corresponding antibodies** or **agglutinins** in the plasma and named them anti-A or α antibody and anti-B or β antibody.

However, a particular agglutinogen and the corresponding agglutinin cannot be present together. If present, it causes clumping of the blood. Based on this, Landsteiner classified the blood groups. Later it has become the 'Landsteiner's Law' for grouping the blood.

■ LANDSTEINER'S LAW

Landsteiner's law states that:

1. If a particular antigen (agglutinogen) is present in the RBCs, corresponding antibody (agglutinin) must be absent in the serum.
2. If a particular antigen is absent in the RBCs, the corresponding antibody must be present in the serum.

Though the second part of Landsteiner's law is a fact, it is not applicable to Rh factor.

■ ABO SYSTEM

Based on the presence or absence of antigen A and antigen B, blood is divided into four groups:

1. 'A' group.
2. 'B' group.
3. 'AB' group.
4. 'O' group.

Blood having antigen A is called A group. This group has β antibody in the serum. The blood with antigen B and α antibody is called B group. If both the antigens are present, the blood group is called AB group and serum of

TABLE 16.1: Antigen and antibody present in ABO blood groups.

Group	Antigen in RBC	Antibody in serum
A	A	Anti-B (β)
B	B	Anti-A (α)
AB	A and B	No antibody
O	No antigen	Anti-A and Anti-B

this group does not contain any antibody. If both antigens are absent, the blood group is called O group and both α and β antibodies are present in the serum. The antigens and antibodies present in different groups of ABO system are given in **Table 16.1**.

'A' group has two subgroups namely 'A_1' and 'A_2'. Similarly, 'AB' group has two subgroups namely 'A_1B' and 'A_2B'.

■ DETERMINATION OF ABO GROUP

Determination of the ABO group is also called blood grouping, blood typing or blood matching.

Principle of Blood Typing: Agglutination

The blood typing is done on the basis of agglutination. **Agglutination** means the collection of separate particles like RBCs into clumps or masses. Agglutination occurs if an antigen is mixed with its corresponding antibody which is called **isoagglutinin**. Agglutination occurs when A antigen is mixed with anti-A or when B antigen is mixed with anti-B.

Requisites for Blood Typing

To determine the blood group of a person, a suspension of his RBC and testing antisera are required. Suspension of RBC is prepared by mixing blood drops with isotonic saline (0.9%).

Test sera are:

1. Antiserum A, containing anti-A.
2. Antiserum B, containing anti-B.

Procedure

1. One drop of antiserum A is placed on one end of a glass slide (or a tile) and one drop of antiserum B on other end of slide.
2. One drop of RBC suspension is mixed with each antiserum. The slide is slightly rocked for 2 minutes. The presence or absence of agglutination is observed by naked eyes and if necessary, it is confirmed by using microscope.
3. Presence of agglutination is confirmed by the presence of clumping of RBCs.
4. Absence of agglutination is confirmed by clear mixture with dispersed RBCs.

Results

1. *If agglutination occurs with antiserum A:* The antiserum A contains anti-A or α antibody. The agglutination

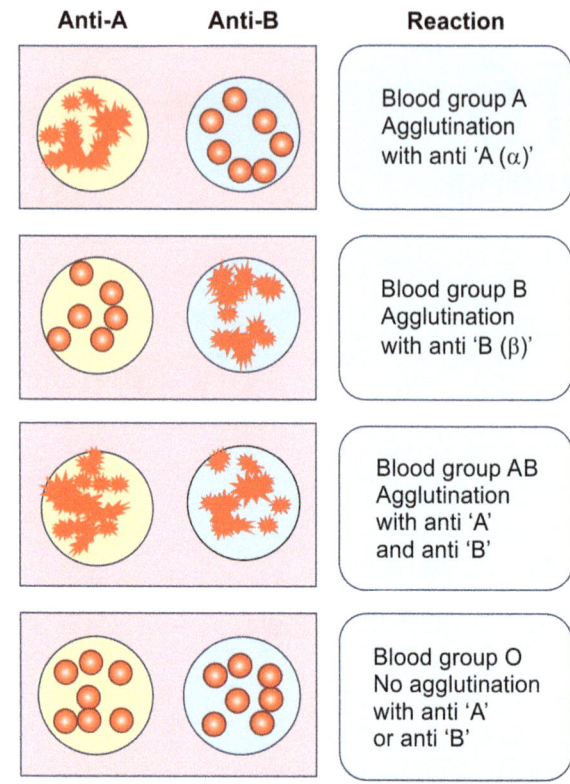

FIGURE 16.1: Determination of blood group.

occurs if the RBC contains A antigen. So, the blood group is A **(Fig. 16.1)**.
2. *If agglutination occurs with antiserum B:* The antiserum B contains anti-B or β antibody. The agglutination occurs if the RBC contains B antigen. So, the blood group is B.
3. *If agglutination occurs with both antisera A and B:* The RBC contains both A and B antigens to cause agglutination. And, the blood group is AB.
4. *If agglutination does not occur either with antiserum A or antiserum B:* The agglutination does not occur if the RBC does not contain any antigen. The blood group is O.

■ IMPORTANCE OF ABO GROUPS IN BLOOD TRANSFUSION

During blood transfusion, only compatible blood must be used. The one who gives blood is called the donor and the one who receives the blood is called recipient. RBC of 'O' group has no antigen and so agglutination does not occur with any other group of blood. So, 'O' group blood can be given to any blood group persons and the people of this group blood are called **universal donors**.

Plasma of AB group blood has no antibody. This does not cause agglutination of RBC from any other group of blood. The people of AB group can receive blood from any blood group persons. So, people with this group blood are called **universal recipients**.

■ MATCHING AND CROSSMATCHING

Blood matching or **blood typing** is a laboratory test done to determine the blood group of a person. When the person needs blood transfusion, another test called crossmatching is done after the blood is typed. It is done to find out whether the person's body will accept the donor's blood or not.

For blood matching, RBC of the individual (recipient) and test sera are used. Crossmatching is done by mixing the serum of the recipient and the RBCs of donor. Crossmatching is always done before blood transfusion. If agglutination of RBCs from a donor occurs during crossmatching, the blood from that person is not used for transfusion.

Matching = Recipient's RBC + Test sera
Crossmatching = Recipient's serum + Donor's RBC

■ Rh FACTOR

Rh factor is an antigen present in RBC. The antigen was discovered by Landsteiner and Wiener. It was first discovered in **rhesus monkey** and hence the name Rh factor. There are many Rh antigens but only the D is more antigenic in human.

The persons having **D antigen** are called Rh positive and those without D antigen are called Rh negative. Among Asian population, 85% of people are Rh positive and 15% are Rh negative.

Rh group system is different from ABO group system because, the antigen D does not have corresponding natural antibody (anti-D). However, if Rh positive blood is transfused to a Rh negative person for the first time, then anti-D is formed in that person. On the other hand, there is no risk of complications if Rh positive person receives Rh negative blood.

■ APPLIED PHYSIOLOGY

■ TRANSFUSION REACTIONS DUE TO ABO INCOMPATIBILITY

Transfusion reactions are the adverse reactions in the body which occur due to transfusion of incompatible (mismatched) blood. The reactions may vary from fever and hives (skin disorder characterized by itching) to renal failure, shock and death.

In mismatched transfusion, the transfusion reactions occur between donor's RBC and recipient's plasma. So, if the donor's plasma contains antibody against recipient's RBC, agglutination does not occur because these antibodies are diluted in recipient's blood.

But, if recipient's plasma contains antibodies against donor's RBCs, the immune system launches a response against the new blood cells. Donor RBCs are agglutinated and hemolyzed.

Signs and Symptoms of Transfusion Reactions

Non-hemolytic transfusion reaction

Non-hemolytic transfusion reaction develops within a few minutes to hours after the commencement of blood transfusion. Common symptoms are fever, breathing difficulty and itching.

Hemolytic transfusion reaction

Hemolytic transfusion reaction may be acute or delayed. The acute hemolytic reaction occurs within few minutes of transfusion. It develops because of rapid hemolysis of donor's RBCs. Symptoms include fever, chills, increased heart rate, low blood pressure, shortness of breath, bronchospasm, nausea, vomiting, red urine, chest pain, back pain and rigor. Some patients may develop pulmonary edema and congestive cardiac failure.

Delayed hemolytic reaction occurs from 1 to 5 days after transfusion. The hemolysis of RBCs results in release of large amount of hemoglobin into the plasma. This leads to the following complications.

1. *Jaundice*: Normally, hemoglobin released from destroyed RBC is degraded and bilirubin is formed from it. When the serum bilirubin level increases above 2 mg/dL, jaundice occurs (Chapter 29).
2. *Cardiac shock*: Simultaneously, the hemoglobin released into the plasma increases the viscosity of blood. This increases the workload on the heart leading to cardiac shock.
3. *Renal shutdown*: Dysfunction of kidneys is called renal shutdown. It occurs due to the toxic substances released from hemolyzed cells **(Fig. 16.2)**.

■ TRANSFUSION REACTIONS DUE TO Rh INCOMPATIBILITY

When a person with Rh negative blood receives Rh positive blood for the first time, he is not affected much, since the reactions do not occur immediately. But the Rh antibodies develop within one month. The transfused RBCs, which are still present in recipient's blood are agglutinated. These agglutinated cells are lysed by macrophages. So, a delayed transfusion reaction occurs. But it is usually mild and does not affect the recipient. However, antibodies developed in the recipient remain in the body forever. So, when this person receives Rh positive blood for the second time, the donor RBCs are agglutinated and severe transfusion reactions occur

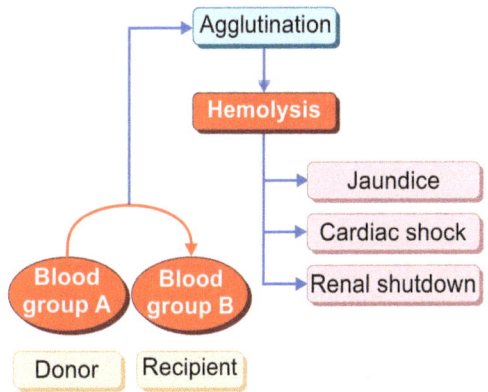

FIGURE 16.2: Complications of mismatched blood transfusion.

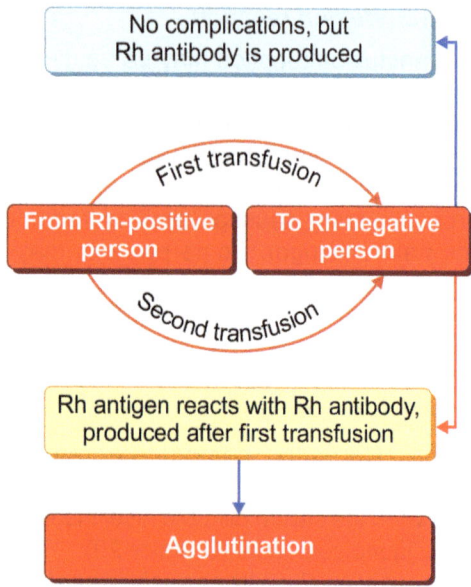

FIGURE 16.3: Rh incompatibility.

immediately (Fig. 16.3). These reactions are similar to the reactions of ABO incompatibility (see above).

Hemolytic Disease of Fetus and Newborn: Erythroblastosis Fetalis

Hemolytic disease is the disease in fetus and newborn characterized by abnormal hemolysis of RBCs. It is due to Rh incompatibility. Hemolytic disease leads to erythroblastosis fetalis.

Erythroblastosis fetalis is a disorder in fetus characterized by the presence of **erythroblasts** in blood. When a mother is Rh negative and fetus is Rh positive (the Rh factor being inherited from the father), first child of the lady escapes the complications of Rh incompatibility. This is because the Rh antigen cannot pass from fetal blood into the mother's blood through the placental barrier.

However, at the time of parturition (delivery of the child) the Rh antigen from fetal blood may leak into mother's blood because of placental detachment. During postpartum period, i.e. within a month after delivery, the mother develops Rh antibody in her blood.

When the mother conceives for the second time and if the fetus happens to be Rh positive again, the Rh antibody from mother's blood crosses placental barrier and enters the fetal blood. Thus, the Rh antigen cannot cross the placental barrier whereas Rh antibody can cross it.

The Rh agglutinins which enter the fetus cause agglutination of fetal RBCs resulting in hemolysis.

Severe hemolysis in the fetus causes jaundice. To compensate the hemolysis of greater number of RBCs, there is rapid production of RBCs, not only from bone marrow, but also from spleen and liver. Now, many large and immature cells in **proerythroblastic** stage are released into circulation. Because of this, the disease is called erythroblastosis fetalis.

Complications of Erythroblastosis Fetalis

Ultimately due to excessive hemolysis following complications develop:

1. Severe anemia

Excessive hemolysis results in anemia. And the infant dies when anemia becomes severe.

2. Hydrops fetalis

It is a serious condition in fetus characterized by edema, enlargement of liver and spleen and cardiac failure. When this condition becomes more severe it may lead to intrauterine death of fetus.

3. Bilirubin encephalopathy: Kernicterus

Bilirubin encephalopathy is a neurological disorder characterized by brain damage in infants caused by severe jaundice. If the baby survives anemia in erythroblastosis fetalis (see above), encephalopathy develops because of high bilirubin content.

Bilirubin encephalopathy is often called as kernicterus. The term kernicterus refers to yellow staining of brain tissues caused by bilirubin.

Prevention or Treatment for Erythroblastosis Fetalis

If the baby is born with erythroblastosis fetalis, the treatment is given by means of **exchange transfusion.**

■ IMPORTANCE OF KNOWING BLOOD GROUP

Nowadays, knowledge of blood group is very essential medically and socially.

Importance of knowing blood group is:

1. Medically, it is important during blood transfusions and in tissue transplants to save life.
2. Socially, one should know his/her own blood group and become a member of the Blood Donor's Club so that he/she can be approached for blood donation during emergency conditions.
3. Among the couple, the knowledge of blood groups helps to prevent the complications due to Rh incompatibility and save the child from the disorders like erythroblastosis fetalis.

■ BLOOD TRANSFUSION
■ DEFINITION AND TYPES

Blood transfusion is a process by which blood or blood components are transfused from one person (donor) into the bloodstream of another person (recipient). Transfusion may be done as a **lifesaving procedure** to replace blood cells or blood products lost through bleeding.

Blood transfusion is of four types:

1. *Whole blood transfusion*: Used in hemorrhage.
2. *Red cell transfusion*: Used in anemia.
3. *Platelet transfusion*: Used in bleeding disorders.

Chapter 16: Blood Groups and Blood Transfusion

4. ***Plasma transfusion***: Used during burns, liver diseases and surgical procedures particularly heart surgery.

■ CONDITIONS WHEN BLOOD TRANSFUSION IS NECESSARY

Blood transfusion is essential in the following conditions:

1. Anemia.
2. Hemorrhage.
3. Trauma.
4. Burns.
5. Surgery.

■ PRECAUTIONS TO BE TAKEN

Precautions to be Taken Before Transfusion of Blood

1. Donor must be healthy, without any diseases such as sexually transmitted diseases like syphilis and diseases caused by virus like hepatitis, AIDS, etc.
2. Only compatible blood must be transfused. Rh compatibility also must be confirmed.
3. Both matching and crossmatching must be done.

Precautions to be Taken While Transfusing Blood

1. Apparatus for transfusion must be sterile.
2. Temperature of blood to be transfused must be same as body temperature.
3. Transfusion of blood must be slow. Sudden rapid infusion of blood into the body increases the load on the heart resulting in many complications.

■ BLOOD SUBSTITUTES

Blood substitutes are the substances infused as a replacement for blood or to expand blood volume.

Commonly used blood substitutes are:

1. Human plasma.
2. 0.9% sodium chloride solution (saline)
3. 5% glucose.
4. Colloids like gum acacia, isinglass, albumin and animal gelatin.

■ EXCHANGE TRANSFUSION

Exchange transfusion is the procedure which involves removal of patient's blood and replacement with fresh blood or plasma from a donor. It is otherwise known as **replacement transfusion**. It is carried out in conditions such as severe jaundice, sickle cell anemia, erythroblastosis fetalis, etc.

■ AUTOLOGOUS BLOOD TRANSFUSION

Autologous blood transfusion is the collection and reinfusion of patient's own blood. It is also called self blood donation. The conventional transfusion of blood that is collected from persons other than the patient is called allogeneic or **heterologous blood transfusion**.

Chapter 17: Reticuloendothelial System, Tissue Macrophage and Spleen

CHAPTER OUTLINE

- **DEFINITION AND DISTRIBUTION**
  - RETICULOENDOTHELIAL SYSTEM OR TISSUE MACROPHAGE SYSTEM
  - TISSUE MACROPHAGE
- **CLASSIFICATION OF RETICULOENDOTHELIAL CELLS**
  - FIXED RETICULOENDOTHELIAL CELLS: TISSUE MACROPHAGES
- **WANDERING RETICULOENDOTHELIAL CELLS**
- **FUNCTIONS OF RETICULOENDOTHELIAL SYSTEM**
- **SPLEEN**
  - FUNCTIONAL ANATOMY
  - FUNCTIONS
  - APPLIED PHYSIOLOGY

DEFINITION AND DISTRIBUTION

RETICULOENDOTHELIAL SYSTEM OR TISSUE MACROPHAGE SYSTEM

Reticuloendothelial system or tissue macrophage system is the system of primitive phagocytic cells which play important role in defense mechanism of the body.

Structures having Reticuloendothelial Cells

1. Endothelial lining of vascular and lymph channels.
2. Connective tissue and some organs such as spleen, liver, lungs, lymph nodes, bone marrow, etc.

Reticular cells in these tissues form the tissue macrophage system.

TISSUE MACROPHAGE

Macrophage is a large phagocytic cell, derived from monocyte (Chapter 11). Monocytes leave the blood and enter tissues and transform into larger macrophages. Tissue macrophages have long lifespan ranging from months to years.

CLASSIFICATION OF RETICULOENDOTHELIAL CELLS

Reticuloendothelial cells are classified into two types called fixed reticuloendothelial cells or tissue macrophages and wandering reticuloendothelial cells.

FIXED RETICULOENDOTHELIAL CELLS: TISSUE MACROPHAGES

Fixed reticuloendothelial cells are also called the tissue macrophages or fixed histiocytes, because these cells are usually located in the tissues.

Tissue macrophages are present in the following areas.

1. *Connective tissue*: Reticuloendothelial cells in connective tissues and in serous membranes like pleura, omentum and mesentery are called the fixed macrophages of connective tissue.
2. *Endothelium of blood sinusoid*: Endothelium of blood sinusoid in bone marrow, liver, spleen, lymph nodes, adrenal glands and pituitary glands also contain fixed cells. **Kupffer cells** present in liver belong to this category.
3. *Reticulum*: Reticulum of spleen, lymph node and bone marrow contain fixed reticuloendothelial cells.
4. *Central nervous system*: **Meningocytes** of meninges and microglia form the tissue macrophages of brain.
5. *Lungs*: Tissue macrophages are present in the alveoli of lungs.
6. *Subcutaneous tissue*: Fixed reticuloendothelial cells are present in subcutaneous tissue also.

WANDERING RETICULOENDOTHELIAL CELLS

Wandering reticuloendothelial cells are also called free histiocytes. Wandering reticuloendothelial cells are of two types:

1. Free Histiocytes of Blood

i. Neutrophils.
ii. Monocytes, which become macrophages and migrate to the site of injury or infection.

2. Free Histiocytes of Solid Tissue

During emergency, the fixed histiocytes from connective tissue and other organs become wandering cells and enter the circulation.

■ FUNCTIONS OF RETICULOENDOTHELIAL SYSTEM

Reticuloendothelial system plays an important role in the defense mechanism of the body. Most of the functions of the reticuloendothelial system are carried out by the tissue macrophages.

■ 1. PHAGOCYTIC FUNCTION

Macrophages play an important role in defense of the body by phagocytosis. When any foreign body invades, macrophages ingest them by phagocytosis and liberate the antigen from the organism. Antigens activate the helper T lymphocytes and B lymphocytes.

■ 2. ANTIGEN PRESENTATION

Macrophages play an important role in development of immunity by presenting the antigenic substances to helper T cells (Chapter 12).

■ 3. SECRETION OF BACTERICIDAL AGENTS

In addition to proteolytic enzymes tissue macrophages secrete many bactericidal agents, which kill the bacteria. Important bactericidal agents secreted by macrophages are the **free radicals**. Free radicals are also called **reactive oxygen species** (ROS).

Free Radicals Secreted by Macrophages

i. Superoxide (O^-)
ii. Hydrogen peroxide (H_2O_2).
iii. Hydroxyl ions (OH^-).

These radicals are the most potent bactericidal agents. So, even the bacteria which cannot be digested by lysosomal enzymes are degraded by these oxidants.

■ 4. SECRETION OF INTERLEUKINS

Tissue macrophages secrete interleukin 1, 6 and 12 which help in immunity.

■ 5. SECRETION OF TUMOR NECROSIS FACTORS

Tissue macrophages secrete tumor necrosis factor-α and tumor necrosis factor-β which cause necrosis of tumor.

■ 6. SECRETION OF TRANSFORMING GROWTH FACTOR

Tissue macrophages secrete transforming growth factor, which prevents rejection of transplanted tissues or organs by immunosuppression.

■ 7. SECRETION OF COLONY-STIMULATING FACTOR

Macrophages secrete the colony-stimulating factor (MCSF) which accelerates growth of granulocytes, monocytes and macrophages.

■ 8. SECRETION OF PLATELET-DERIVED GROWTH FACTOR

Tissue macrophages secrete the platelet-derived growth factor (PDGF), which accelerates repair of damaged blood vessel and wound healing.

■ 9. REMOVAL OF CARBON PARTICLES AND SILICON

Macrophages ingest the substances like carbon dust particles and silicon which enter the body.

■ 10. DESTRUCTION OF SENILE RBC

Reticuloendothelial cells, particularly those in spleen destroy the senile RBCs and release hemoglobin (Chapter 9).

■ 11. DESTRUCTION OF HEMOGLOBIN

Hemoglobin released from broken senile RBCs is degraded by the reticuloendothelial cells (Chapter 9).

■ SPLEEN

■ FUNCTIONAL ANATOMY

Spleen is the largest lymphoid organ in the body and it is highly vascular. It also contains reticuloendothelial cells.

■ FUNCTIONS OF SPLEEN

1. Formation of Blood Cells

Spleen has hemopoietic function in embryo. During the hepatic stage, spleen produces blood cells along with liver. In myeloid stage, it produces the blood cells along with liver and bone marrow.

2. Destruction of Blood Cells

Older RBCs, lymphocytes and thrombocytes are destroyed in the spleen. When the RBCs become old (120 days), the cell membrane becomes more fragile. Diameter of most of the capillaries is less or equal to that of RBC. Fragile old cells are destroyed while trying to squeeze through the capillaries because these cells cannot withstand the stress of squeezing.

Destruction occurs in the capillaries of spleen because the splenic capillaries have a thin lumen. So, the spleen is known as **graveyard of RBCs**.

3. Blood Reservoir Function

In animals, spleen stores large amount of blood. However, this function is not significant in humans. But, a large number of RBCs are stored in spleen. RBCs are released from spleen into circulation during the emergency conditions like hypoxia and hemorrhage.

4. Role in Defense of Body

Spleen filters the blood by removing the microorganisms. Macrophages in splenic pulp destroy the microorganisms and other foreign bodies by phagocytosis. Spleen contains about 25% of T lymphocytes and 15% of B lymphocytes and forms the site of antibody production.

■ APPLIED PHYSIOLOGY

Splenomegaly and Hypersplenism

Splenomegaly refers to enlargement of spleen. Increase in the activities of spleen is called hypersplenism.

Diseases such as malaria, typhoid, tuberculosis and rheumatoid arthritis cause splenomegaly resulting in hypersplenism.

Hyposplenism and Asplenia

Hyposplenism or **hyposplenia** refers to diminished functioning of spleen. It occurs after partial removal of spleen due to trauma or cyst. Asplenia means absence of spleen. Functional asplenia means absence of splenic functions.

Chapter 18

Lymphatic System, Lymph, Tissue Fluid and Edema

CHAPTER OUTLINE

- **LYMPHATIC SYSTEM**
  - ORGANIZATION
  - DRAINAGE
- **LYMPH NODES**
  - STRUCTURE
  - FUNCTIONS
  - APPLIED PHYSIOLOGY
- **LYMPH**
  - DEFINITION
  - FORMATION
- RATE OF FLOW
- COMPOSITION
- FUNCTIONS
- **TISSUE FLUID**
  - FUNCTIONS
  - FORMATION
- **EDEMA**
  - TYPES

LYMPHATIC SYSTEM

Lymphatic system is a closed system of **lymph channels** or **lymph vessels** through which lymph flows. It is a one-way system and allows the lymph flow from tissue spaces towards the blood.

ORGANIZATION OF LYMPHATIC SYSTEM

Lymphatic system arises from tissue spaces as a meshwork of **lymph capillaries**. These capillaries arise from tissue spaces as enlarged blind-ended terminals called **capillary bulbs**. These bulbs contain valves, which allow flow of lymph in only one direction.

DRAINAGE OF LYMPHATIC SYSTEM

Larger lymph vessels ultimately form the **right lymphatic duct** and **thoracic duct**. Right lymphatic duct opens into right subclavian vein and the thoracic duct opens into left subclavian vein. Thoracic duct drains the lymph from more than two-third of the tissue spaces in the body **(Fig. 18.1)**.

LYMPH NODES

Lymph nodes or **lymph glands** are small glandular structures located in the course of lymph vessels.

STRUCTURE OF LYMPH NODES

Each lymph node constitutes masses of lymphatic tissue, covered by a dense connective tissue capsule. The structures are arranged in three layers namely cortex, paracortex and medulla **(Fig. 18.2)**.

Lymphatic Vessels to Lymph Node

Lymph node receives lymph through one or two lymphatic vessels called afferent vessels. Afferent vessels divide into small channels. Lymph passes through afferent vessels and small channels and reaches the cortex. It circulates through cortex, paracortex and medulla of the lymph node. From medulla, the lymph leaves the node via one or two efferent vessels.

Distribution of Lymph Nodes

Lymph nodes are present along the course of lymphatic vessels in elbow, axilla, knee and groin. Lymph nodes are also present in certain points in abdomen, thorax and neck, where many lymph vessels join.

FUNCTIONS OF LYMPH NODES

Lymph nodes serve as filters which filter bacteria and toxic substances from the lymph.

Functions of the lymph nodes:

1. When lymph passes through lymph nodes, it is filtered, i.e. the water and electrolytes are removed. But proteins and lipids are retained in the lymph.
2. Bacteria and other toxic substances are destroyed by macrophages of lymph nodes. Because of this, lymph nodes are called defense barriers.

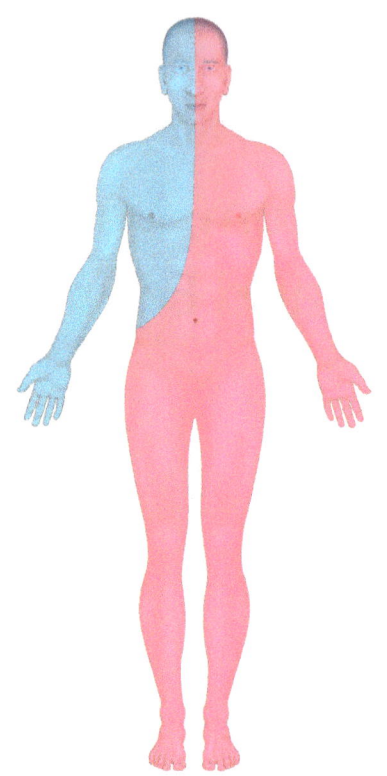

FIGURE 18.1: Lymph drainage. Blue area = Drained by right lymphatic duct. Pink area = Drained by thoracic duct.

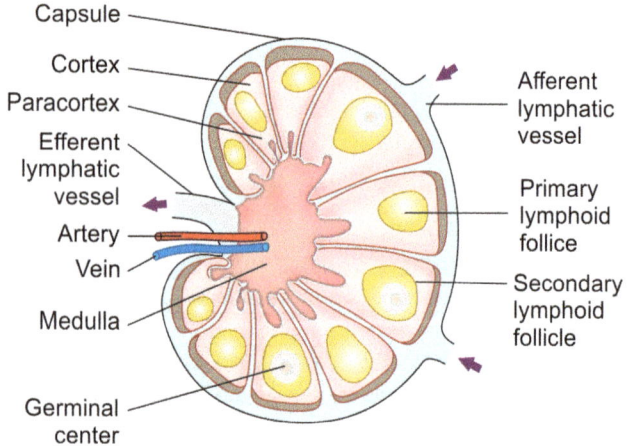

FIGURE 18.2: Structure of a lymph node.

APPLIED PHYSIOLOGY: SWELLING OF LYMPH NODES

During infection or any other processes in a particular region of the body, activities of the lymph nodes in that region increase. This causes swelling of the lymph nodes. Sometimes, the swollen lymph nodes cause pain.

When the body recovers from infection, the lymph nodes restore their original size gradually, in 1 or 2 weeks.

LYMPH

DEFINITION

Lymph is an alkaline clear fluid that is derived from interstitial fluid and flowing to bloodstream through lymphatic vessels.

FORMATION OF LYMPH

Lymph is formed from interstitial fluid, due to the permeability of lymph capillaries. When blood passes via blood capillaries in the tissues, 9/10th of fluid passes into venous end of capillaries from arterial end. And, the remaining 1/10th of the fluid passes into lymph capillaries, which have more permeability than blood capillaries.

So, when lymph passes through lymph capillaries, the composition of lymph is more or less similar to that of interstitial fluid including protein content. Proteins present in the interstitial fluid cannot enter the blood capillaries because of their larger size. So, these proteins enter lymph vessels, which are permeable to large particles also.

Addition of Proteins and Fats

Tissue fluid in liver and gastrointestinal tract (GIT) contains more protein and lipid substances. So, proteins and lipids enter the lymph vessels of liver and GIT in large quantities. Thus, lymph in larger vessels has more proteins and lipids.

Concentration of Lymph

When the lymph passes through the lymph nodes, it is concentrated because of absorption of water and the electrolytes. However, the proteins and lipids are not absorbed.

RATE OF LYMPH FLOW

About 120 mL of lymph flows into blood per hour. Out of this, about 100 mL/h flows through thoracic duct and 20 mL/h flows through the right lymphatic duct.

COMPOSITION OF LYMPH

Usually, lymph is a clear and colorless fluid. It is formed by 96% water and 4% solids. Some blood cells are also present in lymph (**Fig. 18.3**).

FUNCTIONS OF LYMPH

1. Important function of lymph is to return proteins from tissue spaces into the blood.
2. Lymph flow plays an important role in redistribution of fluid in the body.
3. Through lymph, bacteria, toxins and other foreign bodies are removed from tissues.
4. Lymph flow is responsible for the maintenance of structural and functional integrity of tissue. Obstruction to lymph flow affects various types of tissues, particularly myocardium, nephrons and the hepatic cells.
5. Lymph flow serves as an important route for intestinal fat absorption. This is the reason for the milky appearance of lymph after fatty meal.
6. Lymph plays an important role in immunity by transport of lymphocytes.

TISSUE FLUID

Tissue fluid is the medium in which cells are bathed. It is otherwise known as **interstitial fluid**. It forms about 20% of ECF.

Chapter 18: Lymphatic System, Lymph, Tissue Fluid and Edema

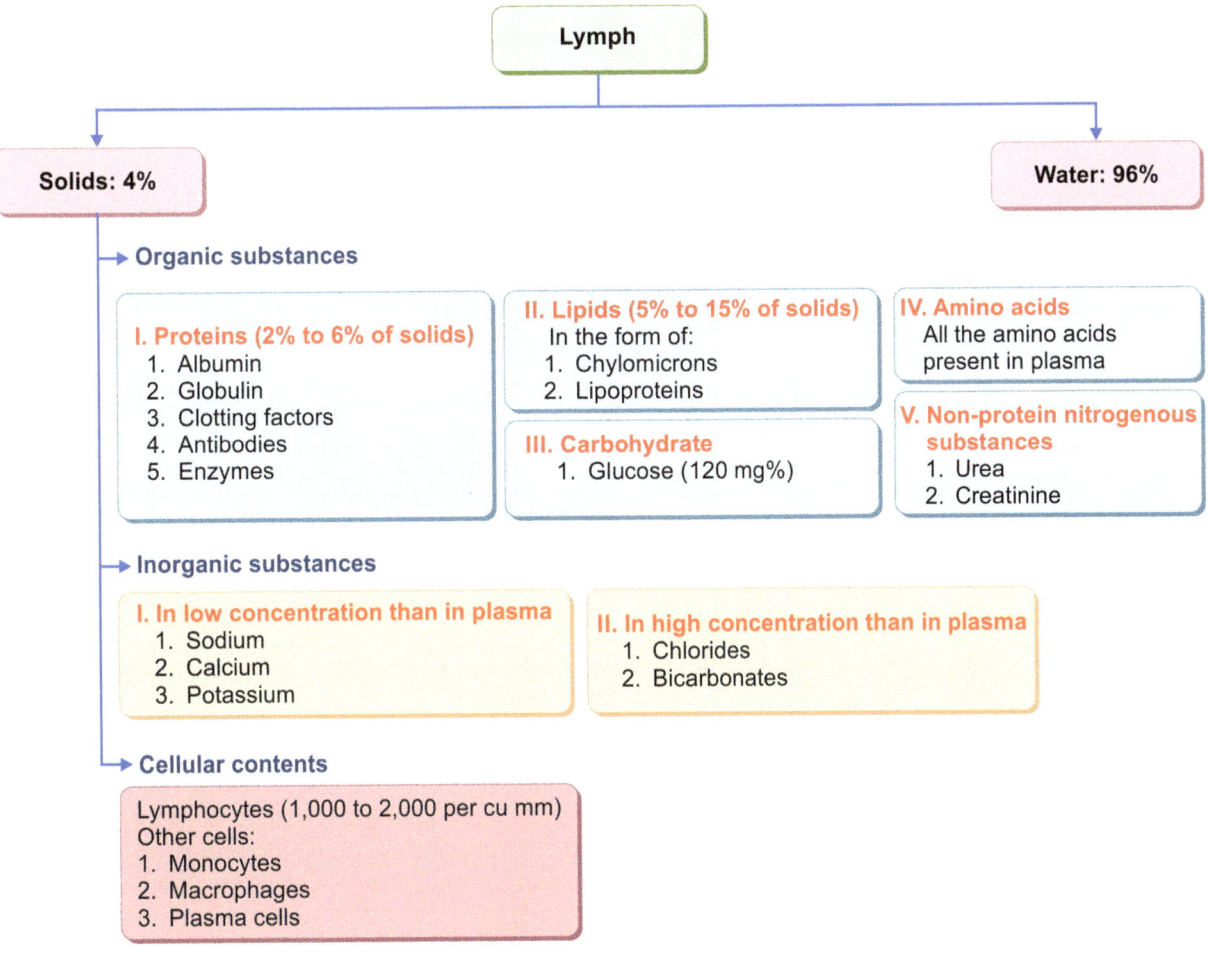

FIGURE 18.3: Composition of lymph.

FUNCTIONS OF TISSUE FLUID

Because of the capillary membrane, there is no direct contact between blood and cells. And the tissue fluid acts as a medium for exchange of various substances between the cells and the blood in the capillary loop. Oxygen and nutritive substances diffuse from the arterial end of capillary through the tissue fluid and reach the cells. Carbon dioxide and waste materials diffuse from the cells into the venous end of capillary through this fluid.

FORMATION OF TISSUE FLUID

Formation of tissue fluid involves two processes, filtration and reabsorption.

Tissue fluid is formed by the process of filtration. Normally, blood pressure (also called hydrostatic pressure) in arterial end of the capillary is about 30 mm Hg. This hydrostatic pressure is the driving force for filtration of water and other substances from blood into tissue spaces (Fig. 18.4).

Fluid filtered at the arterial end of capillaries is reabsorbed back into the blood at the venous end of capillaries. Here also, the pressure gradient plays an important role. At the venous end of capillaries, the hydrostatic pressure is less (15 mm Hg) and the **oncotic pressure** is more (25 mm Hg). Due to the pressure gradient of 10 mm Hg, the fluid is reabsorbed along with waste materials from the tissue fluid into the capillaries. About 10% of filtered fluid enters the lymphatic vessels.

Reabsorption at the venous end helps to maintain the volume of tissue fluid.

EDEMA

Edema is defined as the swelling caused by excess accumulation of fluid in tissues. It may be generalized or local. Edema that involves the entire body is called **generalized edema**. **Local edema** is the one that occurs in specific areas of the body such as abdomen, lungs and extremities like feet, ankles and legs. Accumulation of fluid may be inside or outside the cell.

TYPES OF EDEMA

Edema is classified into two types, intracellular edema and extracellular edema.

Intracellular Edema

Intracellular edema is the accumulation of fluid inside the cell. It occurs because of malnutrition, poor metabolism and inflammation of tissue.

Extracellular Edema

Extracellular edema is defined as the accumulation of fluid outside the cell. Common conditions which leads

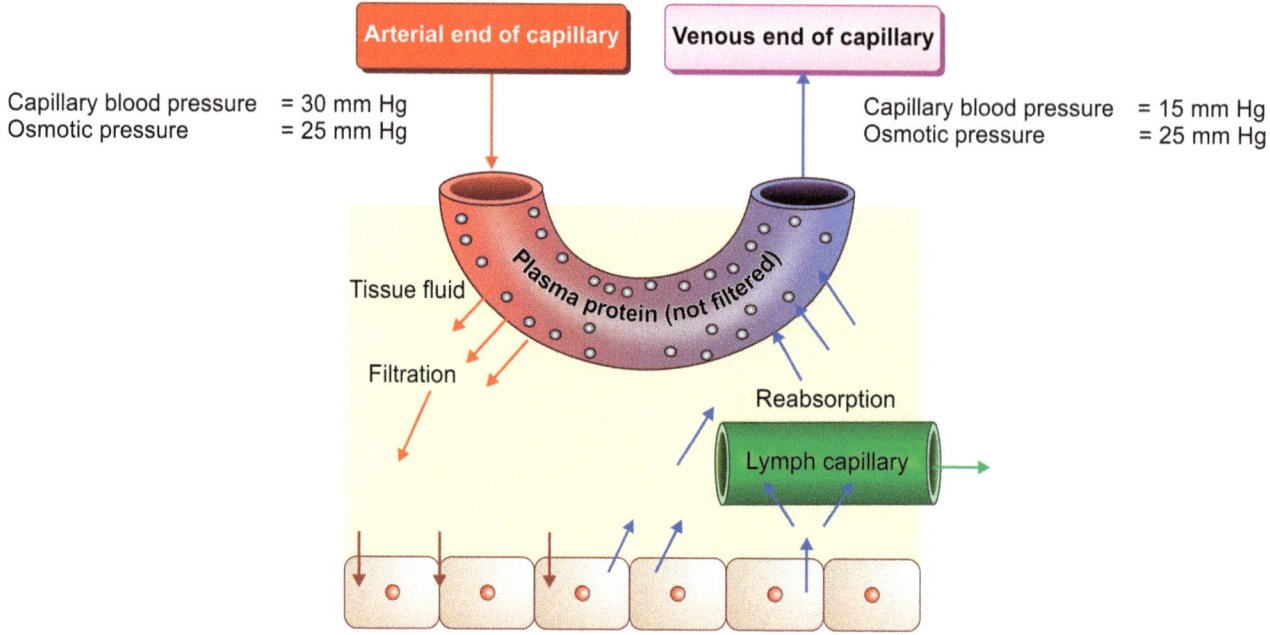

FIGURE 18.4: Formation of tissue fluid. Plasma proteins remain inside the blood capillary, as the capillary membrane is not permeable to plasma proteins.

to extracellular edema are heart failure, renal disease, decreased plasma proteins and lymphatic obstruction.

Pitting and Non-pitting Edema

Interstitial fluid is present in the form of a gel that is almost like a semisolid substance. It is because the interstitial fluid is not present in fluid form, but is bound in a **proteoglycan meshwork**. It does not allow any free space for the movement of fluid.

When interstitial fluid volume increases, most of the fluid becomes free fluid that is not bound to proteoglycan meshwork. It flows freely through tissue spaces, producing a swelling called edema. This type of edema is known as pitting edema, because when this area is pressed with the finger, displacement of fluid occurs producing a depression or pit. When the finger is removed, the pit remains for few seconds, sometimes as long as 1 minute, till the fluid flows back into that area.

Edema also develops due to swelling of the cells or clotting of interstitial fluid in the presence of fibrinogen. This is called non-pitting edema, because it is hard and a pit is not formed while pressing.

MODEL QUESTIONS IN BLOOD AND BODY FLUIDS

■ LONG QUESTIONS

1. What is indicator dilution technique? How is it applied in the measurement of total body water? Describe dehydration briefly.
2. Give a detailed account of erythropoiesis.
3. Define erythropoiesis. List the different stages of erythropoiesis. Describe the changes, which take place in each stage and the factors necessary for erythropoiesis.
4. Describe the morphology, development and functions of leukocytes.
5. Describe the development of cell-mediated immunity.
6. Describe the development of humoral immunity.
7. Enumerate the factors involved in blood coagulation and describe the intrinsic mechanism of coagulation.
8. Give an account of extrinsic mechanism of coagulation of blood. Give a brief description of bleeding disorders.

■ SHORT QUESTIONS

1. Dye or indicator dilution technique.
2. Measurement of total body water.
3. Measurement of ECF volume.
4. Measurement of plasma / blood volume.
5. Dehydration.
6. Water intoxication.
7. Functions of blood.
8. Plasma proteins.
9. Polycythemia.
10. Factors necessary for erythropoiesis.
11. Abnormal hemoglobin derivatives.
12. Erythrocyte sedimentation rate.
13. Packed cell volume or hematocrit.
14. Hemolysis and fragility of RBC.
15. Morphology of WBCs.
16. Functions of WBCs.
17. Role of macrophages in immunity.
18. Immunoglobulins or antibodies.
19. Immune deficiency diseases.
20. Autoimmune diseases.
21. Properties and functions of platelets.
22. Hemostasis.
23. Fibrinolysis.
24. Tests for coagulation.
25. Anticoagulants.
26. Purpura.
27. ABO blood groups.
28. Rh factor.
29. Transfusion reactions due to ABO incompatibility.
30. Transfusion reactions due to Rh incompatibility.
31. Erythroblastosis fetalis.
32. Tissue macrophage.
33. Lymph nodes.
34. Tissue fluid.
35. Edema.

■ VERY SHORT ANSWER QUESTIONS

1. Formula for indicator dilution method.
2. Measurement of volume of interstitial fluid and intracellular fluid.
3. Hematocrit value.
4. Therapeutic plasma exchange.
5. Advantages of biconcave shape of RBCs.
6. Functions of RBCs.
7. Fate of RBCs.
8. Important changes taking place during erythropoiesis.
9. Reticulocytes.
10. Erythropoietin.
11. Types of normal and abnormal hemoglobin.
12. Destruction of hemoglobin.
13. Sickle cell anemia.
14. Thalassemia.
15. Iron deficiency anemia.
16. Pernicious anemia.
17. Granulocytes.
18. Monocytes.
19. Types of T lymphocytes and B lymphocytes.
20. Macrophage.
21. Antigen presentation.
22. NK cell.
23. AIDS.
24. Vaccines.
25. Toxoids.
26. Properties of platelets.
27. Blood clot.
28. Heparin.
29. Procoagulants.
30. Hemophilia.
31. von Willebrand factor and disease.
32. Landsteiner's law.
33. Cross matching.
34. Bilirubin encephalopathy/Kernicterus.
35. Exchange transfusion/Autologous transfusion.
36. Functions of spleen.
37. Functions of lymph.
38. Formation of tissue fluid.
39. Pitting edema.
40. Non-pitting edema.

SECTION 3 MUSCLE PHYSIOLOGY

Chapter 19: Classification of Muscles

CHAPTER OUTLINE

- CLASSIFICATION OF MUSCLES
- CLASSIFICATION DEPENDING UPON STRIATIONS
- CLASSIFICATION DEPENDING UPON CONTROL
- CLASSIFICATION DEPENDING UPON SITUATION

CLASSIFICATION OF MUSCLES

Human body has more than 600 muscles. Muscles perform many useful functions and help us in doing everything in day to day life.

Muscles are classified by three different methods based on different factors:

I. Depending upon presence or absence of striations.
II. Depending upon control.
III. Depending upon function.

CLASSIFICATION OF MUSCLES DEPENDING UPON STRIATIONS

Depending upon presence or absence of cross striations, the muscles are divided into two groups:

1. Striated muscle.
2. Non-striated muscle.

1. STRIATED MUSCLE

Striated muscle is the muscle which has a large number of cross striations (transverse lines). **Skeletal muscle** and **cardiac muscle** belong to this category.

2. NON-STRIATED MUSCLE

Muscle which does not have cross striations is called non-striated muscle. It is also called **plain muscle** or **smooth muscle**. It is found in the wall of the visceral organs.

CLASSIFICATION OF MUSCLES DEPENDING UPON CONTROL

Depending upon control, the muscles are classified into two types:

1. Voluntary muscle.
2. Involuntary muscle.

1. VOLUNTARY MUSCLE

Voluntary muscle is the muscle that is controlled by our will. Skeletal muscles are the voluntary muscles. Voluntary muscles are innervated by somatic nerves.

2. INVOLUNTARY MUSCLE

Muscle that cannot be controlled by our will is called involuntary muscle. Cardiac muscle and our muscle are involuntary muscles. Involuntary muscles are innervated by autonomic nerves.

CLASSIFICATION OF MUSCLES DEPENDING UPON SITUATION

Depending upon situation, the muscles are classified into three types:

1. Skeletal muscle.
2. Cardiac muscle.
3. Smooth muscle.

1. SKELETAL MUSCLE

Skeletal muscles are situated in association with bones forming the skeletal system. Skeletal muscles constitute 40% to 50% of body mass. These muscles are **striated** and **voluntary**. Skeletal muscles are supplied by somatic nerves.

Fibers of the skeletal muscles are arranged in parallel. In most of the skeletal muscles, the muscle fibers are attached to tendons on either end. Skeletal muscles are anchored to the bones by the tendons.

2. CARDIAC MUSCLE

Cardiac muscle forms the musculature of the heart. These muscles are **striated** and **involuntary**. Cardiac muscles are supplied by autonomic nerve fibers.

3. SMOOTH MUSCLE

Smooth muscle is situated in association with viscera. It is also called visceral muscle. Smooth muscle is **non-striated** and **involuntary**. It is different from skeletal and cardiac muscles because of the absence of cross striations, hence the name smooth muscle. Smooth muscles are supplied by autonomic nerve fibers. Smooth muscles form the main contractile units of wall of the various visceral organs.

Features of skeletal, cardiac and smooth muscles are given in **Table 19.1**.

TABLE 19.1: Features of skeletal, cardiac and smooth muscle fibers.

Features	Skeletal muscle	Cardiac muscle	Smooth muscle
Location	In association with bones	In the heart	In the visceral organs
Shape	Cylindrical and unbranched	Branched	Spindle shaped, unbranched
Length	1 cm to 4 cm	80 μ to 100 μ	50 μ to 200 μ
Diameter	10 μ to 100 μ	15 μ to 20 μ	2 μ to 5 μ
Number of nucleus	> 1	1	1
Cross-striations	Present	Present	Absent
Myofibrils	Present	Present	Absent
Sarcomere	Present	Present	Absent
Troponin	Present	Present	Absent
Sarcotubular system	Well developed	Well developed	Poorly developed
T-tubules	Long and thin	Short and broad	Absent
Depolarization	Upon stimulation	Spontaneous	Spontaneous
Fatigue	Possible	Not possible	Not possible
Summation	Possible	Not possible	Possible
Tetanus	Possible	Not possible	Possible
Resting membrane potential	Stable	Stable	Unstable
To trigger contraction, calcium binds with	Troponin	Troponin	Calmodulin
Source of calcium	Sarcoplasmic reticulum	Sarcoplasmic reticulum	Extracellular fluid
Speed of contraction	Quick	Intermediate	Slow
Neuromuscular junction	Well defined	Ill defined	Ill defined
Action	Voluntary action	Involuntary action	Involuntary action
Control of action	Neurogenic	Myogenic	Neurogenic and myogenic
Nerve supply	Somatic nerves	Autonomic nerves	Autonomic nerves

Chapter 20: Structure of Skeletal Muscle

CHAPTER OUTLINE

- MUSCLE MASS
- MUSCLE FIBER
- MYOFIBRIL
  - MICROSCOPIC STRUCTURE
- SARCOMERE
  - COMPONENTS
  - ELECTRON MICROSCOPIC STUDY
- CONTRACTILE ELEMENTS (PROTEINS) OF MUSCLE
- MYOSIN MOLECULE
- ACTIN MOLECULE
- TROPOMYOSIN
- TROPONIN
- OTHER PROTEINS OF THE MUSCLE
- SARCOTUBULAR SYSTEM
  - STRUCTURES
  - FUNCTIONS
- COMPOSITION OF MUSCLE

■ MUSCLE MASS

Muscle mass (or tissue) is made up of many individual **muscle cells** or **myocytes** or **muscle fibers.**

Muscle mass is separated from neighboring tissues by **fascia**. Beneath this fascia, the muscle is covered by **epimysium**. In each muscle, the muscle fibers are arranged in different groups called the bundles or **fasciculi**. Each fasciculus is called **perimysium**. Each muscle fiber is covered by **endomysium (Figs. 20.1 and 20.2)**.

■ MUSCLE FIBER

Each muscle fiber is cylindrical in shape with a length of 1 cm to 4 cm depending upon length of the muscle. Diameter of the muscle fiber varies from 10 µ to 100 µ. Muscle fibers are attached to bone by **tendon**.

Each muscle fiber is enclosed by a cell membrane called **sarcolemma** that lies beneath the endomysium **(Fig. 20.3)**. Cytoplasm of muscle fiber is known as **sarcoplasm**. Many structures are embedded within the sarcoplasm namely, nuclei, myofibril, Golgi apparatus, mitochondria, sarcoplasmic reticulum, ribosomes, glycogen droplets and occasional lipid droplets

Each muscle fiber has got one or more nuclei. In long muscle fibers, many nuclei are seen. Nuclei are oval or elongated and situated just beneath the sarcolemma. Usually in other cells, nucleus is in the interior of cell.

■ MYOFIBRIL

Myofibrils or **myofibrillae** are very fine filaments arranged parallelly in cytoplasm of muscle fibers. Myofibrils run through the entire length of the muscle fiber.

■ MICROSCOPIC STRUCTURE OF A MYOFIBRIL

Light microscopic studies show that, each myofibril consists of a number of two alternating bands called light band or 'I' band and dark band or 'A' band.

Light Band or 'I' Band

Light band in myofibril is called 'I' band because it is isotropic to **polarized light**. When a polarized light is passed through the muscle fiber at this area, all the light rays are refracted at the same angle.

Dark Band or 'A' Band

Dark band is called 'A' band because it is anisotropic to polarized light. When a polarized light is passed through the muscle fiber at this area, the light rays are refracted at different directions (an = not, iso = it, trops = turning).

In an intact muscle fiber, 'I' band and 'A' band of adjacent myofibrils are placed side by side. It gives the appearance of characteristic cross striations in muscle fiber. 'I' band is divided into two portions by a narrow dark line called '**Z' line** or 'Z' disk (in German zwischenscheibe = between disks). The 'Z' line is formed by a protein disk

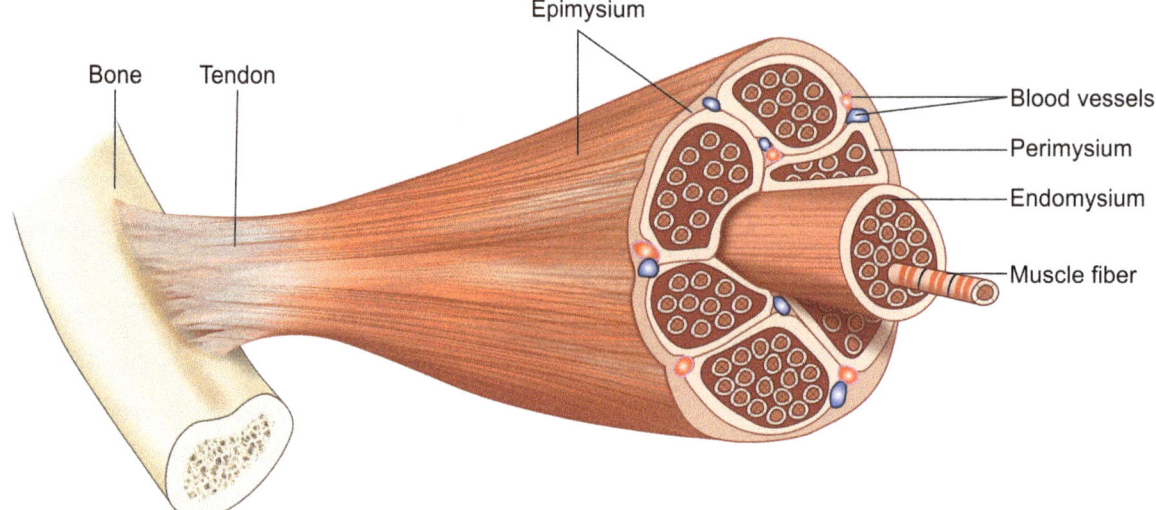

FIGURE 20.1: Structure of a skeletal muscle.

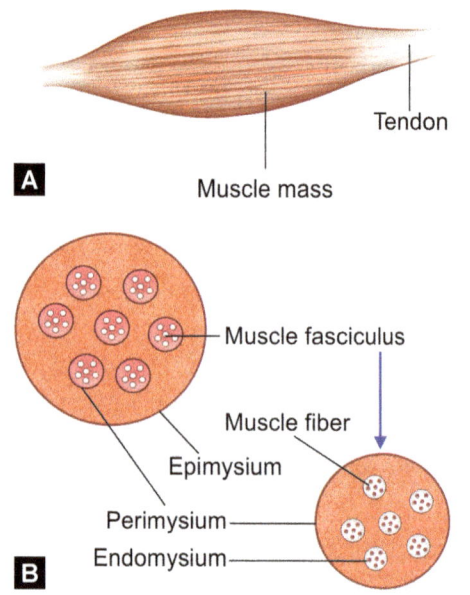

FIGURE 20.2: Diagram showing: **A.** Skeletal muscle mass. **B.** Cross-section of muscle. **C.** One muscle fasciculus.

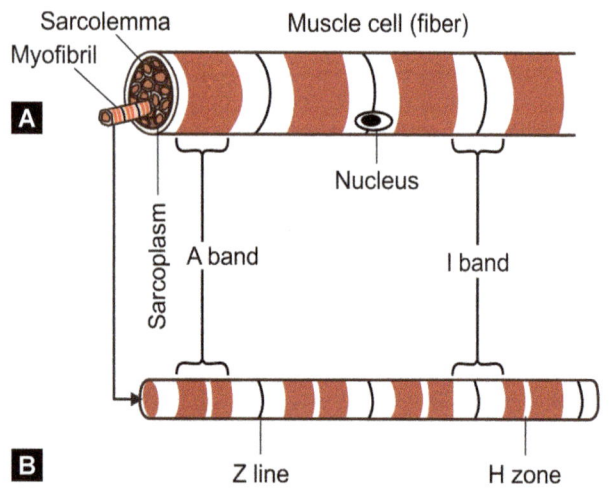

FIGURE 20.3: Diagram showing: **A.** One muscle cell. **B.** One myofibril.

which does not permit passage of light. The portion of myofibril in between two 'Z' lines is called sarcomere.

■ SARCOMERE

Sarcomere is the structural and functional unit of the skeletal muscle. Each sarcomere extends between two 'Z' lines of myofibril. Thus, each myofibril contains many sarcomeres arranged in series throughout its length. When the muscle is in relaxed state, average length of each sarcomere is 2 to 3 microns.

■ COMPONENTS OF SARCOMERE

Each sarcomere consists of:

1. One half of light 'I' band.
2. One dark 'A' band.
3. One half of light 'I' band.

In the middle of 'A' band, there is a light area called '**H' zone** (H indicates hell which means light in German).

In the middle of 'H' zone lies the middle part of myosin filament. This is called '**M' line** (M = middle). 'M' line is formed by myosin binding proteins **(Fig. 20.4)**.

■ ELECTRON MICROSCOPIC STUDY OF SARCOMERE

Electron microscopic studies reveal that the sarcomere consists of many thread-like structures called myofilaments.

Myofilaments are of two types, actin filaments and myosin filaments.

Actin Filaments

Actin filaments are thin filaments that extend from either side of the 'Z' lines, run through 'I' band and enter into 'A' band up to 'H' zone. Each actin filament has a diameter of 20 Å and a length of 1 µ.

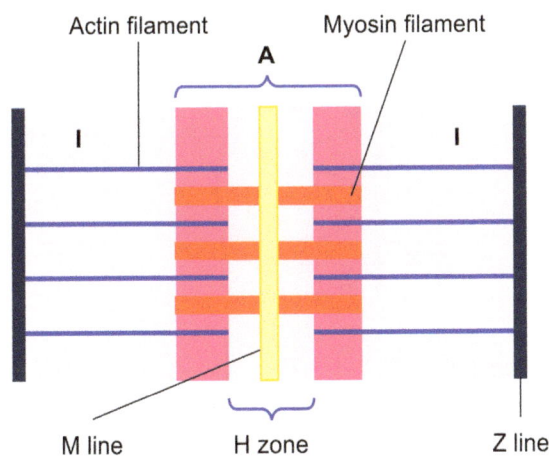

FIGURE 20.4: One sarcomere. A = A band. I = I band.

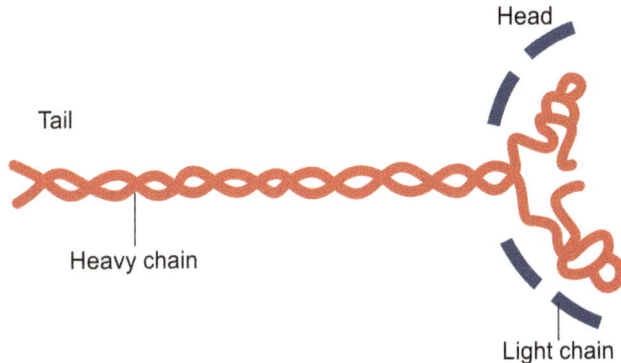

FIGURE 20.5: Myosin molecule formed by two heavy chains and four light chains of polypeptides.

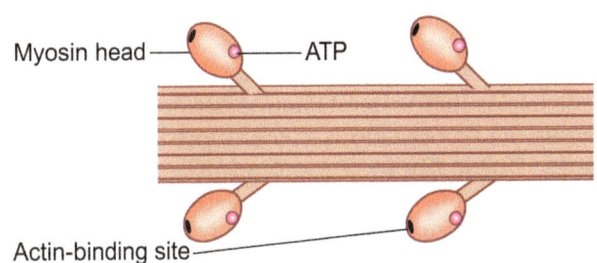

FIGURE 20.6: Diagram showing myosin filament. ATP = Adenosine triphosphate.

Myosin Filaments

Myosin filaments are thick filaments and are situated in 'A' band. Each myosin filament has a diameter of 115 Å and a length of 1.5 μ.

Some lateral processes (projections) or **cross bridges** arise from myosin filaments. These bridges have enlarged structures called myosin heads at their tips. Myosin heads attach themselves to actin filaments. These heads pull the actin filaments during contraction of the muscle by means of a mechanism called sliding mechanism or ratchet mechanism (Chapter 22).

■ CONTRACTILE ELEMENTS (PROTEINS) OF MUSCLE

Myosin filaments are formed by one type of protein namely myosin molecules. However, actin filaments are formed by three types of proteins called actin, tropomyosin and troponin. These four proteins together constitute the muscle proteins or the contractile elements of the muscle.

In addition to the contractile proteins, the sarcomere contains some more proteins.

■ MYOSIN MOLECULE

Each myosin filament consists of about 200 myosin molecules. Myosin is a globulin which is made up of 6 polypeptide chains (2 heavy chains and 4 light chains). Each myosin molecule has a head portion and a tail portion. **Myosin head** has two attachment sites. One site is for actin filament and the other one is for one ATP molecule **(Figs. 20.5** and **20.6)**. In the central part of the myosin filament, i.e. in the 'H' zone, the myosin head is absent.

■ ACTIN MOLECULE

Each actin molecule is called **F-actin.** There are about 300 to 400 actin molecules in each actin filament. Each F-actin molecule has an active site to which the myosin head is attached.

■ TROPOMYOSIN

There are about 40 to 60 tropomyosin molecules situated along actin filament. In relaxed condition of the muscle, the tropomyosin molecules cover all the active sites of F-actin molecules **(Fig. 20.7)**.

■ TROPONIN

Troponin is formed by three subunits:

1. Troponin I which is attached to F-actin.
2. Troponin T which is attached to tropomyosin.
3. Troponin C which is attached to calcium ions.

■ SARCOTUBULAR SYSTEM

Sarcotubular system is a system of membranous structures in the form of vesicles and tubules in sarcoplasm of the muscle fiber. It surrounds the myofibrils embedded in the sarcoplasm.

Sarcotubular system is formed mainly by two types of structures, T-tubules and L-tubules or sarcoplasmic reticulum.

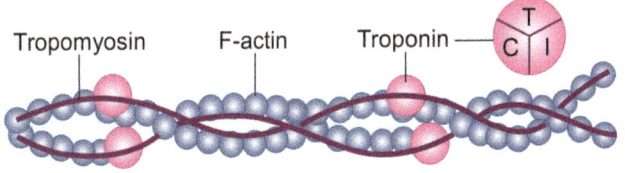

FIGURE 20.7: Part of actin filament. Troponin has three subunits T, C and I.

T-TUBULES

T-tubules or **transverse tubules** are formed by invagination of the sarcolemma. T-tubules penetrate all the way from one side of the muscle fiber to other side. Because of their origin from sarcolemma, T-tubules open to the exterior of the muscle cell. Therefore, the ECF runs through their lumen.

T-tubules are responsible for rapid transmission of action potential from sarcolemma to the myofibrils.

L-TUBULES OR SARCOPLASMIC RETICULUM

L-tubules or **longitudinal tubules** are the closed tubules that run in long axis of muscle fiber forming sarcoplasmic reticulum. These tubules form a closed tubular system around each myofibril and do not open to exterior like T-tubules.

At regular intervals, throughout the length of the myofibrils, the L-tubules dilate to form a pair of lateral sacs called **terminal cisternae**. Each pair of terminal cisternae is in close contact with T-tubule. T-tubule along with the cisternae on either side is called the **triad of skeletal muscle**. Calcium ions are stored in L-tubule and the amount of calcium ions is more in cisternae **(Fig. 20.8)**.

L-tubules store a large quantity of calcium ions.

COMPOSITION OF MUSCLE

Skeletal muscle is formed by 75% of water and 25% of solids. Solids are 20% of proteins and 5% of organic substances other than proteins and inorganic substances **(Fig. 20.9)**.

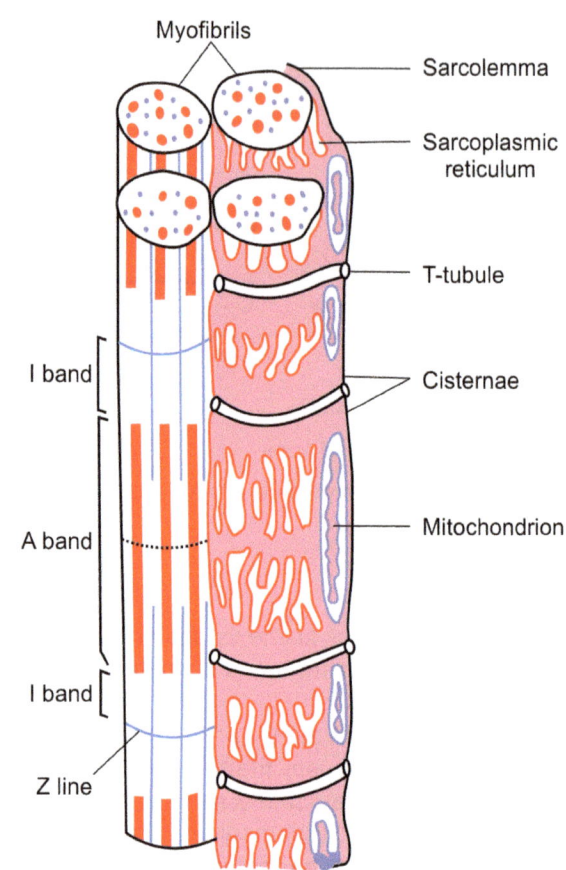

FIGURE 20.8: Diagram showing the relation between sarcotubular system and parts of sarcomere. Only few myofilaments are shown in the myofibril drawn on the right side of the diagram.

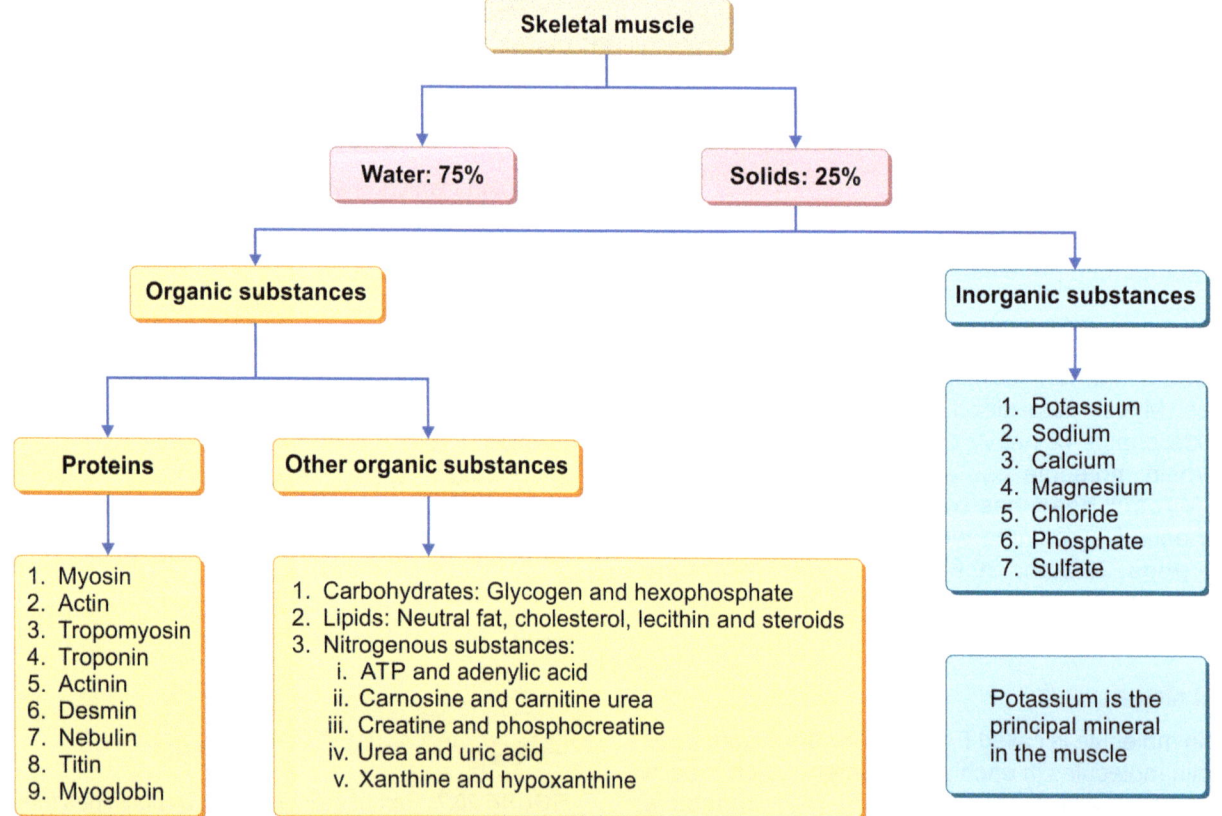

FIGURE 20.9: Composition of skeletal muscle.

Chapter 21

Properties of Skeletal Muscle

CHAPTER OUTLINE

- **EXCITABILITY**
  - DEFINITION
  - TYPES OF STIMULUS
  - QUALITIES OF STIMULUS
  - EXCITABILITY CURVE OR STRENGTH-DURATION CURVE
- **CONTRACTILITY**
  - TYPES OF CONTRACTION
  - SIMPLE MUSCLE CONTRACTION
  - CONTRACTION TIME: RED MUSCLE AND PALE MUSCLE
- FACTORS AFFECTING FORCE OF CONTRACTION
- REFRACTORY PERIOD
- **MUSCLE TONE**
  - DEFINITION
  - MAINTENANCE OF MUSCLE TONE
- **APPLIED PHYSIOLOGY: DISEASES INVOLVING MUSCLE TONE**
  - HYPERTONIA
  - HYPOTONIA
  - MYOTONIA

EXCITABILITY

DEFINITION

Excitability

Excitability is defined as the reaction or response of a tissue to irritation or stimulation. It is a **physicochemical** change.

Stimulus

Stimulus is the change in environment. It is defined as an agent or influence or act which causes the response in an excitable tissue.

TYPES OF STIMULUS

Stimuli, which can excite a living tissue are of four types:

1. Mechanical stimulus (pinching).
2. Electrical stimulus (electric shock).
3. Thermal stimulus (by applying heated glass rod or ice piece).
4. Chemical stimulus (by applying chemical substances like acids).

Electrical stimulus is commonly used for experimental purposes.

QUALITIES OF STIMULUS

To excite a tissue, the stimulus must possess two characters:

I. Intensity or strength
II. Duration.

Intensity of Stimulus

Intensity or strength of a stimulus is of five types:

1. Subminimal stimulus.
2. Minimal stimulus.
3. Submaximal stimulus.
4. Maximal stimulus.
5. Supramaximal stimulus.

The stimulus whose strength (or voltage) is sufficient to excite the tissue is called **threshold** or liminal or minimal stimulus.

Duration of Stimulus

Whatever may be the strength, the stimulus, must be applied for a minimum duration to excite the tissue. However, the duration of a stimulus depends upon the strength of the stimulus. For a weak stimulus, duration is longer and for a stronger stimulus, the duration is shorter.

The relationship between the strength and duration of stimulus is demonstrated by means of excitability curve.

EXCITABILITY CURVE OR STRENGTH-DURATION CURVE

Excitability curve or strength-duration curve is the graph that demonstrates the relationship between strength and duration of a stimulus **(Fig. 21.1)**. In this curve, the strength of the stimulus is plotted (in volts) vertically in Y axis and the duration (in milliseconds) is plotted horizontally in X axis.

Three important features are to be observed in excitability curve.

1. Rheobase

Rheobase is the **minimum strength** (voltage) of stimulus which can excite the tissue. Voltage below this cannot excite the tissue, whatever may be the duration of stimulus. Rheobasic strength is also called **threshold strength.**

2. Utilization Time

Utilization time is the **minimum time** required for rheobasic strength of stimulus (threshold strength) to excite the tissue.

3. Chronaxie

Chronaxie is the **minimum time** required for a stimulus with double the rheobasic strength (voltage) to excite the tissue.

Importance of chronaxie

Measurement of chronaxie determines the **excitability** of the tissues. It is used to compare the excitability in different tissues. Longer the chronaxie, lesser is the excitability.

CONTRACTILITY

Contractility is the response of the skeletal muscle to a stimulus by change in either length or tension of muscle fibers.

TYPES OF CONTRACTION

Muscular contraction is classified into two types based on change in length of muscle fibers or tension of muscle, namely isotonic contraction and isometric contraction.

1. Isotonic Contraction

Isotonic contraction is the type of muscular contraction in which tension remains the same and length of the muscle fiber is altered (Iso = same, Tonic = tension). For example, during simple flexion of arm, there is shortening of muscle fibers occurs but the tension does not change.

2. Isometric Contraction

Isometric contraction is the type of muscular contraction in which length of muscle fibers remains the same and tension is increased. Example is pulling any heavy object when muscles become stiff and strained with increased tension but the length does not change.

SIMPLE MUSCLE CONTRACTION

Contractile property of the muscle is studied by using **gastrocnemius-sciatic preparation** from frog. It is also called muscle-nerve preparation. When a **threshold stimulus** is applied, the muscle contracts and then relaxes. These activities are recorded graphically by using suitable instruments. Contraction is recorded as upward deflection from the base line. And, relaxation is recorded as downward deflection back to the baseline **(Fig. 21.2)**.

Simple contraction of the muscle is called **simple muscle twitch** and the graphical recording of this is called **simple muscle curve**.

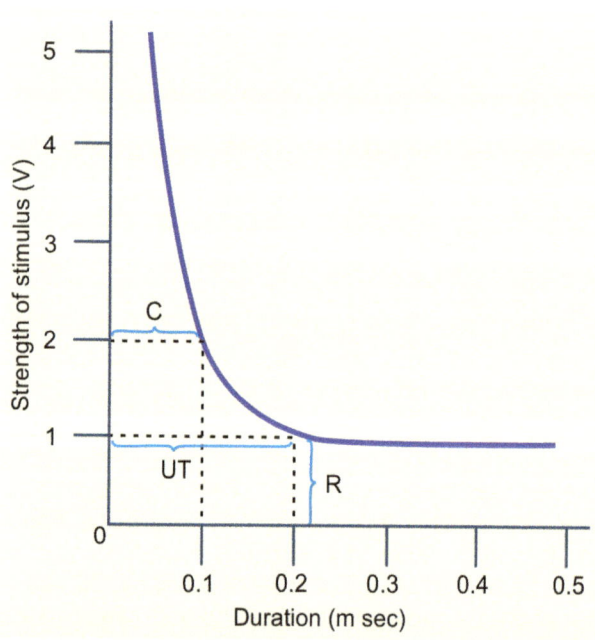

FIGURE 21.1: Strength-duration curve. R = Rheobase. UT = Utilization time. C = Chronaxie.

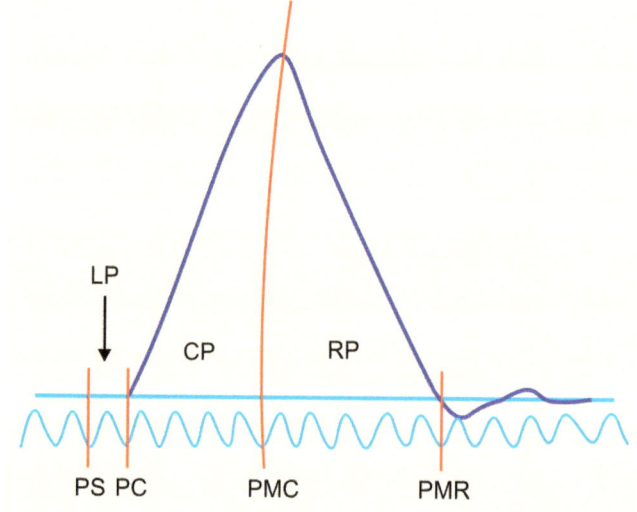

FIGURE 21.2: Isotonic simple muscle curve. PS = Point of stimulus. PC = Point of contraction. PMC = Point of maximum contraction. PMR = Point of maximum relaxation. LP = Latent period (0.01 sec). CP = Contraction period (0.04 sec). RP = Relaxation period (0.05 sec).

Important Points in Simple Muscle Curve

Four points are to be observed in simple muscle curve:

1. *Point of stimulus (PS):* Time when the stimulus is applied.
2. *Point of contraction (PC):* Time when the muscle begins to contract.
3. *Point of maximum contraction (PMC):* Point up to which the muscle contracts. It also indicates the beginning of relaxation of the muscle.
4. *Point of maximum relaxation (PMR):* Point when muscle relaxes completely.

Periods of Simple Muscle Curve

All the four points mentioned above divide the entire simple muscle curve into three periods:

1. Latent period

Latent period (LP) is the time interval between the point of stimulus and point of contraction. Muscle does not show any mechanical activity during this period.

2. Contraction period

Contraction period (CP) is the interval between point of contraction and point of maximum contraction. Muscle contracts during this period.

3. Relaxation period

Relaxation period (RP) is the interval between point of maximum contraction and point of maximum relaxation. Muscle relaxes during this period.

Duration of different periods in a typical simple muscle curve:

Latent period	: 0.01 sec
Contraction period	: 0.04 sec
Relaxation period	: 0.05 sec
Total twitch period	**: 0.10 sec**

Contraction period is always shorter than relaxation period. It is because the contraction is an active process and relaxation is a passive process.

Causes of Latent Period

1. Latent period is the time taken by the impulse to travel along the nerve from place of stimulation to muscle.
2. It is the time taken for the onset of initial chemical changes in the muscle.
3. It is due to the delay in the conduction of impulse at the neuromuscular junction.
4. It is due to the resistance offered by viscosity of the muscle.
5. It is also due to the inertia of the recording instrument.

■ CONTRACTION TIME: RED MUSCLE AND PALE MUSCLE

Based on contraction time, the **skeletal muscles** are classified into two types, red muscles and pale muscles.

1. Red Muscles

Red muscles are the muscles which contain large quantity of myoglobin. These muscles have large number of **type I fibers.** Red muscles are also called **slow muscles** or slow twitch muscles. Contraction time is longer in this type of muscles. Examples are back muscles and gastrocnemius muscles.

2. Pale Muscles

Pale or **white muscles** are the muscles which contain less quantity of myoglobin. Pale muscles have large number of **type II fibers**. These muscles are also called **fast muscles** or fast twitch muscles. Contraction time is shorter in this type of muscles. Examples are hand muscles and ocular muscles.

■ FACTORS AFFECTING FORCE OF CONTRACTION

Force of contraction of the skeletal muscle is affected by the following factors:

A. Strength of stimulus.
B. Number of stimulus.
C. Temperature.
D. Load.

A. Effect of Strength of Stimulus

Force of contraction is directly proportional to strength of stimulus.

B. Effect of Number of Stimulus

Contractility of the muscle varies, depending upon the number of stimuli. If a single stimulus is applied, muscle contracts once (simple muscle twitch). Two or more than two (multiple) stimuli produce two different effects.

When a muscle is stimulated by multiple stimuli, two types of effects are obtained depending upon the frequency of stimuli viz. fatigue and tetanus.

1. Fatigue

Fatigue is defined as the decrease in muscular activity due to repeated stimuli. When the stimuli are applied continuously, after some time, the muscle does not show any response to the stimulus. This condition is called fatigue.

Causes for fatigue

i. Exhaustion of acetylcholine in motor endplate.
ii. Accumulation of metabolites like lactic acid and phosphoric acid.
iii. Lack of nutrients like glycogen.
iv. Lack of oxygen.

Site (seat) of Fatigue

In intact body, sites of fatigue are in the following order:

i. **Betz cells** (pyramidal cells) in cerebral cortex.
ii. Anterior gray horn cells (motor neurons) of spinal cord.
iii. Neuromuscular junction.
iv. Muscle.

2. Tetanus

Tetanus is defined as the **sustained contraction** of muscle due to repeated stimuli with high frequency. When the multiple stimuli are applied at a higher frequency in such a way that the successive stimuli fall during contraction period of previous twitch, the muscle remains in state of tetanus, i.e. all the contractions are fused. Muscle relaxes only after stoppage of stimulus or when the muscle is fatigued.

If the frequency of stimuli is less, partial fusion of contractions takes place leading to **incomplete tetanus** or **clonus**.

Frequency of stimuli necessary to cause tetanus and clonus

In gastrocnemius muscle of human being, the frequency required to cause tetanus is 60/second. And for clonus, the frequency of stimuli necessary is 55/second.

C. Effect of Variations in Temperature

If the temperature of muscle is altered, the force of contraction is also affected.

Warm temperature

At warm temperature of about 40°C, force of contraction increases because of the following reasons:

1. Excitability of muscle increases.
2. Chemical processes involved in muscular contraction are accelerated.
3. Viscosity of muscle decreases.

Cold temperature

At cold temperature of about 10°C, force of contraction decreases because of the following reasons:

1. Excitability of muscle decreases.
2. Chemical processes are slowed or delayed.
3. Viscosity of the muscle increases.

High or hot temperature: Heat rigor

At high temperatures, heat rigor occurs in the muscle. **Rigor** refers to shortening and stiffening of muscle fibers. Heat rigor is the rigor that occurs due to increased temperature above 60°C. Cause of heat rigor is the coagulation of muscle proteins actin and myosin. It is an irreversible phenomenon.

Other types of rigors are:

1. **Cold rigor** that occurs due to the exposure to severe cold. It is a reversible phenomenon.
2. **Calcium rigor** which is due to increased calcium content. It is also reversible.
3. Rigor mortis which develops after death.

Rigor mortis

Rigor mortis is the after-death condition of body which is characterized by stiffness of muscles and joints. Rigor (Latin) means stiff. It occurs due to stoppage of aerobic respiration, which causes changes in the muscles.

Soon after death, the cell membrane becomes highly permeable to calcium. So, a large number of calcium ions enters the muscle fibers and promotes formation of actomyosin complex resulting in contraction of the muscles. Few hours after death, all the muscles of body undergo severe contraction and become rigid. Joints also become stiff and locked. Muscles remain in contracted state until the onset of decomposition.

Rigor mortis has **medicolegal importance.** It is useful in determining the time of death.

D. Effect of Load

Load acting on muscle is of two types called after load and free load.

After load

After load is the load, that acts on the muscle after the beginning of muscular contraction. Example of after load is lifting any object from the ground. Load acts on muscles of arm only after lifting the object off the ground, i.e. only after beginning of the muscular contraction.

Free load

Free load is the load, which acts on muscle freely, even before onset of contraction of the muscle. It is otherwise called **fore load**. Example of free load is filling water from a tap by holding the bucket in hand.

Muscle in free loaded condition works better than the muscle in after loaded condition. It is because, in free loaded condition, the muscle fibers are stretched and initial length of muscle fibers is increased. So, force of contraction and work done by the muscles are increased. It is in accordance with Frank-Starling law.

Frank-Starling law

Frank-Starling law states that the force of contraction is directly proportional to initial length of muscle fibers within physiological limits.

■ REFRACTORY PERIOD

Refractory period is the period at which the muscle does not show any response to a stimulus. It is because already one action potential is in progress and the muscle is in depolarized state during this period. Muscle is unexcitable to further stimulation until it is repolarized. Refractory period is of two types.

1. Absolute Refractory Period

Absolute refractory period is the period during which the muscle does not show any response at all, whatever may be the strength of stimulus.

2. Relative Refractory Period

Relative refractory period is the period, during which the muscle shows some response if the strength of stimulus is increased to maximum.

MUSCLE TONE

DEFINITION

Muscle tone is defined as continuous and partial contraction of the muscles with certain degree of vigor and tension. More details on muscle tone are given in Chapter 88.

MAINTENANCE OF MUSCLE TONE

In Skeletal Muscle

Maintenance of tone in skeletal muscle is neurogenic. It is due to continuous discharge of impulses from **gamma motor neurons** in anterior gray horn of spinal cord. Gamma motor neurons in spinal cord are controlled by higher centers in brain.

In Cardiac Muscle

In cardiac muscle, maintenance of tone is purely myogenic, i.e. the muscles themselves control the tone. The tone is not under nervous control in cardiac muscle.

In Smooth Muscle

In smooth muscle, tone is myogenic. It depends upon calcium level and number of cross bridges.

APPLIED PHYSIOLOGY: DISEASES INVOLVING MUSCLE TONE

1. HYPERTONIA

Hypertonia or hypertonicity is a muscular disease characterized by increased muscle tone and inability of the muscle to stretch. Hypertonia occurs in upper motor neuron lesion (Chapter 82). During upper motor neuron lesion, inhibition of lower motor neurons (gamma motor neurons) is lost. It causes exaggeration of lower motor neuron activity, resulting in hypertonia.

Hypertonia and Spasticity

Hypertonia may be related to spasticity, but it is present with or without spasticity. **Spasticity** is a motor disorder characterized by stiffness of certain muscles due to continuous contraction. Hypertonicity is one of the major symptoms of spasticity. **Paralysis** (complete loss of function) of the muscle with hypertonicity is called **spastic paralysis**.

2. HYPOTONIA

Hypotonia is the muscular disease characterized by decreased muscle tone. Tone of the muscle is decreased or lost. Muscle offers very little resistance to stretch. Muscle becomes flaccid (lack of firmness) and the condition is called **flaccidity**.

Major cause for hypotonia is lower motor neuron lesion (Chapter 82). Paralysis of muscle with hypotonicity is called **flaccid paralysis** and it results in **muscle wastage**.

3. MYOTONIA

Myotonia is a congenital disease characterized by continuous contraction of muscle and slow relaxation even after the cessation of voluntary act. Main feature of this disease is the muscle stiffness, which is sometimes referred as **cramps**. Muscle relaxation is delayed. Muscular stiffness with delayed relaxation causes discomfort during simple actions like walking, grasping and chewing. Muscles are enlarged (hypertrophy) because of continuous contraction.

Myotonia is caused by mutation in the genes of channel proteins in sarcolemma. Such disorders are called **channelopathies**.

Chapter 22: Changes During Muscular Contraction

CHAPTER OUTLINE

- **CHANGES TAKING PLACE DURING MUSCULAR CONTRACTION**
- **ELECTRICAL CHANGES**
  - RESTING MEMBRANE POTENTIAL
  - IONIC BASIS OF RESTING MEMBRANE POTENTIAL
  - ACTION POTENTIAL
  - ACTION POTENTIAL CURVE
  - IONIC BASIS OF ACTION POTENTIAL
- TYPES OF ACTION POTENTIAL
- GRADED POTENTIAL
- **PHYSICAL CHANGES**
- **HISTOLOGICAL OR MOLECULAR CHANGES**
  - ACTOMYOSIN COMPLEX
  - MOLECULAR BASIS OF MUSCULAR CONTRACTION
- **CHEMICAL CHANGES**
- **THERMAL CHANGES**

CHANGES TAKING PLACE DURING MUSCULAR CONTRACTION

Muscle contracts when it is stimulated. Contraction of the muscle is a **physical or mechanical** event. In addition, several other changes occur in the muscle when it is stimulated.

Changes taking place during muscular contraction are:

1. Electrical changes.
2. Physical changes.
3. Histological or molecular changes.
4. Chemical changes.
5. Thermal changes.

ELECTRICAL CHANGES DURING MUSCULAR CONTRACTION

When the muscle is in resting condition, the electrical potential is called resting membrane potential (RMP). When the muscle is stimulated, action potential develops.

RESTING MEMBRANE POTENTIAL

Resting membrane potential or **transmembrane potential** is the electrical **potential difference** (voltage) across the cell membrane (between inside and outside of the cell) under **resting condition**.

Resting muscle shows negativity inside and positivity outside. This condition of the muscle during resting membrane potential is called **polarized state**. In human skeletal muscle, the resting membrane potential is – 90 mV.

IONIC BASIS OF RESTING MEMBRANE POTENTIAL

In a muscle fiber or a neuron, resting membrane potential is developed and maintained by movement of ions, which produce ionic imbalance across the cell membrane. This results in the development of positivity outside and negativity inside the cell.

Ionic imbalance is produced by two factors:

1. Sodium-Potassium Pump

Sodium and potassium ions are actively transported in opposite directions across the cell membrane by the electrogenic pump called sodium-potassium pump. It moves three sodium ions out of the cell and two potassium ions inside the cell by using energy from ATP. Since more positive ions (cations) are pumped outside, a net deficit of positive ions occurs inside the cell. It leads to negativity inside and positivity outside the cell. More details of this pump are given in Chapter 3.

2. Selective Permeability of Cell Membrane

Permeability of cell membrane depends largely on the transport channels. Transport channels are selective for movement of some specific ions. Most of the channels are gated channels and the specific ions can move across the membrane only when these gated channels are opened.

Channels for major anions (negatively charged substances)

Channels for some of the negatively charged large substances such as proteins, organic phosphate and sulfate compounds are absent or closed. So, such substances remain inside the cell and cause development and maintenance of negativity inside the cell (resting membrane potential).

■ ACTION POTENTIAL

Action potential is defined as a series of electrical changes that occur in the membrane potential when the muscle or nerve is stimulated.

Action potential occurs in two phases:

1. Depolarization.
2. Repolarization.

Depolarization

Depolarization is the initial phase of action potential in which inside of the muscle becomes positive and outside becomes negative. That is, the polarized state (resting membrane potential) is abolished resulting in depolarization.

Repolarization

Repolarization is the phase of action potential in which the muscle reverses back to the resting membrane potential. That is, within a short time after depolarization, the inside of muscle becomes negative and outside becomes positive. So, the polarized state of the muscle is re-established.

Properties of Action Potential

Properties of action potential are listed in **Table 22.1**.

■ ACTION POTENTIAL CURVE

Action potential curve is the graphical registration of electrical activity that occurs in an excitable tissue after stimulation.

Action potential curve has three major segments:

1. Latent period.
2. Depolarization.
3. Repolarization.

TABLE 22.1: Properties of action potential and graded potential.

Action potential	Graded potential
Propagative	Non-propagative
Long-distance signal	Short-distance signal
Consists of both depolarization and repolarization	Consists of either depolarization or hyperpolarization
Obeys all-or-none law	Does not obey all-or-none law
Summation is not possible	Summation is possible
Has refractory period	Has no refractory period

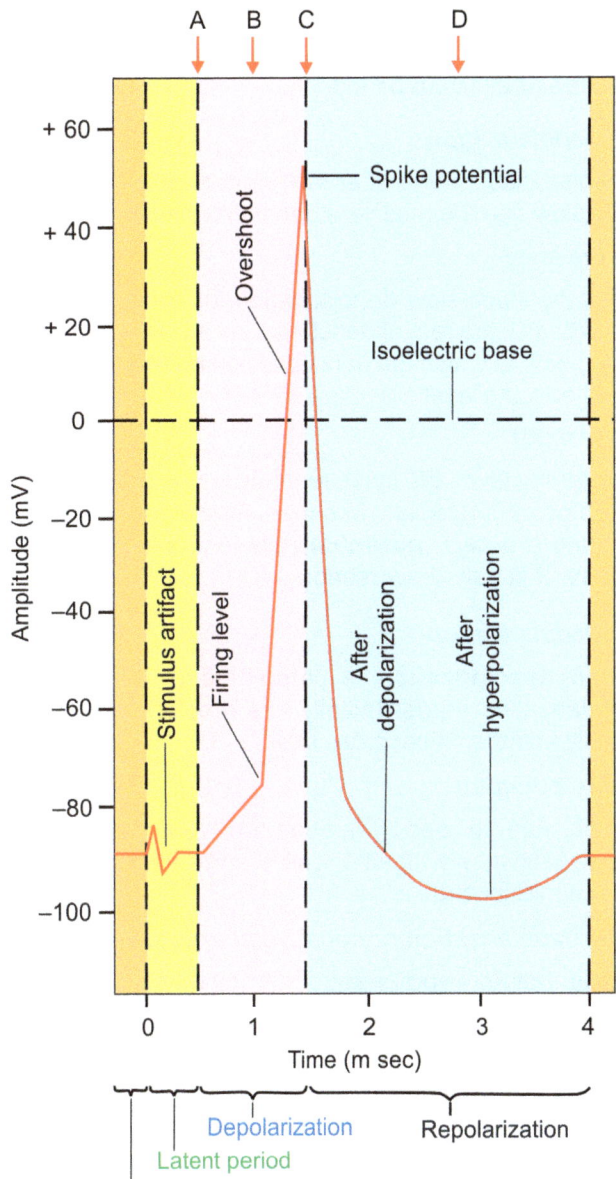

FIGURE 22.1: Action potential in a skeletal muscle.
A = Opening of few Na^+ channels.
B = Opening of many Na^+ channels.
C = Closure of Na^+ channels and opening of K^+ channels.
D = Closure of K^+ channels.

Resting membrane potential in skeletal muscle is – 90 mV and it is recorded as a straight baseline **(Fig. 22.1)**.

1. Latent Period

Latent period is the period during which no change occurs in the electrical potential immediately after applying the stimulus. It is a very short period with duration of 0.5 to 1 millisecond.

Stimulus artifact

Resting membrane potential is recorded as a straight baseline at – 90 mV **(Fig. 22.1)**. When a stimulus is applied, there is a slight irregular deflection of baseline for a very short period. This is called stimulus artifact.

This artifact is due to leakage of current from stimulating electrode to the recording electrode. The stimulus artifact is followed by latent period.

2. Depolarization

Depolarization starts after the latent period. Initially, it is very slow and the muscle is depolarized for about 15 mV.

Firing level

After the initial slow depolarization for about 15 mV (up to – 75 mV), the rate of depolarization increases suddenly. This point, at which the depolarization increases suddenly is called firing level.

Overshoot

From firing level, the curve reaches **isoelectric potential** (zero potential) rapidly and then shoots up (overshoots) beyond the **zero potential** (isoelectric base) up to + 55 mV. It is called overshoot.

3. Repolarization

When depolarization is completed (+ 55 mV), the repolarization starts. Initially, the repolarization occurs rapidly and then it becomes slow.

Spike potential

Rapid rise in depolarization and the rapid fall in repolarization are together called spike potential. It lasts for 0.4 millisecond.

Afterdepolarization or negative afterpotential

Rapid fall in repolarization is followed by a **slow repolarization**. It is called negative afterpotential. Its duration is 2 to 4 milliseconds.

Afterhyperpolarization or positive afterpotential

After reaching the resting level (– 90 mV), it becomes more negative beyond resting level leading to hyperpolarization. It is followed by slow rise in the curve towards resting level. This is called afterhyperpolarization or positive after potential. This lasts for more than 50 milliseconds. After this, the normal RMP is restored slowly.

IONIC BASIS OF ACTION POTENTIAL

Voltage-gated Na^+ channels and voltage-gated K^+ channels play important role in the development of action potential.

Depolarization

During the onset of depolarization, voltage-gated Na^+ channels open and there is slow influx of Na^+. When depolarization reaches 7 to 10 mV, the voltage-gated Na^+ channels start opening at a faster rate. It is called **Na^+ channel activation**. When the firing level is reached, the influx of Na^+ is very great and it leads to overshoot.

Repolarization

The Na^+ transport is short lived. It is because of rapid inactivation of Na^+ channels. Thus, the Na^+ channels open and close quickly. At the same time, K^+ channels start opening. This leads to efflux of K^+ out of the cell, causing repolarization.

Unlike Na^+ channels, K^+ channels remain open for longer duration. These channels remain opened for longer duration after completion of repolarization. It causes efflux of greater number of K^+ producing more negativity inside. It is the cause for hyperpolarization.

TYPES OF ACTION POTENTIAL

Action potential is of three types.

1. Monophasic Action Potential

Monophasic action potential is the series of electrical changes occurring in a single phase when a muscle or a nerve is stimulated. It is characterized by either positive deflection or negative deflection.

2. Biphasic Action Potential

Biphasic or diphasic action potential is the series of electrical changes occurring in two phases when a muscle or a nerve is stimulated. It is characterized by both positive and negative deflections.

3. Compound Action Potential

Compound action potential is the algebraic summation of all action potentials produced by all nerve fibers. Each nerve is made up of thousands of nerve fibers (axons). While stimulating the whole nerve, all nerve fibers are activated and produce action potential.

GRADED POTENTIAL

Graded potential is a mild local change in the membrane potential that develops in receptors, synapse or neuromuscular junction when stimulated. Graded potential is different from action potential and the properties of these two potentials are given in **Table 22.1**.

Examples of graded potentials are:

1. Endplate potential in neuromuscular junction (Chapter 23).
2. Receptor potential (Chapter 79).
3. Excitatory postsynaptic potential (Chapter 79).
4. Inhibitory postsynaptic potential (Chapter 79).

PHYSICAL CHANGES DURING MUSCULAR CONTRACTION

Physical change, which takes place during muscular contraction, is the change in length of muscle fibers or change in tension developed in the muscle. Depending upon this, the muscular contraction is classified into two types, namely **isotonic contraction** and **isometric contraction**. Refer Chapter 21 for details.

HISTOLOGICAL OR MOLECULAR CHANGES DURING MUSCULAR CONTRACTION

ACTOMYOSIN COMPLEX

Actomyosin complex is a complex protein in skeletal muscle formed by actin and myosin. During relaxed state of the muscle, thin actin filaments from opposite ends of the sarcomere are away from each other leaving a broad 'H' zone.

During contraction of the muscle, actin (thin) filaments glide over the myosin (thick) filaments and form actomyosin complex.

■ MOLECULAR BASIS OF MUSCULAR CONTRACTION

Molecular mechanism is responsible for formation of actomyosin complex that results in muscular contraction. It includes three stages:

1. Excitation-contraction coupling.
2. Role of troponin and tropomyosin.
3. Sliding mechanism.

1. Excitation-Contraction Coupling

Excitation-contraction coupling is the process that occurs in between the excitation and contraction of the muscle. This process involves series of activities which are responsible for the contraction of the excited muscle.

When the impulse passes through a motor neuron and reaches the neuromuscular junction, **acetylcholine** is released from motor endplate of neuromuscular junction. Acetylcholine causes opening of ligand-gated sodium channels. So, sodium ions enter the neuromuscular junction. It leads to the development of **endplate potential**. Endplate potential causes generation of action potential in the muscle fiber.

Action potential spreads over sarcolemma and also into the muscle fiber through T-tubules. T-tubules are responsible for rapid spread of action potential into the muscle fiber. When action potential reaches the cisternae of L-tubules, these cisternae are excited. Now, calcium ions stored in cisternae are released into the sarcoplasm. Calcium ions from the sarcoplasm move towards actin filaments to produce the muscular contraction.

Role of calcium ion

Thus, calcium ion forms the link or coupling material between excitation and contraction of muscle. Hence, the calcium ions are said to form the basis of excitation contraction coupling.

2. Role of Troponin and Tropomyosin

Normally, head of myosin molecules has a strong tendency to get attached with active site of F-actin. However, in relaxed condition, the active site of F-actin is covered by the tropomyosin. Therefore, the myosin head cannot combine with actin molecule.

Large number of calcium ions, which are released from L-tubules during excitation of the muscle, bind with troponin 'C'. Loading of troponin 'C' with calcium

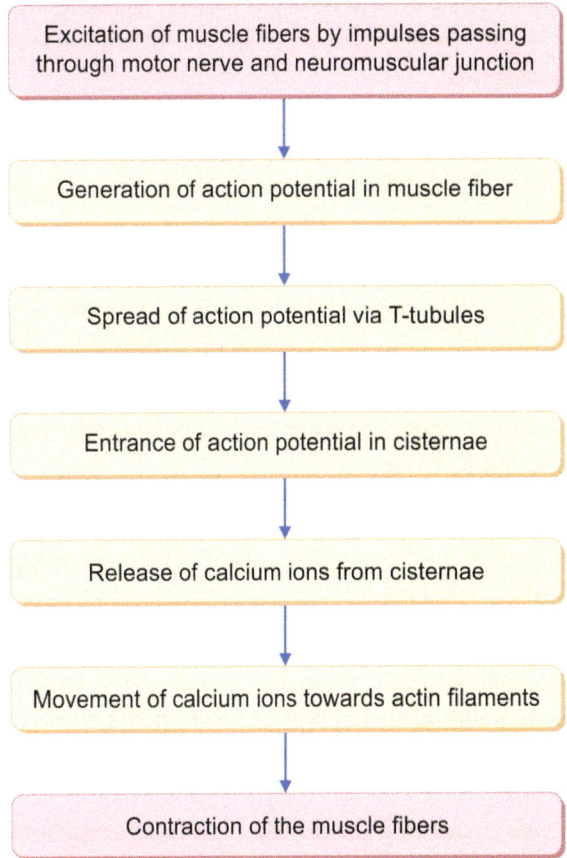

FIGURE 22.2: Excitation-contraction coupling.

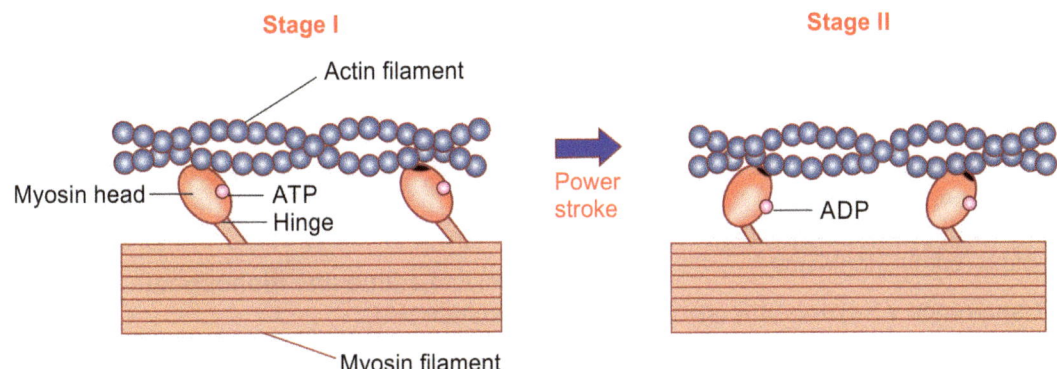

FIGURE 22.3: Diagram showing power stroke by myosin head. Stage I: Myosin head binds with actin. Stage II: Tilting of myosin head (power stroke) drags the actin filament.
ATP = Adenosine triphosphate. ADP = Adenosine diphosphate.

ions produces some change in the position of troponin molecule. It in turn, pulls tropomyosin molecule away from F-actin. Due to the movement of tropomyosin, active site of F-actin is uncovered and immediately the head of myosin gets attached to actin **(Fig. 22.2)**.

3. Sliding Mechanism and Formation of Actomyosin Complex: Sliding Theory

Sliding theory explains how actin filaments slide over myosin filaments and form the actomyosin complex during muscular contraction. It is also called **ratchet theory** or **walk along theory**.

Each **cross bridge** from the myosin filaments has got three components namely, a hinge, an arm and a head.

Power stroke

After binding with active site of F-actin, myosin head is tilted towards the arm, so that the actin filament is dragged along with it **(Fig. 22.3)**. This tilting of head is called power stroke.

Formation of actomyosin complex

After tilting, the head immediately breaks away from the active site and returns to the original position. Now, it combines with a new active site on the actin molecule. And tilting movement occurs again. Thus, the head of cross bridge bends back and forth, and pulls the actin filament towards center of sarcomere.

In this way, all the actin filaments of both ends of sarcomere are pulled. So, the actin filaments of opposite sides overlap and form actomyosin complex. Formation of actomyosin complex results in contraction of the muscle.

When the muscle shortens further, actin filaments from opposite ends of the sarcomere approach each other. So, the 'H' zone becomes narrow. And, the two 'Z' lines come closer with reduction in length of the sarcomere. However, the length of 'A' band is not altered. But, the length of 'I' band decreases.

Changes in sarcomere during muscular contraction

When the muscular contraction becomes severe, the actin filaments from opposite ends overlap and, the 'H' zone disappears.

Following changes occur in sarcomere during muscular contraction:

1. Length of all the sarcomeres decreases, as 'Z' lines come close to each other.
2. Length of 'I' band decreases, since the actin filaments from opposite side overlap.
3. 'H' zone either decreases or disappears.
4. Length of 'A' band remains the same.

Summary of sequence of events during muscular contraction by sliding mechanism is given in **Figure 22.4**.

Energy for Muscular Contraction

Energy for movement of myosin head (power stroke) is obtained by breakdown of **adenosine triphosphate** (ATP) into **adenosine diphosphate** (ADP) and inorganic phosphate (Pi).

Relaxation of the Muscle

Relaxation of the muscle occurs when calcium ions are pumped back into the L-tubules. When calcium ions enter the L-tubules, calcium content in sarcoplasm decreases

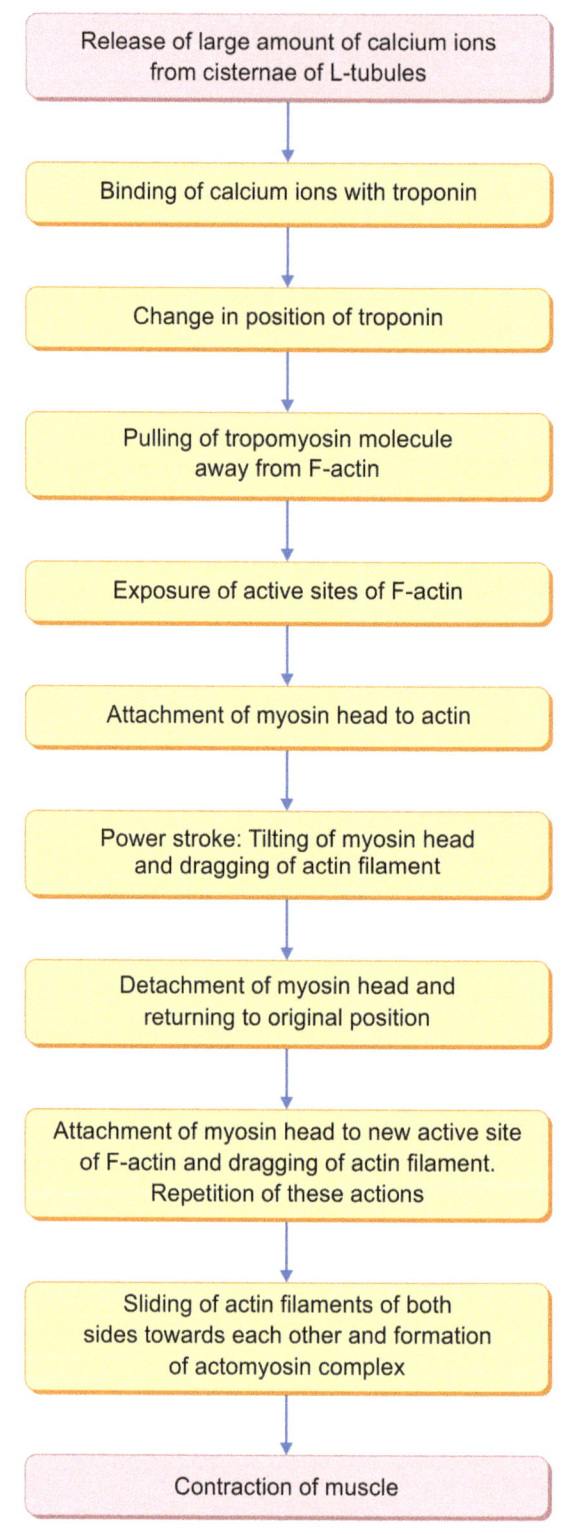

FIGURE 22.4: Muscle contraction by sliding mechanism.

leading to the release of calcium ions from the troponin. It causes detachment of myosin from actin followed by relaxation of the muscle. Detachment of myosin from actin obtains energy from breakdown of ATP.

CHEMICAL CHANGES DURING MUSCULAR CONTRACTION

LIBERATION OF ENERGY

Energy necessary for muscular contraction is liberated during process of breakdown and resynthesis of ATP.

Breakdown of ATP

During muscular contraction, the energy is supplied from breakdown of ATP. ATP is broken into ADP and Pi and energy is liberated:

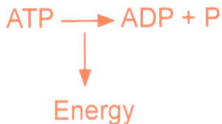

Energy liberated by breakdown of ATP is responsible for the following activities during muscular contraction:

1. Spread of action potential into the muscle.
2. Liberation of calcium ions from cisternae of L-tubules into the sarcoplasm.
3. Movements of myosin head.
4. Sliding mechanism.

Resynthesis of ATP

Adenosine diphosphate, which is formed during ATP breakdown, is immediately utilized for the resynthesis of ATP. But, for resynthesis of ATP, the ADP cannot combine with Pi. It should combine with a **high-energy phosphate** radical. There are two sources from which the high-energy phosphate is obtained namely, **creatine phosphate** and carbohydrate metabolism.

THERMAL CHANGES DURING MUSCULAR CONTRACTION

During muscular contraction, heat is produced. Not all the heat is liberated at a time.

Heat is released in three stages:

1. *Resting heat*: Heat produced in the muscle during resting condition. It is due to basal metabolic process in the muscle.
2. *Initial heat*: Heat produced during initiation of muscular contraction and during muscular contraction.
3. *Recovery heat*: Heat produced after muscular contraction.

Chapter 23

Neuromuscular Junction

CHAPTER OUTLINE

- **DEFINITION AND STRUCTURE**
  - DEFINITION
  - STRUCTURE
- **NEUROMUSCULAR TRANSMISSION**
  - RELEASE OF ACETYLCHOLINE
  - ACTION OF ACETYLCHOLINE
  - DEVELOPMENT OF ENDPLATE POTENTIAL
  - DEVELOPMENT OF MINIATURE ENDPLATE POTENTIAL
  - DESTRUCTION OF ACETYLCHOLINE
- **NEUROMUSCULAR BLOCKERS**
- **DRUGS STIMULATING NEUROMUSCULAR JUNCTION**
- **MOTOR UNIT**
  - DEFINITION
  - NUMBER OF MUSCLE FIBERS IN MOTOR UNIT
- **APPLIED PHYSIOLOGY: DISORDERS OF NEUROMUSCULAR JUNCTION**
  - MYASTHENIA GRAVIS
  - LAMBERT-EATON MYASTHENIC SYNDROME

DEFINITION AND STRUCTURE

DEFINITION

Neuromuscular junction is the junction between the terminal branch of nerve fiber and muscle fiber.

STRUCTURE

Skeletal muscle fibers are innervated by the motor nerve fibers. Each nerve fiber (axon) divides into many terminal branches. Each terminal branch innervates one muscle fiber through the neuromuscular junction **(Fig. 23.1)**.

Axon Terminal and Motor Endplate

Terminal branch of nerve fiber is called axon terminal. When the axon comes close to the muscle fiber, it loses the myelin sheath. So, the axis cylinder is exposed. This portion of the axis cylinder is expanded like a bulb which is called **motor endplate**.

Axon terminal contains **mitochondria** and **synaptic vesicles**. Synaptic vesicles contain the neurotransmitter substance, **acetylcholine**. Acetylcholine is synthesized by mitochondria present in the axon terminal and stored in the vesicles. Mitochondria contain ATP which is the source of energy for the synthesis of acetylcholine.

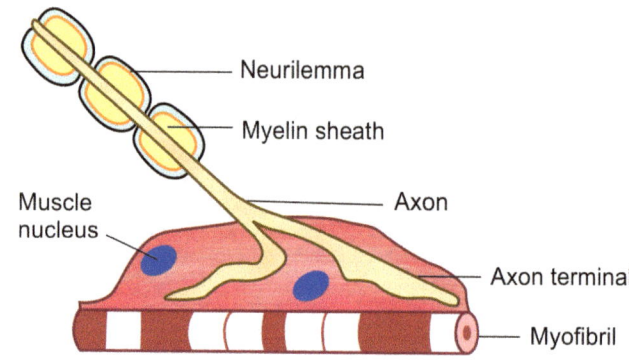

FIGURE 23.1: Longitudinal section of neuromuscular junction.

Synaptic Trough or Gutter

Motor endplate invaginates inside the muscle fiber and forms a depression which is known as synaptic trough or synaptic gutter. Membrane of the muscle fiber below the motor endplate is thickened.

Synaptic Cleft

Membrane of the nerve ending is called the **presynaptic membrane**. Membrane of the muscle fiber is called **postsynaptic membrane**. Space between these two is called synaptic cleft. Synaptic cleft contains **basal lamina**.

It is a thin layer of spongy reticular matrix through which, the extracellular fluid diffuses. Large quantity of an enzyme called **acetylcholinesterase** is attached to the matrix of basal lamina.

Subneural Clefts

Postsynaptic membrane is the membrane of the muscle fiber. It is thrown into numerous folds called subneural clefts. Postsynaptic membrane contains the receptors called nicotinic **acetylcholine receptors (Fig. 23.2)**.

■ NEUROMUSCULAR TRANSMISSION

Neuromuscular transmission is defined as the transfer of information from motor nerve ending to the muscle fiber through neuromuscular junction. It is the mechanism by which the motor nerve impulses initiate muscle contraction.

Series of **five events** take place in the neuromuscular junction during this process **(Fig. 23.3)**.

■ 1. RELEASE OF ACETYLCHOLINE

When action potential reaches axon terminal, it opens the **voltage-gated calcium channels** in membrane of the axon terminal. Calcium ions enter the axon terminal from extracellular fluid and cause bursting of synaptic vesicles. Now, acetylcholine is released from the vesicles and diffuses through presynaptic membrane and enters the synaptic cleft by **exocytosis**.

Each vesicle contains about 10,000 acetylcholine molecules. And, at a time, about 300 vesicles open and release acetylcholine.

■ 2. ACTION OF ACETYLCHOLINE

After entering synaptic cleft, the acetylcholine molecules bind with **nicotinic receptors** present in postsynaptic membrane and form **acetylcholine-receptor complex**. This complex opens the ligand-gated channels for sodium in the postsynaptic membrane. Now, sodium ions from extracellular fluid enter the neuromuscular junction through these channels. And there, the sodium ions produce an electrical potential called endplate potential.

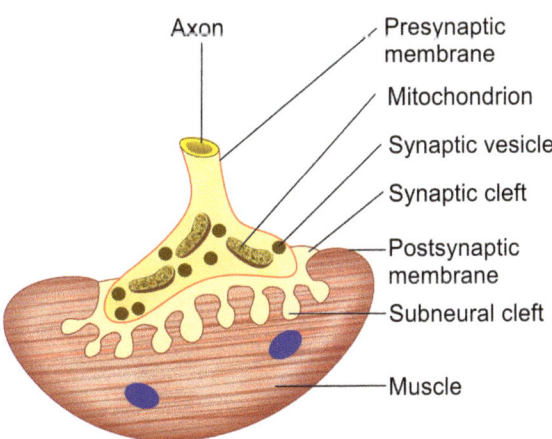

FIGURE 23.2: Structure of neuromuscular junction.

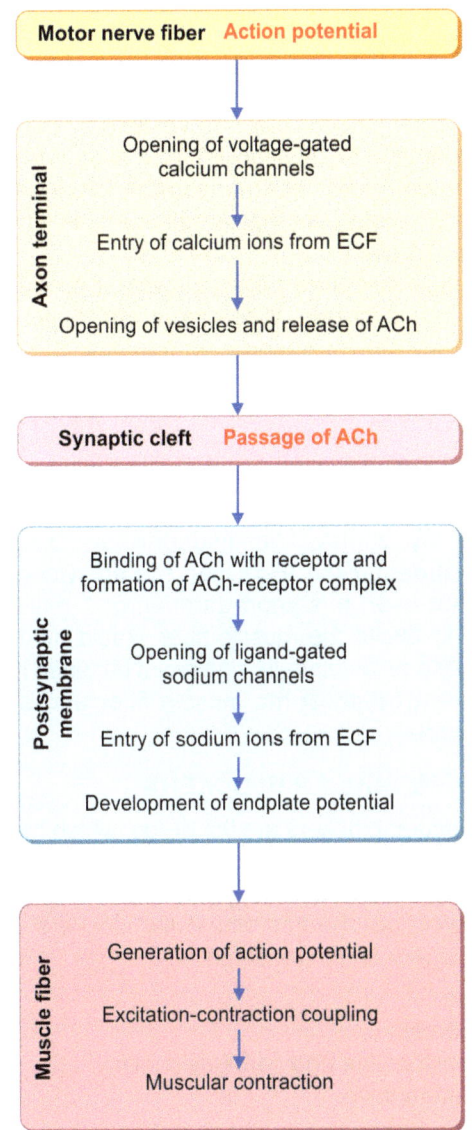

FIGURE 23.3: Sequence of events during neuromuscular transmission.
ACh = Acetylcholine, ECF = Extracellular fluid.

■ 3. DEVELOPMENT OF ENDPLATE POTENTIAL

Endplate potential is the change in the resting membrane potential when an impulse reaches the neuromuscular junction. Resting membrane potential at the neuromuscular junction is – 90 mV. When sodium ions enter inside, slight depolarization occurs up to – 60 mV which is called endplate potential.

Properties of Endplate Potential

Endplate potential is a **graded potential** and it is not action potential. Refer Table 22.1 for properties of graded potential.

Significance of Endplate Potential

Endplate potential is non-propagative. But it causes the development of action potential in the muscle fiber.

4. DEVELOPMENT OF MINIATURE ENDPLATE POTENTIAL

Miniature endplate potential is a weak endplate potential in neuromuscular junction that is developed by the release of a small quantity of acetylcholine from axon terminal. And, each quantum of this neurotransmitter produces a weak miniature endplate potential. Amplitude of this potential is only up to 0.5 mV.

Miniature endplate potential cannot produce action potential in the muscle. When more and more quanta of acetylcholine are released continuously, the miniature endplate potentials are added together and finally produce endplate potential resulting in action potential in the muscle.

5. DESTRUCTION OF ACETYLCHOLINE

Acetylcholine released into the synaptic cleft is destroyed very quickly within 1 millisecond by the enzyme, **acetylcholinesterase**. However, the acetylcholine is so potent, that even this short duration of 1 millisecond is sufficient to excite the muscle fiber. Rapid destruction of acetylcholine is functionally significant because it prevents repeated excitation of the muscle fiber and allows the muscle to relax.

NEUROMUSCULAR BLOCKERS

Neuromuscular blockers are the drugs, which can prevent the transmission of impulses from nerve fiber to muscle fiber through neuromuscular junctions.

Following are the neuromuscular blockers commonly used in surgery and in research.

1. Curare.
2. Bungarotoxin.
3. Succinylcholine and carbamylcholine
4. Botulinum toxin.

DRUGS STIMULATING NEUROMUSCULAR JUNCTION

Neuromuscular junction can be stimulated by some drugs like **neostigmine**, **physostigmine** and diisopropyl fluorophosphate. These drugs inactivate the enzyme, acetylcholinesterase. So, acetylcholine is not hydrolyzed. It leads to repeated stimulation and continuous contraction of the muscle. These drugs are also called **cholinesterase inhibitors**.

MOTOR UNIT
DEFINITION

One single motor neuron, its axon terminals and the muscle fibers innervated by it are together called motor unit. Each motor neuron activates a group of muscle fibers through the axon terminals. Stimulation of a motor neuron causes contraction of all the muscle fibers innervated by that neuron.

NUMBER OF MUSCLE FIBERS IN MOTOR UNIT

Number of muscle fibers is small in the motor units of muscles concerned with fine, graded and precise movements. For examples, ocular muscles have 3 to 6 muscle fibers per motor unit.

Muscles concerned with crude or coarse movements have motor units with large number of muscle fibers. For example, leg muscles have more than 120 muscle fibers per motor unit.

APPLIED PHYSIOLOGY: DISORDERS OF NEUROMUSCULAR JUNCTION
1. MYASTHENIA GRAVIS

Myasthenia gravis is an autoimmune disorder of neuromuscular junction caused by antibodies to cholinergic receptors. It is characterized by grave weakness of the muscle due to the inability of neuromuscular junction to transmit impulses from nerve to the muscle.

2. LAMBERT-EATON MYASTHENIC SYNDROME

Lambert-Eaton myasthenic syndrome is also an autoimmune disorder of neuromuscular junction. It is caused by antibodies to calcium channels in axon terminal. This disease is characterized by features of myasthenia gravis. In addition, the patients have blurred vision and dry mouth.

Chapter 24: Smooth Muscle

CHAPTER OUTLINE

- DISTRIBUTION
- FUNCTIONS
- STRUCTURE
- TYPES
- ELECTRICAL ACTIVITY IN SINGLE-UNIT SMOOTH MUSCLE
- ELECTRICAL ACTIVITY IN MULTI-UNIT SMOOTH MUSCLE
- CONTRACTILE PROCESS
- NEUROMUSCULAR JUNCTION
- CONTROL OF SMOOTH MUSCLE ACTIVITIES

DISTRIBUTION SMOOTH MUSCLE

Smooth muscles are **nonstriated** (plain) and **involuntary** muscles present in almost all the organs in the form of sheets, bundles or sheaths around other tissues. These muscles form major contractile tissues of various organs.

STRUCTURES HAVING SMOOTH MUSCLE FIBERS

1. Wall of organs such as esophagus, stomach and intestine in gastrointestinal tract.
2. Ducts of digestive glands.
3. Trachea, bronchial tube and alveolar ducts of respiratory tract.
4. Ureter, urinary bladder and urethra in excretory system.
5. Wall of the blood vessels in circulatory system.
6. Arrector pilorum of skin.
7. Mammary glands, uterus, genital ducts, prostate gland and scrotum in reproductive system.
8. Iris and ciliary body of the eye.

FUNCTIONS OF SMOOTH MUSCLE

Smooth muscles are concerned with very important functions in different parts of the body such as:

IN CARDIOVASCULAR SYSTEM

Smooth muscle fibers around the blood vessels regulate blood pressure and blood flow through different organs and regions of the body.

IN RESPIRATORY SYSTEM

Contraction and relaxation of smooth muscle fibers of the air passage alter the diameter of air passage and regulate the inflow and outflow of air.

IN DIGESTIVE SYSTEM

Smooth muscle fibers in digestive tract help in:

i. Movement of food substances.
ii. Mixing of food substance with digestive juices.
iii. Absorption of digested material.
iv. Elimination of unwanted substances.

Sphincters along the digestive tract regulate the flow of materials.

IN RENAL SYSTEM

Smooth muscle fibers in renal blood vessels regulate renal blood flow and glomerular filtration. Smooth muscles in the ureters propel urine from kidneys to urinary bladder through ureters. Smooth muscles present in urinary bladder help in voiding urine to the exterior.

IN REPRODUCTIVE SYSTEM

In males, smooth muscle fibers facilitate the movement of sperms and secretions from accessory glands along the reproductive tract. In females, these muscles accelerate the movement of sperms through genital tract after sexual act, movement of ovum into uterus through fallopian tube, expulsion of menstrual fluid and delivery of the baby.

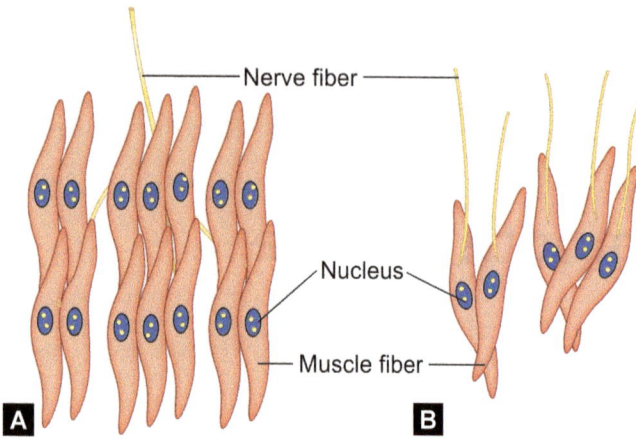

FIGURE 24.1: Smooth muscle fibers. **A.** Single-unit smooth muscle fibers. **B.** Multi-unit smooth muscle fibers.

■ STRUCTURE OF SMOOTH MUSCLE

Smooth muscle fibers are fusiform or elongated cells. Nucleus is single and elongated and it is centrally placed. Nucleus has two or more nucleoli **(Fig. 24.1)**. Smooth muscle fibers are small, with a diameter of 2 to 5 microns and a length of 50 to 200 microns. Tendon is absent in smooth muscle.

Myofibrils and Sarcomere

Well-defined myofibrils and sarcomere are absent in smooth muscles. So, the alternate dark and light bands are absent. Absence of dark and light bands gives the non-striated appearance to the smooth muscle.

Myofilaments and Contractile Proteins

Contractile proteins in smooth muscle fiber are actin, myosin and tropomyosin. But troponin or troponin-like substance is absent. Thick and thin filaments are present in smooth muscle. However, these filaments are not arranged in orderly fashion as in skeletal muscle. Thick filaments are formed by myosin molecules and have many numbers of cross bridges than in skeletal muscle. Thin filaments are formed by actin and tropomyosin molecules.

Dense Bodies

Dense bodies are the special structures of smooth muscle fibers to which the actin and tropomyosin molecules of thin filaments are attached.

Sarcotubular System

Sarcotubular system in smooth muscle fibers is in the form of network. T-tubules are absent and L-tubules are poorly developed.

■ TYPES OF SMOOTH MUSCLE FIBERS

Smooth muscle fibers are of two types, namely single-unit or visceral smooth muscle fibers and multi-unit smooth muscle fibers.

■ SINGLE-UNIT OR VISCERAL SMOOTH MUSCLE FIBERS

Single-unit smooth muscle fibers or visceral smooth muscle fibers are the fibers with interconnecting **gap junctions**. Gap junctions allow rapid spread of action potential throughout the tissue so that all the muscle fibers show synchronous contraction as a single-unit.

Features of Single-unit Smooth Muscle Fibers

i. Muscle fibers are arranged in sheets or bundles.
ii. Cell membrane of adjacent fibers fuses at many points to form **gap junctions**. Through the gap junctions, ions move freely from one cell to the other. Thus, a functional **syncytium** is developed. Syncytium contracts as a single-unit. In this way, the visceral smooth muscle resembles cardiac muscle more than the skeletal muscle.

Single-unit smooth muscle fibers are present in the walls of the organs such as gastrointestinal organs, uterus, ureters, respiratory tract, etc.

■ MULTI-UNIT SMOOTH MUSCLE FIBERS

Multi-unit smooth muscle fibers are the muscle fibers without interconnecting gap junctions. These smooth muscle fibers resemble the skeletal muscle fibers in many ways.

Features of Multi-unit Smooth Muscle Fibers

i. Muscle fibers are individual fibers.
ii. Each muscle fiber is innervated by a single nerve ending.
iii. Each muscle fiber has got an outer membrane made up of glycoprotein, which helps to insulate and separate the muscle fibers from one another.
iv. Control of the muscle fibers is mainly by nerve signals.
v. Smooth muscle fibers do not exhibit spontaneous contractions.

Multi-unit muscle fibers are present in ciliary muscles of the eye, iris of the eye, arrector pili and smooth muscles of the blood vessels and urinary bladder.

■ ELECTRICAL ACTIVITY IN SINGLE-UNIT SMOOTH MUSCLE

Usually 30 to 40 smooth muscle fibers are simultaneously depolarized which leads to development of **selfpropagating** action potential. It is possible because of gap junctions and syncytial arrangements of single-unit smooth muscles.

■ RESTING MEMBRANE POTENTIAL

Resting membrane potential in single-unit smooth muscle fiber is very much unstable and ranges between – 50 and – 75 mV. Sometimes, it reaches low level of – 25 mV.

■ CAUSE FOR UNSTABLE RESTING MEMBRANE POTENTIAL: SLOW-WAVE RHYTHM

Unstable resting membrane potential in single-unit smooth muscle fiber is caused by appearance of some wave-like fluctuations called **slow waves**. These slow waves occur in a rhythmic fashion at a frequency of 4 to 10 per minute with the amplitude of 10 to 15 mV **(Fig. 24.2)**. **Slow-wave rhythm** may be due to the rhythmic modulations in the activities of sodium-potassium pump. Slow wave is not action potential and it cannot cause contraction of the muscle. But it initiates the action potential (see below).

■ ACTION POTENTIAL

Three types of action potential occur in single-unit smooth muscle fibers:

1. Spike potential.
2. Spike potential initiated by slow-wave rhythm.
3. Action potential with plateau.

1. Spike Potential

Spike potential in single-unit smooth muscle is different from that in skeletal muscles. In smooth muscle, the average duration of spike potential varies between 30 and 50 milliseconds. Its amplitude is very low and it does not reach the isoelectric base. It is due to nervous and other stimuli and it leads to contraction of the muscle.

2. Spike Potential Initiated by Slow-wave Rhythm

Sometimes the slowwave rhythm of resting membrane potential initiates the spike potentials, which lead to contraction of the muscle. Spike potentials appear rhythmically at a rate of about one or two spikes at the peak of each slow wave. These potentials initiated by the slowwave rhythm cause rhythmic contractions of smooth muscles. This type of potentials appears mostly in smooth muscles, which are selfexcitatory and contract themselves without any external stimuli. So, the spike potentials initiated by slowwave rhythm are otherwise called **pacemaker waves**. Smooth muscles showing rhythmic contractions are present in some of the visceral organs such as intestine.

3. Action Potential with Plateau

This type of action potential starts with rapid depolarization as in the case of skeletal muscle. But repolarization does not occur immediately. Muscle remains depolarized for a long period. This forms the plateau (stable period) in action potential and it lasts for about 100 to 1,000 milliseconds. This type of action potential is responsible

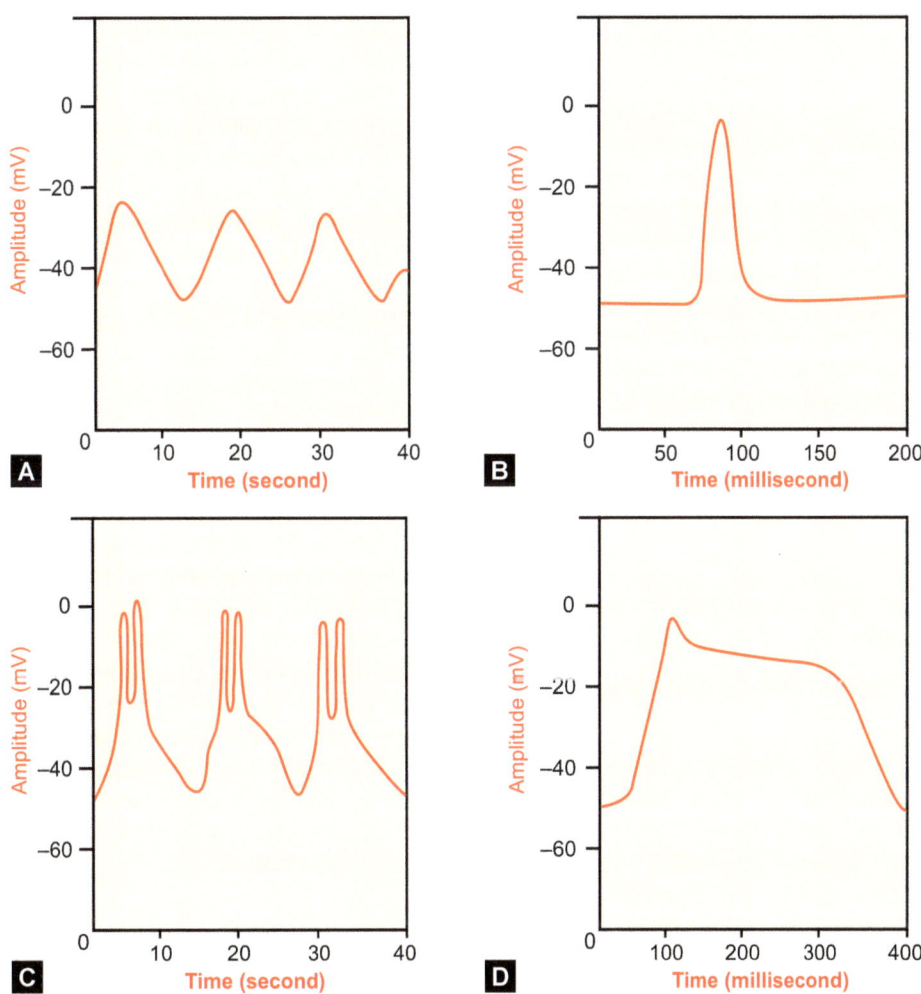

FIGURE 24.2: Electrical activities in smooth muscle.
A = Slow-wave rhythm of resting membrane potential. **B** = Spike potential.
C = Spike potential initiated by slow-wave rhythm. **D** = Action potential with plateau.

for sustained contraction of smooth muscle fibers. After long depolarized state, slow repolarization occurs.

TONIC CONTRACTION OF SMOOTH MUSCLE WITHOUT ACTION POTENTIAL

Smooth muscles of some visceral organs maintain a state of partial contraction called **tonus** or **tone**. It is due to the tonic contraction of the muscle that occurs without any action potential or any stimulus. Sometimes, the tonic contraction occurs due to the action of some hormones.

IONIC BASIS OF ACTION POTENTIAL

Important difference between the action potential in skeletal muscle and single-unit smooth muscle lies in the ionic basis of depolarization. In skeletal muscle, the depolarization occurs due to opening of sodium channels and entry of sodium ions from extracellular fluid into the muscle fiber. But in single-unit smooth muscle, the depolarization is due to entry of calcium ions rather than sodium ions. Unlike the fast sodium channels, the calcium channels open and close slowly. It is responsible for the prolonged action potential with plateau in smooth muscles. Calcium ions play an important role during the contraction of the smooth muscle.

ELECTRICAL ACTIVITY IN MULTI-UNIT SMOOTH MUSCLE

Electrical activity in multi-unit smooth muscle is different from that in the single-unit smooth muscle. Electrical changes leading to contraction of multi-unit smooth muscle are triggered by nervous stimuli. Nerve endings secrete neurotransmitters such as acetylcholine and noradrenaline. These neurotransmitters depolarize the membrane of smooth muscle fiber slightly leading to contraction. Action potential does not develop. This type of depolarization is called **local depolarization** of **junctional potential**. Local depolarization travels throughout the entire smooth muscle fiber and causes contraction. Local depolarization is developed because the multi-unit smooth muscle fibers are too small to develop action potential.

CONTRACTILE PROCESS IN SMOOTH MUSCLE

Compared to skeletal muscles, in smooth muscles, the contraction and relaxation processes are slow.

MOLECULAR BASIS OF SMOOTH MUSCLE CONTRACTION

Process of excitation and contraction is very slow in smooth muscles is because of poor development of L-tubules (sarcoplasmic reticulum). So, the calcium ions, which are responsible for **excitation-contraction coupling**, must be obtained from the extracellular fluid. It makes the process of excitation-contraction coupling slow.

Calcium-calmodulin Complex

Stimulation of ATPase activity of myosin in smooth muscle is different from that in the skeletal muscle. In smooth muscle, the myosin has to be phosphorylated for the

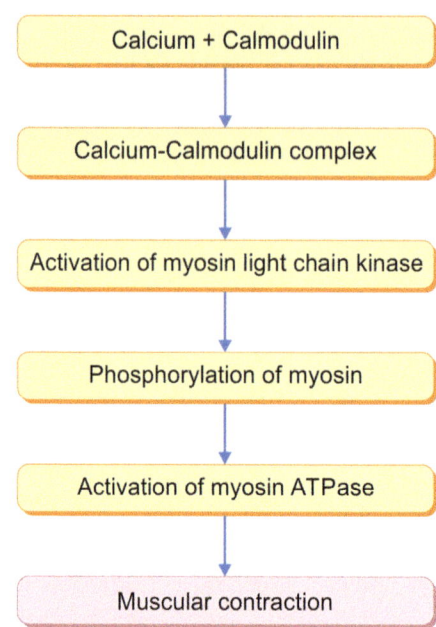

FIGURE 24.3: Molecular basis of smooth muscle contraction.

activation of **myosin ATPase**. **Phosphorylation** of myosin occurs in the following manner **(Fig. 24.3)**.

Calcium, which enters the sarcoplasm from the extracellular fluid combines with a protein called **calmodulin** and forms calcium-calmodulin complex. It activates an enzyme called calmodulin-dependent myosin light chain kinase. This enzyme in turn causes phosphorylation of myosin followed by activation of myosin ATPase. Now, the sliding of actin filaments starts.

The phosphorylated myosin gets attached to the actin molecule for longer period. It is called **latchbridge mechanism** and it is responsible for the sustained contraction of the muscle with expenditure of little energy.

Relaxation of the muscle occurs due to the dissociation of calcium-calmodulin complex.

Length-Tension Relationship: Plasticity

Smooth muscle fibers have the property of plasticity. Plasticity is the adaptability of smooth muscle fibers to a wide range of lengths. If the smooth muscle fiber is stretched, it adapts to this new length and contracts when stimulated. This adaptability exists to a wide range of lengths. Because of this property, tension produced in the muscle fiber is not directly proportional to resting length of the muscle fiber. In other words, **Starling's law** is not applicable to smooth muscle. In skeletal and cardiac muscles, Starling's law is applicable and the tension or force of contraction is directly proportional to initial length of the muscle fibers.

NEUROMUSCULAR JUNCTION IN SMOOTH MUSCLE

Well-defined neuromuscular junctions are absent in smooth muscle. Nerve fibers (axons) do not end in the form of endplate. Instead, these nerve fibers end on smooth muscle fibers in three different ways:

1. In some smooth muscles, nerve fibers diffuse on the sheet of smooth muscle fibers without making any direct contact with the muscle. These **diffused nerve fibers** form **diffused junctions** which contain neurotransmitters.
2. In some smooth muscle fibers, axon terminal ends in the form of many **varicosities** (bulged or enlarged ends) which contain the neurotransmitter.
3. In some of the multi-unit smooth muscle fibers, a gap is present between varicosities and the membrane of smooth muscle fibers which resembles the synaptic cleft in skeletal muscle. This gap is called **contact junction** and it functions as neuromuscular junction of skeletal muscle.

■ CONTROL OF SMOOTH MUSCLE ACTIVITIES

Smooth muscle fibers are controlled by nervous factors and humoral factors.

■ NERVOUS FACTORS

Single-unit smooth muscle and multi-unit smooth muscle are innervated by nerves of both the divisions of autonomic nervous system. Al these nerves initiate the contraction of multi-unit smooth muscles only. Nerves supplying single-unit smooth muscles do not initiate contraction. But these nerves can modify or regulate the rate and force of contraction.

■ HUMORAL FACTORS

Activity of smooth muscle is also controlled by humoral factors which include hormones, neurotransmitters and other humoral factors.

Action of the hormones and neurotransmitters depends upon the type of receptors present in membrane of smooth muscle fibers in particular area. The receptors are of two types, excitatory and inhibitory receptors.

If excitatory receptors are present, the hormones or the neurotransmitters contract the muscle by producing depolarization. If inhibitory receptors are present, the hormones or the neurotransmitters relax the muscles by producing hyperpolarization.

Humoral Factors which Cause Contraction of Smooth Muscles

1. Acetylcholine.
2. Antidiuretic hormone (ADH).
3. Adrenaline.
4. Angiotensin II, III and IV.
5. Endothelin.
6. Histamine.
7. Noradrenaline.
8. Oxytocin.
9. Serotonin.

Humoral Factors which Cause Relaxation of Smooth Muscles

1. Lack of oxygen.
2. Excess of carbon dioxide.
3. Increase in hydrogen ion concentration.
4. Adenosine.
5. Lactic acid.
6. Excess of potassium ion.
7. Decrease in calcium ion.
8. Nitric oxide (NO), the endothelium-derived relaxing factor (EDRF).

MODEL QUESTIONS IN MUSCLE PHYSIOLOGY

■ LONG QUESTIONS

1. Enumerate the properties of muscles and give an account of contractile property of the skeletal muscle.
2. Explain the molecular basis of contraction.
3. Describe the electrical changes during muscular contraction.
4. Explain the ionic basis of electrical events during contraction of skeletal muscle.
5. Describe the neuromuscular junction with a suitable diagram. Add a note on neuromuscular transmission.

■ SHORT QUESTIONS

1. Classify muscles by different methods.
2. Sarcomere.
3. Muscle proteins.
4. Sarcotubular system.
5. Composition of muscle.
6. Differences between pale and red muscles.
7. Rigor.
8. Effects of repeated stimuli on skeletal muscle.
9. Fatigue.
10. Tetanus.
11. Refractory period.
12. Resting membrane potential.
13. Action potential in skeletal muscle.
14. Actomyosin complex.
15. Excitation-contraction coupling.
16. Sliding theory of muscular contraction.
17. Electrical activity in smooth muscle.
18. Molecular basis of smooth muscular contraction.
19. Neuromuscular junction.
20. Neuromuscular transmission.

■ VERY SHORT ANSWER QUESTIONS

1. Compare skeletal muscle and cardiac muscle.
2. Compare skeletal muscle and smooth muscle.
3. Microscopic structure of myofibril.
4. Contractile elements of the muscle.
5. Composition of skeletal muscle.
6. Sarcoplasmic reticulum.
7. Define excitability and stimulus.
8. Strength-duration curve
9. Types of muscular contraction.
10. Latent period and its causes.
11. Types of (red and pale) skeletal muscle. Give examples for each type.
12. Free load and afterload.
13. Starling's law of muscle.
14. Define muscle tone. How it is maintained in different types of muscles?
15. Name the changes taking place during muscular contraction.
16. Resting membrane potential.
17. Graded potentials.
18. Actomyosin complex.
19. Endplate potential.
20. Neuromuscular blockers.
21. Motor unit.
22. Disorders of neuromuscular junction.
23. Types of smooth muscle.
24. Myasthenia gravis.
25. Hypotonia.
26. Hypertonia.
27. Myotonia.

SECTION 4: DIGESTIVE SYSTEM

Chapter 25: Overview of Digestive System

CHAPTER OUTLINE

- **DIGESTION AND DIGESTIVE PROCESS**
- **FUNCTIONAL ANATOMY**
  - GASTROINTESTINAL TRACT
  - ACCESSORY DIGESTIVE ORGANS
- **WALL OF GASTROINTESTINAL TRACT**
  - MUCUS LAYER
  - SUBMUCUS LAYER
- **MUSCULAR LAYER**
- **SEROUS OR FIBROUS LAYER**
- **NERVE SUPPLY TO GASTROINTESTINAL TRACT**
  - INTRINSIC NERVE SUPPLY
  - EXTRINSIC NERVE SUPPLY

DIGESTION AND DIGESTIVE PROCESS

Digestion is defined as the process by which food is broken down into simple substances that can be absorbed and utilized as nutrients by the body. Most of the substances in diet cannot be utilized as such. These substances must be broken into smaller particles. Then only these substances can be absorbed into blood and distributed to various parts of the body for utilization. Digestive system is responsible for these functions.

FUNCTIONS OF DIGESTIVE SYSTEM

1. Ingestion or consumption of food substances.
2. Breaking them into small particles.
3. Secretion of necessary enzymes and other substances for digestion.
4. Digestion of food particles.
5. Absorption of digested products (nutrients).
6. Removal of unwanted substances from body.

FUNCTIONAL ANATOMY OF THE DIGESTIVE SYSTEM

Digestive system is made up of **gastrointestinal tract** (GI tract) or **alimentary canal** and **accessory digestive organs** (Fig. 25.1).

GASTROINTESTINAL TRACT

GI tract is a tubular structure extending from the mouth to anus with a length of about 30 feet. It opens to external environment at both the ends. Gastrointestinal tract includes the **primary digestive organs** where actual digestion takes place.

Primary digestive organs are:

1. Mouth.
2. Pharynx.
3. Esophagus.
4. Stomach.

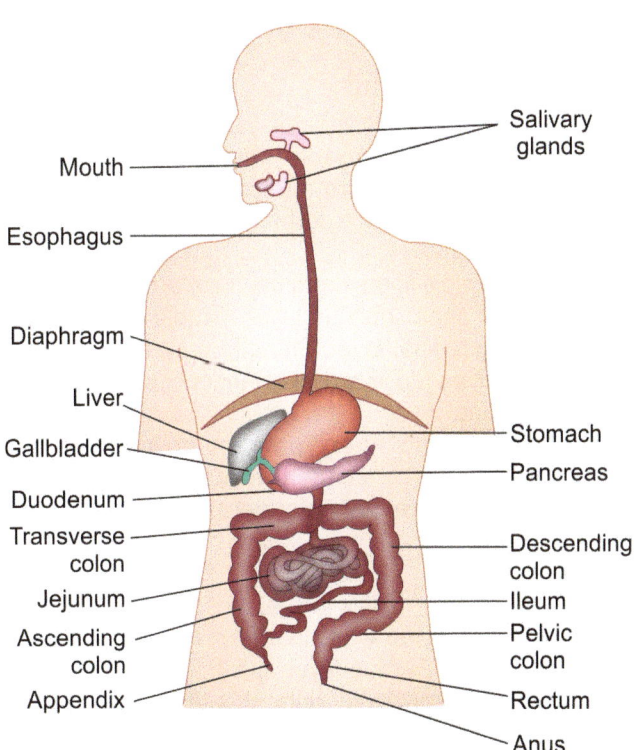

FIGURE 25.1: Gastrointestinal tract.

5. Small intestine.
6. Large intestine.

ACCESSORY DIGESTIVE ORGANS

Accessory digestive organs are the organs which help the primary digestive organs in the process of digestion.

Accessory digestive organs are:
1. Teeth.
2. Tongue.
3. Salivary glands.
4. Exocrine part of pancreas.
5. Liver.
6. Gallbladder.

WALL OF GASTROINTESTINAL TRACT

In general, wall of the GI tract is formed by **four layers**, which are from inside out:

1. MUCUS LAYER

Mucus layer or **gastrointestinal mucosa** or **mucous membrane** is the innermost layer of the wall of GI tract. It faces the lumen of GI tract.

Mucosa has three layers of structures:
  i. **Epithelial lining**, which is in contact with contents of GI tract.
  ii. **Lamina propria** formed by connective tissue.
  iii. **Muscularis mucosa** formed by smooth muscle fibers.

2. SUBMUCUS LAYER

This layer is present in all parts of GI tract except mouth and pharynx. Submucus layer contains loose collagen fibers, elastic fibers, reticular fibers and few cells of connective tissue. Blood vessels, lymphatic vessels and nerve plexus are present in this layer.

3. MUSCULAR LAYER

Muscular layer in lips, cheeks and wall of pharynx consists of **skeletal muscle** fibers. Esophagus has both skeletal and smooth muscle fibers. Wall of the stomach and intestine is formed by **smooth muscle** fibers only.

Smooth muscle fibers in stomach are arranged in three layers namely, inner oblique layer, middle circular layer and outer longitudinal layer. Smooth muscle fibers in the intestine are arranged in two layers inner circular layer and outer longitudinal layer.

Smooth muscle fibers present in inner circular layer of anal canal constitute **internal anal sphincter**. **External anal sphincter** is formed by skeletal muscle fibers.

4. SEROUS LAYER

Outermost layer of the wall of GI tract is either serous or fibrous in nature. Serous layer is formed by connective tissue and **mesoepithelial cells**. It is also called **serosa** or **serous membrane**.

NERVE SUPPLY TO GASTROINTESTINAL TRACT

GI tract has two types of nerve supply called intrinsic nerve supply and extrinsic nerve supply.

INTRINSIC NERVE SUPPLY: ENTERIC NERVOUS SYSTEM

Enteric nervous system is present within the wall of GI tract from esophagus to anus. Nerve fibers of this system are interconnected and form two major networks called Auerbach's plexus and Meissner's plexus.

These two nerve plexuses contain nerve cell bodies, processes of nerve cells and the receptors. Receptors in the GI tract are **stretch receptors** and **chemoreceptors**. Enteric nervous system is controlled by extrinsic nerves.

1. *Auerbach's Plexus*

It is also known as **myenteric nerve plexus**. It is present in between the inner circular muscle layer and the outer longitudinal muscle layer **(Fig. 25.2)**.

Functions of Auerbach's plexus

Major function of this plexus is to regulate the movements of GI tract. Some nerve fibers of this plexus accelerate the movements by secreting the excitatory neurotransmitter substances such as acetylcholine, serotonin and substance P. Other fibers of this plexus inhibit the GI motility by secreting the inhibitory neurotransmitters such as vasoactive intestinal polypeptide (VIP), neurotensin and enkephalin.

2. *Meissner's Nerve Plexus*

Meissner's plexus or **submucus nerve plexus** is situated in between the muscular layer and submucosal layer of GI tract.

Functions of Meissner's plexus

Meissner's plexus regulates secretory functions of GI tract and also causes constriction of blood vessels of GI tract.

EXTRINSIC NERVE SUPPLY

Extrinsic nerves that control the enteric nervous system are from autonomic nervous system. Both sympathetic

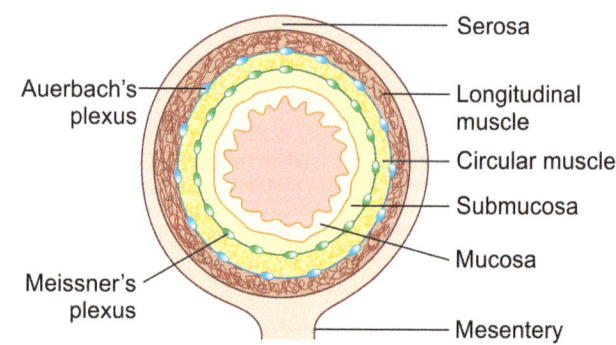

FIGURE 25.2: Structure of intestinal wall with intrinsic nerve plexus.

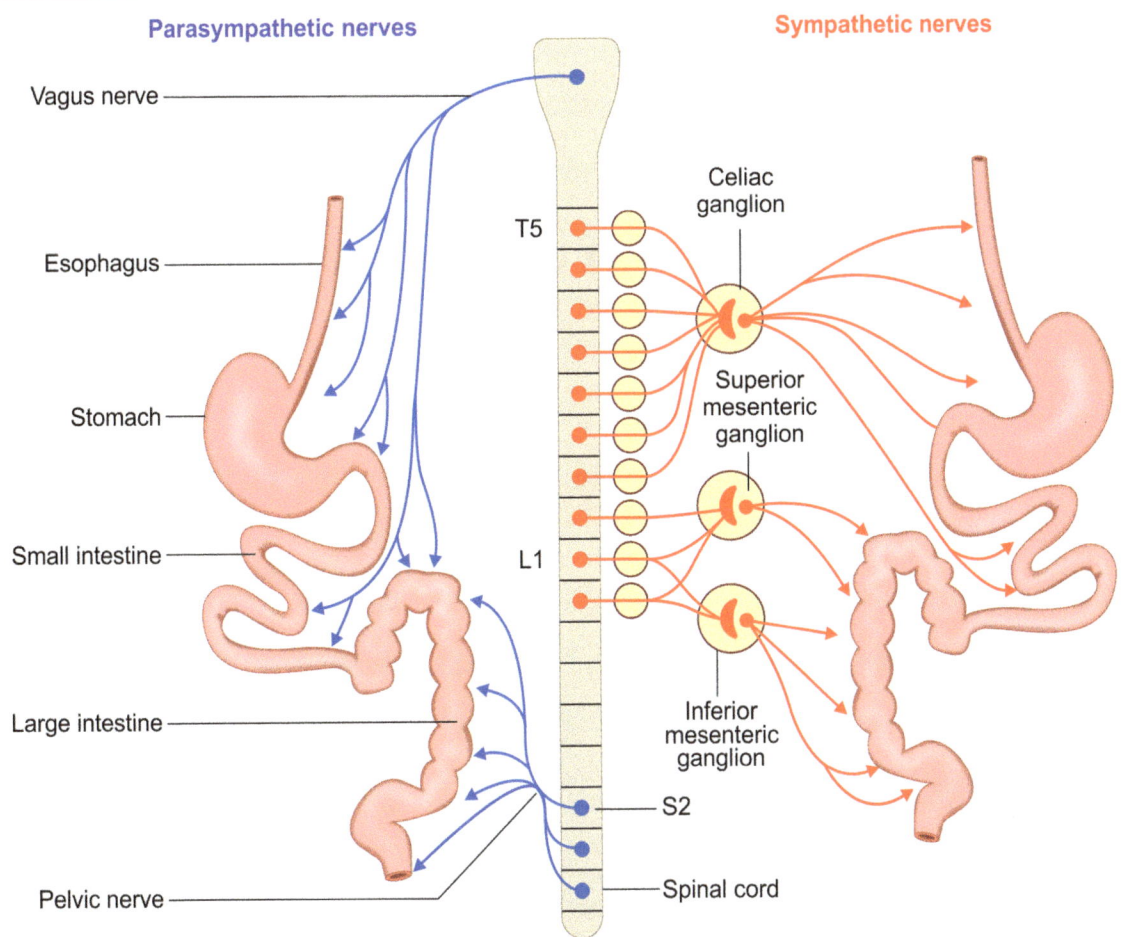

FIGURE 25.3: Extrinsic nerve supply to GI tract.
T5 = 5th thoracic segment of spinal cord, L1 = 1st lumbar segment of spinal cord, S2 = 2nd sacral segment of spinal cord.

and parasympathetic divisions of the autonomic nervous system innervate GI tract **(Fig. 25.3)**.

Sympathetic Nerve Fibers

Preganglionic sympathetic nerve fibers to GI tract arise from lateral horns of spinal cord between fifth thoracic and second lumbar segments (T5 to L2). From here, the fibers leave the spinal cord, pass through the ganglia of sympathetic chain without having any synapse and then terminate in the **celiac ganglion** and **mesenteric ganglia**. The postganglionic fibers from these ganglia are distributed throughout the GI tract.

Functions of sympathetic nerve fibers

Sympathetic nerve fibers inhibit the movements and decrease the secretions of GI tract by secreting the neurotransmitter noradrenaline.

Parasympathetic Nerve Fibers

Parasympathetic nerve fibers to GI tract pass through some of the cranial nerves and sacral nerves. Preganglionic and postganglionic parasympathetic nerve fibers to mouth and salivary glands pass through **facial nerve** and **glossopharyngeal nerve**.

Preganglionic parasympathetic nerve fibers to esophagus, stomach, small intestine and upper part of large intestine pass through **vagus nerve**. Preganglionic nerve fibers to lower part of large intestine arise from second, third and fourth sacral segments (S2, S3 and S4) of spinal cord and pass through **pelvic nerve**. All these preganglionic parasympathetic nerve fibers synapse with the postganglionic nerve cells in the myenteric and submucus plexus.

Functions of parasympathetic nerve fibers

Parasympathetic nerve fibers accelerate movements and increase the secretions of GI tract. Neurotransmitter secreted by the parasympathetic nerve fibers is acetylcholine.

Chapter 26

Mouth and Salivary Secretion

CHAPTER OUTLINE

- FUNCTIONAL ANATOMY OF MOUTH
- FUNCTIONS OF MOUTH
- SALIVARY GLANDS
- PROPERTIES AND COMPOSITION OF SALIVA
- FUNCTIONS OF SALIVA
- REGULATION OF SALIVARY SECRETION
- APPLIED PHYSIOLOGY: DISORDERS OF SALIVARY SECRETION

FUNCTIONAL ANATOMY OF MOUTH

Mouth or **oral cavity** or **buccal cavity** is formed by cheeks, lips and palate. It encloses the teeth, tongue and salivary glands. It opens anteriorly to the exterior through lips and posteriorly through fauces into the pharynx.

Digestive juice present in the mouth is **saliva** which is secreted by the **salivary glands**.

FUNCTIONS OF MOUTH

Primary function of mouth is eating. It has few other important functions also. Refer **Table 26.1** for details.

SALIVARY GLANDS

In humans, saliva is secreted by three pairs of major (larger) salivary glands and some minor (small) salivary glands in the oral and pharyngeal mucous membrane.

MAJOR SALIVARY GLANDS

Major salivary glands are:

1. Parotid glands.
2. Submaxillary or submandibular glands.
3. Sublingual glands.

1. *Parotid Glands*

Parotid glands are the largest of all salivary glands situated at the side of face just below and in front of ear. Secretions from these glands are emptied into the oral cavity by **Stensen's duct** that opens inside the cheek against the upper second molar tooth **(Fig. 26.1)**.

2. *Submaxillary Glands*

Submaxillary glands or **submandibular glands** are located in submaxillary triangle medial to mandible. Saliva from these glands is emptied into the oral cavity by **Wharton's duct**. This duct opens at the side of frenulum of tongue by means of a small opening on the summit of papilla called **caruncula sublingualis**.

3. *Sublingual Glands*

Sublingual glands are the smallest salivary glands situated in the mucosa at the floor of mouth. Saliva from these glands is poured into 5 to 15 small ducts called **ducts of Rivinus**. These ducts open on small papillae beneath the tongue. One of the ducts is larger and it is called **Bartholin's duct (Table 26.2)**. It drains the anterior part of the gland and opens on caruncula sublingualis near the opening of **Wharton's duct**.

MINOR SALIVARY GLANDS

Minor salivary glands are:

1. **Lingual mucous glands** situated in posterior 1/3 of the tongue, behind circumvallate papillae and at the tip and margins of tongue.
2. **Lingual serous glands** located near circumvallate papillae and filiform papillae.
3. **Buccal glands** present between the mucous membrane and buccinator muscle. Four to five of these are larger and situated outside buccinator around terminal part of parotid duct. These glands are called **molar glands**.

Chapter 26: Mouth and Salivary Secretion

TABLE 26.1: Functions of mouth.

Function	Process
1. Mastication	Teeth cut and grind the food Lips and cheeks hold food in the mouth with the help of tongue Muscles of the mouth along with jaw movements help in chewing the food properly and mixing the food with saliva Saliva lubricates and softens the food to facilitate chewing and swallowing
2. Taste	Taste buds present on tongue and other structures of mouth help to appreciate and differentiate the taste of food Saliva helps in appreciation of taste by dissolving the foodstuffs
3. Speech	Mouth coordinates with larynx, pharynx, lips and tongue during speech Saliva helps in speech by moistening and lubricating soft parts of mouth and lips
4. Appearance	Shape of the mouth along with jaws, lips and teeth together contribute to the appearance of face
5. Expression	Facial expressions such as smiling and laughing are mostly centered on mouth along with movements of lips and cheeks
6. Breathing	Occasionally, when nose breathing is inadequate, as in case of running or nasal block, mouth is used for breathing

4. **Labial glands** situated beneath the mucous membrane around the orifice of mouth.
5. **Palatal glands** found beneath the mucous membrane of the soft palate.

■ CLASSIFICATION OF SALIVARY GLANDS

Salivary glands are classified into three types based on the type of secretion.

1. Serous Glands

Serous glands are predominately made up of **serous cells**. Serous glands secrete thin and **watery saliva**. Parotid glands and lingual (serous) glands are the serous glands.

2. Mucous Glands

Mucous glands are made up of mainly the **mucous cells**. These glands secrete thick, **viscus saliva** with high mucin content. Lingual mucous glands, buccal glands and palatal glands belong to this type.

TABLE 26.2: Ducts of major salivary glands.

Gland	Duct
Parotid gland	Stensen's duct
Submaxillary gland	Wharton's duct
Sublingual gland	Ducts of Rivinus / Bartholin's duct

3. Mixed Glands

Mixed glands are made up of both **serous** and **mucus cells**. Submandibular, sublingual and labial glands are the mixed glands.

■ STRUCTURE AND DUCT SYSTEM OF SALIVARY GLANDS

Salivary glands are made up of **acini** or **alveoli**. Each acinus is formed by a small group of cells which surround a central cavity. Central cavity of each acinus is continuous with the lumen of the duct. Fine duct draining each acinus is called **intercalated duct**. Many intercalated ducts join together to form **intralobular duct**. Few intralobular ducts join to form **interlobular ducts**, which unite to form the main duct of the gland **(Fig. 26.2)**. Gland with this type of structure and duct system is called **racemose type** (racemose = bunch of grapes).

■ PROPERTIES AND COMPOSITION OF SALIVA

■ PROPERTIES OF SALIVA

1. *Volume*: 1,000 to 1,500 mL of saliva is secreted per day and it is approximately about 1 mL/min.
   Contribution by each major salivary gland is:
   i. Parotid glands : 25%
   ii. Submaxillary glands : 70%
   iii. Sublingual glands : 5%
2. *Reaction*: Mixed saliva from all the glands is slightly acidic with pH of 6.35 to 6.85.

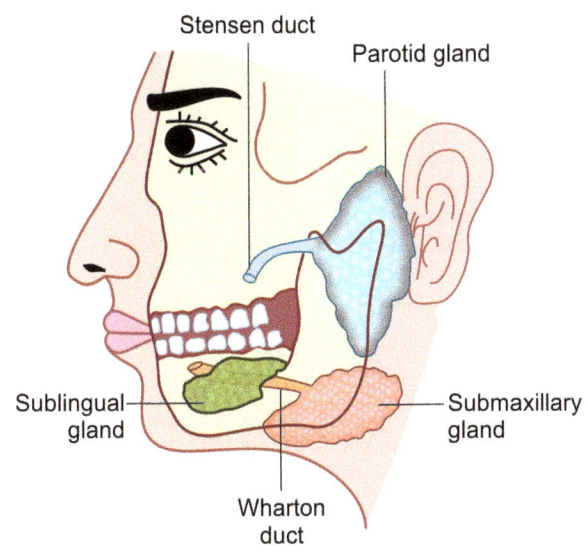

FIGURE 26.1: Major salivary glands.

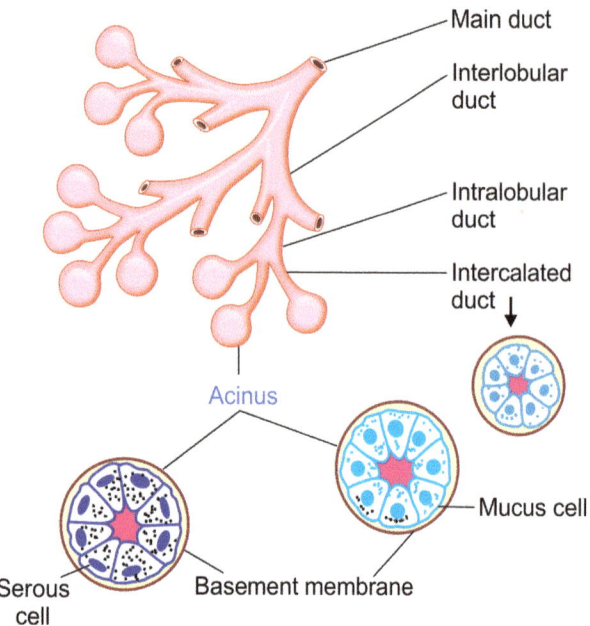

FIGURE 26.2: Diagram showing acini and duct system in salivary glands.

3. *Specific gravity*: It ranges between 1.002 and 1.012.
4. *Tonicity*: Saliva is hypotonic to plasma.

■ COMPOSITION OF SALIVA

Mixed saliva contains 99.5% water and 0.5% solids. Composition of saliva is given in **Figure 26.3**.

■ FUNCTIONS OF SALIVA

Saliva is an essential digestive juice. Since it has many functions, its absence leads to many inconveniences.

■ 1. PREPARATION OF FOOD FOR SWALLOWING

When food is taken into the mouth, it is moistened and dissolved by saliva. Mucous membrane of mouth is also moistened by saliva. It facilitates **chewing**. By the movement of tongue, moistened and masticated food is rolled into a **bolus**. **Mucin** of saliva lubricates the bolus and facilitates swallowing.

■ 2. APPRECIATION OF TASTE

Taste is a chemical sensation. Saliva, by its solvent action, dissolves the solid food substances, so that dissolved substances can stimulate the taste buds. The stimulated taste buds recognize the taste.

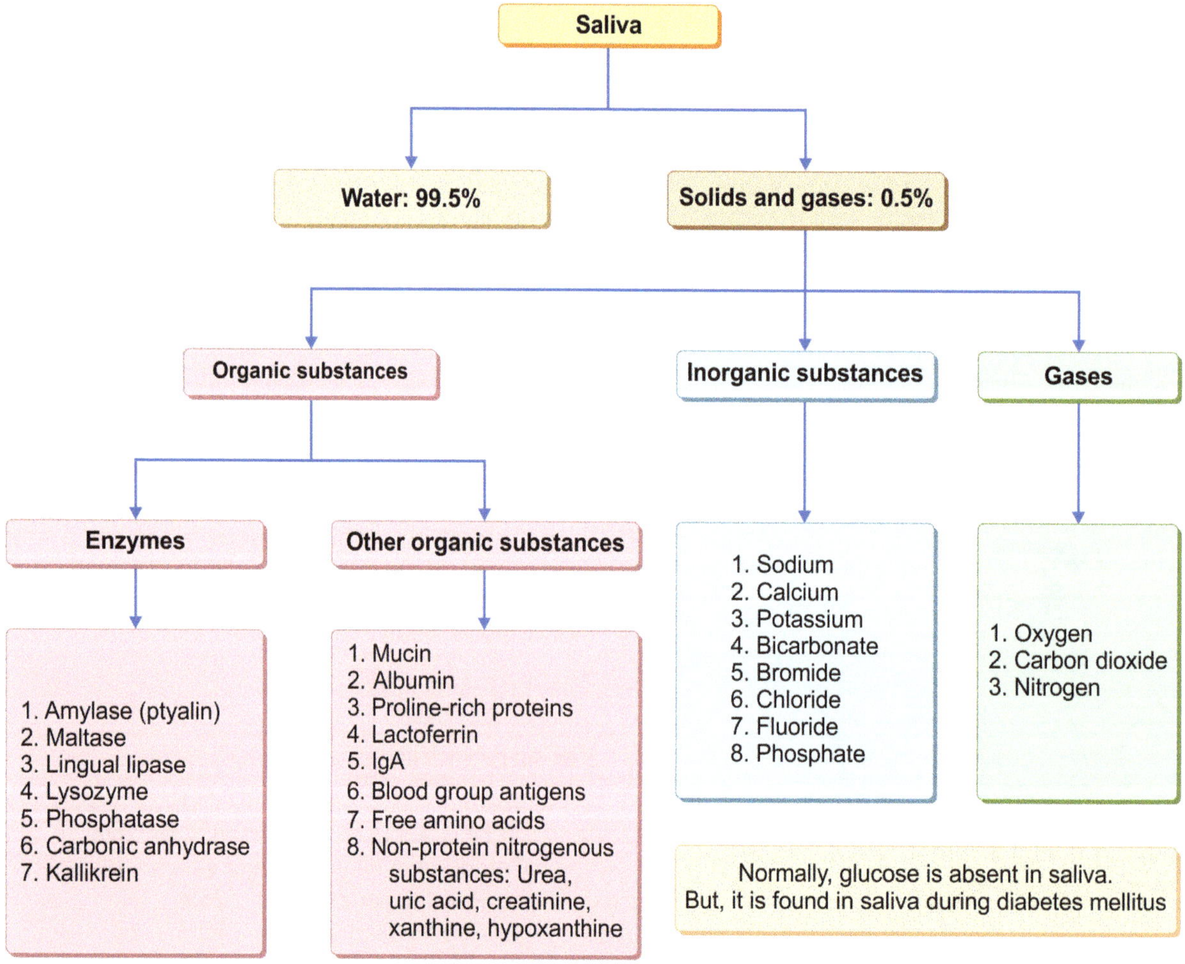

```
                           Saliva
                ┌────────────┴────────────┐
          Water: 99.5%              Solids and gases: 0.5%
                         ┌────────────────┼───────────────┐
                  Organic substances  Inorganic substances  Gases
                   ┌─────┴─────┐
               Enzymes    Other organic substances
```

Enzymes:
1. Amylase (ptyalin)
2. Maltase
3. Lingual lipase
4. Lysozyme
5. Phosphatase
6. Carbonic anhydrase
7. Kallikrein

Other organic substances:
1. Mucin
2. Albumin
3. Proline-rich proteins
4. Lactoferrin
5. IgA
6. Blood group antigens
7. Free amino acids
8. Non-protein nitrogenous substances: Urea, uric acid, creatinine, xanthine, hypoxanthine

Inorganic substances:
1. Sodium
2. Calcium
3. Potassium
4. Bicarbonate
5. Bromide
6. Chloride
7. Fluoride
8. Phosphate

Gases:
1. Oxygen
2. Carbon dioxide
3. Nitrogen

Normally, glucose is absent in saliva. But, it is found in saliva during diabetes mellitus.

FIGURE 26.3: Composition of saliva.

Chapter 26: Mouth and Salivary Secretion

TABLE 26.3: Digestive enzymes of saliva.

Enzyme	Source of secretion	Activation	Action
Salivary amylase	All salivary glands	Acid medium	Converts starch into maltose
Maltase	Major salivary glands	Acid medium	Converts maltose into glucose
Lingual lipase	Lingual glands	Acid medium	Converts triglycerides of milk fat into fatty acids and diacylglycerol

3. DIGESTIVE FUNCTION

Saliva has three digestive enzymes namely, salivary amylase, maltase and lingual lipase **(Table 26.3)**.

Salivary Amylase

Salivary amylase is an **amylolytic enzyme** (carbohydrate digesting enzyme). It acts on cooked or **boiled starch** and converts it into dextrin and maltose. Though starch digestion starts in the mouth, major part of it occurs in the stomach, because food stays only for a short time in the mouth. Salivary amylase cannot act on **cellulose**.

Maltase

Maltase is present only in traces in human saliva. It converts maltose into glucose.

Lingual Lipase

Lingual lipase is a **lipolytic enzyme** (lipid digesting enzyme). It digests **milk fats** which are the **pre-emulsified fats**. It hydrolyzes triglycerides into fatty acids and diacylglycerol **(Table 26.3)**.

4. CLEANSING AND PROTECTIVE FUNCTIONS

i. Due to the constant secretion of saliva, the mouth and teeth are rinsed and kept free of food debris, shed epithelial cells and foreign particles. In this way, saliva prevents bacterial growth by removing materials, which may serve as culture media for the bacterial growth
ii. Enzyme **lysozyme** of saliva kills some bacteria such as *Staphylococcus*, *Streptococcus* and *Brucella*
iii. **Proline-rich proteins** present in saliva have antimicrobial property and neutralize the toxic substances, e.g. tannins. Tannins are present in many food substances including fruits
iv. **Lactoferrin** of saliva also has antimicrobial property
v. Proline-rich proteins and lactoferrin protect the teeth by stimulating enamel formation
vi. Immunoglobulin IgA in saliva also has antibacterial and antiviral actions
vii. **Mucin** present in the saliva protects the mouth by lubricating the mucous membrane of mouth.

5. ROLE IN SPEECH

By moistening and lubricating soft parts of mouth and lips, saliva helps in speech. If the mouth becomes dry, articulation and pronunciation become difficult.

6. EXCRETORY FUNCTION

Many organic and inorganic substances are excreted in saliva. It excretes substances like mercury, potassium iodide, lead and thiocyanate. Saliva also excretes some viruses such as those causing rabies and mumps.

7. REGULATION OF WATER BALANCE

When the body water content decreases, salivary secretion also decreases. This causes dryness of the mouth and induces thirst. When the water is taken, it quenches the thirst and restores the body water content.

REGULATION OF SALIVARY SECRETION

Salivary secretion is regulated only by nervous mechanism. Autonomic nervous system is involved in the regulatory function.

NERVE SUPPLY TO SALIVARY GLANDS

Salivary glands are supplied by parasympathetic and sympathetic divisions of autonomic nervous system.

Parasympathetic Fibers

When the parasympathetic fibers of salivary glands are stimulated, a large quantity of watery saliva is secreted with less quantity of organic constituents. It is because, parasympathetic fibers activate acinar cells and cause vasodilation in salivary glands by secreting **acetylcholine**.

Sympathetic Fibers

Stimulation of sympathetic fibers causes less secretion of saliva, which is thick and rich in mucus. It is because these fibers activate the acinar cells and cause vasoconstriction in salivary glands by secreting **noradrenaline**.

REFLEX REGULATION OF SALIVARY SECRETION

Salivary secretion is regulated by nervous mechanism through reflex action. Salivary reflexes are of two types, unconditioned reflex and conditioned reflex.

1. Unconditioned Reflex

Unconditioned reflex is the inborn reflex that is present since birth. It does not need any previous experience. This reflex induces salivary secretion when any substance is placed in the mouth. It is due to the stimulation of nerve endings in mucous membrane of the oral cavity.

2. Conditioned Reflex

Conditioned reflex is acquired by experience and it needs previous experience (Chapter 90). Presence of food in the mouth is not necessary to elicit this reflex. Stimulus for this reflex is the sight, smell, hearing or thought of food. It is due to the impulses arising from eyes, nose, ears, etc.

■ APPLIED PHYSIOLOGY: DISORDERS OF SALIVARY SECRETION

■ HYPOSALIVATION

Hyposalivation is the reduction in secretion of saliva. Temporary hyposalivation occurs in fever, dehydration and emotional condition such as fear. Permanent hyposalivation occurs in the following conditions:

 i. **Sialolithiasis:** Obstruction of salivary duct by salivary stone.
 ii. **Congenital absence** salivary glands.
 iii. **Bell's palsy**: Paralysis of facial nerve.

■ HYPERSALIVATION

Hypersalivation is the excess secretion of saliva. Physiological condition when hypersalivation occurs is pregnancy. Hypersalivation in pathological conditions is called **ptyalism** or **sialorrhea**

Hypersalivation occurs in the following conditions:

1. Decay of tooth or **neoplasm** (abnormal new growth or tumor) in mouth or tongue.
2. Disease of esophagus, stomach and intestine.
3. Neurological disorders such as mental retardation, cerebral stroke and parkinsonism.
4. Some psychological and psychiatric conditions.
5. Nausea and vomiting.

■ OTHER DISORDERS

In addition to hyposalivation and hypersalivation, salivary secretion is also affected by following disorders.

1. Xerostomia

Xerostomia means dry mouth. It is also called **pasties** or **cottonmouth**. It is due to hyposalivation or absence of salivary secretion (**aptyalism**). Xerostomia causes difficulties in mastication, swallowing and speech. It also causes **halitosis** (bad breath).

Common causes for xerostomia are Sjögren's syndrome (see below), radiotherapy, trauma to salivary gland or their ducts and shock.

2. Drooling

Uncontrolled flow of saliva outside the mouth is called drooling. Drooling occurs because of excess production of saliva in association with inability to retain saliva within the mouth.

Drooling occurs in conditions such as upper respiratory tract infection or nasal allergies in children and tonsillitis. It also occurs during teeth eruption in children.

3. Chorda Tympani Syndrome

Chorda tympani syndrome is the condition characterized by sweating while eating. During trauma or surgical procedure, some of the parasympathetic nerve fibers to salivary glands may be severed. And during regeneration, some of these nerve fibers, which run along with chorda tympani branch of facial nerve, may deviate and join with the nerve fibers supplying sweat glands. So when food is placed in the mouth, salivary secretion is associated with sweat secretion.

4. Mumps

Mumps is the acute viral infection affecting parotid glands. The virus causing this disease is **paramyxovirus**. It is common in children who are not immunized. It occurs in adults also. Features of mumps are puffiness of cheeks (due to swelling of parotid glands), fever, sore throat and weakness. Mumps affects meninges, gonads and pancreas also.

5. Sjögren's Syndrome

It is an autoimmune disorder in which the immune cells destroy exocrine glands such as salivary glands. It is characterized by dryness of the mouth due to lack of saliva (xerostomia), persistent cough and dryness of eyes.

Chapter 27: Stomach and Gastric Secretion

CHAPTER OUTLINE

- FUNCTIONAL ANATOMY OF STOMACH
- GLANDS OF STOMACH
- NERVE SUPPLY TO STOMACH
- FUNCTIONS OF STOMACH
- PROPERTIES AND COMPOSITION OF GASTRIC JUICE
- FUNCTIONS OF GASTRIC JUICE
- SECRETION OF GASTRIC JUICE
- REGULATION OF GASTRIC SECRETION
- COLLECTION OF GASTRIC JUICE
- GASTRIC FUNCTION TESTS: GASTRIC ANALYSIS
- APPLIED PHYSIOLOGY: GASTRIC DISORDERS

■ FUNCTIONAL ANATOMY OF STOMACH

Stomach is a hollow organ situated just below diaphragm on the left side in abdominal cavity.

■ PARTS OF STOMACH

In humans, stomach has four parts:

1. Cardiac Region

Cardiac region or **cardiac end** of stomach is the upper part of stomach where esophagus opens. Opening of esophagus is guarded by a sphincter called **cardiac sphincter** which opens only towards stomach. **Sphincter** is a circular muscle that surrounds and closes a tube or an opening in the body.

2. Fundus

Fundus is a small dome-shaped structure. It is elevated above the level of esophageal opening.

3. Body or Corpus

Body or corpus of the stomach is the largest part of stomach forming about 75% to 80% of the whole stomach. It extends esophagus from just below the fundus up to the pyloric region **(Fig. 27.1)**.

4. Pyloric Region

Pyloric region has two parts, **antrum** and **pyloric canal**. Body of the stomach ends in antrum. The junction between body and antrum is marked by an angular notch called incisura angularis. Antrum is continued as the narrow canal which is called **pylorus** or **pyloric canal** or pyloric end. Pyloric canal opens into first part of small intestine called duodenum. The opening of pyloric canal is guarded by a sphincter called **pyloric sphincter**. It opens towards duodenum.

Stomach has two curvatures. One on the right side is lesser curvature and other one on the left side is greater curvature.

■ STRUCTURE OF STOMACH WALL

Wall of stomach is formed by four layers of structures:

1. Outer serous layer formed by **peritoneum**.
2. Muscular layer made up of three layers of smooth muscle fibers namely, inner oblique, middle circular and outer longitudinal layers.

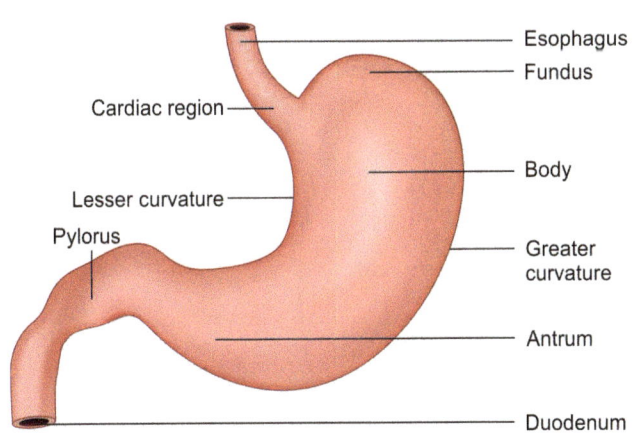

FIGURE 27.1: Parts of stomach.

3. Submucus layer formed by areolar tissue, blood vessels and lymph vessels.
4. Inner mucus layer lined by mucus-secreting columnar epithelial cells. Gastric glands are situated in this layer. Inner surface of mucus layer is covered by 2 mm thick **mucus**.

GLANDS OF STOMACH

Glands of the stomach or **gastric glands** are tubular structures made up of different types of cells. These glands open into the stomach cavity through **gastric pits**.

CLASSIFICATION OF GLANDS OF THE STOMACH

Gastric glands are classified into three types depending upon their situation:

A. Fundic glands situated in body and fundus of stomach.
B. Pyloric glands present in pyloric part of stomach.
C. Cardiac glands located in cardiac region of stomach.

STRUCTURE OF GASTRIC GLANDS

Fundic Glands

Fundic glands or **oxyntic glands** of the stomach are considered as typical gastric glands **(Fig. 27.2)**. These glands are long and tubular glands. Each fundic gland has three parts, viz. body, neck and isthmus.

Cells present in fundic glands

Fundic gland is formed by the following types of cell:

1. **Chief cells** or **pepsinogen cells**
2. Parietal cells or **oxyntic cells**
3. **Mucus neck cells**
4. **Enteroendocrine cells**
5. **Enterochromaffin cells** (EC cells) or **Kulchitsky cells**
6. **Enterochromaffin-like cells** (ECL cells)
7. Stem cells.

Stem cells divide and replace other cells in gastric glands. Secretory functions of other cells mentioned above are given in **Table 27.1**.

TABLE 27.1: Secretory functions of cells in gastric glands.

Cells	Secretory products
Chief cells or pepsinogen cells	Pepsinogen Rennin Lipase Gelatinase Urase
Parietal cells or oxyntic cells	Hydrochloric acid Intrinsic factor of Castle
Mucus neck cells	Mucin
Enterochromaffin (EC) cells	Serotonin
Enterochromaffin-like (ECL) cells	Histamine
Enteroendocrine cells	
G cells	Gastrin
D cells	Somatostatin
A cells	Glucagon
Ghrelin producing cells	Ghrelin
Unnamed cells	Vasoactive intestinal polypeptide

Vasoactive intestinal polypeptide is also secreted by nerve endings in stomach.

Parietal cells are different from other cells of the gland because of the presence of **canaliculi** (singular = canaliculus). Parietal cells empty their secretions into the lumen of the gland through the canaliculi. But other cells empty their secretions directly into lumen of the gland.

Pyloric Glands

Pyloric glands of stomach are short and tortuous in nature. Pyloric glands are formed by **G cells**, mucus cells, EC cells and ECL cells.

Cardiac Glands

Cardiac glands of the stomach are also short and tortuous in structure with many mucus cells. EC cells, ECL cells and chief cells are also present in the cardiac glands.

Enteroendocrine cells, enterochromaffin cells and enterochromaffin like cells

Enteroendocrine cells, enterochromaffin cells and enterochromaffin-like cells are the hormone-secreting cells present in glands or mucosa of gastrointestinal tract particularly stomach and intestine. Secretory functions of these types of cells in glands of the stomach are given in **Table 27.1**.

NERVE SUPPLY TO STOMACH

Stomach receives sympathetic fibers through **splanchnic nerve**. Parasympathetic fibers to stomach pass through branches of anterior and posterior **vagal trunks**.

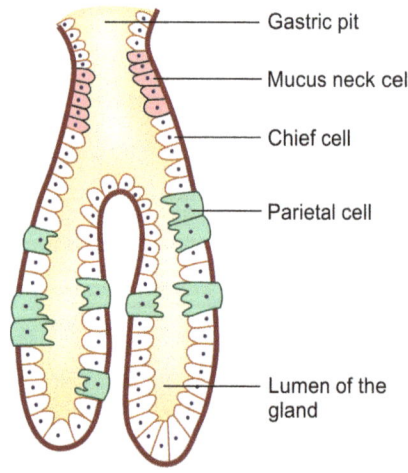

FIGURE 27.2: Gastric glands.

FUNCTIONS OF STOMACH

1. MECHANICAL FUNCTION

i. Storage Function

Food is stored in the stomach for a long period, i.e. for 3 to 4 hours and emptied into the intestine slowly. The maximum capacity of stomach is up to 1.5 L. Slow emptying of stomach provides enough time for proper digestion and absorption of food substances in the small intestine.

ii. Formation of Chyme

Peristaltic movements of stomach mix the bolus with gastric juice and convert it into the semisolid material known as chyme.

2. DIGESTIVE FUNCTION

Refer functions of gastric juice.

3. PROTECTIVE FUNCTION

Refer functions of gastric juice.

4. HEMOPOIETIC FUNCTION

Refer functions of gastric juice.

5. EXCRETORY FUNCTION

Many substances like toxins, alkaloids and metals are excreted through gastric juice.

PROPERTIES AND COMPOSITION OF GASTRIC JUICE

Gastric juice is the mixture of secretions from different gastric glands.

PROPERTIES OF GASTRIC JUICE

Volume : 1,200 to 1,500 mL/day
Specific gravity : 1.002 to 1.004
Reaction : Gastric juice is highly acidic with pH of 0.9 to 1.2 due to hydrochloric acid

COMPOSITION OF GASTRIC JUICE

Gastric juice contains 99.5% water and 0.5% solids. The solids are organic and inorganic substances. Refer **Figure 27.3** for composition of gastric juice.

FUNCTIONS OF GASTRIC JUICE

1. DIGESTIVE FUNCTION

Gastric juice acts mainly on proteins. **Proteolytic enzymes** of the gastric juice are pepsin and **rennin (Table 27.2)**. Gastric juice also contains some other enzymes like gastric lipase, gelatinase, urase and gastric amylase.

Pepsin

Pepsin is secreted as inactive **pepsinogen**. Pepsinogen is converted into pepsin by hydrochloric acid. Optimum pH for activation of pepsinogen is below 6.

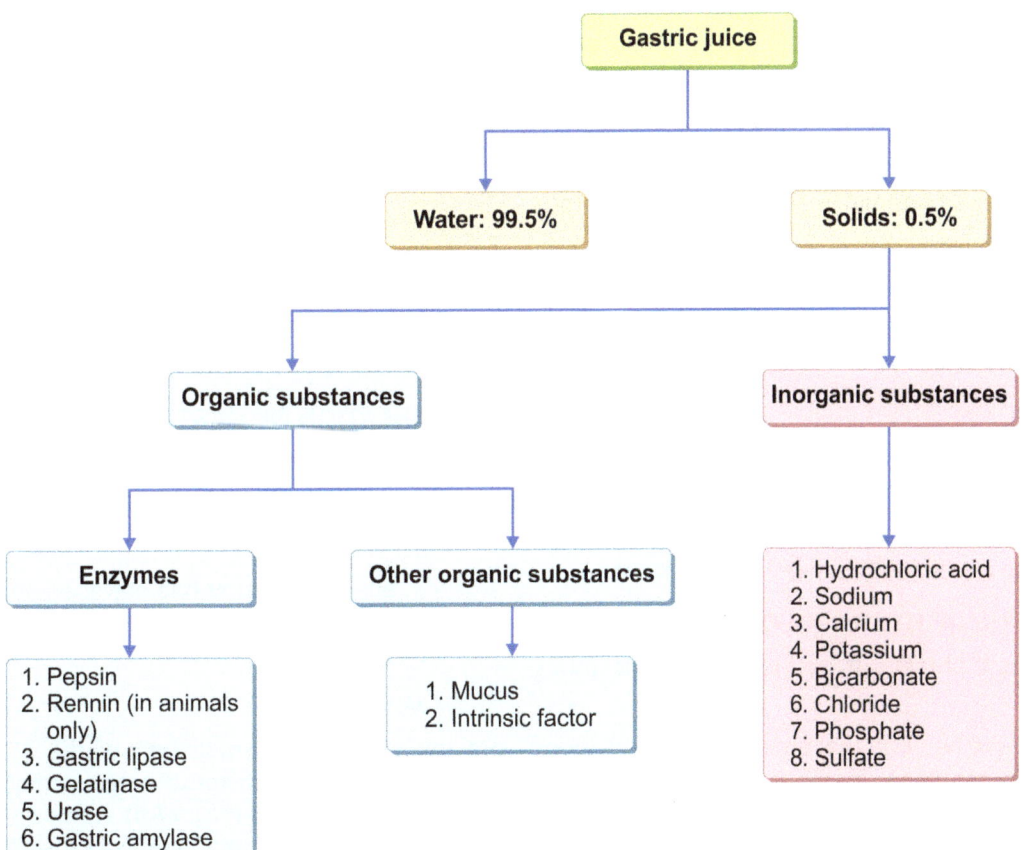

FIGURE 27.3: Composition of gastric juice.

TABLE 27.2: Digestive enzymes of gastric juice.

Enzyme	Activator	Substrate	End products
Pepsin	Hydrochloric acid	Proteins	Proteoses, peptones and polypeptides
Gastric lipase	Acid medium	Triglycerides of butter	Fatty acids and glycerols
Gastric amylase	Acid medium	Starch	Dextrin and maltose (negligible action)
Gelatinase	Acid medium	Gelatin and collagen of meat	Peptides
Urase	Acid medium	Urea	Ammonia

Pepsin converts proteins into proteoses, peptones and polypeptides. Pepsin also causes curdling and digestion of milk (**casein**).

Gastric Lipase

Gastric lipase is a weak **lipolytic enzyme**. To execute its action, gastric lipase needs acidic medium with a pH between 4 and 5. But it becomes inactive when the pH falls below 2.5. Gastric lipase acts on **tributyrin** (**butter fat**) and hydrolyzes it into fatty acids and glycerols.

Other Enzymes of Gastric Juice

i. Gelatinase: Degrades gelatin and collagen into peptides.
ii. Urase: Acts on urea and produces ammonia.
iii. Gastric amylase: Degrades starch (but its action is insignificant).
iv. Rennin: Curdles milk (present in animals only).

2. HEMOPOIETIC FUNCTION

Intrinsic factor of Castle secreted by parietal cells of gastric glands is necessary for absorption of vitamin B_{12} (which is called **extrinsic factor**) from GI tract into the blood. Vitamin B_{12} is an important maturation factor during erythropoiesis. Absence of intrinsic factor in gastric juice causes deficiency of vitamin B_{12} leading to **pernicious anemia** (Chapter 10).

3. PROTECTIVE FUNCTION: FUNCTION OF MUCUS

Mucus present in gastric juice protects gastric wall by the following functions.

i. It protects wall of the stomach from irritation or mechanical injury.
ii. It prevents the digestive action of pepsin on gastric mucosa.
iii. It protects the gastric mucosa from hydrochloric acid of gastric juice because of its alkaline nature.

4. FUNCTIONS OF HYDROCHLORIC ACID

Hydrochloric acid present in gastric juice has following functions:

i. HCl kills some bacteria that enter the stomach along with food substances.
ii. It activates pepsinogen into pepsin.
iii. HCl provides acid medium necessary for the action of hormones.

SECRETION OF GASTRIC JUICE
SECRETION OF PEPSINOGEN

Pepsinogen is synthesized from amino acids in the ribosomes in chief cells. Pepsinogen molecules are packed into **zymogen granules** by Golgi apparatus.

When zymogen granule is secreted into stomach from chief cells, the granule is dissolved and pepsinogen is released into gastric juice. Pepsinogen is activated into **pepsin** by hydrochloric acid.

SECRETION OF HYDROCHLORIC ACID

Hydrochloric acid secretion is an active process that takes place in the canaliculi of parietal cells in gastric glands.

In parietal cells, the carbon dioxide is formed from metabolic activity. It is also derived from blood. Carbon dioxide combines with water to form **carbonic acid** in the presence of **carbonic anhydrase**. This enzyme is present in high concentration in **parietal cells**. Carbonic acid is the most unstable compound and immediately it splits into hydrogen ion and bicarbonate ion. Hydrogen ion is actively pumped into the canaliculus of parietal cell.

Simultaneously, the chloride ion is also pumped into canaliculus actively. Chloride is derived from sodium chloride in the blood. Now, the hydrogen ion combines with chloride ion to form hydrochloric acid. To compensate the loss of chloride ion, bicarbonate ion from parietal cell enters the blood and combines with sodium to form sodium bicarbonate. Thus, the entire process is summarized as (**Fig. 27.4**):

$$CO_2 + H_2O + NaCl \longrightarrow HCl + NaHCO_3$$

REGULATION OF GASTRIC SECRETION

Regulation of gastric secretion and intestinal secretion is studied by some experimental procedures.

METHODS OF STUDY

Russian scientist **Pavlov** has designed some methods in dogs during his studies on conditioned reflexes. Important methods followed by Pavlov are:

1. Pavlov Pouch

Pavlov pouch is a small part of the stomach that is incompletely separated from the main portion and made into a small bag-like pouch (**Fig. 27.5**). A small part of muscular coat called isthmus is retained. Isthmus connects the two parts. Pavlov pouch receives parasympathetic (vagus)

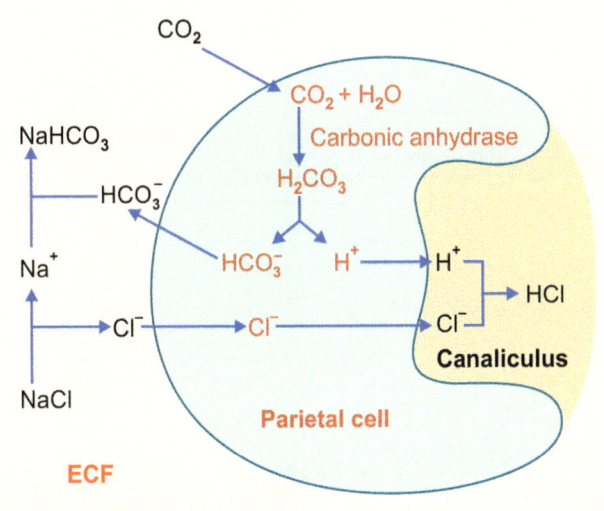

FIGURE 27.4: Secretion of hydrochloric acid in parietal cell of gastric gland.

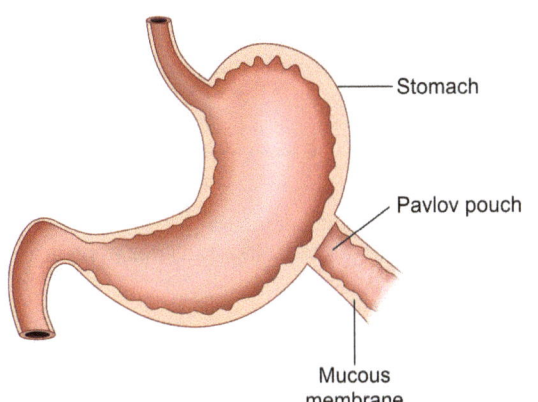

FIGURE 27.5: Pavlov pouch.

nerve fibers through isthmus and sympathetic fibers through blood vessels.

Use of Pavlov pouch

Pavlov pouch is used to demonstrate the different phases of gastric secretion particularly the cephalic phase and used to demonstrate the role of vagus in cephalic phase.

2. Farrell and Ivy Pouch

Farrell and Ivy pouch is prepared by removing the part of Pavlov pouch from the stomach and transplanting it in the subcutaneous tissue of abdominal wall or thoracic wall in the same animal. It is used for experimental purpose, when the new blood vessels are developed.

Uses of Farrell and Ivy pouch

This pouch is useful to study the role of hormones during gastric and intestinal phases of gastric secretion.

3. Sham Feeding

Sham feeding means the false feeding. It is another experimental procedure devised by Pavlov to demonstrate the regulation of gastric secretion.

A hole is made in the neck of an anesthetized dog. Esophagus is transversely cut. The cut ends are drawn out through the hole in the neck. When the dog eats food, it comes out through the cut end of the esophagus. But the dog has the satisfaction of eating the food. It is called sham feeding.

This experimental procedure is supported by the preparation of Pavlov pouch with a fistula from the stomach. The fistula opens to the exterior and it is used to observe the gastric secretion.

Uses of Sham feeding

Sham feeding is useful to demonstrate the secretion of gastric juice during cephalic phase. In the same animal after vagotomy, sham feeding does not induce gastric secretion and this proves the role of vagus nerve during cephalic phase.

■ PHASES OF GASTRIC SECRETION

Gastric juice is secreted in three different phases:

I. Cephalic phase.
II. Gastric phase.
III. Intestinal phase.

In human beings, a fourth phase called interdigestive phase exists. All the phases are regulated by neural mechanism or hormonal mechanism or both.

■ CEPHALIC PHASE

Secretion of gastric juice by the stimuli arising from head region (**cephalus**) is called cephalic phase (**Fig. 27.6**). This phase is regulated by nervous mechanism. During this phase 30% of total amount of gastric juice is secreted.

During this phase, gastric secretion occurs even without the presence of food in the stomach. Quantity of the juice is less but it is rich in enzymes and hydrochloric acid. The nervous mechanism that regulates cephalic phase operates through reflex action.

Two types of reflexes occur, namely unconditioned reflex and conditioned reflex.

Unconditioned Reflex

Unconditioned reflex is the inborn reflex. When food is placed in the mouth, it induces salivary secretion (Chapter 26). Simultaneously, gastric secretion also occurs. This is experimentally proved by Pavlov pouch and sham feeding.

Conditioned Reflex

Conditioned reflex is the reflex acquired by previous experience (Chapter 90). Presence of food in the mouth is not necessary to elicit this reflex. Sight, smell, hearing or thought of food which induce salivary secretion also induce gastric secretion. Conditioned reflex of gastric secretion is proved by Pavlov pouch and bell dog experiment (Chapter 90).

■ GASTRIC PHASE

Secretion of gastric juice when food enters the stomach is called gastric phase. This phase is regulated by both

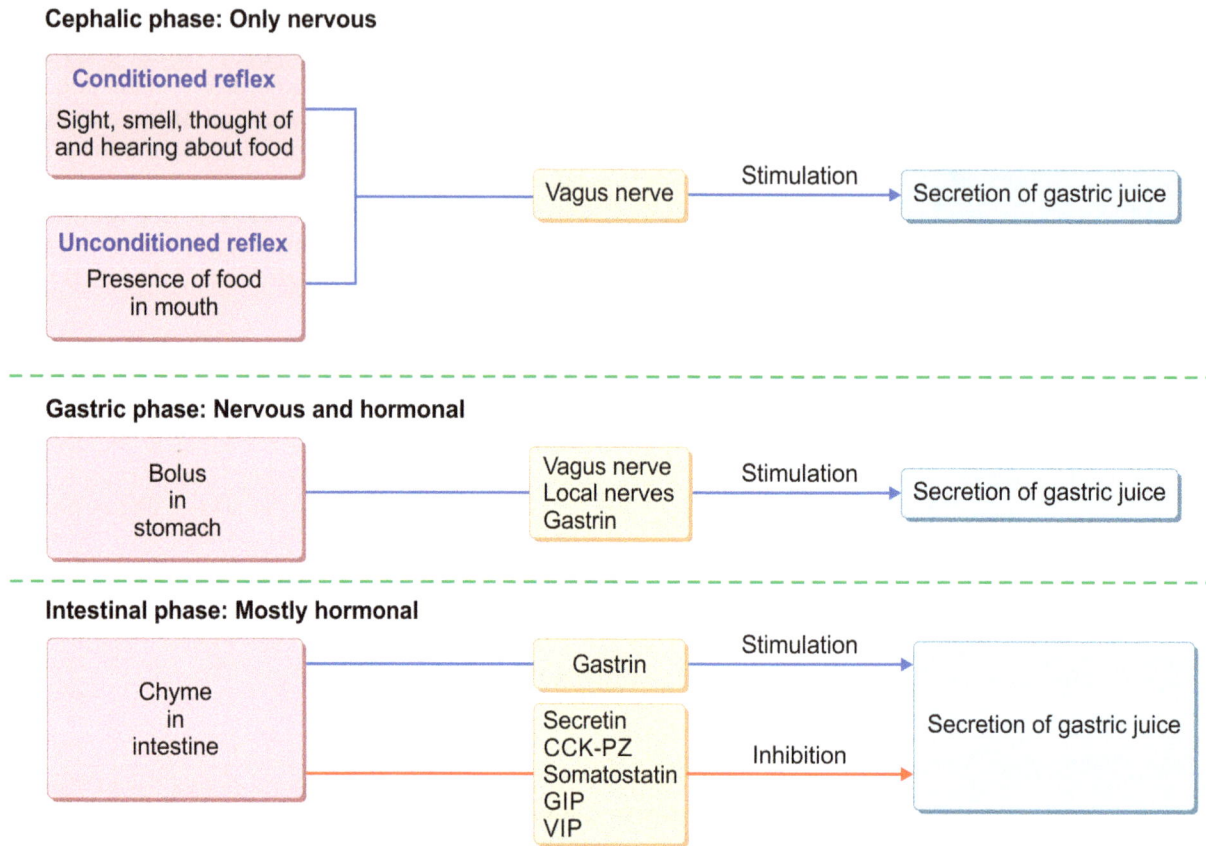

FIGURE 27.6: Schematic diagram showing the regulation of gastric secretion. CCK-PZ = Cholecystokinin-pancreozymin. GIP = Gastric inhibitory peptide. VIP = Vasoactive intestinal peptide.

nervous and hormonal mechanisms. Gastric juice secreted during this phase is rich in pepsinogen and hydrochloric acid. During gastric phase 60% of total amount of gastric juice is secreted.

Mechanisms involved in this phase are nervous mechanism and hormonal mechanism.

1. Nervous Mechanism

Nervous mechanism controls the secretion during gastric phase through local myenteric reflex and vagovagal reflex.

Local myenteric reflex

After entering stomach, food particles stimulate the local nerve plexus (Chapter 25) present in the wall of the stomach. These nerve fibers release acetylcholine which stimulates the gastric glands to secrete a large quantity of gastric juice. It also stimulates **G cells** to secrete gastrin (see below).

Vagovagal reflex

Vagovagal reflex is the reflex in which both afferent and efferent vagal fibers are involved. Presence of food in stomach stimulates the sensory (afferent) nerve endings of vagus which generate sensory impulses. These sensory impulses are transmitted to the brainstem via sensory fibers of vagus. Brainstem in turn sends efferent impulses through the motor (efferent) fibers of vagus back to stomach and cause secretion of gastric juice. Since, both afferent and efferent impulses pass through vagus, this reflex is called vagovagal reflex.

Nervous mechanism of gastric secretion during gastric phase is proved by Pavlov pouch.

2. Hormonal Mechanism: Gastrin

Gastrin is released when food enters stomach. Gastrin is a gastrointestinal hormone secreted by the G cells of pyloric glands of stomach. Gastrin stimulates the secretion of pepsinogen and hydrochloric acid by the gastric glands.

Hormonal mechanism of gastric secretion is proved by Farrell and Ivy pouch.

■ INTESTINAL PHASE

When chyme enters the intestine initially gastric secretion increases and later it stops. Intestinal phase of gastric secretion is under both nervous and hormonal control. Intestinal phase of gastric secretion is demonstrated by Farrell and Ivy pouch.

Initial Stage of Intestinal Phase

Chyme entering intestine stimulates the duodenal mucosa to release gastrin which is transported to stomach through blood. Gastrin increases gastric secretion. During this phase 10% of total amount of gastric juice is secreted.

Later Stage of Intestinal Phase

After the initial increase, there is decrease or complete stoppage of secretion of gastric juice.

Two factors are responsible for the inhibition viz, enterogastric reflex and **gastrointestinal hormones** (GI hormones).

1. Enterogastric reflex

It is a reflex that inhibits the secretion and movements of stomach due to distention or irritation of intestinal mucosa. It is mediated by myenteric nerve (Auerbach's) plexus and vagus.

2. GI hormones

Presence of chyme in intestine stimulates the secretion of many GI hormones. All these hormones inhibit the gastric secretion.

GI hormones which inhibit gastric secretion:

  i. Secretin.
  ii. Cholecystokinin.
  iii. Gastric inhibitory peptide (GIP).
  iv. Vasoactive intestinal polypeptide (VIP)
  v. Peptide YY.
  vi. Pancreatic somatostatin.

■ INTERDIGESTIVE PHASE

Secretion of small amount of gastric juice in between meals (or during period of fasting) is called interdigestive phase. Gastric secretion during this phase is due to gastrin. This phase of gastric secretion is demonstrated by Farrell and Ivy pouch.

■ COLLECTION OF GASTRIC JUICE

In human beings, gastric juice is collected by using **Ryle tube.** This tube is made out of rubber or plastic. It is passed through nostril or mouth and through esophagus into the stomach. A line is marked in the tube. Entrance of the tip of the tube into stomach is indicated when this line comes near the mouth. Then, the contents of stomach are collected by means of aspiration

■ GASTRIC FUNCTION TESTS: GASTRIC ANALYSIS

For analysis, gastric juice is collected from patient only in the morning. Analysis of the gastric juice is done for the diagnosis of ulcer and other disorders of stomach.

Gastric juice is analyzed for the following:

1. Measurement of **peptic activity**.
2. Measurement of **gastric acidity**: Total acid, free acid (hydrochloric acid) and combined acid.

Fractional Test Meal (FTM): Fractional Gastric Analysis

Fractional gastric analysis is the common method of gastric analysis. It is carried out with fractional test meal.

After overnight fasting, gastric juice is collected. Then, the patient takes a small test meal called fractional test meal. After the ingestion of a test meal, gastric juice is collected at every 15th minute for a period of 2½ hours. All these samples are analyzed for peptic activity and acidity.

■ APPLIED PHYSIOLOGY: GASTRIC DISORDERS
■ 1. GASTRITIS

Inflammation of gastric mucosa is called gastritis. It may be acute or chronic. Common causes of gastritis are infection, alcohol, long-term use of **non-steroidal anti-inflammatory drugs** (NSAIDs) and autoimmune disease.

Common Features of Gastritis

  i. Abdominal upset or pain.
  ii. Nausea and vomiting.
  iii. **Anorexia** (loss of appetite).
  iv. Indigestion.
  v. **Belching** (process to relieve swallowed air that is accumulated in stomach).

■ 2. GASTRIC ATROPHY

Gastric atrophy is the condition in which muscles of the stomach shrink and become weak. Gastric glands also shrink resulting in the deficiency of gastric juice. Gastric atrophy is caused by chronic gastritis and autoimmune disease.

Features of Gastric Atrophy

Gastric atrophy causes **achlorhydria** (absence of hydrochloric acid in gastric juice) and pernicious anemia. Some patients develop **gastric cancer**.

■ 3. PEPTIC ULCER

Ulcer means erosion of the surface of any organ due to shedding or sloughing of inflamed necrotic tissue that lines the organ. Peptic ulcer means an ulcer in the wall of stomach or duodenum caused by digestive action of gastric juice. If peptic ulcer is found in stomach, it is called **gastric ulcer** and if found in duodenum it is called **duodenal ulcer**.

Common Causes of Peptic Ulcer

  i. Increased peptic activity.
  ii. Hyperacidity of gastric juice.
  iii. Reduced alkalinity of duodenal content.
  iv. Decreased mucin content in gastric juice.
  v. Stress.
  vi. Food with excess spices or smoking.
  vii. Long-term use of NSAIDs (see above).
  viii. Chronic inflammation of stomach wall by *Helicobacter pylori*.

Features of Peptic Ulcer

Most common feature of peptic ulcer is severe burning pain in epigastric region. In gastric ulcer, pain occurs while eating or drinking. In duodenal ulcer, pain is felt 1 or 2 hours after food intake and during night.

Other symptoms of peptic ulcer accompanying pain sensation are:

 i. Nausea.
 ii. Vomiting.
 iii. **Hematemesis** (vomiting blood).
 iv. **Heartburn** (burning pain in chest due to regurgitation of acid from stomach into esophagus).
 v. **Anorexia** (loss of appetite).
 vi. Loss of weight.

■ 4. ZOLLINGER-ELLISON SYNDROME

Zollinger-Ellison syndrome is a gastric disorder characterized by secretion of excess hydrochloric acid in the stomach. It is caused by **pancreatic tumor** which produces a large quantity of gastrin. Gastrin increases the hydrochloric acid secretion in stomach by stimulating the parietal cells.

Common features of this syndrome are abdominal pain, **diarrhea** (frequent and watery, loose bowel movements) and difficulty in eating.

Chapter 28

Pancreas and Pancreatic Secretion

CHAPTER OUTLINE

- DUAL FUNCTIONS OF PANCREAS
- FUNCTIONAL ANATOMY OF EXOCRINE PART OF PANCREAS
- NERVE SUPPLY TO PANCREAS
- PROPERTIES AND COMPOSITION OF PANCREATIC JUICE
- FUNCTIONS OF PANCREATIC JUICE
- REGULATION OF PANCREATIC SECRETION
- COLLECTION OF PANCREATIC JUICE
- PANCREATIC EXOCRINE FUNCTION TESTS
- APPLIED PHYSIOLOGY: DISORDERS OF PANCREAS

■ DUAL FUNCTIONS OF PANCREAS

Pancreas is a dual organ having two functions namely endocrine function and exocrine function. **Endocrine function** is concerned with production of the hormones. Refer Chapter 47 for details. **Exocrine function** is concerned with secretion of digestive juice called pancreatic juice and it is explained in this chapter.

■ FUNCTIONAL ANATOMY OF EXOCRINE PART OF PANCREAS

Exocrine part of pancreas is made up of **acini** or **alveoli** like salivary glands. Each acinus has a single layer of acinar cells with a lumen in the center. **Acinar cells** contain **zymogen granules**, which possess digestive enzymes.

Duct System in Pancreas

A small duct arises from lumen of each alveolus. Some of these ducts from neighboring alveoli unite to form **intralobular duct**. All the intralobular ducts unite to form the main pancreatic duct or **Wirsung's duct**. Pancreatic duct joins **common bile duct** to form **ampulla of Vater**, which opens into duodenum (Refer **Fig. 29.3**).

■ NERVE SUPPLY TO PANCREAS

Pancreas is supplied by both sympathetic and parasympathetic nerve fibers. Sympathetic nerve fibers are supplied through **splanchnic nerve** and parasympathetic nerve fibers are supplied through **vagus nerve**.

■ PROPERTIES AND COMPOSITION OF PANCREATIC JUICE

■ PROPERTIES OF PANCREATIC JUICE

Volume : 500 to 800 mL/day
Reaction : Highly alkaline with pH of 8 to 8.3
Specific gravity : 1.010 to 1.018

■ COMPOSITION OF PANCREATIC JUICE

Pancreatic juice contains 99.5% of water and 0.5% of solids. Solids are the organic and inorganic substances. Composition of pancreatic juice is given in **Figure 28.1**.

Bicarbonate content is very high in pancreatic juice. It is about 110 to 150 mEq/L. This high concentration of **bicarbonate** is responsible for the **alkalinity** of pancreatic juice.

■ FUNCTIONS OF PANCREATIC JUICE

Pancreatic juice has digestive functions and neutralizing action.

■ DIGESTIVE FUNCTIONS OF PANCREATIC JUICE

Pancreatic juice plays an important role in the digestion of proteins and lipids. It also has mild action on carbohydrate digestion.

■ DIGESTION OF PROTEINS

Major **proteolytic enzymes** of pancreatic juice are trypsin and chymotrypsin. Other proteolytic enzymes are carboxypeptidases, nuclease, elastase and collagenase.

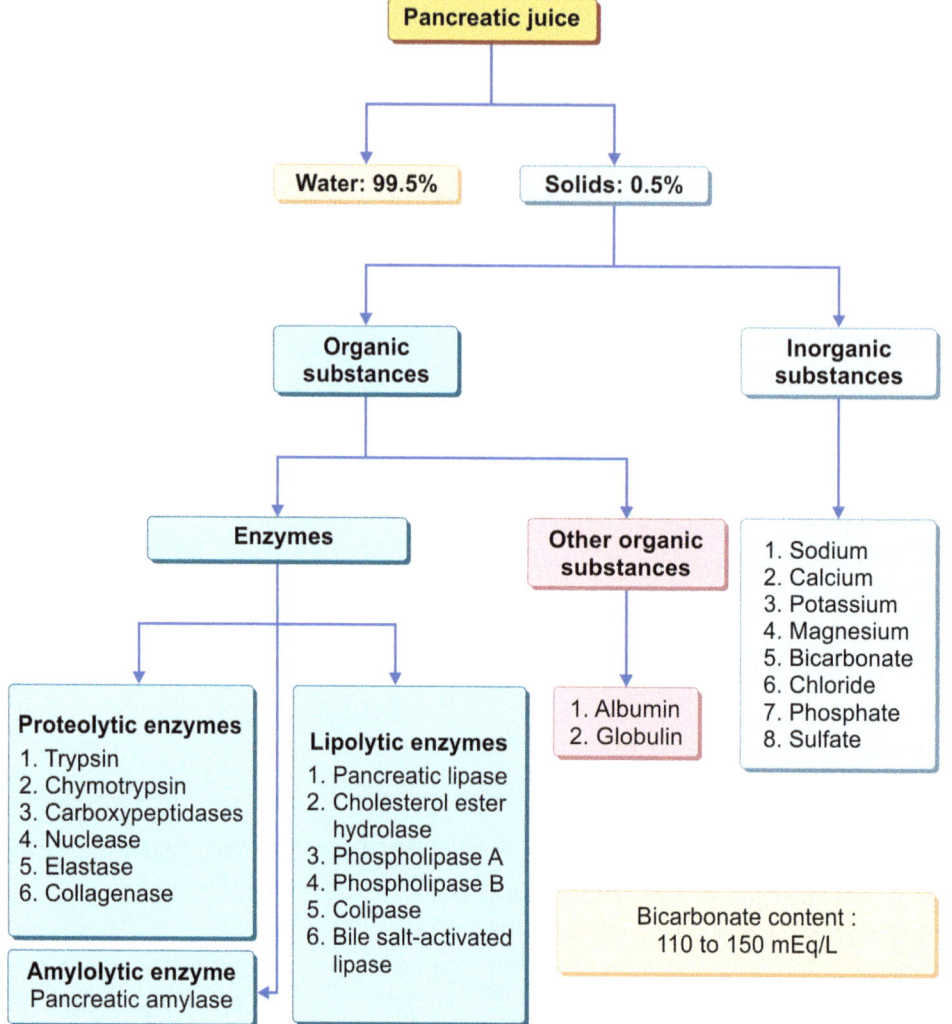

FIGURE 28.1: Composition of pancreatic juice.

1. Trypsin

Trypsin is a single polypeptide with a molecular weight of 25,000. It contains 229 amino acids.

It is secreted as inactive **trypsinogen** which is converted into active trypsin by **enterokinase**. Enterokinase or **enteropeptidase** is secreted in duodenum.

Actions of trypsin

i. *Digestion of proteins*: Trypsin is the most powerful **proteolytic enzyme**. It is an **endopeptidase** and breaks the interior bonds of protein molecules. And it converts proteins into proteoses and polypeptides.
ii. *Curdling of milk*: It converts **caseinogens** in the milk into casein.
iii. It accelerates blood clotting.
iv. It activates other enzymes of pancreatic juice:
    a. Chymotrypsinogen into chymotrypsin.
    b. Procarboxypeptidases into carboxypeptidases.
    c. Proelastase into elastase.
    d. Procolipase into colipase.

Trypsin also activates collagenase, phospholipase A and phospholipase B.

Autocatalytic or autoactive action of Trypsin

Once formed trypsin itself converts trypsinogen into trypsin. This action is called autocatalytic or autoactive action.

2. Chymotrypsin

Chymotrypsin is a polypeptide with a molecular weight of 25,700 and 246 amino acids. It is secreted as inactive **chymotrypsinogen** and activated into chymotrypsin by trypsin.

Actions of chymotrypsin

i. *Digestion of proteins*: Chymotrypsin is also an **endopeptidase** and it breaks the proteins into polypeptides.
ii. *Digestion of milk*: Chymotrypsin digests casein faster than trypsin.

3. Carboxypeptidases

Carboxypeptidases are carboxypeptidase A and carboxypeptidase B. These two enzymes are secreted as procarboxypeptidase A and procarboxypeptidase

B. Inactive **procarboxypeptidases** are activated into carboxypeptidases by trypsin.

Actions of carboxypeptidases

Carboxypeptidases are **exopeptidases** and split the polypeptides and other proteins into amino acids.

4. Nucleases

Nucleases of pancreatic juice are ribonuclease and deoxyribonuclease, which are responsible for the digestion of nucleic acids. These enzymes convert the ribonucleic acid (RNA) and deoxyribonucleic acid (DNA) into mononucleotides.

5. Elastase

Elastase is secreted as inactive **proelastase** and is activated into active elastase by trypsin. It digests the elastic fibers.

6. Collagenase

Collagenase is secreted as inactive **procollagenase** and is activated into active collagenase by trypsin. It digests collagen.

■ DIGESTION OF LIPIDS

Lipolytic enzymes present in pancreatic juice are pancreatic lipase, cholesterol ester hydrolase, phospholipase A, phospholipase B and a coenzyme called colipase.

1. Pancreatic Lipase

Pancreatic lipase is a powerful **lipolytic enzyme**. It digests the triglycerides into monoglycerides and fatty acids. Activity of pancreatic lipase is accelerated in the presence of bile. Optimum pH required for activity of this enzyme is 7 to 9.

2. Cholesterol Ester Hydrolase

Cholesterol ester hydrolase or cholesterol esterase converts cholesterol ester into free cholesterol and fatty acid by hydrolysis.

3. Phospholipase A

It is activated by trypsin. Phospholipase A digests phospholipids namely **lecithin** and **cephalin** and converts them into **lysolecithin** and **lysocephalin** respectively.

4. Phospholipase B

Phospholipase B is also activated by trypsin. This enzyme converts lysolecithin and lysocephalin into **phosphorylcholine** and free fatty acids.

5. Colipase

Colipase is a small **coenzyme**, which facilitates the hydrolysis of fats by pancreatic lipase.

6. Bile Salt-activated Lipase

This enzyme has a weak lipolytic action. It digests a variety of lipids like phospholipids, cholesterol esters and triglycerides. Since it is activated bile salt it is known as bile salt-activated lipase **(Table 28.1)**.

■ DIGESTION OF CARBOHYDRATES

Pancreatic amylase is the **amylolytic enzyme** present in pancreatic juice. Like salivary amylase, the pancreatic amylase also converts **starch** into dextrin and maltose.

■ NEUTRALIZING ACTION OF PANCREATIC JUICE

When acid chyme enters intestine from stomach, pancreatic juice with large quantity of bicarbonate is released into intestine. Presence of large quantity of **bicarbonate ions** makes the pancreatic juice highly alkaline. This alkaline pancreatic juice neutralizes acidity of chyme in the intestine.

Neutralizing action is an important function of pancreatic juice, because it protects the intestine from the destructive action of acid in the chyme.

■ REGULATION OF PANCREATIC SECRETION

Pancreatic secretion occurs in three stages:

  I. Cephalic phase.
  II. Gastric phase.
  III. Intestinal phase.

Each phase is regulated by nervous mechanism or hormonal mechanism or both.

■ CEPHALIC PHASE

As in case of gastric secretion, cephalic phase of pancreatic secretion is regulated by nervous mechanism through **reflex action**. During this phase, 20% of total amount pancreatic juice is secreted. Two types of reflexes occur.

1. Unconditioned Reflex

Unconditioned reflex is the inborn reflex. When food is placed in the mouth, it induces salivary secretion (Chapter 26), gastric secretion (Chapter 27). Simultaneously it induces pancreatic secretion also.

2. Conditioned Reflex

Conditioned reflex is the reflex response acquired by previous experience (Chapter 90). Presence of food in the mouth is not necessary to elicit this reflex. Sight, smell, hearing or thought of food which induce salivary secretion and gastric secretion also induces pancreatic secretion **(Fig. 28.2)**.

■ GASTRIC PHASE

Secretion of pancreatic juice when food enters the stomach is known as gastric phase. This phase of pancreatic secretion is under **hormonal control**. Hormone involved is **gastrin**.

When food enters stomach, gastrin is secreted from stomach (Chapter 27). When gastrin is transported to pancreas through blood, it stimulates the pancreatic secretion. Pancreatic juice secreted during gastric phase is **rich in enzymes**. During gastric phase, only 10% of pancreatic juice is secreted.

TABLE 28.1: Digestive enzymes of pancreatic juice.

Enzyme	Activator	Acts on (substrate)	End products
Trypsin	Enterokinase Trypsin	Proteins	Proteoses Polypeptides
Chymotrypsin	Trypsin	Proteins	Polypeptides
Carboxypeptidases	Trypsin	Polypeptides	Amino acids
Nucleases	Trypsin	RNA and DNA	Mononucleotides
Elastase	Trypsin	Elastin	Amino acids
Collagenase	Trypsin	Collagen	Amino acids
Pancreatic lipase	Alkaline medium	Triglycerides	Monoglycerides Fatty acids
Cholesterol ester hydrolase	Alkaline medium	Cholesterol ester	Cholesterol Fatty acids
Phospholipase A	Trypsin	Phospholipids	Lysophospholipids
Phospholipase B	Trypsin	Lysophospholipids	Phosphorylcholine Free fatty acids
Colipase	Trypsin	Facilitates action of pancreatic lipase	-
Bile salt-activated lipase	Bile salt	Phospholipids	Lysophospholipids
		Cholesterol esters	Cholesterol Fatty acids
		Triglycerides	Monoglycerides Fatty acids
Pancreatic amylase	Acid medium	Starch	Dextrin Maltose

■ INTESTINAL PHASE

Intestinal phase is the secretion of pancreatic juice when the chyme enters the intestine. This phase is also under **hormonal control**. In this phase, 70% of total amount of pancreatic juice is secreted.

When **chyme** enters the intestine, many hormones are released. Some hormones stimulate the pancreatic secretion and some hormones inhibit the pancreatic secretion.

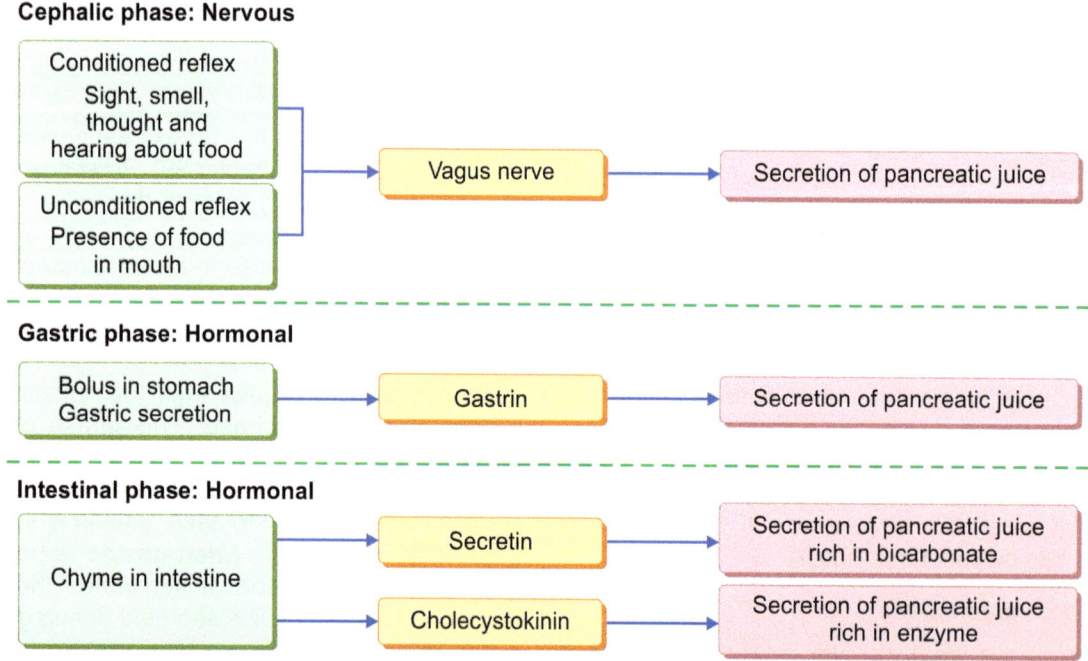

FIGURE 28.2: Schematic diagram showing the regulation of pancreatic secretion.

Hormones Stimulating Pancreatic Secretion

1. Secretin

Secretin is produced by **S cells** of mucous membrane in duodenum and jejunum. It is produced in an inactive **prosecretin** which is activated into secretin by acid chyme.

Secretin stimulates the secretion of watery pancreatic juice which contains high concentration of **bicarbonate** ion.

2. Cholecystokinin

Cholecystokinin (CCK) is also called **cholecystokinin-pancreozymin** (CCK-PZ). It is secreted by **I cells** in duodenal and jejunal mucosa.

Cholecystokinin stimulates the secretion of pancreatic juice which is rich in enzyme and less in volume.

Hormones Inhibiting Pancreatic Secretion

1. **Pancreatic polypeptide** secreted by **PP cells** in islets of Langerhans of pancreas.
2. **Somatostatin** secreted by **D cells** in islets of Langerhans of pancreas.
3. **Peptide YY** secreted by intestinal mucosa.
4. Peptides such as **ghrelin** and **leptin**.

■ COLLECTION OF PANCREATIC JUICE

Pancreatic juice is collected by a **multilumen tube**. This tube is inserted through nose or mouth, till tip of the tube reaches intestine near the **ampulla of Vater**. The tube has a marking. Entrance of the tip of tube into the intestine near the ampulla is indicated when this line comes near mouth.

This tube has three lumens. Small balloons are attached to the two outer lumens. When balloons are inflated by air, the intestine near the ampulla is enlarged. Now, the pancreatic juice is collected through the middle lumen by means of aspiration.

■ PANCREATIC EXOCRINE FUNCTION TESTS

1. Blood tests:
    i. Amylase test.
    ii. Serum lipase test.
2. Lundh test: After giving a test meal, duodenal content is aspirated and tested for trypsin activity.
3. Stool tests.

■ APPLIED PHYSIOLOGY: DISORDERS OF PANCREAS

■ PANCREATITIS

Pancreatitis is the inflammation of pancreatic acini resulting in absence of pancreatic enzymes. Common causes of pancreatitis are long-time consumption of alcohol, congenital abnormalities of pancreatic duct and **malnutrition** (poor nutrition).

Features of Pancreatitis

1. Steatorrhea.
2. Severe abdominal pain.
3. Nausea and vomiting.
4. Loss of appetite and weight.
5. Fever.
6. Shock.

■ STEATORRHEA

Steatorrhea is the formation of bulky, foul smelling, frothy and clay colored stools with large quantity of undigested fat because of impaired digestion and absorption of fat.

Causes of Steatorrhea

1. Lack of pancreatic lipase.
2. Liver disease affecting secretion of bile.
3. **Celiac disease:** Autoimmune disease characterized by damage of villi in small intestine. It is caused by gluten intake.
4. **Cystic fibrosis:** Genetic disorder affecting the functions of many organs such as lungs, pancreas and biliary system and immune system. It is characterized by production of abnormal thick secretions which impair the functions of organs particularly lungs and pancreas.

Chapter 29

Liver and Biliary System

CHAPTER OUTLINE

- DUAL FUNCTIONS OF LIVER
- FUNCTIONAL ANATOMY OF LIVER AND BILIARY SYSTEM
- BLOOD SUPPLY TO LIVER
- NERVE SUPPLY TO LIVER
- PROPERTIES AND COMPOSITION OF BILE
- SECRETION OF BILE
- STORAGE OF BILE
- BILE SALTS
- BILE PIGMENTS
- FUNCTIONS OF BILE
- FUNCTIONS OF LIVER
- GALLBLADDER
- REGULATION OF BILE SECRETION
- LIVER FUNCTION TESTS
- APPLIED PHYSIOLOGY: DISORDERS OF LIVER AND GALLBLADDER

■ DUAL FUNCTIONS OF LIVER

Liver is a dual organ having dual functions. It has both secretory and excretory functions.

■ FUNCTIONAL ANATOMY OF LIVER AND BILIARY SYSTEM

■ LIVER

Liver is the largest gland in the body weighing about 1.5 kg in man. It is situated in upper and right side of the abdominal cavity immediately beneath diaphragm.

Liver is made up of many lobes called **hepatic lobes** (Fig. 29.1). Each lobe consists of many lobules called **hepatic lobules**.

Hepatic lobule is the structural and functional unit of liver. It is a honeycomb-like structure and it is made up of liver cells called **hepatocytes**. Hepatocytes are arranged in **hepatic plates**. Each plate is made up of two columns of cells. In between the two columns of each plate lies a **bile canaliculus (Fig. 29.2)**.

In between the neighboring plates, a blood space called **sinusoid** is present. Sinusoid is lined by the endothelial cells. In between the endothelial cells, macrophages called **Kupffer cells** are present.

Portal Triads

Each hepatic lobule is surrounded by many portal triads.

Each portal triad consists of three vessels:

1. A branch of hepatic artery.
2. A branch of portal vein.
3. A tributary of bile duct.

Branches of hepatic artery and portal vein open into the sinusoid. Sinusoid opens into the central vein. Central vein empties into hepatic vein. Bile is secreted by hepatic cells and emptied into **bile canaliculus**. From canaliculus, the bile enters the tributary of bile duct.

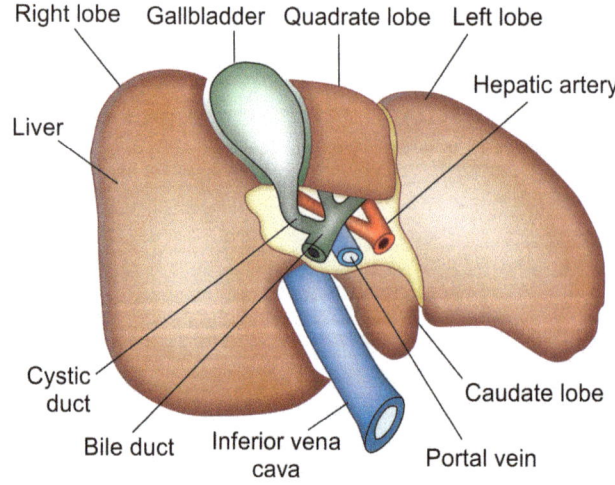

FIGURE 29.1: Posterior surface of liver.

Chapter 29: Liver and Biliary System   131

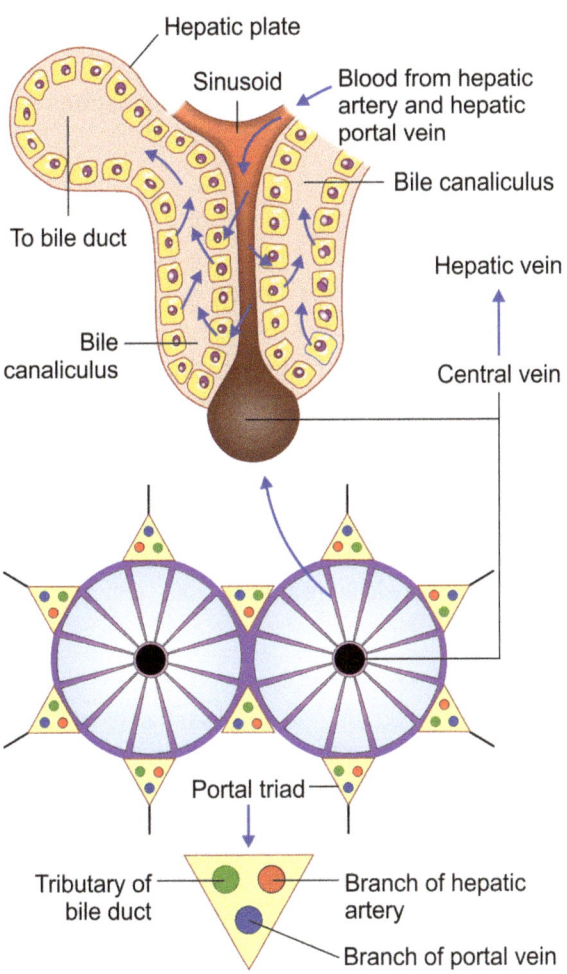

FIGURE 29.2: Hepatic lobule.

Tributaries of bile duct from canaliculi of neighboring lobules unite to form small **bile ducts**. These small bile ducts join together and finally form left and right **hepatic ducts** which emerge out of liver.

■ BILIARY SYSTEM

Biliary system or **extrahepatic biliary apparatus** is formed by gallbladder and the extrahepatic bile ducts (bile ducts outside the liver). Right and left hepatic bile ducts which come out of liver join to form **common hepatic duct**. It unites with the **cystic duct** from gallbladder to form **common bile duct (Fig. 29.3)**.

Common bile duct unites with pancreatic duct to form the common hepatopancreatic duct or **ampulla of Vater** which opens into the duodenum. There is a sphincter called **sphincter of Oddi** at the lower part of common bile duct, before it joins the pancreatic duct. It is formed by smooth muscle fibers of common bile duct.

■ BLOOD SUPPLY TO LIVER

Liver receives the maximum blood supply of about 1,500 mL/min. It receives blood from two sources, namely the hepatic artery and portal vein.

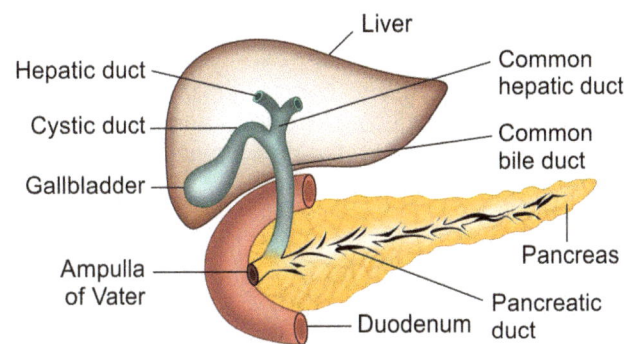

FIGURE 29.3: Biliary system.

■ HEPATIC ARTERY

Hepatic artery arises directly from aorta and supplies **oxygenated blood** to liver.

■ HEPATIC PORTAL VEIN

Hepatic portal vein is formed by superior mesenteric vein and splenic vein. It brings **deoxygenated blood** from stomach, intestine, spleen and pancreas to liver. Blood from hepatic artery mixes with the blood from portal vein in the hepatic sinusoids. Hepatic cells obtain oxygen and nutrients from the sinusoid.

■ HEPATIC VEIN

Venous drainage from liver is through right and left hepatic veins which open into inferior vena cava.

■ ENTEROHEPATIC CIRCULAITON

Enterohepatic circulation is the circulation of substances such as bile salts and bilirubin that are absorbed from intestine and transported to liver through hepatic portal vein. These substances are excreted or secreted in bile and enter intestine again **(Fig. 29.4)**.

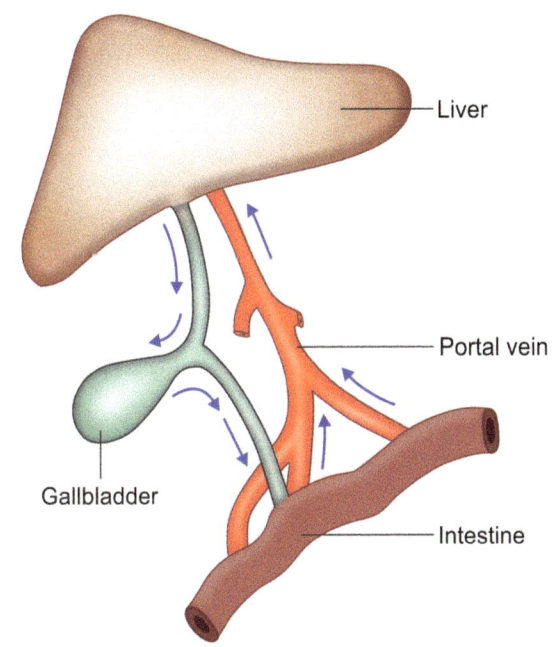

FIGURE 29.4: Enterohepatic circulation.

Significance of Enterohepatic Circulation

Enterohepatic circulation is responsible for recycling of both metabolized and nonmetabolized substances. Many substances including **bile salts** and **bile pigments** that are secreted or excreted by liver into small intestine through bile are brought back to liver via enterohepatic circulation.

■ NERVE SUPPLY TO LIVER

Parenchyma of liver is supplied by sympathetic fibers from **celiac plexus** and parasympathetic fibers anterior and posterior trunks of **vagus**.

■ PROPERTIES AND COMPOSITION OF BILE

Bile is a golden yellow or greenish fluid. It enters the digestive tract along with pancreatic juice through ampulla of Vater.

Properties of Bile

Volume : 800 to 1,200 mL/day
Reaction : Alkaline
pH : 8 to 8.6
Specific gravity : 1.010 to 1.011

Composition of Bile

Bile contains 97.6% of water and 2.4% of solids. Solids include organic and inorganic substances. Refer **Figure 29.5** for details.

■ SECRETION OF BILE

Bile is secreted by **hepatocytes**. Initial bile secreted by hepatocytes contains large quantity of bile acids, bile pigments, cholesterol, lecithin and fatty acids. From hepatocytes, bile passes through canaliculi and hepatic ducts to reach common hepatic duct. From here it may enter the intestine or gallbladder.

■ STORAGE OF BILE

Most of the bile from liver enters the gallbladder where it is stored. It is released from gallbladder into the intestine whenever it is required.

Changes Taking Place in Bile during Storage at Gallbladder

When bile is stored in gallbladder, it undergoes many changes both in quality and quantity such as:

1. Volume is reduced because of absorption of large amount of water and electrolytes (except calcium and potassium).
2. Concentration of bile salts, bile pigments, cholesterol, fatty acids and lecithin is increased because of absorption of water.
3. The pH is slightly decreased.
4. Specific gravity is increased.
5. Mucin is added.

■ BILE SALTS

Bile salts are the sodium and potassium salts of bile acids, which are conjugated with glycine or taurine. Bile salts are formed in liver and released into intestine.

About 90% to 95% of bile salts from intestine are transported to liver through **enterohepatic circulation**. Remaining 5% to 10% of the bile salts enter large intestine. Here, the bile salts are converted into **deoxycholate** and **lithocholate** and excreted in feces.

■ FUNCTIONS OF BILE SALTS

Bile salts are required for digestion and absorption of fats in the intestine. Functions of bile salts are:

1. Emulsification of Fats: Detergent Action

Emulsification is the process by which fat globules are broken down into minute droplets and made in the form of a milky fluid called **emulsion**. Emulsification of fats occurs in small intestine by the action of bile salts.

Fats cannot be digested directly by lipolytic enzymes of GI tract, because the fats are insoluble in water due to the surface tension. Bile salts reduce the **surface tension of fats** due to their **detergent action**. Because of this, the lipid granules are broken into minute particles which can be easily digested by lipolytic enzymes. Emulsification of fats by bile salts needs the presence of lecithin from bile.

2. Absorption of Fats

Bile salts help in the absorption of digested fats from intestine into blood. Bile salts combine with fats and make complexes of fats called **micelles**. Fats in the form of micelles can be absorbed easily.

3. Choleretic Action

Bile salts stimulate the secretion of bile from liver. This action is called choleretic action.

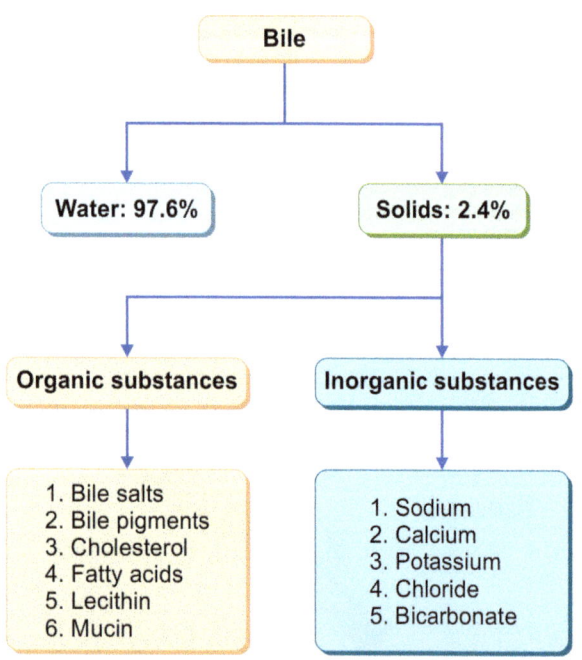

FIGURE 29.5: Composition of bile.

4. Cholagogue Action

Cholagogue is an agent, which causes contraction of gallbladder and release of bile into the intestine. Bile salts act as cholagogues indirectly by stimulating the secretion of hormone cholecystokinin. This hormone causes contraction of gallbladder resulting in release of bile.

5. Laxative Action

Laxative is an agent which induces **defecation**. Bile salts act as laxatives by stimulating peristaltic movements of the intestine.

6. Prevention of Gallstone Formation

Bile salts prevent formation of gallstone by keeping the cholesterol and lecithin in solution. In the absence of bile salts, cholesterol precipitates along with lecithin and forms gallstone.

■ BILE PIGMENTS

Bile pigments are the **excretory products** in bile. Bile pigments are bilirubin and biliverdin. And, bilirubin is the major bile pigment in human being.

■ FORMATION, CIRCULATION AND EXCRETION OF BILE PIGMENTS

Bile pigments are formed during the breakdown of hemoglobin, which is released from the destroyed RBCs in the reticuloendothelial system. First formed pigment **biliverdin** is reduced to **bilirubin**. Bilirubin is released into blood from reticuloendothelial cells.

Bilirubin circulating in the blood is called **free bilirubin** or **unconjugated bilirubin**. When it is taken up by the liver cells, it is conjugated with glucuronic acid to form **conjugated bilirubin** or **direct bilirubin**. Conjugated bilirubin is then excreted into intestine through bile.

In the intestine, 50% of conjugated bilirubin is converted into **urobilinogen** by intestinal bacteria. Remaining 50% of conjugated bilirubin enters the liver through **enterohepatic circulation**. From liver, it is re-excreted in bile.

Most of the urobilinogen from intestine enters liver via enterohepatic circulation. Later, it is re-excreted through bile. About 5% of urobilinogen is excreted by kidney through urine. Some of the urobilinogen is excreted in feces as **stercobilinogen**.

■ NORMAL PLASMA LEVELS OF BILIRUBIN

Normal bilirubin (total bilirubin) content in plasma is 0.5 to 1.5 mg/dL. When it exceeds 1 mg/dL, the condition is called **hyperbilirubinemia**. When it exceeds 2 mg/dL, **jaundice** occurs.

■ FUNCTIONS OF BILE

Most of the functions of bile are due to the bile salts.

■ 1. DIGESTIVE FUNCTION

Bile salts are responsible for digestion of fats by lipolytic enzymes of GI tract. Refer functions of bile salts for details.

■ 2. ABSORPTIVE FUNCTIONS

Bile salts are responsible for absorption of digested fats from intestine into blood. Refer functions of bile salts for details.

■ 3. EXCRETORY FUNCTIONS

Bile pigments are the major excretory products of the bile. Other substances excreted in bile are:

i. Heavy metals such as copper and iron.
ii. Some bacteria such as typhoid bacteria.
iii. Some toxins.
iv. Cholesterol.
v. Lecithin.
vi. Alkaline phosphatase.

■ 4. LAXATIVE ACTION

Bile salts act as laxatives (see above).

■ 5. ANTISEPTIC ACTION

Bile inhibits the growth of certain bacteria in the lumen of intestine by its natural detergent action.

■ 6. CHOLERETIC ACTION

Bile salts have the choleretic action (see above).

■ 7. MAINTENANCE OF PH IN GASTROINTESTINAL TRACT

As the bile is highly alkaline, it neutralizes acid chyme which enters the intestine from stomach. Thus, an optimum pH is maintained for the action of digestive enzymes.

■ 8. PREVENTION OF GALLSTONE FORMATION

Refer function of bile salts.

■ 9. LUBRICATION FUNCTION

Mucin in bile acts as a lubricant for the chyme in intestine.

■ 10. CHOLAGOGUE ACTION

Bile salts act as cholagogues (see above).

■ FUNCTIONS OF LIVER

Liver is the largest gland and one of the vital organs of the body. It performs many vital metabolic and homeostatic functions, which are summarized below.

■ 1. METABOLIC FUNCTION

Liver is the organ where maximum metabolic reactions are carried out such as metabolism of carbohydrates, proteins, fats, vitamins and many hormones.

■ 2. STORAGE FUNCTION

Many substances like glycogen, amino acids, iron, folic acid and vitamins A, B_{12}, and D are stored in liver.

■ 3. SYNTHETIC FUNCTION

Liver produces glucose by gluconeogenesis. It synthesizes all the plasma proteins and other proteins (except immunoglobulins) such as clotting factors, complement factors and hormone-binding proteins. It also synthesizes steroids, somatomedin and heparin.

■ 4. SECRETION OF BILE

Liver secretes bile, which contains bile salts, bile pigments, cholesterol, fatty acids and lecithin. Functions of bile are mainly due to the bile salts. Bile salts are required for digestion and absorption of fats in the intestine. Bile helps to carry away waste products and breakdown fats, which are excreted through feces or urine.

■ 5. EXCRETORY FUNCTION

Liver excretes cholesterol, bile pigments, heavy metals (such as lead, arsenic and bismuth), toxins, bacteria and virus through bile.

■ 6. HEAT PRODUCTION

Liver is the organ where maximum heat is produced because of the metabolic reactions.

■ 7. HEMOPOIETIC FUNCTION

In fetus (hepatic stage), liver produces the blood cells (Chapter 8). It stores vitamin B_{12} necessary for erythropoiesis and iron necessary for synthesis of hemoglobin. Liver produces **thrombopoietin** that promotes production of thrombocytes.

■ 8. HEMOLYTIC FUNCTION

Senile RBCs after the lifespan of 120 days are destroyed by reticuloendothelial cells (Kupffer cells) of liver (Chapter 7).

■ 9. INACTIVATION OF HORMONES AND DRUGS

Liver catabolizes the hormones such as growth hormone, parathormone, cortisol, insulin, glucagon and estrogen. It also inactivates the drugs particularly fat-soluble drugs. Fat-soluble drugs are converted into water-soluble substances, which are excreted through bile or urine.

■ 10. DEFENSIVE AND DETOXIFICATION FUNCTIONS

Kupffer cells (reticuloendothelial cells) of the liver play an important role in the defense of the body. Foreign bodies such as bacteria or antigens are swallowed and digested by reticuloendothelial cells of liver by means of phagocytosis.

Liver cells are also involved in removal of toxic property of various harmful substances. Removal of toxic property of the harmful agent is known as detoxification.

■ GALLBLADDER

Bile secreted from liver is stored in gallbladder. Capacity of gallbladder is approximately 50 mL.

■ FUNCTIONS OF GALLBLADDER

Major functions of gallbladder are the storage and concentration of bile.

1. *Storage of Bile*

Bile is continuously secreted from liver. But it is released into intestine only intermittently and most of the bile is stored in gallbladder till it is required.

2. *Concentration of Bile*

Bile is concentrated while it is stored in gallbladder. Mucosa of gallbladder rapidly reabsorbs water and electrolytes except calcium and potassium. But the bile salts, bile pigments, cholesterol and lecithin are not reabsorbed. So, the concentration of these substances in bile increases 5 to 10 times.

3. *Alteration of pH of Bile*

The pH of bile decreases from 8 – 8.6 to 7 – 7.6 and it becomes less alkaline when it is stored in gallbladder.

4. *Secretion of Mucin*

Gallbladder secretes mucin into the bile. Mucin acts as a lubricant for movement of chyme in the intestine.

5. *Maintenance of Pressure in Biliary System*

Due to the concentrating capacity, gallbladder maintains a pressure of about 7 cm H_2O in biliary system. This pressure in the biliary system is essential for the release of bile into the intestine.

■ REGULATION OF BILE SECRETION

Bile secretion is a continuous process though the amount secreted may be less during fasting. It starts increasing 3 hours after the meals. Secretion of bile from the liver and release of bile from the gallbladder are influenced by some chemical factors which are categorized into three groups:

1. *Choleretics*

Choleretic is the substance, which increases the secretion of bile from liver. Effective choleretic agents are, acetylcholine, secretin, cholecystokinin, acid chyme in intestine and bile salts.

2. *Cholagogues*

Cholagogue is an agent, which increases the release of bile from gallbladder into intestine by contracting the gallbladder. Common cholagogues are bile salts, calcium, fatty acids and amino acids.

All these substances stimulate the secretion of cholecystokinin, which in turn causes contraction of gallbladder and flow of bile into intestine.

3. *Hydrocholeretic Agents*

Hydrocholeretic agent is a substance, which causes secretion of bile from liver with large amount of water and less quantity of solids. Hydrochloric acid is a hydrocholeretic agent.

■ LIVER FUNCTION TESTS

Liver function tests or hepatic function tests are the group of blood tests to assess the health and normal functioning of liver.

Following are the liver functions tests.

1. Total bilirubin.
2. Total protein.
3. Total albumin.
4. Albumin/Globulin ratio.
5. Alkaline phosphatase (ALP).
6. Alanine transaminase (ALT).
7. Aspartate aminotransferase (ALP).
8. Gamma glutamyl transferase (GGT).

■ APPLIED PHYSIOLOGY: DISORDERS OF LIVER AND GALLBLADDER

■ JAUNDICE OR ICTERUS

Jaundice or icterus is the condition characterized by yellow coloration of the skin, mucous membrane and deeper tissues due to increased bilirubin level in blood. The word jaundice is derived from the French word 'jaune' meaning yellow.

Normal serum bilirubin level is 0.5 to 1.5 mg/dL. Jaundice occurs when bilirubin level exceeds 2 mg/dL.

Types of Jaundice

Jaundice is classified into three types:

1. Prehepatic or hemolytic jaundice.
2. Hepatic or hepatocellular jaundice.
3. Posthepatic or obstructive jaundice.

1. Prehepatic or Hemolytic Jaundice

Hemolytic jaundice is the type of jaundice that occurs because of excess destruction of RBCs resulting in increased blood level of free (unconjugated) bilirubin. Function of liver is normal. Since the quantity of bilirubin increases enormously, liver cells cannot excrete that much bilirubin rapidly. So, bilirubin accumulates in the blood resulting in jaundice **(Fig. 29.6)**.

Common causes of hemolytic jaundice are:

i. Liver failure.
ii. Renal disorder.
iii. Hypersplenism.
iv. Burns.
v. Infections such as malaria.
vi. Hemoglobin abnormalities such as sickle cell anemia or thalassemia.
vii. Drugs or chemical substances causing red cell damage.
viii. Autoimmune diseases.

2. Hepatic or Hepatocellular or Cholestatic Jaundice

This is the type of jaundice that occurs due to damage of hepatic cells. Because of the damage, bilirubin from liver cannot be excreted and it returns to blood.

Causes of hepatic jaundice are hepatitis, cirrhosis of liver, alcoholism and exposure to toxic materials.

3. Posthepatic or Obstructive or Extrahepatic Jaundice

This type of jaundice occurs because of the obstruction of bile flow at any level of the biliary system. The bile cannot

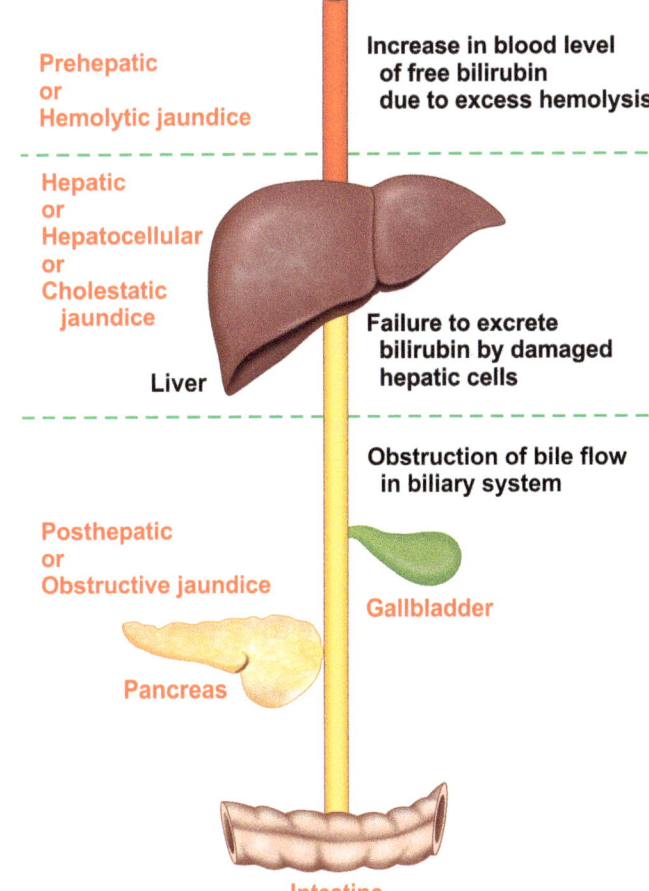

FIGURE 29.6: Types of jaundice.

be excreted into small intestine. So, bile salts and bile pigments enter the circulation.

Causes of posthepatic jaundice are gallstones and cancer of biliary system or pancreas.

Jaundice in Newborn Babies

In newborn babies, because of high count, RBCs are destroyed in large numbers. This increases blood level of bilirubin. And, they develop jaundice because their liver is not fully developed to excrete that much of bilirubin. Refer **Box 29.1** for details of jaundice in newborn babies.

■ HEPATITIS

Hepatitis is the liver damage characterized by swelling and inadequate functioning of liver. It is caused by several factors such as viral infection, bacterial infection and excess alcohol.

Common features of hepatitis are fever, nausea, vomiting, diarrhea, loss of appetite and jaundice. Liver failure and death occur in severe conditions.

■ CIRRHOSIS OF LIVER

Cirrhosis of liver refers to inflammation and damage of parenchyma of liver resulting in degeneration of hepatic cells and dysfunction of liver. It is caused by infection,

BOX 29.1: Jaundice in newborn babies.
Physiological jaundice
Physiological jaundice develops if bilirubin level increases between 6 to 8 mg/L within 48 to 72 hours after birth (Chapter 7)
Physiological jaundice lasts only for few days
Pathological jaundice
High bilirubin level results in pathological jaundice
When bilirubin level increases above 15 mg/dL, immediate treatment is required
Treatment includes: 1. Phototherapy   2. Administration of IgG (antibody against Rh antigen)   3. Exchange blood transfusion in severe cases (Chapter 16).
Pathological jaundice in infants may lead to bilirubin encephalopathy and kernicterus (Chapter 16).

obstruction of biliary system and liver enlargement due to intoxication.

Features of cirrhosis of liver are fever, nausea and vomiting, jaundice, portal hypertension, muscular weakness and wasting of muscles. Coma occurs in advanced stages.

■ GALLSTONES

Definition and Formation of Gallstone

Gallstone is a solid crystal deposit that is formed by cholesterol, calcium ions and bile pigments in the gallbladder or bile duct. **Cholelithiasis** is the presence of gallstones in gallbladder.

Normally, cholesterol is water soluble. Under some abnormal conditions, it precipitates resulting in the formation of crystals in the mucosa of gallbladder. Bile pigments and calcium are attached to these crystals resulting in formation of gallstones.

Causes for Gallstone Formation

1. Reduction in bile salts.
2. Excess of cholesterol.
3. Excess of calcium ions.
4. Damage or infection of gallbladder.
5. Obstruction of bile flow from the gallbladder.

Features of Gallstone

Common feature of gallstone is the pain in stomach area or in upper right part of the belly under the ribs. Other features include nausea, vomiting, abdominal bloating and indigestion.

Chapter 30

Small Intestine, Large Intestine and their Secretions

CHAPTER OUTLINE

- **SMALL INTESITNE**
  - FUNCTIONAL ANATOMY
  - INTESTINAL VILLI AND GLANDS
  - PROPERTIES AND COMPOSITION OF SUCCUS ENTERICUS
  - FUNCTIONS OF SUCCUS ENTERICUS
  - FUNCTIONS OF SMALL INTESTINE
  - REGULATION OF SECRETION OF SUCCUS ENTERICUS
- APPLIED PHYSIOLOGY: DISORDERS OF SMALL INTESTINE
- **LARGE INTESTINE**
  - FUNCTIONAL ANATOMY
  - LARGE INTESTINAL JUICE
  - FUNCTIONS OF LARGE INTESTINAL JUICE
  - FUNCTIONS OF LARGE INTESTINE
  - APPLIED PHYSIOLOGY: DISORDERS OF LARGE INTESTINE

■ SMALL INTESTINE

■ FUNCTIONAL ANATOMY OF SMALL INTESTINE

Small intestine is the part of GI tract extending between pyloric sphincter of stomach and ileocecal valve, which opens into large intestine. It is called small intestine because, its diameter is smaller than that of large intestine. But it is longer than large intestine. Its length is about 6 meters.

Functional importance of small intestine is absorption. Maximum absorption of digested food products takes place in small intestine.

Parts of Small Intestine

Small intestine consists of three portions:

1. Proximal part known as duodenum.
2. Middle part known as jejunum.
3. Distal part known as ileum.

Ileum of small intestine opens into cecum of large intestine through **ileocecal valve**. Ileocecal valve is a sphincter like structure present in **ileocecal junction**. Wall of the small intestine has all the four layers as in stomach (Chapter 27).

■ INTESTINAL VILLI AND GLANDS OF SMALL INTESTINE

Intestinal Villi

Mucous membrane of small intestine is covered by minute projections called **villi**. These villi are lined by columnar cells, called **enterocytes**. Each enterocyte gives rise to hair-like projections called **microvilli**. Within each villus, there is a central channel called **lacteal**. The lacteal opens into lymphatic vessels. It contains blood vessels also.

Crypts of Lieberkühn or Intestinal Glands

Crypts of Lieberkühn or intestinal glands are simple tubular glands of intestine. These glands open into lumen of intestine between the villi. Intestinal glands are lined by columnar cells. Lining of each gland is continuous with epithelial lining of the villi (**Fig. 30.1**).

Epithelial cells lining the intestinal glands undergo division by mitosis at a faster rate. Newly formed cells push the older cells upward over the lining of villi. The cells which move to villi are called **enterocytes**.

Enterocytes secrete the enzymes. Old enterocytes are continuously shed into lumen along with enzymes.

Types of cells in intestinal glands

Different types of cells are interposed between columnar cells of intestinal glands. Types of cells present in intestinal glands and their secretory functions are given in **Table 30.1**.

Three types of cells are interposed between columnar cells of the glands:

1. **Argentaffin cells** or **enterochromaffin cells** secrete intrinsic factor that is essential for the absorption of vitamin B_{12}.
2. **Goblet cells** which secrete mucus.

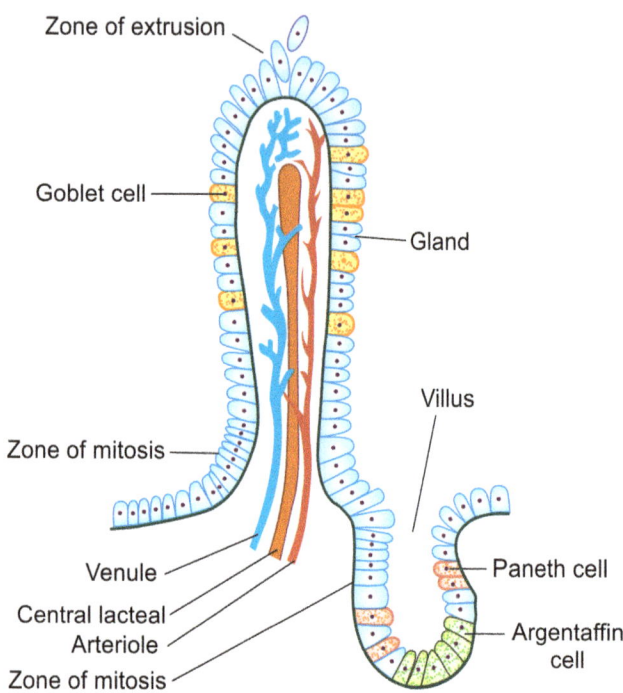

FIGURE 30.1: Gland and villus in small intestine.

3. **Paneth cells** which secrete the cytokines called defensins.

Brunner's Glands

In addition to intestinal glands, the first part of duodenum contains some mucus glands, which are called Brunner's glands. Brunner's glands secrete mucus and traces of enzymes.

■ PROPERTIES AND COMPOSITION OF SUCCUS ENTERICUS

Secretion from small intestine is called succus entericus.

Properties of Succus Entericus

Volume : 1,800 mL/day
Reaction : Alkaline
pH : 8.3

Composition of Succus Entericus

Succus entericus contains water (99.5%) and solids (0.5%). Solids include organic and inorganic substances. Refer **Figure 30.2** for details. Bicarbonate concentration is slightly high in succus entericus.

■ FUNCTIONS OF SUCCUS ENTERICUS

1. Digestive Function

Enzymes of succus entericus act on the partially digested food and convert them into final digestive products.

Proteolytic enzymes

Proteolytic enzymes in succus entericus are the **peptidases** which convert peptides into amino acids **(Table 30.2)**.

Amylolytic enzymes

Amylolytic enzymes of succus entericus are listed in **Figure 30.2**. **Lactase**, **sucrase** and **maltase** convert the disaccharides (lactose, sucrose and maltose) into two molecules of monosaccharides **(Table 30.2)**. **Dextrinase** converts dextrin, maltose and maltotriose into glucose. **Trehalase** or **trehalose glucohydrolase** causes hydrolysis of trehalose (carbohydrate present in mushrooms and yeast) and converts it into glucose.

Lipolytic enzyme

Lipolytic enzyme in small intestine is called **intestinal lipase**. It acts on triglycerides and converts them into fatty acids.

2. Protective Function

Mucus present in the succus entericus protects intestinal wall from the acid chyme, which enters the intestine from stomach; thereby it prevents the intestinal ulcer.

Paneth cells of intestinal glands secrete **defensins** which are the antimicrobial peptides.

3. Activator Function

Enterokinase present in intestinal juice activates trypsinogen into trypsin. Trypsin which in turn activates other enzymes (Chapter 28).

TABLE 30.1: Secretory function of cells in glands of small intestine.

Cells	Secretory products
Enterocytes (columnar cells)	Pepsinogen Rennin Lipase Gelatinase Urase
Argentaffin cells	Intrinsic factor of Castle
Goblet cells	Mucus
Paneth cells	Cytokines: Defensins Lysosomal enzymes
Enterochromaffin (EC) cells	Serotonin
Enterochromaffin-like (ECL) cells	Histamine
Enteroendocrine cells	
G cells	Gastrin
S cells	Secretin
I cells	Cholecystokinin
K cells	Glucose-dependent insulinotropic hormone or gastric inhibitory peptide
M cells	Motilin
L cells	Glucagon-like polypeptide-1 Glucagon-like polypeptide-2 Peptide YY
Unnamed cells	Vasoactive intestinal polypeptide

Nerve endings in small intestine secrete vasoactive intestinal polypeptide and substance P.

Chapter 30: Small Intestine, Large Intestine and their Secretions

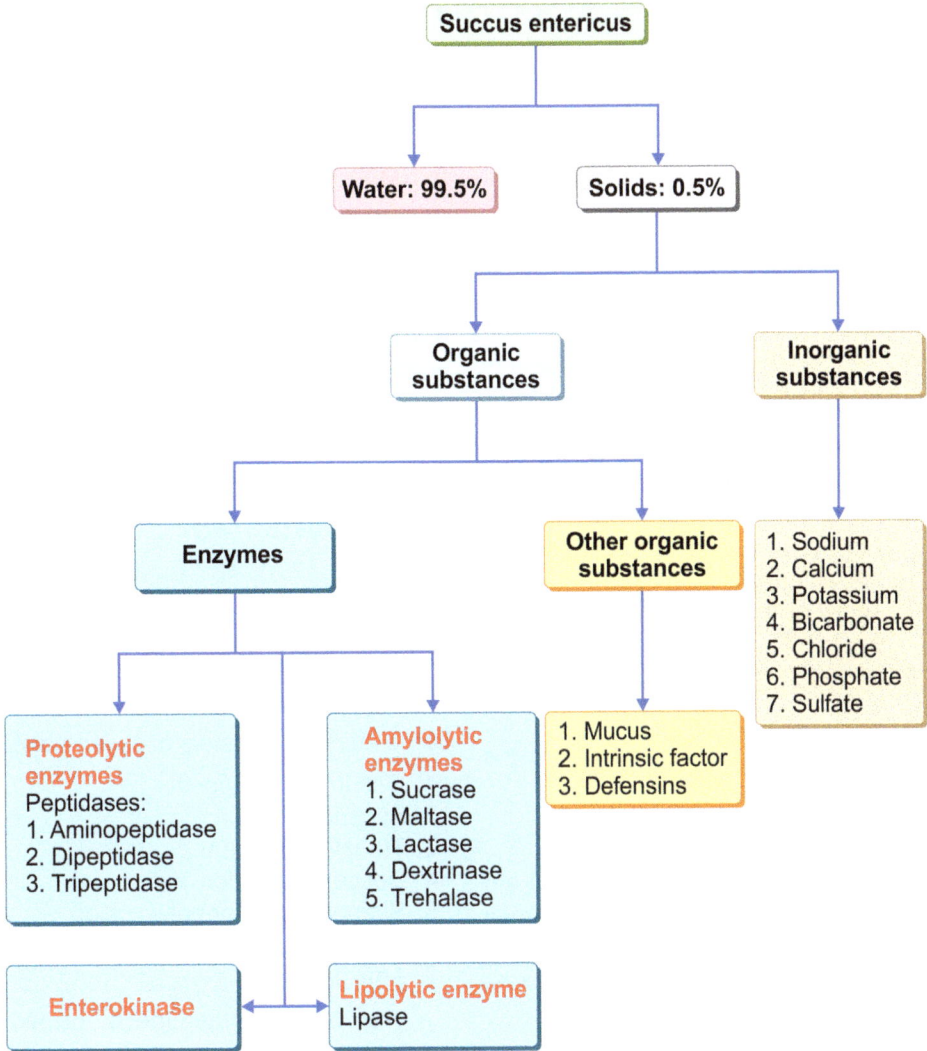

FIGURE 30.2: Composition of succus entericus.

4. Hemopoietic Function

The **intrinsic factor of Castle**, which is present in the intestine, plays an important role in erythropoiesis (Chapter 9).

5. Hydrolytic Process

Intestinal juice helps in all the enzymatic reactions of digestion.

FUNCTIONS OF SMALL INTESTINE

1. Mechanical Function

The mixing movements of small intestine help in the thorough mixing of chyme with the digestive juices like succus entericus, pancreatic juice and bile.

2. Secretory Function

Small intestine secretes succus entericus, enterokinase and the GI hormones.

3. Hormonal Function

Small intestine secretes many GI hormones such as secretin, cholecystokinin, etc. These hormones regulate the movement of GI tract and secretory activities of small intestine and pancreas.

4. Digestive Function

Refer functions of succus entericus.

TABLE 30.2: Digestive enzymes of succus entericus.

Enzyme	Substrate	End products
Peptidases	Peptides	Amino acids
Sucrase	Sucrose	Fructose Glucose
Maltase	Maltose Maltotriose	Glucose
Lactase	Lactose	Galactose Glucose
Dextrinase	Dextrin Maltose Maltotriose	Glucose
Trehalase	Trehalose	Glucose
Intestinal lipase	Triglycerides	Fatty acids

5. Activator Function
Refer functions of succus entericus.

6. Hemopoietic Function
Refer functions of succus entericus.

7. Hydrolytic Function
Refer functions of succus entericus.

8. Absorptive Functions
Presence of villi and microvilli in small intestinal mucosa increases the surface area of the mucosa. This facilitates the absorptive function of intestine.

Digested products of foodstuffs, proteins, carbohydrates, fats and other nutritive substances such as vitamins, minerals and water are absorbed mostly in small intestine. From the lumen of intestine, these substances pass through lacteal of villi, cross the mucosa and enter the blood directly or through lymphatics.

REGULATION OF SECRETION OF SUCCUS ENTERICUS
Secretion of succus entericus is regulated by both the nervous and hormonal mechanisms.

Nervous Regulation
Secretion of succus entericus is regulated mainly by the local nervous reflexes. When chyme enters the small intestine, the mucosa is stimulated by tactile stimuli or irritation. It causes development of local nervous reflexes, which stimulate the glands of intestine.

Hormonal Regulation
When the chyme enters the small intestine, the intestinal mucosa secretes enterocrinin, secretin and cholecystokinin which promote the secretion of succus entericus by stimulating the intestinal glands.

APPLIED PHYSIOLOGY: DISORDERS OF SMALL INTESTINE

1. Malabsorption
Malabsorption is the failure to absorb nutrients, such as proteins, carbohydrates, fats and vitamins. Malabsorption affects growth and development of the body. It also causes some specific diseases (see below).

2. Malabsorption Syndrome
Malabsorption syndrome is the condition characterized by the failure of digestion and absorption in small intestine.

3. Inflammatory Bowel Disease
Inflammatory bowel disease (IBD) is a group of intestinal disorders characterized by chronic inflammation of digestive tract. Common types of IBD are **Crohn's disease** which involves inflammation of small intestine and **ulcerative colitis** which involves inflammation of large intestine.

4. Tropical Sprue
Tropical sprue is a malabsorption syndrome affecting the residents of or visitors of tropical areas where the disease is epidemic.

5. Steatorrhea
Steatorrhea is the condition caused by deficiency of pancreatic lipase resulting in malabsorption of fat. Refer Chapter 29 for details.

6. Celiac Disease
Celiac disease is an autoimmune disease caused by gluten intake and it leads to damage of villi in small intestine resulting in impaired digestion and absorption. It is also known as gluten-sensitive enteropathy or celiac sprue.

LARGE INTESTINE
FUNCTIONAL ANATOMY OF LARGE INTESTINE
Large intestine is also known as **colon**. It extends from **ileocecal valve** up to **anus** (Fig. 30.1).

Parts of Large Intestinal Juice
Large intestine consists of seven parts:
1. Cecum with appendix.
2. Ascending colon.
3. Transverse colon.
4. Descending colon.
5. Sigmoid colon or pelvic colon.
6. Rectum.
7. Anal canal.

Wall of large intestine is formed by four layers of structures like any other part of the digestive system (Chapter 25).

LARGE INTESTINAL JUICE
Large intestinal juice is a watery fluid with pH of 8.0.

Composition of Large Intestinal Juice
Large intestinal juice contains 99.5% of water and 0.5% of solids. Refer **Figure 30.3** for details.

Digestive enzymes are absent and concentration of bicarbonate is high in large intestinal juice.

FUNCTIONS OF LARGE INTESTINAL JUICE
1. Neutralization of Acids
Strong acids formed by bacterial action in large intestine are neutralized by the alkaline nature of large intestinal juice. Alkalinity of this juice is mainly due to the presence of large quantity of bicarbonate.

2. Lubrication Activity
Mucin present in secretion of large intestine lubricates the mucosa of large intestine and bowel contents, so that the movement of bowel is facilitated.

Mucin also protects mucous membrane of large intestine by preventing the damage caused by mechanical injury or chemical substances.

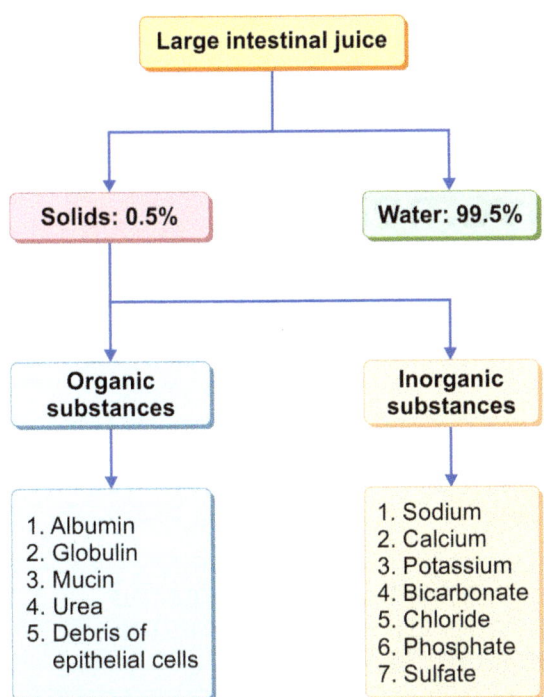

FIGURE 30.3: Composition of large intestinal juice

■ FUNCTIONS OF LARGE INTESTINE

1. Absorptive Function

Large intestine plays an important role in the absorption of various substances such as water, electrolytes and organic substances like glucose, alcohol and drugs like anesthetic agents, sedatives and steroids.

2. Formation of Feces

After the absorption of nutrients, water and other substances, unwanted substances in the large intestine form feces, which is excreted out.

3. Excretory Function

Large intestine excretes heavy metals like mercury, lead, bismuth and arsenic through feces.

4. Secretory Function

Large intestine secretes mucin and inorganic substances like chlorides and bicarbonates.

5. Synthetic Function

Bacterial flora of large intestine synthesizes folic acid, vitamin B_{12} and vitamin K.

By this function, large intestine contributes in erythropoietic activity and blood clotting mechanism.

■ APPLIED PHYSIOLOGY: DISORDERS OF LARGE INTESTINE

1. Diarrhea

Diarrhea is the frequent and profuse discharge of intestinal contents in loose and fluid form. It occurs due to the increased movement of intestine. It may be acute or chronic.

Causes of diarrhea

   i. Intake of contaminated water or food, artificial sweeteners found in food, spicy food, etc.
  ii. Indigestion.
 iii. Infections by bacteria, viruses and parasites.
  iv. Reaction to medicines like antibiotics, laxatives.
   v. Intestinal diseases.

Features of diarrhea

Severe diarrhea results in loss of excess water and electrolytes leading to **dehydration** and **electrolyte imbalance**. Chronic diarrhea results in **hypokalemia** and **metabolic acidosis**. Other features of diarrhea are abdominal pain, nausea and **bloating** (a condition in which the subject feels the abdomen full and tight due to excess intestinal gas).

2. Constipation

Constipation is the failure of voiding of feces, which produces discomfort. It is due to the lack of movements necessary for defecation (Chapter 31). Due to absence of mass movement in colon, feces remain in the large intestine for a longtime resulting in absorption of fluid. So, the feces become hard and dry.

Causes of constipation

   i. Lack of fiber or lack of liquids in diet.
  ii. Irregular bowel habit.
 iii. Spasm of sigmoid colon.
  iv. Many types of diseases.
   v. Drugs such as diuretics, pain relievers, antihypertensive drugs antiparkinsonian drugs, antidepressants and anticonvulsants.
  vi. Dysfunction of myenteric plexus in large intestine called megacolon.

3. Megacolon

Megacolon is a condition characterized by distension and hypertrophy of colon associated with constipation. It is caused by the absence or damage of ganglionic cells in myenteric plexus, which causes dysfunction of myenteric plexus. It leads to accumulation of large quantity of feces in colon. Colon is distended to a diameter of 4 to 5 inches. It also results in **hypertrophy of colon**.

4. Appendicitis

Appendix is a small, finger-like pouch projecting from cecum of ascending colon. Inflammation of appendix is known as appendicitis. The cause for appendicitis is not known. It may occur by viral infection of the gastrointestinal (GI) tract or if the connection between appendix and large intestine is blocked.

Major symptom of appendicitis is the pain, which starts around the umbilicus and then spreads to the lower right side of the abdomen. This pain becomes severe within 6 to 12 hours. Other features are nausea, vomiting, constipation, diarrhea and abdominal swelling.

If not treated immediately, appendix may rupture and the inflammation will spread to the whole body leading to severe complications, sometimes even death.

CHAPTER 31

Movements of Gastrointestinal Tract

CHAPTER OUTLINE

- MASTICATION
- DEGLUTITION
- MOVEMENTS OF STOMACH
- FILLING AND EMPTYING OF STOMACH
- VOMITING
- MOVEMENTS OF SMALL INTESTINE
- MOVEMENTS OF LARGE INTESTINE
- DEFECATION

■ MASTICATION

Mastication or **chewing** is the first mechanical process in GI tract by which the food substances are torn or cut into small particles and crushed or ground into a soft **bolus**.

Significances of Mastication

1. Breakdown of foodstuffs into smaller particles.
2. Mixing of saliva with food substances thoroughly.
3. Lubrication and moistening of dry food by saliva so that the bolus can be easily swallowed.
4. Appreciation of taste of the food.

■ MUSCLES AND THE MOVEMENTS OF MASTICATION

Muscles of Mastication

1. Masseter muscle.
2. Temporal muscle.
3. Pterygoid muscles.
4. Buccinator muscle.

Movements of Mastication

1. Opening and closure of mouth.
2. Rotational movements of jaw.
3. Protraction and retraction of jaw.

■ CONTROL OF MASTICATION

Action of mastication is mostly a reflex process. It is carried out voluntarily also. Center for mastication is situated in medulla and cerebral cortex. Muscles of mastication are supplied by mandibular division of **trigeminal nerve** (V cranial nerve).

■ DEGLUTITION

Definition

Deglutition or **swallowing** is the process by which food passes from mouth into stomach.

Stages of Deglutition

Deglutition occurs in three stages:

I. Oral stage, when food moves from mouth to pharynx.
II. Pharyngeal stage, when food moves from pharynx to esophagus.
III. Esophageal stage, when food moves from esophagus to stomach.

■ I. ORAL STAGE OR FIRST STAGE

Oral stage is a voluntary stage. In this stage, the bolus from oral cavity passes into the pharynx by means of series of actions.

Sequence of Events during Oral Stage

1. Bolus is placed over posterodorsal surface of the tongue. It is called the preparatory position.
2. Anterior part of tongue is retracted and depressed.
3. Posterior part of tongue is elevated and retracted against hard palate. This pushes the bolus backwards into pharynx.
4. Forceful contraction of tongue against the palate produces a positive pressure in the posterior part of oral cavity which pushes the food into pharynx **(Fig. 31.1)**.

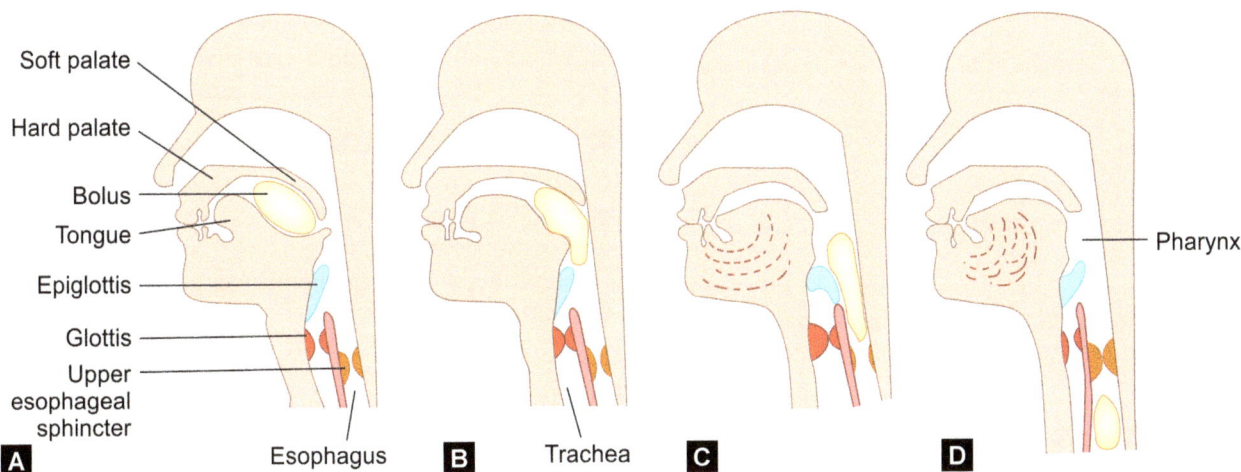

FIGURE 31.1: Stages of deglutition. A. Preparatory stage. B. Oral stage. C. Pharyngeal stage. D. Esophageal stage.

II. PHARYNGEAL STAGE OR SECOND STAGE

Pharyngeal stage is an involuntary stage. In this stage, the bolus is pushed from pharynx into the esophagus. Pharynx is a common passage for food and air. It divides into larynx and esophagus. Larynx lies anteriorly and continues as respiratory passage. Esophagus lies behind the larynx and continues as GI tract. Since pharynx communicates with mouth, nose, larynx and esophagus, during this stage of deglutition, the **bolus** from pharynx can enter into **four paths**:

1. It can come back into mouth.
2. It can go upwards into nasopharynx.
3. It can move forwards into larynx.
4. It can move downwards into esophagus.

However, due to various coordinated movements, bolus is made to enter only into the esophagus. Entrance of bolus through other paths is prevented. Entrance of bolus into esophagus occurs by the combined effects of various factors.

Sequence of Events during Entrance of Bolus into Esophagus

i. Upward movement of larynx stretches the opening of esophagus.
ii. Simultaneously, upper 3 to 4 cm of esophagus relaxes. This part of esophagus is formed by **cricopharyngeal muscle** and it is called **upper esophageal sphincter** or pharyngoesophageal sphincter.
iii. At the same time, peristaltic contractions start in pharynx due to the contraction of pharyngeal muscles.
iv. Elevation of larynx also lifts the glottis away from food passage.

All the factors mentioned above act together so that bolus moves easily into the esophagus. Whole process takes place within 1 to 2 seconds. And this process is purely involuntary.

Deglutition Apnea

Apnea refers to temporary arrest of breathing. Deglutition apnea or **swallowing apnea** is the arrest of breathing during pharyngeal stage of deglutition.

Choking

Choking is the inability to breathe due to obstruction or compression of respiratory passage. Sometimes during second stage of swallowing, solid food particles may enter larynx resulting in obstruction and choking. However, it may be prevented automatically by **gag reflex** (Chapter 80).

III. ESOPHAGEAL STAGE OR THIRD STAGE

It is also an involuntary stage. In esophageal stage food from stomach enters esophagus. Function of esophagus is to transport the bolus from pharynx to stomach. Movements of esophagus called **peristaltic waves** are specifically organized for this function. **Peristalsis** means a wave of contraction followed by a wave of relaxation of muscle fibers of GI tract, which travel in aboral direction (away from mouth). By this type of movement, the contents are propelled down along the GI tract.

Role of Lower Esophageal Sphincter

Lower esophageal sphincter is constricted always. When bolus enters this part of the esophagus, this sphincter relaxes so that the contents enter stomach. After entry of bolus into the stomach, this sphincter constricts and closes the lower end of esophagus.

Relaxation and constriction of lower esophageal sphincter occur in sequence with the arrival of peristaltic contractions of esophagus.

DEGLUTITION REFLEX

Though the beginning of swallowing is a voluntary act, later it becomes involuntary and it is carried out by a reflex action called deglutition reflex. This reflex occurs during the pharyngeal and esophageal stages.

Stimulus

When the bolus enters oropharyngeal region, the receptors present in this region are stimulated.

Afferent Fibers

Afferent impulses from the oropharyngeal receptors pass via glossopharyngeal nerve fibers to deglutition center.

Center

Deglutition center is at the floor of fourth ventricle in medulla oblongata of brain.

Efferent Fibers

Impulses from deglutition center travel through glossopharyngeal and vagus nerves.

Response

This reflex causes passage of bolus into esophagus. Now, peristalsis occurs in esophagus pushing the bolus into stomach.

■ SWALLOWING IN BABIES

Swallowing hard and solid food by babies below 6 months is prevented by **gag reflex** or **pharyngeal reflex** (Chapter 80). Gag reflex prevents choking.

■ MOVEMENTS OF STOMACH

Movements of the stomach are:
1. Hunger contractions.
2. Receptive relaxation.
3. Peristalsis of stomach.

■ 1. HUNGER CONTRACTIONS

Hunger contractions are the movements of empty stomach. These contractions are related to the sensations of hunger.

Hunger contractions are strong peristaltic contractions associated with hunger pain. This type of peristaltic contractions is different from the **digestive peristaltic contractions** (see below). Digestive peristaltic contractions usually occur in body and pyloric parts of the stomach. But hunger contractions of empty stomach involve the entire stomach.

■ 2. RECEPTIVE RELAXATION

Receptive relaxation is the relaxation of upper portion of stomach when bolus enters the stomach from esophagus. It involves fundus and upper part of the body of stomach. Its significance is to accommodate the food easily without much increase in pressure inside the stomach. This process is called **accommodation of stomach**.

■ 3. PERISTALSIS OF STOMACH

When the food enters the stomach, peristaltic contraction or peristaltic wave appears with a frequency of 3/min. It starts from the lower part of the body of stomach, passes through pylorus till the pyloric sphincter.

This type of peristaltic contraction is called **digestive peristalsis** because it is responsible for the grinding of food particles and mixing them with gastric juice for digestive activities.

■ FILLING AND EMPTYING OF STOMACH

■ FILLING OF STOMACH

While taking food, it arranges itself in the stomach in different layers. First eaten food is placed against the greater curvature in fundus and body of the stomach. Successive layers of food particles lie nearer the lesser curvature until the last portion of food eaten lies near upper end of lesser curvature, adjacent to cardiac sphincter.

■ EMPTYING OF STOMACH

Gastric emptying is a process by which chyme from stomach is emptied into intestine. Food that is swallowed enters the stomach and remains there for about 3 hours. During this period, digestion takes place. Partly digested food becomes the chyme.

Chyme

Chyme is a semisolid mass of partially digested food that is formed in the stomach. It is acidic in nature. Acid chyme is emptied from stomach into intestine slowly with the help of peristaltic contractions. It takes about 3 to 4 hours for emptying of the chyme. This slow emptying is necessary to facilitate the final digestion and maximum (about 80%) absorption of digested food materials from small intestine.

Gastric emptying occurs due to peristaltic waves in the body and pyloric part of stomach and simultaneous relaxation of pyloric sphincter.

■ VOMITING

Vomiting or **emesis** is the abnormal emptying of stomach and upper part of intestine through esophagus and mouth.

■ CAUSES OF VOMITING

Common causes of vomiting are:

1. Any gastrointestinal disorder.
2. Mechanical stimulation of pharynx.
3. Excess intake of alcohol.
4. Nauseating sight, odor or taste.
5. Unusual stimulation of labyrinthine apparatus as in the case of sea sickness, air sickness, car sickness or swinging.
6. Metabolic disturbances such as carbohydrate starvation and ketosis during **pregnancy**, acidosis during **diabetes** and uremia.

■ MECHANISM OF VOMITING

Nausea

Vomiting is always preceded by nausea. Nausea is unpleasant sensation which induces the desire for vomiting. It is characterized by secretion of large amount of saliva containing more amount of mucus.

Retching

Strong involuntary movements in GI tract start even before actual vomiting and intensify the feeling of vomiting. This condition is called retching (try to vomit). And, vomiting occurs few minutes after this.

Act of Vomiting

Act of vomiting involves series of movements that takes place in GI tract. **Antiperistalsis** develops in ileum and runs towards mouth through intestine and it pushes the intestinal contents into stomach.

This is followed by contraction of diaphragm and abdominal muscles so that stomach is compressed between diaphragm and abdominal wall. This leads to rise in intragastric pressure. Simultaneously there is relaxation of lower esophageal sphincter, esophagus and upper esophageal sphincter.

Deep inspiration occurs followed by temporary cessation of breathing. And gastric contents (vomitus) are expelled forcefully through esophagus, pharynx and mouth.

VOMITING REFLEX

Vomiting is a reflex act. Sensory impulses for vomiting arise from the irritated or distended part of GI tract or other organs and are transmitted to vomiting center through vagus and sympathetic fibers.

Vomiting center is situated in medulla oblongata near the nucleus tractus solitarius.

Motor impulses from the vomiting center are transmitted through V, VII, IX, X and XII cranial nerves to the upper part of GI tract; and through spinal nerves to diaphragm and abdominal muscles.

MOVEMENTS OF SMALL INTESTINE

Movements of small intestine are essential for mixing the chyme with digestive juices, propulsion of food and absorption.

Movements of small intestine are of four types:

1. Mixing movements:
    i. Segmentation movements.
    ii. Pendular movements.
2. Propulsive movements:
    i. Peristaltic movements.
    ii. Peristaltic rush.
3. Peristalsis in fasting: Migrating motor complex.
4. Movements of villi.

MIXING MOVEMENTS

Mixing movements of small intestine are responsible for proper mixing of chyme with digestive juices such as pancreatic juice, bile and intestinal juice. Mixing movements of small intestine are segmentation contractions and pendular movements.

Segmentation Contractions

Segmentation contractions are the common type of movements of small intestine, which occur regularly or irregularly but in a rhythmic fashion. So, these movements are also called rhythmic segmentation contractions.

Contractions occur at regularly spaced intervals along a section of intestine. Segment of the intestine involved in each contraction is about 1 to 5 cm long. Segments of intestine in between the contracted segments are relaxed. Length of the relaxed segments is same as that of the contracted segments. These alternate segments of contraction and relaxation give appearance of rings resembling the chain of sausages.

After sometime, contracted segments are relaxed and the relaxed segments are contracted (**Fig. 31.2**). Therefore, segmentation contractions chop the chyme many times. This helps in mixing of chyme with digestive juices.

Pendular Movement

Pendular movement is the sweeping movement of small intestine resembling movements of pendulum of clock. Small portions of intestine (loops) sweep forward and backward or upward and downward. It helps in mixing of chyme with digestive juices.

PROPULSIVE MOVEMENTS

Propulsive movements are movements of small intestine which push the chyme in aboral direction through intestine. Propulsive movements are peristaltic movements and peristaltic rush.

Peristaltic Movements

Peristalsis (see above for details) travels from point of stimulation in both directions. But under normal conditions, the progress of contraction in an oral direction is inhibited quickly and the contractions disappear. Only the contraction that travels in an aboral direction persists.

Peristaltic Rush

Sometimes, small intestine shows a powerful peristaltic contraction. It is caused by excessive irritation of intestinal mucosa or extreme distention of the intestine. This type of powerful contraction begins in duodenum and passes through entire length of small intestine and reaches the

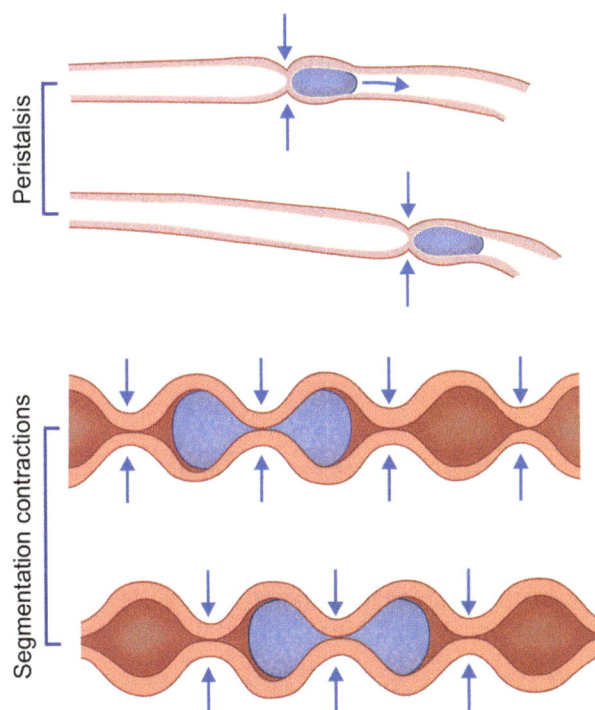

FIGURE 31.2: Movements of small intestine.

ileocecal valve within few minutes. This is called peristaltic rush or rush waves.

Peristaltic rush sweeps the contents of intestine into colon. Thus, it relieves the small intestine off either irritants or excessive distention.

■ PERISTALSIS IN FASTING: MIGRATING MOTOR COMPLEX

It is a type of peristaltic contraction, which occurs in stomach and small intestine during the periods of fasting for several hours. It is different from regular peristalsis because, a large portion of stomach or intestine is involved in this contraction. Contraction extends to about 20 cm to 30 cm of the stomach or intestine. This type of movement occurs once in every 1½ to 2 hours.

Significance of Peristalsis in Fasting

Peristalsis in fasting sweeps the excess digestive secretions into colon and prevents the accumulation of secretions in stomach and intestine. It also sweeps the residual undigested materials into colon.

■ MOVEMENTS OF VILLI

Intestinal villi also show movements simultaneously along with intestinal movements. Movements of villi are shortening and elongation, which occur alternatively and help in emptying lymph from the central lacteal into the lymphatic system. Surface area of villi is increased during elongation. This helps absorption of digested food particles from the lumen of intestine.

Movements of villi are caused by local nervous reflexes, which are initiated by the presence of chyme in small intestine.

■ MOVEMENTS OF LARGE INTESTINE

Large intestine shows sluggish movements. Still these movements are important for mixing, propulsive and absorptive functions. Large intestine shows two types of movements:

■ MIXING MOVEMENTS: SEGMENTATION CONTRACTIONS

Large circular constrictions, which appear in the colon, are called mixing segmentation contractions. The contractions occur at regular distance in colon. Length of the portion of colon involved in each contraction is nearly about 2.5 cm.

■ PROPULSIVE MOVEMENTS: MASS PERISTALSIS

Mass peristalsis or mass movement propels the feces from colon towards anus. Usually, this movement occurs only a few times every day. Duration of mass movement is about 10 minutes in the morning before or after breakfast. This is because of the neurogenic factors like gastrocolic reflex (see below) and parasympathetic stimulation.

■ DEFECATION

Voiding of feces is known as defecation. **Feces** is formed in the large intestine and stored in **sigmoid colon**. By the influence of an appropriate stimulus, it is expelled out through anus. This is prevented by tonic constriction of anal sphincters, in the absence of the stimulus.

■ DEFECATION REFLEX

Mass movement drives the feces into sigmoid or pelvic colon. Feces is stored in the sigmoid colon. Desire for defecation occurs when some feces enters rectum due to the mass movement. Usually, the desire for defecation is elicited by an increase in **intrarectal pressure** to about 20 to 25 cm H_2O.

Usual stimulus for defecation is intake of liquid like coffee or tea or water. But it differs from person to person.

Act of Defecation

Act of defecation is preceded by voluntary efforts like assuming an appropriate posture, voluntary relaxation of external sphincter and the compression of abdominal contents by voluntary contraction of abdominal muscles.

Usually, the rectum is empty. During development of mass movement, the feces is pushed into rectum and the defecation reflex is initiated. Process of defecation involves the contraction of rectum and relaxation of internal and external anal sphincters.

Internal anal sphincter is made up of smooth muscle and it is innervated by parasympathetic nerve fibers via pelvic nerve. **External anal sphincter** is composed of skeletal muscle and it is controlled by somatic nerve fibers, which pass through pudendal nerve. Pudendal

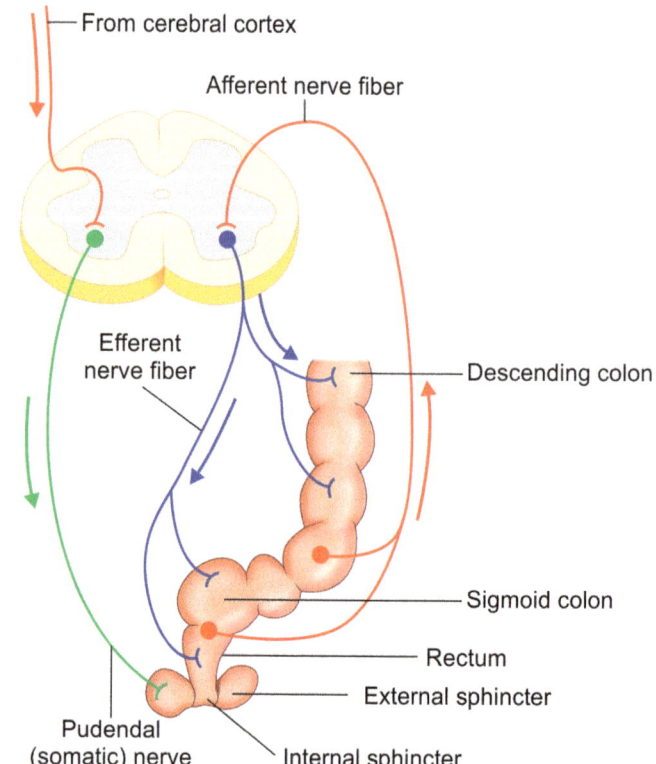

FIGURE 31.3: Defecation reflex. Afferent and efferent fibers of the reflex pass through pelvic (parasympathetic) nerve. Voluntary control of defecation is by pudendal (somatic) nerve. Defecation center is in the sacral segments of spinal cord.

nerve always keeps the external sphincter constricted and the sphincter can relax only when the pudendal nerve is inhibited.

Failure of voiding of feces is called **constipation** (Chapter 30).

Gastrocolic Reflex

Gastrocolic reflex is the contraction of rectum followed by desire for defecation caused by distention of stomach by food. It is mediated by intrinsic nerve fibers of GI tract. This reflex causes only a weak contraction of rectum. But it initiates defecation reflex.

■ PATHWAY FOR DEFECATION REFLEX

When rectum is distended due to the entry of feces by mass movement, sensory nerve endings are stimulated. Impulses from the nerve endings are transmitted via afferent fibers of **pelvic nerve** to the defecation center, situated in sacral segments (center) of spinal cord.

The center, in turn sends motor impulses to the descending colon, sigmoid colon and rectum via efferent nerve fibers of pelvic nerve. Motor impulses cause strong contraction of descending colon, sigmoid colon and rectum and relaxation of internal sphincter.

Simultaneously, voluntary relaxation of external sphincter occurs. It is due to the inhibition of **pudendal nerve** by impulses arising from cerebral cortex **(Fig. 31.3)**.

MODEL QUESTIONS IN DIGESTIVE SYSTEM

■ LONG QUESTIONS

1. What are the different types of salivary glands? Describe the composition, functions and regulation of secretion of saliva.
2. Describe the different phases of gastric secretion with experimental evidences.
3. Explain the composition, functions and regulation of secretion of pancreatic juice.
4. Describe the composition, functions and regulation of secretion of bile. Add a note on enterohepatic circulation.

■ SHORT QUESTIONS

1. Enteric nerve supply to GI tract.
2. Properties and composition of saliva.
3. Functions of saliva.
4. Glands of stomach.
5. Functions of stomach.
6. Properties and composition of gastric juice.
7. Functions of gastric juice.
8. Mechanism of secretion of hydrochloric acid in stomach.
9. Cephalic phase of gastric secretion.
10. Gastrin.
11. Peptic ulcer.
12. Properties and composition of pancreatic juice.
13. Functions of pancreatic juice.
14. Regulation of exocrine function of pancreas.
15. Hormones affecting pancreatic secretion.
16. Composition of bile.
17. Functions of bile.
18. Bile salts/bile pigments.
19. Functions of liver.
20. Functions of gallbladder.
21. Jaundice.
22. Properties and composition of succus entericus.
23. Functions of small intestine.
24. Functions of large intestine.
25. Mastication.
26. Swallowing.
27. Movements of stomach.
28. Filling and emptying of stomach.
29. Vomiting.
30. Movements of small intestine.

■ VERY SHORT ANSWER QUESTIONS

1. Functions of sympathetic and parasympathetic nerves on GI tract.
2. Functions of mouth.
3. Classify salivary glands with examples.
4. Structure and duct system of salivary glands.
5. Mention ducts of major salivary glands.
6. Properties of saliva.
7. Reflexes regulating salivary secretion.
8. Hypersalivation.
9. Hyposalivation.
10. Xerostomia.
11. Drooling.
12. Chorda tympani syndrome.
13. Cells present in glands of stomach and their secretory products.
14. Pavlov's pouch.
15. Sham feeding.
16. Local myenteric reflex.
17. Vagovagal reflex.
18. Duct system in pancreas.
19. Trypsin/chymotrypsin/peptidase/ pancreatic lipase.
20. Neutralizing action of pancreatic juice.
21. Steatorrhea.
22. Secretin.
23. Cholecystokinin.
24. Choleretics and cholagogues.
25. Biliary system.
26. Blood supply to liver.
27. Enterohepatic circulation.
28. Properties of bile.
29. Jaundice in newborn babies.
30. Gallstones.
31. Malabsorption and malabsorption syndrome.
32. Deglutition reflex.
33. Deglutition apnea.
34. Choking.
35. Gag reflex.
36. Receptive relaxation.
37. Migrating motor complex.
38. Movements of large intestine.
39. Constipation.
40. Diarrhea.

SECTION 5 RENAL PHYSIOLOGY AND SKIN

CHAPTER 32

Overview of Renal System

CHAPTER OUTLINE

- **EXCRETION AND RENAL SYSTEM**
- **FUNCTIONAL ANATOMY OF KIDNEY**
  - **DIFFERENT LAYERS OF KIDNEY**
  - **TUBULAR STRUCTURES OF KIDNEY**
- **FUNCTIONS OF KIDNEY**
  - **ROLE IN HOMEOSTASIS**
  - **HEMATOPOIETIC FUNCTION**
- **ENDOCRINE FUNCTION**
- **REGULATION OF BLOOD PRESSURE**
- **REGULATION OF BLOOD CALCIUM LEVEL**

■ EXCRETION AND RENAL SYSTEM

Excretion is the process by which unwanted substances and metabolic wastes are eliminated from the body.

Although various organs such as GI tract, liver, skin and lungs are involved in removal of wastes from the body, renal system has maximum capacity of excretory function.

Renal system includes:

1. A pair of kidneys which produce urine.
2. Ureters which transport urine to urinary bladder.
3. Urinary bladder that stores urine till it is voided (emptied).
4. Urethra through which urine is voided from bladder **(Fig. 32.1)**.

■ FUNCTIONAL ANATOMY OF KIDNEY

Kidney is a compound tubular gland covered by a connective tissue capsule. There is a depression on the medial border of kidney called **hilum**, through which renal artery, renal veins, nerves and ureter pass.

■ DIFFERENT LAYERS OF KIDNEY

Components of kidney are arranged in **three layers**:

1. Outer Cortex

Cortex is dark and granular in appearance. It contains **renal corpuscles** and **convoluted tubules (Fig. 32.2)**. At intervals, cortical tissue penetrates medulla in the form of columns, which are called **renal columns** or **columns of Bertin**.

2. Inner Medulla

Medulla contains tubular and vascular structures arranged in parallel radial lines. It is divided into 8 to 18 **Malpighian pyramids** or **medullary pyramids**. Broad base of each pyramid is in contact with cortex and the apex projects into minor calyx.

3. Renal Sinus

Renal sinus consists of the following structures:

i. Upper expanded part of ureter called **renal pelvis**.

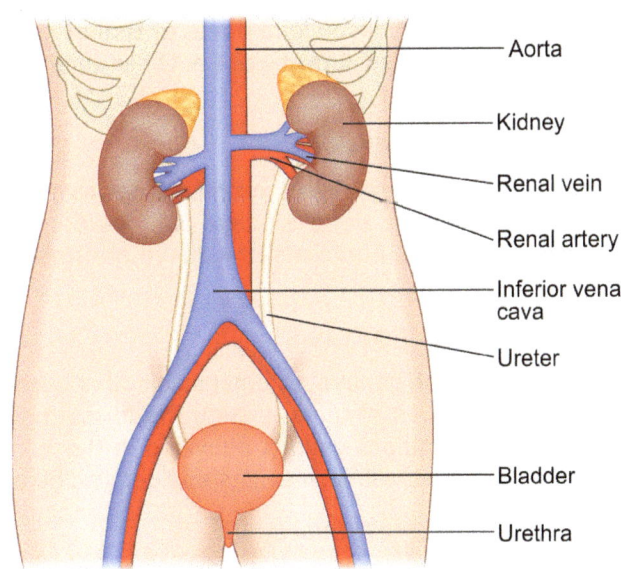

FIGURE 32.1: Urinary system.

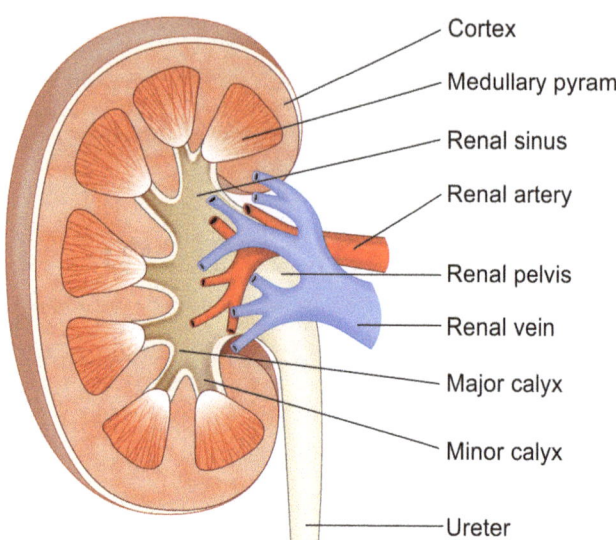

FIGURE 32.2: Longitudinal section of kidney.

ii. Subdivisions of pelvis, 2 or 3 **major calyces** and about 8 **minor calyces**.
iii. Branches of nerves and arteries and tributaries of veins.
iv. Loose connective tissues and fat.

■ TUBULAR STRUCTURES OF KIDNEY

Kidney is made up of very closely arranged tubular structures called uriniferous tubules. Blood vessels and interstitial connective tissues are interposed between these tubules.

Parts of Uriniferous Tubules

Uriniferous tubules have two parts:

1. Terminal or secretary tubules called nephrons, which are concerned with formation of urine.
2. Collecting ducts or tubules which are concerned with transport of urine from nephrons to pelvis of ureter.

Collecting ducts unite to form **ducts of Bellini**, which open into minor calyces through papilla. Other details are given in Chapter 33.

■ FUNCTIONS OF KIDNEY

Kidneys perform several vital functions besides formation of urine. By excreting urine, kidneys play the principal role in homeostasis. Functions of kidneys are detailed below.

■ 1. ROLE IN HOMEOSTASIS

Primary function of kidneys is homeostasis. It is carried out by the formation of urine. During the formation of urine, kidneys regulate various activities in the body, which are concerned with homeostasis as detailed below.

i. Excretion of Waste Products

Kidneys excrete the unwanted waste products which are formed during metabolic activities. Examples of waste products are urea, uric acid, creatinine, bilirubin. Kidneys also excrete harmful foreign chemical substances such as toxins, drugs, heavy metals and pesticides.

ii. Maintenance of Water Balance

Kidneys maintain the water balance in the body by conserving water when it is decreased and excreting water when it is excess in the body.

iii. Maintenance of Electrolyte Balance

Kidneys are involved in the maintenance of electrolyte balance, especially sodium is in relation to water balance. Kidneys retain sodium if the osmolarity of body water decreases and eliminate sodium when osmolarity increases.

iv. Maintenance of Acid-base Balance

The pH of blood and body fluids should be maintained within narrow range for healthy living. Body is under constant threat to develop acidosis, because of production of lot of acids during metabolic activities. However, it is prevented by kidneys, lungs and blood buffers, which eliminate these acids. Among these organs, kidneys play major role in preventing acidosis.

■ 2. HEMATOPOIETIC FUNCTION

Kidneys stimulate the production of erythrocytes by secreting **erythropoietin**. Erythropoietin is an important stimulating factor for erythropoiesis (Chapter 8). Kidneys also secrete another factor called **thrombopoietin**, which stimulates the production of thrombocytes (Chapter 13).

■ 3. ENDOCRINE FUNCTION

Kidneys secrete many hormonal substances in addition to erythropoietin and thrombopoietin (Chapter 50).

Hormones secreted by kidneys are:

i. Erythropoietin.
ii. Thrombopoietin.
iii. Renin.
iv. 1,25-dihydroxycholecalciferol (calcitriol).
v. Prostaglandins.

■ 4. REGULATION OF BLOOD PRESSURE

Kidneys are involved in long-term regulation of arterial blood pressure (Chapter 63) by two ways: by regulating ECF volume and through renin-angiotensin mechanism.

■ 5. REGULATION OF BLOOD CALCIUM LEVEL

Kidneys regulates blood calcium level by activating 1,25-dihydroxycholecalciferol into vitamin D. Vitamin D is necessary for the absorption of calcium from intestine (Chapter 46).

Chapter 33

Nephron

CHAPTER OUTLINE

- DEFINITION AND PARTS
- RENAL CORPUSCLE
  - SITUATION OF RENAL CORPUSCLE AND TYPES OF NEPHRON
  - STRUCTURE
- TUBULAR PORTION
  - PROXIMAL CONVOLUTED TUBULE
- LOOP OF HENLE
- DISTAL CONVOLUTED TUBULE
- COLLECTING DUCT
- PASSAGE OF URINE

DEFINITION AND PARTS OF NEPHRONS

Nephron is defined as the structural and functional unit of kidney. Each kidney consists of 1 to 1.3 million nephrons. Number of nephrons decreases in old age.

Each nephron is formed by two parts:

1. A blind end called renal corpuscle or Malpighian corpuscle.
2. A tubular portion called renal tubule.

RENAL CORPUSCLE

Renal corpuscle or **Malpighian corpuscle**. It is a spheroidal and slightly flattened structure with a diameter of about 200 µ (**Fig. 33.1**). Function of renal corpuscle is filtration of blood which forms the first phase of urine formation.

SITUATION OF RENAL CORPUSCLE AND TYPES OF NEPHRON

Renal corpuscle is situated in cortex of kidney either near the periphery or near medulla. Based on the situation of renal corpuscle, nephrons are classified into two types.

1. Cortical Nephrons

Cortical nephrons are the nephrons, which have their corpuscles in outer cortex of kidney near the periphery (**Fig. 33.2**). In human kidneys 85% nephrons are cortical nephrons.

2. Juxtamedullary Nephrons

Juxtamedullary nephrons are the nephrons which have their corpuscles in the inner cortex near medulla or **corticomedullary junction**.

STRUCTURE OF RENAL CORPUSCLE

Renal corpuscle is formed by two structures namely glomerulus and Bowman's capsule.

1. Glomerulus

Glomerulus is a tuft of capillaries called glomerular capillaries which are enclosed by Bowman's capsule. The vascular system in glomerulus is purely arterial (**Fig. 33.3**).

Glomerular capillaries arise from the **afferent arteriole**. After entering Bowman's capsule, afferent arteriole divides into many small capillaries. These small capillaries irregular capillary loops and form anastomosis. All the smaller capillaries finally reunite to form **efferent arteriole** which leaves the Bowman's capsule.

Diameter of efferent arteriole is less than that of afferent arteriole. This difference in diameter has functional significance.

Glomerular capillaries are made up of single layer of endothelial cells which are attached to a basement membrane. Endothelium has many pores called **fenestra** or **filtration pores**. Diameter of each pore is 0.1 µ. Presence of the fenestra is evidence of filtration function of the glomerulus.

2. Bowman's Capsule

Bowman's capsule encloses the glomerulus. Structure of Bowman's capsule is similar to a funnel with filter paper. Its diameter is 200 µ. Bowman's capsule is formed by two layers, the inner visceral layer and outer parietal layer.

Visceral layer covers the glomerular capillaries. It is continued as parietal layer at the visceral pole. **Parietal**

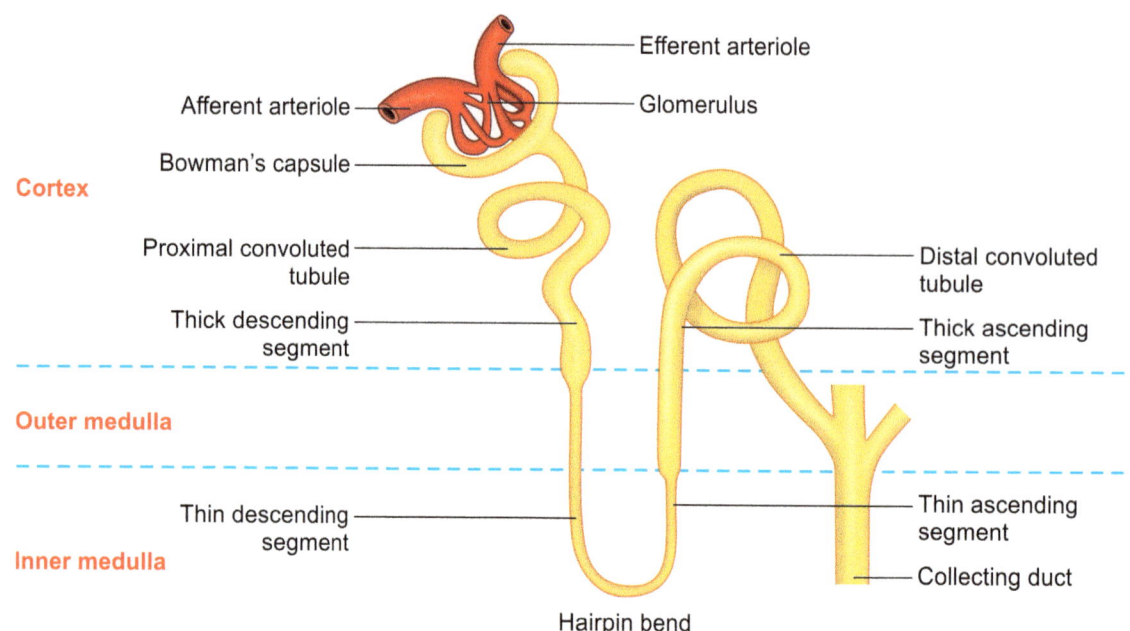

FIGURE 33.1: Structure of nephron.

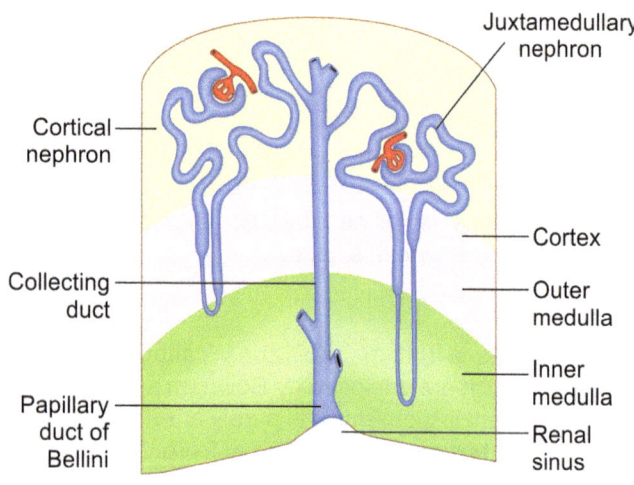

FIGURE 33.2: Types of nephron.

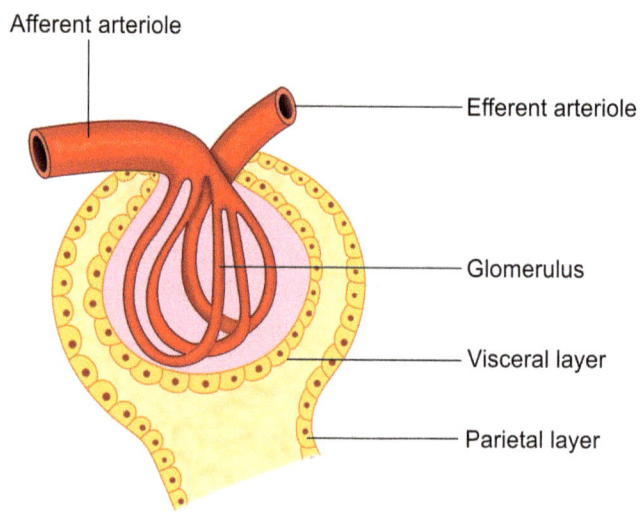

FIGURE 33.3: Renal corpuscle.

layer is continued with wall of the tubular portion of nephron. Cleft like space between visceral and parietal layers is continued as the lumen of tubular portion.

Both the layers of Bowman's capsule are composed of a single layer of flattened epithelial cells resting on a basement membrane.

■ TUBULAR PORTION OF NEPHRON

Tubular portion of nephron is the continuation of Bowman's capsule.

It is made up of three parts:

1. Proximal convoluted tubule.
2. Loop of Henle.
3. Distal convoluted tubule.

■ 1. PROXIMAL CONVOLUTED TUBULE

Proximal convoluted tubule is the coiled portion arising from Bowman's capsule. It is situated in renal cortex. It is continued as descending limb of loop of Henle. Length of this tubule is 14 mm. And its diameter is 55 μ.

Proximal convoluted tubule is formed by single layer of **brush bordered** cuboidal epithelial cells.

■ 2. LOOP OF HENLE

Loop of Henle consists of **three portions**:

i. *Descending Limb*

Descending limb of loop of Henle is made up of thick descending segment and thin descending segment. Thick descending segment is the direct continuation of proximal convoluted tubule. It descends down into medulla. It has a length of 6 mm and a diameter of 55 μ. Thick descending segment of Henle's loop is continued as thin descending segment **(Fig. 33.4)**.

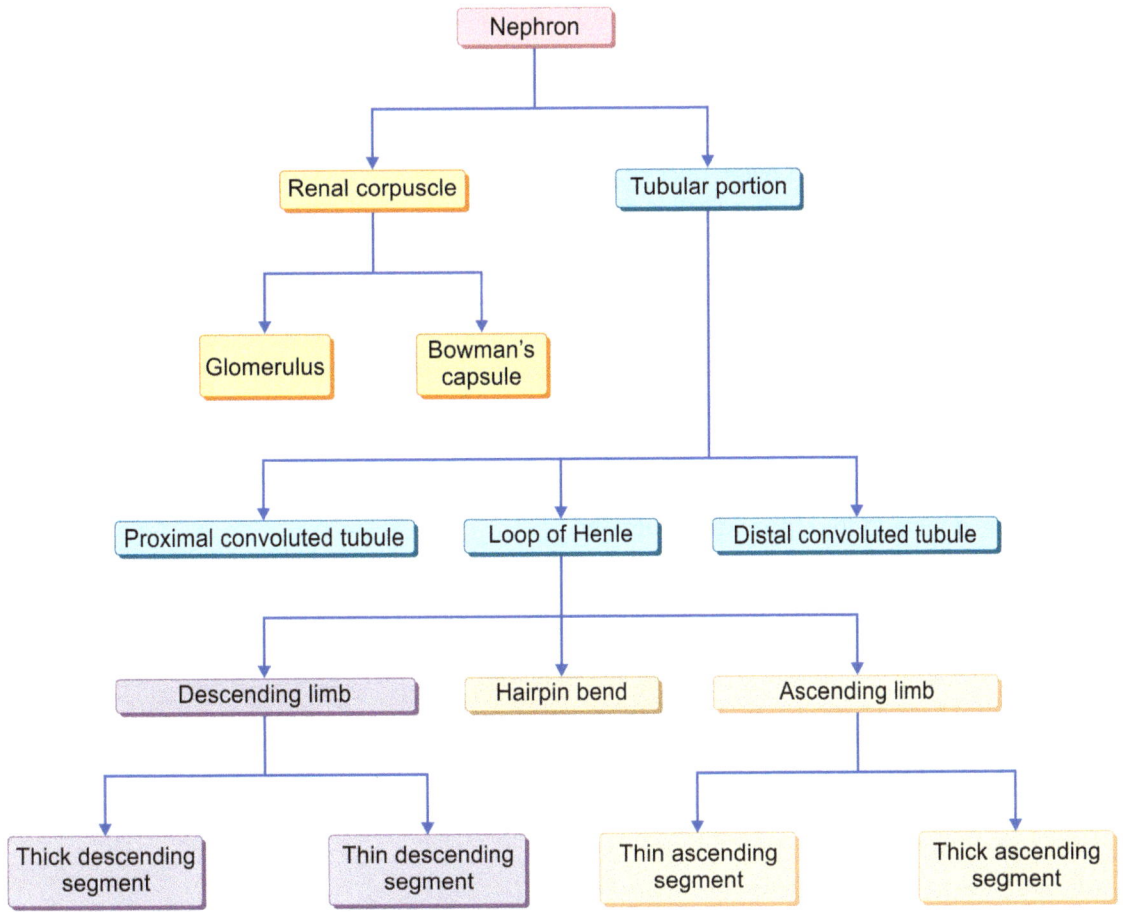

FIGURE 33.4: Parts of nephron.

ii. Hairpin Bend

Thin descending segment is continued as hairpin bend of the loop. Hairpin bend is continued as the ascending segment of loop of Henle.

iii. Ascending Limb

Ascending limb of Henle's loop has two parts, thin ascending segment and thick ascending segment. Thin ascending segment is the continuation of hairpin bend.

Total length of thin descending segment, hairpin bend and thin ascending segment of Henle's loop 10 mm to 15 mm and the diameter is 15 μ **(Table 33.1)**.

Thin ascending segment is continued as thick ascending segment. It is about 9 mm long with a diameter of 30 μ. Thick ascending segment ascends to the cortex and continues as distal convoluted tubule.

■ 3. DISTAL CONVOLUTED TUBULE

Distal convoluted tubule is the continuation of thick ascending segment and it occupies the cortex of kidney. It is continued as collecting duct. Length of the distal convoluted tubule is 14.5 mm to 15 mm. It has a diameter of 22 μ to 50 μ.

Distal convoluted tubule is lined by single layer of cuboidal epithelial cells without brush border. Epithelial

TABLE 33.1: Epithelium, length and diameter and different parts of nephron and collecting duct.

Segment	Epithelium	Length (mm)	Diameter (μ)
Bowman's capsule	Flattened epithelium	–	200
Proximal convoluted tubule	Cuboidal cells with brush border	14	55
Thick descending segment	Cuboidal cells with brush border	6	55
Thin descending segment, hairpin bend and thin ascending segment	Flattened epithelium	10 to 15	15
Thick ascending segment	Cuboidal epithelium without brush border	9	30
Distal convoluted tubule	Cuboidal epithelium without brush border	14.5 to 15	22 to 50
Collecting duct	Cuboidal epithelium without brush border	20 to 22	40 to 200

cells in distal convoluted tubule are called **intercalated cells** or **I cells**.

■ COLLECTING DUCT

Distal convoluted tubule continues as the initial or arched collecting duct, which is in cortex. Lower part of the collecting duct lies in medulla. 7 to 10 initial collecting ducts unite to form the straight collecting duct, which passes through medulla. Length of the collecting duct is 20 mm to 22 mm. Its diameter varies between 40 µ and 200 µ.

Collecting duct is formed by cuboidal or columnar epithelial cells. Epithelial cells of collecting duct are of two types, viz. **Principal** or **P cells** and intercalated or I cells.

■ PASSAGE OF URINE

At the inner zone of medulla, straight **collecting ducts** from each medullary pyramid unite to form **papillary ducts** or **ducts of Bellini** or papillary ducts of Bellini, which open into a 'V-shaped' area called **papilla**. Urine from each medullary pyramid is collected in the papilla. From here it is drained into a **minor calyx.** Three or four minor calyces unite to form one **major calyx**. Each kidney has got about 8 minor calyces and 2 to 3 major calyces.

From minor calyces, urine passes through major calyces, which open into the **pelvis of the ureter** (renal pelvis). Pelvis is the expanded portion of ureter present in the renal sinus.

From **renal pelvis**, urine passes through remaining portion of **ureter** and reaches **urinary bladder**.

Chapter 34

Juxtaglomerular Apparatus

CHAPTER OUTLINE

- **DEFINITION**
- **STRUCTURE**
  - MACULA DENSA
  - EXTRAGLOMERULAR MESANGIAL CELLS
  - JUXTAGLOMERULAR CELLS
- **FUNCTIONS**
  - SECRETION OF RENIN
  - SECRETION OF OTHER SUBSTANCES
  - REGULATION OF GLOMERULAR BLOOD FLOW AND GLOMERULAR FILTRATION RATE

DEFINITION

Juxtaglomerular apparatus is a specialized organ situated near the glomerulus of each nephron (juxta means near).

STRUCTURE OF JUXTAGLOMERULAR APPARATUS

Juxtaglomerular apparatus is formed by **three structures:**

1. MACULA DENSA

Macula densa is the terminal portion of thick ascending segment that runs in between afferent and efferent arterioles of the same nephron. Actually, it is very close to afferent arteriole **(Fig. 34.1)**. Macula densa is made up of specialized epithelial cells which are packed closely.

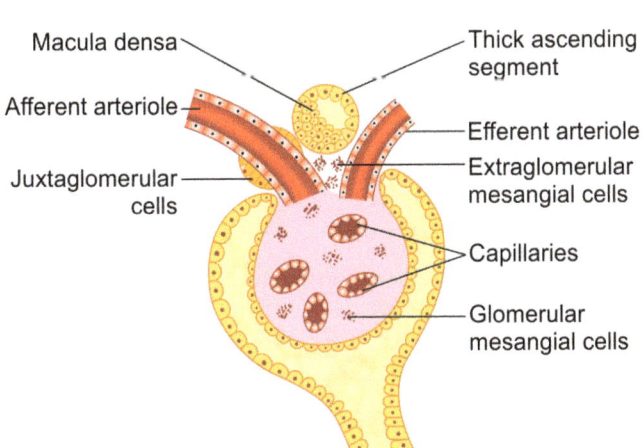

FIGURE 34.1: Juxtaglomerular apparatus.

2. EXTRAGLOMERULAR MESANGIAL CELLS

Extraglomerular cells are situated in the triangular region bound by afferent arteriole, efferent arteriole and macula densa. These cells are also called **agranular cells, lacis cells, Polkissen cells** or **Goormaghtigh cells.**

Glomerular mesangial cells or intraglomerular mesangial cells are situated in between glomerular capillaries and form a cellular network which supports the capillary loops. These cells are contractile in nature and regulate the glomerular filtration.

3. JUXTAGLOMERULAR CELLS

Juxtaglomerular cells or **granular cells** are specialized **smooth muscle cells** situated in the wall of afferent arteriole just before it enters the Bowman's capsule. Juxtaglomerular cells form a thick cuff called **polar cushion** or **Polkissen** around the afferent arteriole before it enters the Bowman's capsule.

FUNCTIONS OF JUXTAGLOMERULAR APPARATUS

1. SECRETION OF RENIN

Juxtaglomerular cells secrete renin. Renin is a peptide with 340 amino acids. Along with angiotensins, renin forms the renin-angiotensin system which is a hormone system that is involved in the maintenance of blood pressure (Chapter 63).

Secretion of renin is stimulated by four factors:

1. Fall in arterial blood pressure.
2. Reduction in the ECF volume.

3. Increased sympathetic activity.
4. Decreased load of sodium and chloride in macula densa.

Renin-Angiotensin System

When renin is released into the blood, it acts on **angiotensinogen** or renin substrate which α2 globulin in nature. Renin converts angiotensinogen into **angiotensin I**. Angiotensin I is converted into **angiotensin II** by the activity of **angiotensin-converting enzyme (ACE)** secreted from lungs. Most of the conversion of angiotensin I into angiotensin II takes place in lungs.

Angiotensin II is rapidly degraded into **angiotensin III** by **angiotensinases** present in RBCs and vascular beds in many tissues. Angiotensin III is converted into **angiotensin IV** (Fig. 34.2).

Actions of Angiotensins

Angiotensin I

Angiotensin I physiologically inactive and serves only as a precursor of angiotensin II.

Angiotensin II

Angiotensin II is the most active form. Its actions are given below:

1. On blood vessels:

Angiotensin II increases arterial blood pressure by causing vasoconstriction.

2. On adrenal cortex:

Angiotensin II stimulates zona glomerulosa of adrenal cortex to secrete aldosterone which increases retention of sodium by kidney. This is also responsible for elevation of blood pressure.

3. On kidney:

i. Angiotensin II regulates glomerular filtration rate by two ways:
   a. It constricts the efferent arteriole which causes decrease in filtration after an initial increase (Chapter 36).
   b. It contracts the glomerular mesangial cells leading to decrease in surface area of glomerular capillaries and filtration.
ii. It increases sodium reabsorption from renal tubules.

4. On brain:

i. Angiotensin II inhibits baroreceptor reflex and thereby indirectly increases the blood pressure. Baroreceptor reflex is responsible for decreasing the blood pressure (Chapter 63).
ii. It increases water intake by stimulating the thirst center.
iii. It increases the secretion of corticotropinreleasing hormone (CRH) from hypothalamus. CRH in turn-increases secretion of adrenocorticotropic hormone (ACTH) from pituitary.
iv. It increases secretion of antidiuretic hormone (ADH) from hypothalamus.

5. Other actions:

Angiotensin II acts as a growth factor in heart.

Angiotensin III

Angiotensin III increases the blood pressure and stimulates aldosterone secretion from adrenal cortex.

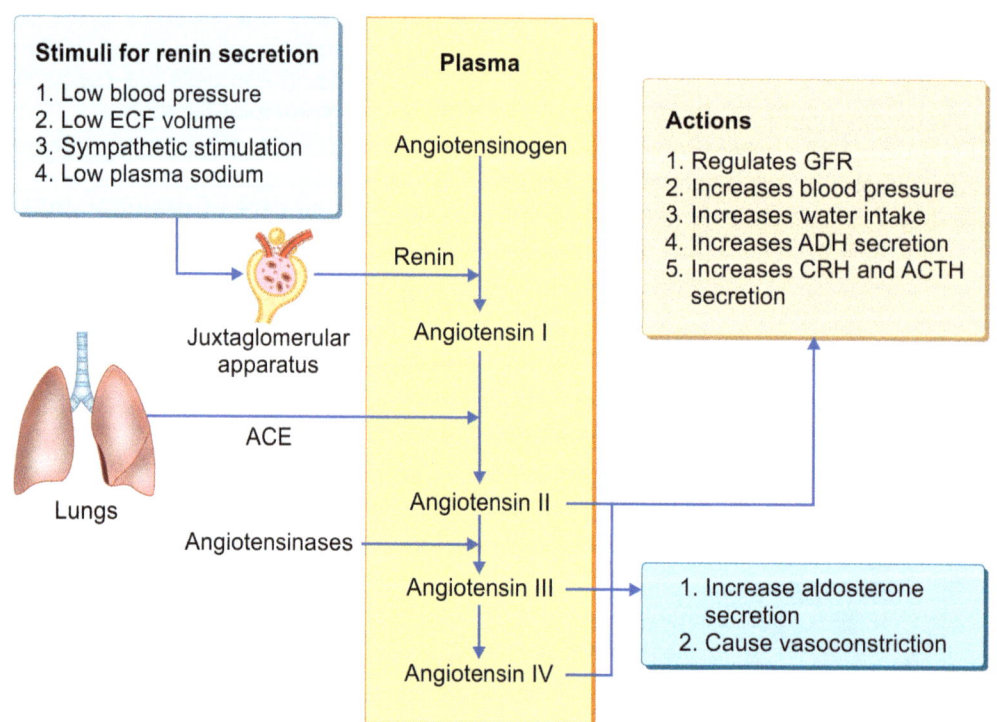

FIGURE 34.2: Renin-angiotensin system.
ECF = Extracellular fluid, ACE = Angiotensin-converting enzyme, GFR = Glomerular filtration rate, ADH = Antidiuretic hormone, CRH = Corticotropin-releasing hormone, ACTH = Adrenocorticotropic hormone.

Angiotensin IV

Angiotensin IV also has adrenal cortical stimulating and vasopressor activities.

■ 2. SECRETION OF OTHER SUBSTANCES

Extraglomerular mesangial cells of juxtaglomerular apparatus secrete prostaglandin.

Macula densa secretes thromboxane A_2.

■ 3. REGULATION OF GLOMERULAR BLOOD FLOW AND GLOMERULAR FILTRATION RATE

Macula densa of juxtaglomerular apparatus is responsible for tubuloglomerular feedback mechanism which regulates of renal blood flow and glomerular filtration rate. Refer Chapter 36 for details.

Chapter 35

Renal Circulation

CHAPTER OUTLINE

- RENAL BLOOD FLOW
- RENAL BLOOD VESSELS
- MEASUREMENT OF RENAL BLOOD FLOW
- REGULATION OF RENAL BLOOD FLOW
- SALIENT FEATURES OF RENAL CIRCULATION

■ RENAL BLOOD FLOW

Blood vessels of kidneys are highly specialized to facilitate the functions of nephrons in the formation of urine. Kidneys are supplied by renal arteries.

In adults, during resting conditions both the kidneys receive 1,300 mL of blood per minute or about 26% of cardiac output. Kidneys are the second organs to receive maximum blood flow, the first organ being liver which receives 1,500 mL per minute.

■ RENAL BLOOD VESSELS

Renal Artery

Renal artery arises directly from abdominal aorta and enters the kidney through the hilus.

Segmental Artery

While passing through renal sinus, renal artery divides into many segmental arteries, which subdivide into interlobar arteries **(Fig. 35.1)**.

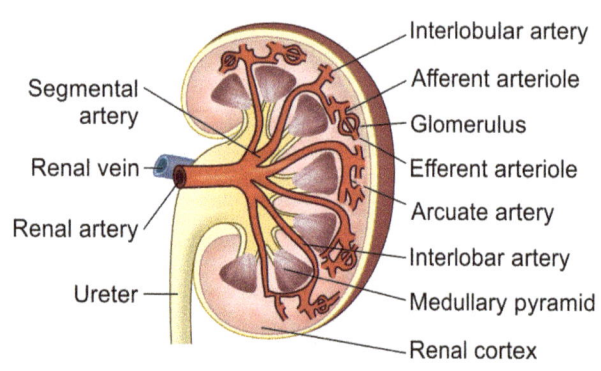

FIGURE 35.1: Renal blood vessels.

Interlobar Artery

Each interlobar artery passes in between the medullary pyramids. At the base of pyramid, it turns and runs parallel to the base of pyramid forming arcuate artery.

Arcuate Artery

Each arcuate artery gives rise to interlobular arteries.

Interlobular Artery

Interlobular arteries run through the renal cortex perpendicular to arcuate artery. From each interlobular artery, numerous afferent arterioles arise.

Afferent Arteriole

Afferent arteriole enters the Bowman's capsule and forms glomerular capillary tuft. After entering the Bowman's capsule, the afferent arteriole divides into 4 or 5 large capillaries.

Glomerular Capillaries

Large capillary divides into small glomerular capillaries, which form the loops. And, **capillary loops** unite to form efferent arteriole, which leaves the Bowman's capsule.

Efferent Arteriole

Efferent arterioles form a second capillary network called peritubular capillaries, which surround the tubular portions of nephrons. Thus, renal circulation forms a **portal system** by the presence of two sets of capillaries, namely glomerular capillaries and peritubular capillaries.

Peritubular Capillaries and Vasa Recta

Peritubular capillaries are found around the tubular portion of cortical nephrons only. Tubular portion of

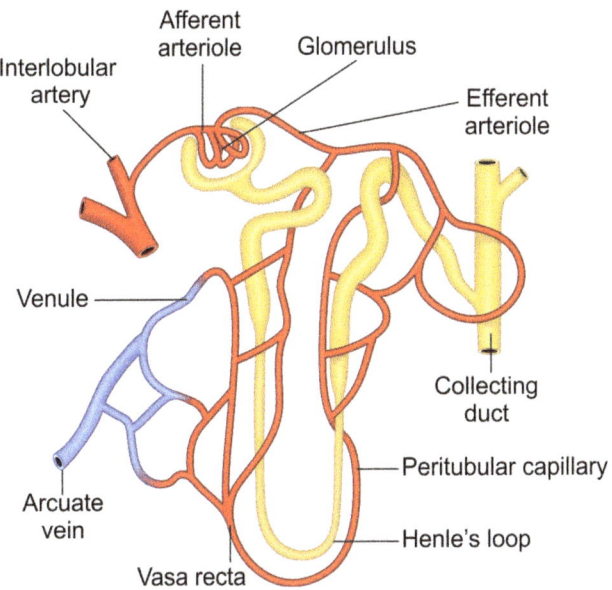

FIGURE 35.2: Renal capillaries.

juxtamedullary nephrons is supplied by some specialized capillaries called vasa recta (singular = vas rectum). These capillaries are straight blood vessels hence the name vasa recta. Vasa recta arise directly from efferent arteriole of the juxtamedullary nephrons and run parallel to renal tubule into the medulla and ascend up towards cortex **(Fig. 35.2)**.

Venous System

Peritubular capillaries and vasa recta drain into the venous system. Venous system starts with peritubular venules and continues as interlobular veins, arcuate veins, interlobar veins, segmental veins and finally the renal vein.

Renal vein leaves the kidney through the hilus and joins **inferior vena cava**.

■ MEASUREMENT OF RENAL BLOOD FLOW

Blood flow to kidneys is measured by using plasma clearance of **para-aminohippuric acid** (Chapter 39).

■ REGULATION OF RENAL BLOOD FLOW

Renal blood flow is regulated mostly by autoregulation. Nerves innervating renal blood vessels have no significant role in regulation of blood flow.

■ AUTOREGULATION

Autoregulation is the intrinsic ability of an organ to regulate its own blood flow. Autoregulation is present in some vital organs in the body such as brain, heart and kidneys. It is highly significant and more efficient in kidneys.

Renal Autoregulation

Renal autoregulation is important to maintain the glomerular filtration rate (GFR). Blood flow to kidneys remains normal even when the mean arterial blood pressure varies widely between 60 mm Hg and 180 mm Hg. This helps to maintain normal GFR.

Two mechanisms are involved in renal autoregulation:

1. Myogenic Response

Whenever blood flow to kidneys increases, elastic wall of afferent arteriole stretches. Stretch of the vessel wall increases flow of calcium ions from extracellular fluid into the cells. Influx of calcium ions leads to the contraction of smooth muscles in afferent arteriole which causes constriction of afferent arteriole. So, the blood flow is decreased.

2. Tubuloglomerular Feedback

Macula densa plays an important role in tubuloglomerular feedback which controls the renal blood flow and GFR. Refer Chapter 36 for details.

■ SALIENT FEATURES OF RENAL CIRCULATION

1. Renal arteries arise directly from the aorta. So, the pressure in aorta is very high and it facilitates a high blood flow to the renal parenchyma.
2. Kidneys receive about 1,300 mL of blood per minute, i.e. about 26% of cardiac output. Kidneys are the second organs to receive maximum blood flow, the first organ being the liver which receives 1,500 mL per minute, i.e. about 30% of cardiac output.
3. Whole amount of blood which flows to kidney has to pass through the glomerular capillaries before entering the venous system. Because of this, blood is completely filtered at the renal glomeruli.
4. Renal circulation has a **portal system**, i.e. a double network of capillaries namely glomerular capillaries and peritubular capillaries.
5. Renal glomerular capillaries form **high pressure bed** with a pressure of 60 mm Hg to 70 mm Hg. It is much greater than the capillary pressure elsewhere in the body, which is only about 25 mm Hg to 30 mm Hg. High pressure is maintained in the glomerular capillaries because the diameter of afferent arteriole is more than that of efferent arteriole. High capillary pressure augments glomerular filtration.
6. Peritubular capillaries form **low pressure bed** with a pressure of 8 mm Hg to 10 mm Hg. This low pressure helps tubular reabsorption.
7. Autoregulation of renal blood flow is well established.

CHAPTER 36

Urine Formation

CHAPTER OUTLINE

- **URINE FORMATION**
- **GLOMERULAR FILTRATION**
  - DEFINITION
  - FILTRATION MEMBRANE
  - PROCESS OF GLOMERULAR FILTRATION
  - GLOMERULAR FILTRATION RATE
  - FILTRATION FRACTION
  - PRESSURES DETERMINING FILTRATION
  - FACTORS REGULATING (AFFECTING) GFR
- **TUBULAR REABSORPTION**
  - SELECTIVE REABSORPTION
  - MECHANISM OF REABSORPTION
- SITE OF REABSORPTION
- ROUTES OF REABSORPTION
- REGULATION OF TUBULAR REABSORPTION
- TRANSPORT MAXIMUM: Tm VALUE
- RENAL THRESHOLD
- REABSORPTION OF IMPORTANT SUBSTANCES
- **TUBULAR SECRETION**
  - SUBSTANCES SECRETED IN DIFFERENT SEGMENTS OF RENAL TUBULES

URINE FORMATION

Urine formation is the blood-cleansing function in which kidneys excrete the unwanted substances along with water from the blood as urine. **Urinary output** in a normal person is 1 to 1.5 L/day.

Processes of Urine Formation

When blood passes through glomerular capillaries, plasma is filtered into the Bowman's capsule. This process is called **glomerular filtration**.

Filtrate from Bowman's capsule passes through tubular portion of the nephron. While passing through tubule, the filtrate undergoes various changes both in quality and in quantity. Many wanted substances like glucose, amino acids, water and electrolytes are reabsorbed from the tubules. This process is called **tubular reabsorption**.

And, some unwanted substances are secreted into the tubule from peritubular blood vessels. This process is called **tubular secretion** or excretion **(Fig. 36.1)**.

Thus, urine formation includes **three processes**:

1. Glomerular filtration.
2. Tubular reabsorption.
3. Tubular secretion.

Among the three processes, filtration is the function of glomerulus. Reabsorption and secretion are the functions of tubular portion of the nephron.

GLOMERULAR FILTRATION

DEFINITION

Glomerular filtration is the process by which blood passing through glomerular capillaries is filtered through filtration membrane. It is the first process of urine formation. Structure of filtration membrane is well suited for this.

FILTRATION MEMBRANE

Filtration membrane is formed by **three layers**:

1. Glomerular Capillary Membrane

Glomerular capillary membrane is formed by single layer of endothelial cells which are attached to the basement membrane. Capillary membrane has many pores called **fenestra** or **filtration pores** with a diameter of 0.1 μ.

2. Basement Membrane

Basement membrane of glomerular capillaries fuses with the basement membrane of visceral layer of Bowman's capsule. Basement membrane separates endothelium of glomerular capillary and epithelium of visceral layer of Bowman's capsule.

3. Visceral Layer of Bowman's Capsule

This is composed of a single layer of flattened epithelial cells resting on a basement membrane. Each cell is connected with the basement membrane by cytoplasmic

Chapter 36: Urine Formation

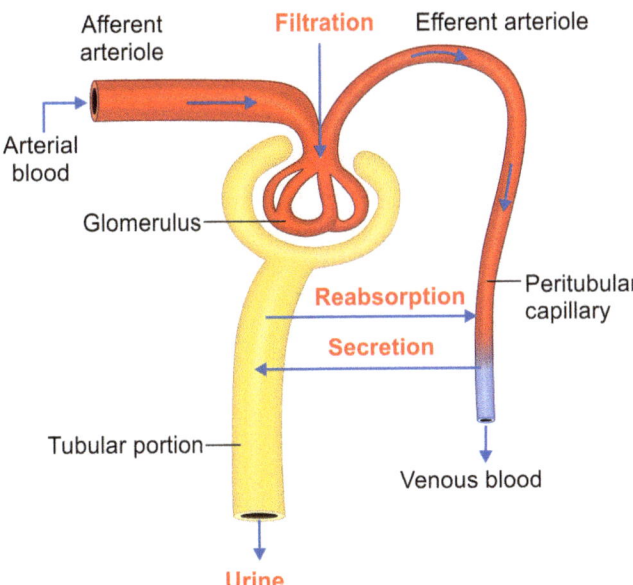

FIGURE 36.1: Events of urine formation.

extensions called **pedicles** or feet. Pedicles are arranged in an interdigitating manner leaving small cleft-like spaces in between. Cleft-like space is called **slit pore**. Filtration takes place through these slit pores. Epithelial cells with pedicles are called **podocytes (Fig. 36.2)**.

■ PROCESS OF GLOMERULAR FILTRATION

When blood passes through glomerular capillaries, plasma is filtered into the Bowman's capsule. All the substances of plasma are filtered, except **plasma proteins**. The filtered fluid is called **glomerular filtrate**.

Glomerular filtration is called **ultrafiltration** because even the minute particles are filtered. But the plasma proteins which have larger molecular size are not filtered. Thus, glomerular filtrate contains all the substances of plasma except the plasma proteins.

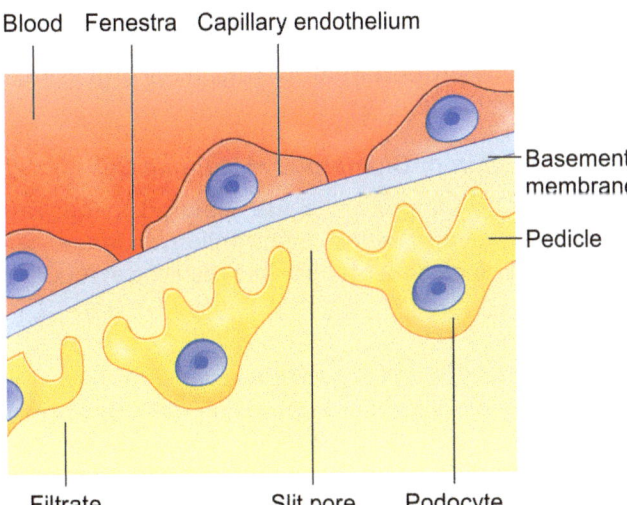

FIGURE 36.2: Filtration membrane in renal corpuscle. It is formed by capillary endothelium on one side (red) and visceral layer of Bowman's capsule (yellow) on the other side.

■ GLOMERULAR FILTRATION RATE

Glomerular filtration rate (GFR) is defined as the total quantity of filtrate formed in all nephrons of both the kidneys in the given unit of time.

Normal GFR is 125 mL per minute or about 180 L per day.

■ FILTRATION FRACTION

Filtration fraction is the fraction (portion) of renal plasma which becomes filtrate. It is the ratio between renal plasma flow and glomerular filtration rate. It is expressed in percentage. Normal filtration fraction varies from 15% to 20%.

■ PRESSURES DETERMINING FILTRATION

Glomerular filtration is determined by **three types of pressures**:

1. *Glomerular Capillary Pressure*

Glomerular capillary pressure is the pressure exerted by blood in glomerular capillaries. It is about 60 mm Hg, and varies between 45 mm Hg and 70 mm Hg. Glomerular capillary pressure is the highest capillary pressure in the body. This pressure **favors filtration**.

2. *Colloidal Osmotic Pressure*

Colloidal osmotic pressure is exerted by plasma proteins in the glomeruli. Plasma proteins are not filtered through the glomerular capillaries and remain in glomerular capillaries. These proteins develop the colloidal osmotic pressure which is about 25 mm Hg. It **opposes filtration**.

3. *Hydrostatic Pressure in Bowman's Capsule*

Hydrostatic pressure in Bowman's capsule is the pressure exerted by the filtrate in Bowman's capsule. It is also called capsular pressure. It is about 15 mm Hg. It also **opposes filtration**.

Net Filtration Pressure

Net filtration pressure or **effective filtration pressure** is the balance between pressure favoring filtration and pressures opposing filtration.

Net filtration pressure =

$$\text{Glomerular capillary pressure} - \left\{ \text{Colloidal osmotic pressure} + \text{Hydrostatic pressure in Bowman's capsule} \right\}$$

$$= 60 - (25 + 15) = 20 \text{ mm Hg}.$$

Normal net filtration pressure is about 20 mm Hg, and it varies between 15 mm Hg and 20 mm Hg.

Starling Hypothesis and Starling Forces of Filtration

Determination of net filtration pressure is based on Starling hypothesis. Starling hypothesis states that the net filtration through capillary membrane is proportional to hydrostatic pressure difference across the membrane minus oncotic pressure difference. Hydrostatic pressure within the glomerular capillaries is the glomerular capillary pressure.

All the pressures involved in determination of filtration are called Starling forces of filtration.

■ FACTORS REGULATING (AFFECTING) GFR

1. Renal Blood Flow

GFR is **directly proportional** to renal blood flow. Renal blood flow itself is controlled by autoregulation. Refer Chapter 35 for details.

2. Tubuloglomerular Feedback

Tubuloglomerular feedback is the mechanism that regulates GFR through renal tubule and macula densa. Macula densa of juxtaglomerular apparatus is sensitive to sodium chloride in the tubular fluid.

When glomerular filtrate passes through the terminal portion of thick ascending segment, macula densa acts like a sensor. It detects the concentration of sodium chloride in tubular fluid and accordingly alters the glomerular blood flow and GFR.

When the concentration of sodium chloride increases in the filtrate

When the concentration of sodium chloride increases in filtrate, macula densa releases **adenosine** from ATP. Adenosine causes constriction of afferent arteriole. So, the blood flow through glomerulus decreases leading to decrease in GFR.

When the concentration of sodium chloride decreases in the filtrate

When the concentration of sodium chloride decreases in the filtrate, macula densa secretes **prostaglandin (PGE$_2$), bradykinin** and **renin**.

PGE$_2$ and bradykinin cause dilatation of afferent arteriole. Renin induces the formation of angiotensin II which causes constriction of efferent arteriole. Dilatation of afferent arteriole and constriction of efferent arteriole leads to increase in glomerular blood flow and GFR.

3. Glomerular Capillary Pressure

Glomerular filtration pressure is **directly proportional** to glomerular capillary pressure. Capillary pressure, in turn depends upon the renal blood flow and arterial blood pressure.

4. Colloidal Osmotic Pressure

GFR is **inversely proportional** to colloidal osmotic pressure which is exerted by plasma proteins in the glomerular capillary blood.

5. Hydrostatic Pressure in Bowman's Capsule

GFR is **inversely proportional** to hydrostatic pressure in Bowman's capsule.

6. Constriction of Afferent Arteriole

Constriction of afferent arteriole reduces the blood flow to glomerular capillaries which in turn reduces GFR.

7. Constriction of Efferent Arteriole

If efferent arteriole is constricted, initially GFR increases because of stagnation of blood in the capillaries. Later when all the substances are filtered from this blood, further filtration does not occur. This is because the efferent arteriolar constriction prevents outflow of blood from glomerulus and no fresh blood enters the glomerulus for filtration.

8. Systemic Arterial Pressure

Renal blood flow or GFR are not affected till the mean arterial blood pressure is between 60 mm Hg and 180 mm Hg. It is due to the autoregulatory mechanism (Chapter 35). Variation in pressure above 180 mm Hg or below 60 mm Hg affects the renal blood flow and GFR accordingly, because the autoregulatory mechanism fails beyond this range.

9. Sympathetic Stimulation

Afferent and efferent arterioles are supplied by sympathetic nerves. Mild or moderate stimulation of sympathetic nerves does not cause any significant change either in renal blood flow or GFR.

Strong sympathetic stimulation causes severe constriction of the blood vessels by releasing the neurotransmitter substance, **noradrenaline**. Effect is more severe on efferent arterioles than on the afferent arterioles. So, initially there is increase in filtration, but later it decreases.

10. Surface Area of Capillary Membrane

GFR is **directly proportional** to the surface area of the capillary membrane.

11. Permeability of Capillary Membrane

GFR is **directly proportional** to permeability of glomerular capillary membrane.

12. Contraction of Glomerular Mesangial Cells

Glomerular mesangial cells are situated in between the glomerular capillaries. Contraction of these cells decreases surface area of capillaries resulting in reduction in GFR.

13. Hormonal and Other Factors

Many hormones and other factors alter GFR by affecting the blood flow through glomerulus. For example, atrial natriuretic peptide, brain natriuretic peptide, dopamine, endothelium-derived nitric oxide and prostaglandin E$_2$ (PGE$_2$) increase GFR by vasodilatation.

Angiotensin II, endothelin, noradrenaline and prostaglandin F$_2$ (PGF$_2$) decrease GFR by vasoconstriction.

TUBULAR REABSORPTION

Tubular reabsorption is the process by which water and other substances are transported from renal tubules back to the blood. When glomerular filtrate flows through the tubular portion of nephron, large quantity of water (more than 99%), electrolytes and other substances are reabsorbed by the tubular epithelial cells. Reabsorbed substances move into peritubular capillaries via interstitial fluid of renal medulla.

SELECTIVE REABSORPTION

Tubular reabsorption is known as selective reabsorption because tubular cells reabsorb only the substances necessary for the body. Essential substances such as glucose, amino acids and vitamins are completely reabsorbed from renal tubule. Whereas the unwanted substances like metabolic waste products are excreted through urine.

MECHANISM OF REABSORPTION

Basic transport mechanisms involved in tubular reabsorption are of **two types**:

1. Active Reabsorption

Active reabsorption is the movement of molecules against the electrochemical gradient. It needs liberation of energy which is derived from ATP. Substances which are reabsorbed actively from the renal tubule are sodium, calcium, potassium, phosphates, sulfates, bicarbonates, glucose, amino acids, ascorbic acid, uric acid and ketone bodies.

2. Passive Reabsorption

Passive reabsorption is the movement of molecules along the electrochemical gradient. This process does not need energy. Substances which are reabsorbed passively are chloride, urea and water.

SITE OF REABSORPTION

Reabsorption of the substances occurs in almost all the segments of tubular portion of nephron.

1. Substances Reabsorbed from Proximal Convoluted Tubule

About 7/8 of the filtrate (about 88%) is reabsorbed in proximal convoluted tubule. Brush border of the epithelial cell in proximal convoluted tubule increases the surface area and facilitates reabsorption.

Substances reabsorbed from proximal convoluted tubule are glucose, amino acids, sodium, potassium, calcium, bicarbonates, chlorides, phosphates, uric acid and water.

2. Substances Reabsorbed from Loop of Henle

Substances reabsorbed from loop of Henle are sodium and chloride.

3. Substances Reabsorbed from Distal Convoluted Tubule

Sodium, calcium, bicarbonate and water are reabsorbed from distal convoluted tubule.

ROUTES OF REABSORPTION

Reabsorption of substances from tubular lumen into the peritubular capillary occurs by two routes:

1. Transcellular Route

In this route, the substances move through the cell. It includes transport of substances:

i. From tubular lumen into tubular cell through apical (luminal) surface of the cell membrane
ii. Tubular cell into interstitial fluid
iii. Interstitial fluid into capillary.

2. Paracellular Route

In this route, the substances move through intercellular space. It includes transport of substances:

i. From tubular lumen into interstitial fluid present in lateral intercellular space through the tight junction between the cells.
ii. From interstitial fluid into capillary **(Fig. 36.3)**.

REGULATION OF TUBULAR REABSORPTION

Tubular reabsorption is regulated by **three factors**:

1. Glomerulotubular Balance

Glomerulotubular balance is the balance between filtration and reabsorption of solutes and water in kidney. When GFR increases, the tubular load of solutes and water in proximal convoluted tubule is increased. It is followed by increase in the reabsorption of solutes and water.

This process helps in constant reabsorption of solute, particularly sodium and water from renal tubule.

2. Hormonal Factors

i. Aldosterone, angiotensin II increase sodium reabsorption. Atrial natriuretic factor and brain natriuretic factor decrease sodium reabsorption.
ii. Antidiuretic hormone increases water reabsorption.
iii. Parathormone increases calcium reabsorption and calcitonin decreases calcium reabsorption.

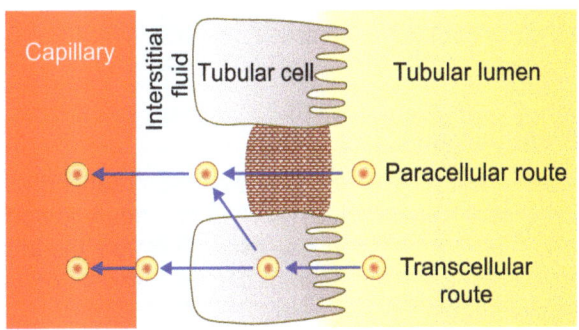

FIGURE 36.3: Routes of reabsorption.

3. Nervous Factor

Activation of sympathetic nervous system increases the tubular reabsorption (particularly of sodium) from renal tubules. It also increases the tubular reabsorption indirectly by stimulating secretion of renin from juxtaglomerular cell. Renin causes formation of angiotensin II which increases the sodium reabsorption (Chapter 34).

■ TRANSPORT MAXIMUM: Tm VALUE

Tubular transport maximum or Tm is the rate at which a substance is reabsorbed from renal tubule. For example, **transport maximum for glucose (TmG)**, is 375 mg/minute in adult males and about 300 mg/minute in adult females.

■ RENAL THRESHOLD

Renal threshold is the plasma concentration at which a substance appears first in urine. Every substance has a threshold level in plasma or blood. Below that threshold level, the substance is completely reabsorbed and does not appear in urine. When concentration of that substance reaches the threshold, excess amount is not reabsorbed and, so it appears in urine. This level is called the renal threshold of that substance.

For example, **renal threshold for glucose** is 180 mg/dL. That is, glucose is completely reabsorbed from tubular fluid, if its concentration in blood is below 180 mg/dL. So, the glucose does not appear in urine. When the blood level of glucose reaches 180 mg/dL, it is not reabsorbed completely and appears in urine.

■ REABSORPTION OF IMPORTANT SUBSTANCES

1. Reabsorption of Sodium

From the glomerular filtrate, 99% of sodium is reabsorbed. Two-thirds of sodium are reabsorbed in proximal convoluted tubule and remaining one third in other segments (except descending limb) and collecting duct.

Sodium reabsorption occurs in three steps:

  i. Transport from lumen of renal tubules into the tubular epithelial cells.
  ii. Transport from tubular cells into the interstitial fluid.
  iii. Transport from interstitial fluid to the blood.

2. Reabsorption of Water

Reabsorption of water occurs from proximal and distal convoluted tubules and in collecting duct.

Reabsorption of water from proximal convoluted tubule: Obligatory water reabsorption

Obligatory reabsorption is the type of water reabsorption in proximal convoluted tubule, which is secondary to sodium reabsorption. When sodium is reabsorbed from the tubule, osmotic pressure decreases. It causes osmosis of water from renal tubule.

Reabsorption of water from distal convoluted tubule and collecting duct: Facultative water reabsorption

Facultative reabsorption is the type of water reabsorption in distal convoluted tubule and collecting duct that occurs by the activity of **antidiuretic hormone**. Normally, distal convoluted tubule and the collecting duct are not permeable to water. But antidiuretic hormone makes these segments become permeable to water and so it is reabsorbed.

Mechanism of action of antidiuretic hormone

Antidiuretic hormone combines with V_2 **receptors** in tubular epithelial membrane and activates adenyl cyclase, to form cyclic AMP. This cyclic AMP increases the permeability of the tubules for water by activating aquaporins which form the water channels.

Aquaporins are the membrane proteins which function as water channels. ADH increases water reabsorption in distal convoluted tubules and collecting ducts by regulating the aquaporins.

3. Reabsorption of Glucose

Glucose is completely reabsorbed in the proximal convoluted tubule. It is transported by secondary active transport (sodium cotransport) mechanism. Glucose and sodium bind to a common carrier protein in the luminal membrane of tubular epithelium and enter the cell. Carrier protein is called **sodium-dependent glucose transporter 2 (SGLT2)**. From tubular cell glucose is transported into medullary interstitium by another carrier protein called **glucose transporter 2 (GLUT2)**.

Renal threshold for glucose

Renal threshold for glucose is 180 mg/dL in venous blood. When the blood level reaches 180 mg/dL glucose is not reabsorbed completely and appears in urine.

Tubular maximum for glucose (TmG)

In adult male, TmG is 375 mg/minute and in adult females, it is about 300 mg/minute (see above).

4. Reabsorption of Bicarbonates

Most of the bicarbonate is reabsorbed actively in proximal tubule. It is reabsorbed in the form of carbon dioxide.

Bicarbonate is mostly present as sodium bicarbonate in the filtrate. Sodium bicarbonate dissociates into sodium and bicarbonate ions in the tubular lumen. Sodium diffuses into tubular cell in exchange of hydrogen. Bicarbonate combines with hydrogen to form carbonic acid. Carbonic acid dissociates into carbon dioxide and water in the presence of carbonic anhydrase. Carbon dioxide and water enter the tubular cell.

In the tubular cells, carbon dioxide combines with water to form carbonic acid. It immediately dissociates into hydrogen and bicarbonate. Bicarbonate from the tubular cell enters the interstitium. There it combines with sodium to form sodium bicarbonate **(Fig. 38.1)**.

5. *Reabsorption of Amino Acids*

Amino acids are also reabsorbed completely in proximal convoluted tubule. Amino acids are reabsorbed actively by the secondary active transport mechanism along with sodium.

■ TUBULAR SECRETION

Tubular secretion is the process by which the substances are transported from blood into renal tubules. It is also called tubular excretion.

■ SUBSTANCES SECRETED IN DIFFERENT SEGMENTS OF RENAL TUBULES

1. Potassium is secreted actively by sodium-potassium pump in proximal and distal convoluted tubules and collecting ducts.
2. Ammonia is secreted in the proximal convoluted tubule.
3. Hydrogen ions are secreted in the proximal and distal convoluted tubules.

Chapter 37: Concentration of Urine

CHAPTER OUTLINE

- **OSMOLARITY OF URINE**
  - FORMATION OF DILUTE URINE
  - FORMATION OF CONCENTRATED URINE
- **MEDULLARY GRADIENT**
  - MEDULLARY HYPEROSMOLARITY
  - DEVELOPMENT AND MAINTENANCE OF MEDULLARY GRADIENT
- **COUNTERCURRENT MECHANISM**
  - COUNTERCURRENT FLOW
  - COUNTERCURRENT MULTIPLIER
  - COUNTERCURRENT EXCHANGER
- **ROLE OF ADH**
- **SUMMARY OF URINE CONCENTRATION**
- **APPLIED PHYSIOLOGY**

OSMOLARITY OF URINE

Everyday 180 L of glomerular filtrate is formed with large quantity of water. If this much of water is excreted in urine, body will face serious threats. So, the concentration of urine is very essential.

Osmolarity of glomerular filtrate is same as that of plasma and it is 300 mOsm/L. But normally urine is concentrated and its osmolarity is four times more than that of plasma, i.e. 1,200 mOsm/L.

Osmolarity of urine depends upon two factors, namely water content in the body and **antidiuretic hormone (ADH)**.

FORMATION OF DILUTE URINE

When, water content in the body increases, kidney excretes dilute urine. This is achieved by **inhibition of ADH** secretion from posterior pituitary (Chapter 44). So, water reabsorption from renal tubules does not take place leading to excretion of large amount of water. This makes the urine dilute.

FORMATION OF CONCENTRATED URINE

When the water content in body decreases, kidney retains water and excretes concentrated urine. Formation of concentrated urine is not as simple as that of dilute urine.

It involves two processes:

1. Development and maintenance of medullary gradient by countercurrent system.
2. Secretion of ADH.

MEDULLARY GRADIENT

MEDULLARY HYPEROSMOLARITY

Interstitial fluid in renal cortex is isotonic to plasma with the osmolarity of 300 mOsm/L. Osmolarity of interstitial fluid near in medulla the cortex also is 300 mOsm/L.

However, while proceeding from outer part towards the inner part of medulla, osmolarity increases gradually and reaches the maximum at the inner most part of medulla near renal sinus. Here, it is 1,200 mOsm/L **(Fig. 37.1)**.

This type of gradual increase in osmolarity of the medullary interstitial fluid is called the **medullary gradient**. It plays an important role in the concentration of urine.

DEVELOPMENT AND MAINTENANCE OF MEDULLARY GRADIENT

Kidney has some unique anatomical arrangements called countercurrent system, which are responsible for the development and maintenance of medullary gradient and hyperosmolarity of interstitial fluid in the inner medulla.

COUNTERCURRENT MECHANISM

COUNTERCURRENT FLOW

A **countercurrent system** is a system of 'U' shaped tubules (tubes) in which the flow of fluid is in opposite direction in two limbs of the U-shaped tubules. In kidney, the structures, which form counter current system, are loop of Henle and vasa recta. In both, the direction of flow of

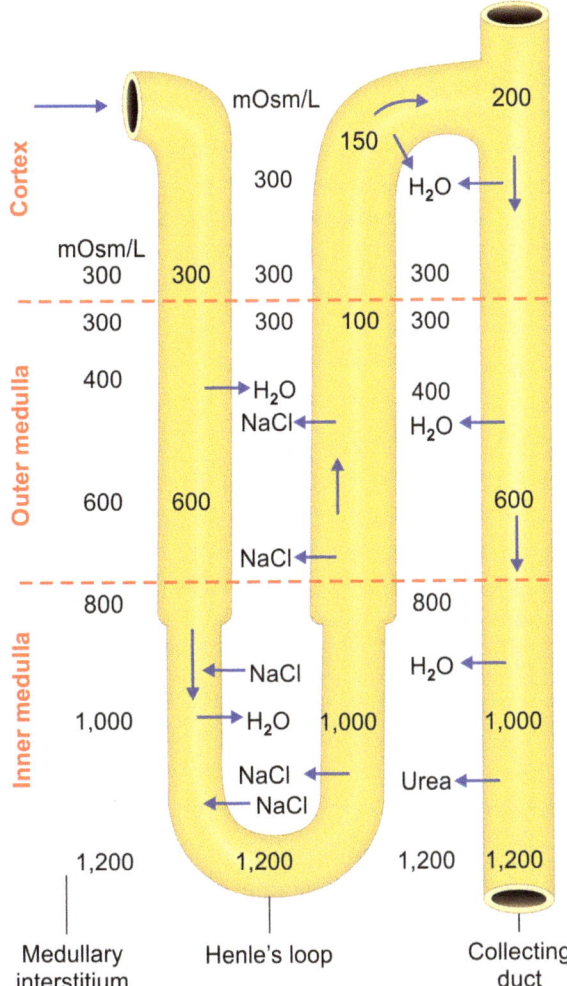

FIGURE 37.1: Countercurrent multiplier. Numerical indicate osmolarity (mOsm/L).

fluid in the descending limb is just opposite to that in the ascending limb.

Divisions of Countercurrent System in Kidney

In kidney, countercurrent system has two divisions:

1. Countercurrent multiplier formed by loop of Henle.
2. Countercurrent exchanger formed by vasa recta.

■ COUNTERCURRENT MULTIPLIER

Loop of Henle functions as countercurrent multiplier. It is responsible for the development of hyperosmolarity of medullary interstitial fluid and medullary gradient. Loop of Henle of juxtamedullary nephrons plays a major role as countercurrent multiplier. It is because the loop of juxtamedullary nephrons is long and extends up to the deeper parts of medulla.

Events during Development of Medullary Gradient by Countercurrent Multiplier

1. Hyperosmolarity of medullary interstitial fluid is due to active reabsorption of sodium chloride and other solutes from ascending limb of Henle's loop into the medullary interstitium.
2. Now, due to the concentration gradient, sodium and chloride ions diffuse from medullary interstitium into the descending limb of Henle's loop. Then it reaches ascending limb again via hairpin bend.
   Thus, the sodium and chlorine ions are repeatedly **recirculated** between descending limb and ascending limb of Henle's loop through medullary interstitial fluid leaving a small portion to be excreted in the urine.
3. Apart from this, there is regular addition of more and more new sodium and chlorine ions into descending limb by constant filtration.
4. Thus, the reabsorption of sodium chloride from ascending limb and addition of new sodium chlorine ions into filtrate multiply the osmolarity of medullary interstitial fluid and medullary gradient. Hence, it is called countercurrent multiplier.

Other Factors Responsible for Hyperosmolarity of Medullary Interstitial Fluid

In addition to countercurrent multiplier action provided by the loop of Henle, two more factors are involved in hyperosmolarity of medullary interstitial fluid:

1. Reabsorption of sodium from collecting duct

Reabsorption of sodium from medullary part of collecting duct into the medullary interstitium, adds to the osmolarity in inner medulla.

2. Recirculation of urea

Urea is completely filtered in the glomeruli. As it is a waste product, it is not reabsorbed from the renal tubule. So, all the filtered urea reach collecting duct. Now, due to concentration gradient, urea diffuses from collecting duct into the inner medullary interstitium. So, the osmolarity increases in the inner medulla.

Due to continuous diffusion, the concentration of urea increases in medullary interstitium. Again, by concentration gradient, urea enters the ascending limb. From here, it passes through distal convoluted tubule and reaches the collecting duct. From here, urea enters medullary interstitium and the cycle repeats. By this way urea recirculates repeatedly, and helps to maintain the hyperosmolarity in the inner medullary interstitium. Only a small amount of urea is excreted in urine.

■ COUNTERCURRENT EXCHANGER

Vasa Recta

Vasa recta functions as countercurrent exchanger. It is responsible for the maintenance of hyperosmolarity of medullary interstitial fluid and the medullary gradient developed by countercurrent multiplier **(Fig. 37.2)**.

Events during Maintenance of Medullary Gradient by Countercurrent Exchanger

1. Sodium chloride is reabsorbed from ascending limb of Henle's loop into medullary interstitium. From here it enters the descending limb of vasa recta.

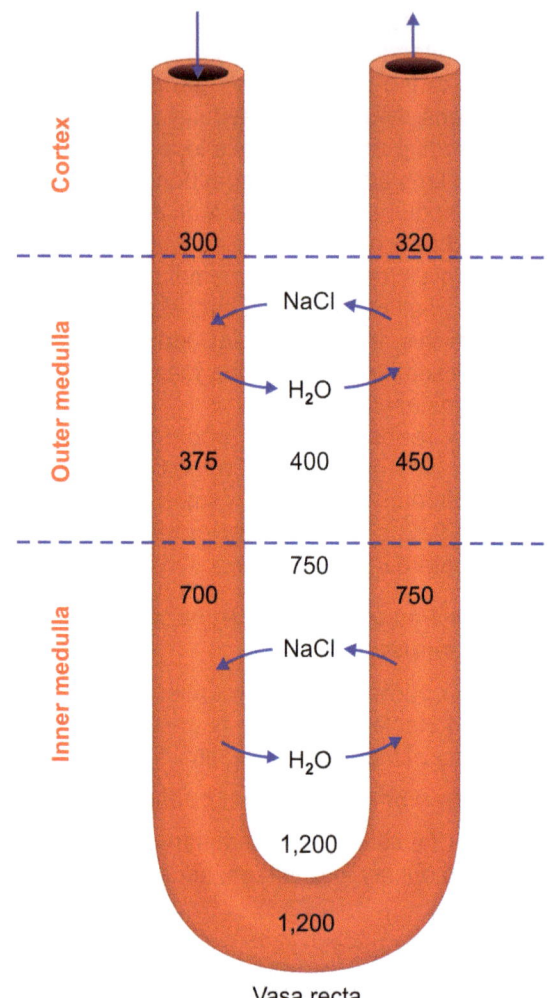

FIGURE 37.2: Countercurrent exchanger. Numerical indicate osmolarity (mOsm/L).

2. Simultaneously water diffuses from descending limb of vasa recta into medullary interstitium.
3. Blood flows very slowly through vasa recta. So, a large quantity of sodium chloride accumulates in descending limb of vasa recta and flows slowly towards ascending limb.
4. By the time the blood reaches the ascending limb of vasa recta, the concentration of sodium chloride increases very much.
5. This causes diffusion of sodium chloride into the medullary interstitium.
6. Simultaneously, water from medullary interstitium enters the ascending limb of vasa recta. And the cycle is repeated.

Thus, when blood passes through the ascending limb of vasa recta, sodium chloride diffuses out of blood and enters the interstitial fluid of medulla and, water diffuses into the blood. Thus, vasa recta retain sodium chloride in the medullary interstitium and removes water from it. So, the hyperosmolarity of medullary interstitium is maintained. Blood passing through the ascending limb of vasa recta may carry very little amount of sodium chloride from the medulla.

Recirculation of urea

Recirculation of urea also occurs through vasa recta. From medullary interstitium, along with sodium chloride, urea also enters the descending limb of vasa recta. When blood passes through ascending limb of vasa recta, urea diffuses back into the medullary interstitium along with sodium chloride.

Thus, **sodium chloride** and **urea** are **exchanged for water** between the ascending and descending limbs of vasa recta, hence this system is called countercurrent exchanger.

ROLE OF ADH

Final concentration of urine is achieved by ADH. Normally, distal convoluted tubule and the collecting duct are not permeable to water. In the presence of ADH, distal convoluted tubule and collecting duct become permeable to water resulting in water reabsorption. The water reabsorption induced by ADH is called **facultative reabsorption** of water (Chapter 36).

A large quantity of water is removed from the fluid while passing through distal convoluted tubule and collecting duct. So, the urine becomes hypertonic with an osmolarity of 1,200 mOsm/L.

SUMMARY OF URINE CONCENTRATION

When the glomerular filtrate passes through renal tubule, its osmolarity is altered in different segments as described below.

1. BOWMAN'S CAPSULE

Glomerular filtrate collected at the Bowman's capsule is **isotonic to plasma**. This is because it contains all the substances of plasma except proteins. Osmolarity of the filtrate at Bowman's capsule is **300 mOsm/L**.

2. PROXIMAL CONVOLUTED TUBULE

When the filtrate flows through proximal convoluted tubule, there is active reabsorption of sodium and chloride followed by obligatory reabsorption of water. So, osmolarity of fluid remains the same as in the case of Bowman's capsule, i.e. **300 mOsm/L**. Thus, in proximal convoluted tubules, the fluid is **isotonic to plasma**.

3. THICK DESCENDING SEGMENT

When the fluid passes into thick descending segment, water is reabsorbed from the tubule into outer medullary interstitium by means of osmosis. It is due to the increased osmolarity in the medullary interstitium, i.e. outside the thick descending tubule. Osmolarity of the fluid inside this segment is between **450 mOsm/L** and **600 mOsm/L**. That means the fluid is **slightly hypertonic to plasma** (Table 37.1).

4. THIN DESCENDING SEGMENT OF HENLE'S LOOP

As the thin descending segment of Henle's loop passes through inner medullary interstitium more water is

TABLE 37.1: Osmolarity of fluid at different parts of nephron.

Parts of nephron	Osmolarity of fluid (mOsm/L)	Comparison to plasma
Bowman's capsule (glomerular filtrate)	300	Isotonic
Proximal convoluted tubule	300	Isotonic
Thick descending segment	450 to 600	Hypertonic
Thin descending segment of Henle's loop (short loop of cortical nephron)	600	Hypertonic
Thin descending segment of Henle's loop (long loop of juxtamedullary nephron)	1,200	Hypertonic
Thin ascending segment of Henle's loop	400	Hypertonic
Thick ascending segment	150 to 200	Hypotonic
While entering distal convoluted tubule	200	Hypotonic
While leaving collecting duct (urine)	1,200	Hypertonic

reabsorbed. So, the osmolarity of tubular fluid becomes equal to that of the surrounding medullary interstitium.

In the short loops of cortical nephrons, osmolarity of fluid at the hairpin bend of loop becomes **600 mOsm/L**. And, in the long loops of juxtamedullary nephrons, at the hairpin bend, osmolarity is **1,200 mOsm/L**. Thus, in this segment the fluid is **hypertonic to plasma**.

■ 5. THIN ASCENDING SEGMENT OF HENLE'S LOOP

When the thin ascending segment of loop ascends upwards through the medullary region, osmolarity decreases gradually. Due to concentration gradient, sodium chloride diffuses out of tubular fluid and osmolarity decreases to **400 mOsm/L**. Fluid in this segment is **slightly hypertonic to plasma**.

■ 6. THICK ASCENDING SEGMENT

Active reabsorption of sodium from this segment decreases the osmolarity of tubular fluid to a greater extent. The osmolarity is between **150 mOsm/L** and **200 mOsm/L**. The fluid inside becomes **hypotonic to plasma**.

■ 7. DISTAL CONVOLUTED TUBULE AND COLLECTING DUCT

In the presence of ADH, distal convoluted tubule and collecting duct become permeable to water resulting in water reabsorption and final concentration of urine.

Reabsorption of large quantity of water increases the osmolarity to **1,200 mOsm/L**. The urine becomes **hypertonic to plasma**.

■ APPLIED PHYSIOLOGY

■ 1. DIURESIS

Diuresis is the excretion of large quantity of water through urine. Diuresis is classified into two types:

1. Osmotic Diuresis

Osmotic diuresis is the diuresis induced by presence of some osmotically active substances such as glucose in renal tubule. Such substances increase osmotic pressure in renal tubules and reduce reabsorption of water resulting in excretion of water through urine.

Osmotic diuresis is common in diabetes mellitus because of high blood glucose level (Chapter 47).

2. Water Diuresis

Water diuresis is the diuresis due to decreased reabsorption of water in renal tubules particularly distal convoluted tubule and collecting duct. It is caused by deficiency of antidiuretic hormone.

Water diuresis is common in diabetes insipidus (Chapter 44).

■ 2. POLYURIA

Polyuria is the increased urinary output with frequent voiding. It is due to osmotic diuresis as in diabetes mellitus or water diuresis as in diabetes insipidus (see above).

■ 3. OLIGURIA

Oliguria is the condition with decreased output of urine. Urine output is <500 mL per day in this condition. It is different from another condition called **anuria** in which urine output is <50 mL per day. Anuria means absence of urine output.

Oliguria occurs in many conditions including acute renal failure, obstruction in urinary tract, infection or trauma of kidneys.

CHAPTER 38

Acidification of Urine and Role of Kidney in Acid-base Balance

CHAPTER OUTLINE

- ACID-BASE BALANCE
- REABSORPTION OF BICARBONATE IONS
- SECRETION OF HYDROGEN IONS
- REMOVAL OF HYDROGEN IONS AND ACIDIFICATION OF URINE
  - BICARBONATE MECHANISM
- PHOSPHATE MECHANISM
- AMMONIA MECHANISM
- APPLIED PHYSIOLOGY: DISTURBANCES OF ACID-BASE STATUS

ACID-BASE BALANCE

Kidney plays an important role in maintenance of acid-base balance by excreting hydrogen ions and retaining bicarbonate ions.

Normally, urine is acidic in nature with a pH of 4.5 to 6. Metabolic activities in the body produce large quantity of acids (with lot of hydrogen ions), which threaten to push the body towards acidosis. However, kidneys prevent this.

Kidneys prevent acidosis by two ways:

1. Reabsorption of bicarbonate ions
2. Secretion of hydrogen ions.

REABSORPTION OF BICARBONATE IONS

About 4,320 mEq of HCO^- is filtered by the glomeruli every day. It is called **filtered load** of HCO^-. Excretion of this much HCO^- in urine will affect the acid-base balance of body fluids. So, HCO_3 must be taken back from the renal tubule by reabsorption.

SECRETION OF HYDROGEN IONS

Reabsorption of filtered HCO^- occurs by the secretion of H^+ in the renal tubules. About 4,380 mEq of H^+ appear every day in the renal tubule by means of filtration and secretion. Not all the H^+ are excreted in urine. Out of 4,380 mEq, about 4,280 to 4,330 mEq of H^+ is utilized for the reabsorption of filtered HCO_3^-. Only the remaining 50 to 100 mEq is excreted. It results in the **acidification of urine**.

REMOVAL OF HYDROGEN IONS AND ACIDIFICATION OF URINE

Role of Kidney in Preventing Metabolic Acidosis

Kidney plays an important role in preventing metabolic acidosis by excreting H^+. Excretion of hydrogen ions occurs by **three mechanisms**:

1. BICARBONATE MECHANISM

All the HCO_3^- filtered into the renal tubules is reabsorbed. About 80% of it is reabsorbed in proximal convoluted tubule; 15% in Henle's loop and 5% in distal convoluted tubule and collecting duct. Reabsorption of HCO_3^- utilizes the H^+ secreted into the renal tubules.

In tubular cells, carbon dioxide combines with water to form carbonic acid. It immediately dissociates into H^+ and HCO_3^-. HCO_3^- from the tubular cell enters the interstitium. Simultaneously Na^+ is reabsorbed from the renal tubule under the influence of **aldosterone**. HCO_3^- combines with Na^+ to form $NaHCO_3$. Now, the H^+ is secreted into the tubular lumen from the cell in exchange for Na^+ **(Fig. 38.1)**.

The H^+ secreted into the renal tubule, combines with filtered HCO_3^- forming carbonic acid. Carbonic acid dissociates into carbon dioxide and water in the presence of carbonic anhydrase. Carbon dioxide and water enter the tubular cell.

Thus, for every hydrogen ion secreted into lumen of tubule, one bicarbonate ion is reabsorbed from the tubule. In this way, kidneys conserve the HCO_3^-. Reabsorption of filtered HCO_3^- is an important factor in maintaining pH of the body fluids.

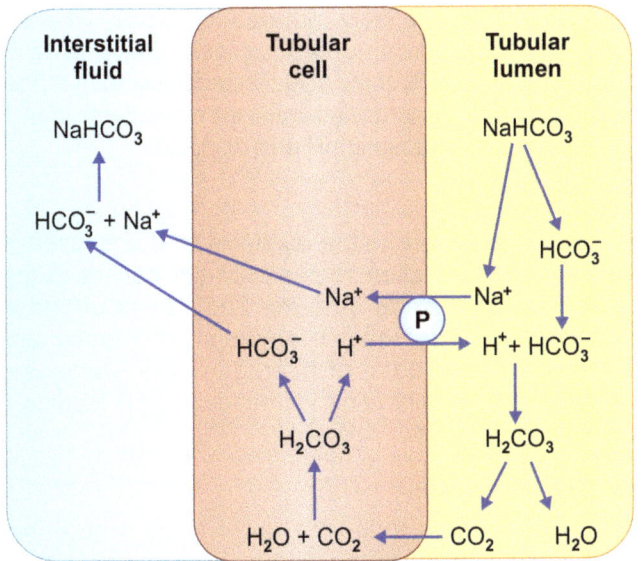

FIGURE 38.1: Reabsorption of bicarbonate ions by secretion of hydrogen ions in renal tubule.
P = Sodium-hydrogen antiport pump.

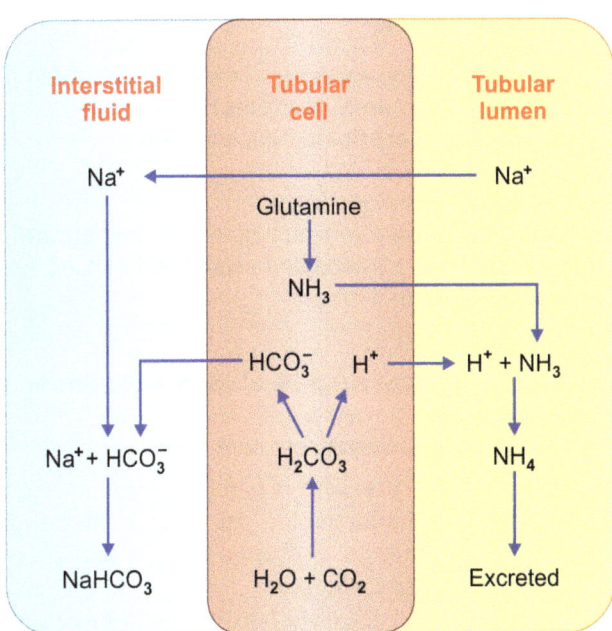

FIGURE 38.3: Excretion of hydrogen in combination with ammonia.

phosphate. Sodium-dihydrogen phosphate is excreted in urine. The H^+, which is added to urine, makes it acidic. It happens mainly in distal tubule and collecting duct because of the presence of large quantity of sodium-hydrogen phosphate in these segments.

■ 3. AMMONIA MECHANISM

This is the most important mechanism by which kidneys excrete H^+ and make the urine acidic. In the tubular epithelial cells, ammonia is formed when the amino acid **glutamine** is converted into **glutamic acid** in the presence of enzyme **glutaminase**. Ammonia is also formed by the deamination of some of the amino acids such as **glycine** and **alanine** (Fig. 38.3).

Ammonia (NH_3) formed in tubular cells is secreted into tubular lumen in exchange for sodium ion. Here, it combines with H^+ to form **ammonium** (NH_4). Tubular cell membrane is not permeable to ammonium. Therefore, it remains in the lumen and combines with **sodium acetoacetate** to form **ammonium acetoacetate**. Ammonium acetoacetate is excreted through urine. Thus, H^+ is added to urine in the form of ammonium compounds resulting in acidification of urine. This process takes place mostly in the proximal convoluted tubule because glutamine is converted into ammonia in the cells of this segment.

Thus, by excreting H^+ and conserving HCO_3^-, kidneys produce acidic urine and help to maintain the acidbase balance of body fluids.

■ APPLIED PHYSIOLOGY: DISTURBANCES OF ACID-BASE STATUS

■ ACIDOSIS

Acidosis is the condition characterized by abnormal increase in acidity of blood and body fluids with reduction in pH below normal range.

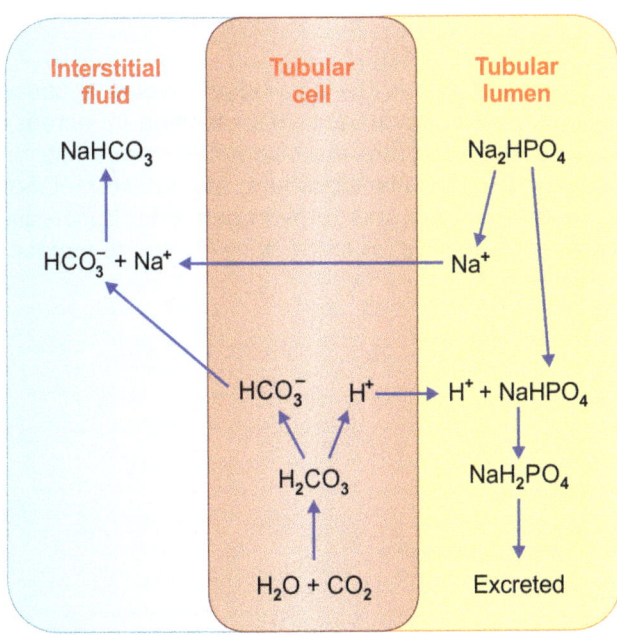

FIGURE 38.2: Excretion of hydrogen ions in combination with phosphate ions.

■ 2. PHOSPHATE MECHANISM

In the tubular cells, carbon dioxide combines with water to form **carbonic acid**. It immediately dissociates into H^+ and HCO_3^-. HCO_3^- from the tubular cell enters the interstitium. Simultaneously, Na^+ is reabsorbed from renal tubule under the influence of aldosterone. Na^+ enters the interstitium and combines with HCO_3^-. The H^+ is secreted into the tubular lumen from the cell in exchange for Na^+ (Fig. 38.2).

The H^+, which is secreted into renal tubules, reacts with **phosphate buffer system**. It combines with sodium-hydrogen phosphate to form sodium-dihydrogen

Acidosis is produced by:

1. Increase in partial pressure of **carbon dioxide** in the body fluids particularly in arterial blood.
2. Decrease in **bicarbonate** concentration.

■ ALKALOSIS

Alkalosis is the condition characterized by abnormal increase in alkalinity of blood and body fluids with increase in pH above the normal range.

Alkalosis is produced by:

1. Decrease in partial pressure of **carbon dioxide** in the arterial blood.
2. Increase in **bicarbonate** concentration.

Since the partial pressure of carbon dioxide in arterial blood is controlled by lungs, the acid-base disturbances produced by the change in arterial carbon dioxide are called **respiratory disturbances**.

On the other hand, the disturbances in acid-base status produced by the change in bicarbonate concentration are called **metabolic disturbances**.

Thus acid-base disturbances are:

1. Respiratory acidosis
2. Respiratory alkalosis
3. Metabolic acidosis
4. Metabolic alkalosis.

■ 1. RESPIRATORY ACIDOSIS

Respiratory acidosis is the acidosis that is caused by alveolar hypoventilation. During hypoventilation, the lungs fail to expel carbon dioxide, which is produced in the tissues. Carbon dioxide is the major end product of oxidation of carbohydrates, proteins and fats.

Carbon dioxide accumulates in blood where it reacts with water to form carbonic acid, which is called **respiratory acid.** Carbonic acid dissociates into hydrogen and bicarbonate. Increased hydrogen concentration in blood leads to decrease in pH and acidosis.

■ 2. RESPIRATORY ALKALOSIS

Respiratory alkalosis is the alkalosis that is caused by alveolar hyperventilation. Hyperventilation causes excess loss of carbon dioxide from the body. Loss of carbon dioxide leads to decreased formation of carbonic acid and decreased release of hydrogen ions. Decreased hydrogen ion concentration increases the pH leading to respiratory alkalosis.

■ 3. METABOLIC ACIDOSIS

Metabolic acidosis is the acid-base imbalance characterized by excess accumulation of **organic acids** in the body, which is caused by abnormal metabolic processes. Organic acids such as lactic acid, ketoacids and uric acid are formed by normal metabolism. The quantity of these acids increases due to abnormality in the metabolism.

■ 4. METABOLIC ALKALOSIS

Metabolic alkalosis is the acid-base imbalance caused by loss of excess hydrogen ions resulting in increased bicarbonate concentration. Some of the endocrine disorders, renal tubular disorders, etc. cause metabolic disorders leading to loss of hydrogen ions. It increases bicarbonate ions and pH in the body leading to metabolic alkalosis.

Chapter 39: Renal Function Tests, Renal Failure, Dialysis and Diuretics

CHAPTER OUTLINE

- **PROPERTIES AND COMPOSITION OF NORMAL URINE**
- **RENAL FUNCTION TESTS**
  - EXAMINATION OF URINE
  - EXAMINATION OF BLOOD
  - EXAMINATION OF BLOOD AND URINE
- **RENAL FAILURE**
  - ACUTE RENAL FAILURE
  - CHRONIC RENAL FAILURE
- **DIALYSIS AND ARTIFICIAL KIDNEY**
- **KIDNEY TRANSPLANTATION**
- **DIURETICS**
  - USES OF DIURETICS
  - TYPES OF DIURETICS

■ PROPERTIES AND COMPOSITION OF NORMAL URINE

■ PROPERTIES OF URINE

Volume : 1,000 to 1,500 mL/day.
Appearance : Clear
Reaction : Slightly acidic with pH of 4.5 to 6.
Specific gravity : 1.010 to 1.025.
Color : Normally, urine is straw colored.
Odor : Fresh urine has light aromatic odor. If stored for some time, the odor becomes stronger due to bacterial decomposition.

■ COMPOSITION OF URINE

Urine consists of water and solids. Solids include organic and inorganic substances **(Fig. 39.1)**.

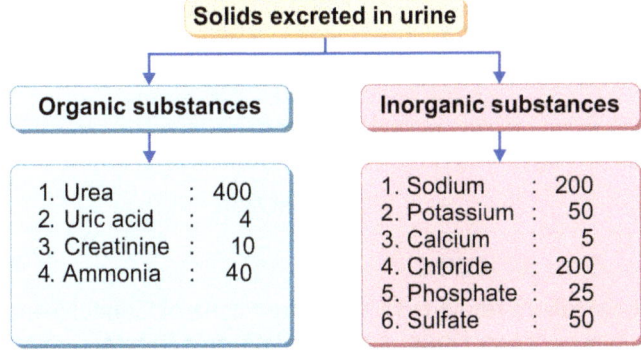

FIGURE 39.1: Quantity of solids excreted in urine (mMol/day).

■ RENAL FUNCTION TESTS

Renal function tests are the group of tests that are performed to assess the functions of kidney.

Renal function tests are of three types:

I. Examination of urine alone.
II. Examination of blood alone.
III. Examination of blood and urine.

■ EXAMINATION OF URINE: URINALYSIS

Routine examination of urine or urinalysis is a group of diagnostic tests performed on the sample of urine.

Urinalysis is done by three tests:

1. Physical Examination of Urine

Physical examination of urine includes volume, appearance, reaction, pH, specific gravity, color and odor of urine.

2. Microscopic Examination of Urine

Microscopic examination reveals the presence of red blood cells, pus cells, epithelial cells, casts and crystals which suggests the renal pathology.

3. Chemical Analysis of Urine

Chemical analysis of urine helps to determine the presence of abnormal constituents of urine or presence of normal constituents in abnormal quantity. Both the findings reveal the presence of renal abnormality.

Chemical analysis is done to determine the following substances:

i. Glucose.
ii. Protein, particularly albumin.
iii. Ketone bodies.
iv. Bilirubin.
v. Urobilinogen.
vi. Bile salts.
vii. Blood.
viii. Hemoglobin.
ix. Nitrite.

■ EXAMINATION OF BLOOD

Level of plasma proteins, urea, uric acid and creatinine are determined in blood. Blood level of these substances is altered in renal failure.

■ EXAMINATION OF BLOOD AND URINE

Plasma Clearance

Plasma clearance is defined as the amount of plasma that is cleared off a substance in a given unit of time. It is also known as **renal clearance**. It is based on Fick's principle (Chapter 61).

To determine the plasma clearance of a particular substance, measurement of the following factors is required:

i. Volume of urine excreted.
ii. Concentration of the substance in urine.
iii. Concentration of the substance in blood.

Formula to calculate clearance value is:

$$C = \frac{UV}{P}$$

Where,
C = Clearance.
U = Concentration of the substance in urine.
V = Volume of urine flow.
P = Concentration of the substance in plasma.

Determination of clearance value for certain substances helps in assessing the following renal functions:

1. Glomerular filtration rate.
2. Renal plasma flow.
3. Renal blood flow.

1. Measurement of Glomerular Filtration Rate

A substance that is completely filtered but neither reabsorbed nor secreted should be used to measure glomerular filtration rate (GFR). Inulin is a substance that is completely filtered. And, it is neither reabsorbed nor secreted. So, **inulin** is the ideal substance used to measure GFR.

Inulin clearance

A known amount of inulin is injected into the body. After sometime, the concentration of inulin in plasma and urine and the volume of urine excreted are estimated.

For example,
Concentration of inulin in urine = 125 mg/dL
Plasma concentration = 1 mg/dL
Volume of urine output = 1 mL/min

Thus,

$$\text{Glomerular filtration rate} = \frac{UV}{P}$$

$$= \frac{125 \times 1}{1}$$

$$= 125 \text{ mL/min}$$

2. Measurement of Renal Plasma Flow

To measure renal plasma flow, a substance, which is filtered and secreted but not reabsorbed, should be used. Such a substance is **para-aminohippuric acid (PAH)**. PAH clearance indicates the amount of plasma passed through kidneys.

A known amount of PAH is injected into the body. After sometime, the concentration of PAH in plasma and urine and the volume of urine excreted are estimated. From these values, renal plasma flow is calculated by using the formula of plasma clearance (see above).

3. Measurement of Renal Blood Flow

To determine renal blood flow, value of the following **two factors** is necessary, renal plasma flow and percentage of plasma volume in the blood.

i. Renal plasma flow

Renal plasma flow is measured by using PAH clearance.

ii. Percentage of plasma volume in the blood

Percentage of plasma volume is indirectly determined by using PCV. For example, if PCV is 45%, the plasma volume in the blood is 100 − 45 = 55%, i.e. 55 mL of plasma is present in every 100 mL of blood.

Renal blood flow is calculated with the values of renal plasma flow and % of plasma in blood by using a formula given below:

$$\text{Renal blood flow} = \frac{\text{Renal plasma flow}}{\text{\% of plasma in blood}}$$

For example,
Renal plasma flow = 660 mL/min
Amount of plasma in blood = 55%

$$\text{Renal blood flow} = \frac{660}{55/100}$$

$$= \frac{660 \times 100}{55}$$

$$= 1,200 \text{ mL/min}$$

■ RENAL FAILURE

Renal failure refers to failure of functions of kidney. Renal failure is of two types, acute and chronic failure.

ACUTE RENAL FAILURE

Acute renal failure is the temporary loss of kidney function. It occurs abruptly or suddenly. It is often reversible within few days to few weeks. Acute renal failure may result in sudden life-threatening reactions in the body with the need for emergency treatment.

Causes of Acute Renal Failure

Common causes of acute renal failure are:

1. **Pyelonephritis**: Inflammation of kidney involving glomeruli, tubules and interstitium.
2. Acute **glomerulonephritis**: Inflammation of glomeruli.
3. Renal ischemia: Inadequate blood supply to kidney.
4. Acute tubular necrosis: Necrosis of tubular cells in kidney.
5. Severe transfusion reactions: Refer Chapter 16 for transfusion reactions.
6. Sudden fall in blood pressure: Due to conditions such as hemorrhage, diarrhea, severe burns and cholera.
7. **Blockage of ureter**: Caused by the formation of calculi (renal stone) or tumor.

Treatment for Acute Renal Failure

Treatment involves use of medications, change in diet and dialysis if necessary.

CHRONIC RENAL FAILURE

Chronic renal failure is the progressive, long standing and irreversible impairment of renal functions. Last stage of chronic renal failure is called **end stage renal disease (ESRD)**.

Causes of Chronic Renal Failure

1. Chronic glomerulonephritis: Long-term inflammation of glomeruli.
2. **Polycystic kidney disease (PKD)**: Development of clusters of cysts in kidneys.
3. Renal calculi.
4. Urethral constriction.
5. Hypertension.
6. Atherosclerosis.
7. Tuberculosis.
8. Slow poisoning by drugs or metals.

Treatment for Chronic Renal Failure

Chronic renal failure is treated by dialysis or kidney transplant.

DIALYSIS AND ARTIFICIAL KIDNEY

Dialysis is the procedure to remove waste materials and toxic substances and to restore normal volume and composition of body fluid in severe **renal failure**. It is also called **hemodialysis**.

Artificial kidney is a machine that is used to carry out hemodialysis during renal failure. Principle of artificial kidney is the diffusion of solutes from an area of higher concentration to the area of lower concentration, through a semipermeable membrane.

Patient's arterial blood is passed continuously or intermittently through the artificial kidney and then back to the body through the vein.

Dialysis is used to treat the patients suffering from acute or chronic renal failure.

In some cases, patient's peritoneal membrane is used as a semipermeable membrane. This technique is called **peritoneal dialysis**. It is also used to treat the patients suffering from renal failure.

KIDNEY TRANSPLANTATION

Kidney or renal transplantation is the surgical procedure to place the healthy kidney into the renal failure patients. Transplanted kidney takes over the functions of diseased kidney and the patient needs no further dialysis. Healthy kidney is taken from either a live donor or a deceased donor.

Kidney transplantation is the treatment of choice for patients suffering from **end stage renal disease (ESRD)**.

DIURETICS

Diuretics or **diuretic agents** are the substances which enhance the urine formation and output. These substances increase the excretion of water, sodium and chloride through urine. Diuretic agents increase the urine formation, by influencing any of the processes involved in urine formation. Diuretics are commonly called '**water pills**'.

USES OF DIURETICS

Diuretics are generally used for the treatment of disorders involving increase in extracellular fluid volume such as hypertension, congestive cardiac failure and edema.

Diuretic agents prevent hypertension, congestive cardiac failure and edema, by increasing the urinary output and reducing extracellular fluid (ECF) volume.

TYPES OF DIURETICS

1. Osmotic Diuretics

Osmotic diuretics are the substances that induce **osmotic diuresis.** When injected in large quantities into the body, these substances increase the osmotic pressure in the tubular fluid. Increased osmotic pressure in the tubular fluid, in turn reduces water reabsorption. It leads to excretion of excess of water through urine. Elevated blood sugar level in diabetes can also cause osmotic diuresis in the same manner. Examples of osmotic diuretics are urea, mannitol, sucrose and glucose.

2. Diuretics Which Inhibit Reabsorption of Electrolytes

Diuretics of this type inhibit the active reabsorption of electrolytes like sodium and potassium from the renal tubular fluid. Inhibition of electrolyte reabsorption causes osmotic diuresis. Common diuretics of this category are loop diuretics

Loop diuretics

Loop diuretics are the substances that inhibit electrolyte reabsorption in **Henle's loop.** These diuretics inhibit the sodium and chloride reabsorption from thick ascending limb of Henle's loop. So, the osmotic pressure in tubular fluid increases, leading to diuresis. Examples are furosemide and torasemide.

3. Diuretics Which Inhibit Action of Aldosterone

Some diuretics inhibit sodium reabsorption and potassium excretion in the distal convoluted tubule and collecting duct, by inhibiting the action of aldosterone. These substances are also called the **potassium-retaining diuretics** or **aldosterone antagonists.** Examples are spironolactone and eplerenone.

4. Diuretics Which Inhibit Activity of Carbonic Anhydrase

Some diuretics inhibit the activity of carbonic anhydrase in proximal convoluted tubules and prevent reabsorption of bicarbonate from renal tubules, resulting in osmotic diuresis. Such diuretic agents are called **carbonic anhydrase inhibitors.** Acetazolamide is a carbonic anhydrase inhibitor.

5. Diuretics Which Increase Glomerular Filtration Rate

Some xanthines (alkaloids, used as mild stimulants) cause diuresis by increasing the glomerular filtration rate and to some extent by decreasing the sodium reabsorption. Examples are caffeine and theophylline.

6. Diuretics which Inhibit Secretion of ADH

Some diuretics produce diuresis by inhibiting the secretion of ADH. Examples are water and ethanol.

7. Diuretics which Inhibit ADH Receptors

The antagonists of V2 receptors cause diuresis by inhibiting the receptors of antidiuretic hormone, thereby preventing the activity of this hormone.

Chapter 40

Micturition

CHAPTER OUTLINE

- DEFINITION
- FUNCTIONAL ANATOMY OF URINARY BLADDER AND URETHRA
  - URINARY BLADDER
  - URETHRA
  - URETHRAL SPHINCTERS
- NERVE SUPPLY TO URINARY BLADDER AND SPHINCTERS
  - SYMPATHETIC NERVE SUPPLY
  - PARASYMPATHETIC NERVE SUPPLY
  - SOMATIC NERVE SUPPLY
- FILLING OF URINARY BLADDER
  - PROCESS OF FILLING
  - CYSTOMETROGRAM
- MICTURITION REFLEX
- APPLIED PHYSIOLOGY: ABNORMALITIES OF MICTURITION
  - ATONIC BLADDER
  - AUTOMATIC BLADDER
  - NOCTURNAL MICTURITION

DEFINITION

Micturition is a process by which urine is voided from the urinary bladder. Knowledge of functional anatomy and nerve supply of urinary bladder, urethra and sphincters is essential to understand the process of micturition.

FUNCTIONAL ANATOMY OF URINARY BLADDER AND URETHRA

URINARY BLADDER

Urinary bladder consists of the body, neck and internal urethral sphincter. Smooth muscle forming the bladder is called **detrusor muscle**. At the posterior surface of the bladder wall, there is a triangular area called **trigone**. At the upper angles of this trigone, two **ureters** enter the bladder.

Lower part of bladder is narrow and forms the neck. Distal end of the bladder is guarded by **internal urethral sphincter**. This sphincter is made up of **detrusor muscle**. It opens towards urethra. At the distal end of urethra, there is **external urethral sphincter**. It is made up of **skeletal muscle** fibers.

URETHRA

Male urethra has both urinary function and reproductive function. It transports urine and semen. Female urethra has only urinary function and it transports only urine. So, male urethra is structurally different from female urethra.

Male Urethra

Male urethra is about 20 cm long. After arising from bladder, it traverses prostate gland and then runs through the penis (Fig. 40.1). Throughout its length, the urethra has mucus glands called **glands of Littre**.

Male urethra is divided into three parts, namely prostatic urethra, membranous urethra and spongy urethra.

Female Urethra

Female urethra is narrower and shorter than male urethra. It is about 3.5 cm to 4 cm long. After arising from bladder, it traverses through urogenital diaphragm and runs along anterior wall of vagina. Then it terminates at external orifice of urethra which is located between clitoris and vaginal opening (Fig. 40.2).

URETHRAL SPHINCTERS

Urinary tract has two urethral sphincters, internal urethral sphincter and external urethral sphincter.

1. Internal Urethral Sphincter

This sphincter is situated between neck of the bladder and upper end of urethra. It is made up of smooth muscle fibers and formed by thickening of detrusor muscle.

2. External Urethral Sphincter

External sphincter is located in the urogenital diaphragm. This sphincter is made up of circular skeletal muscle fibers.

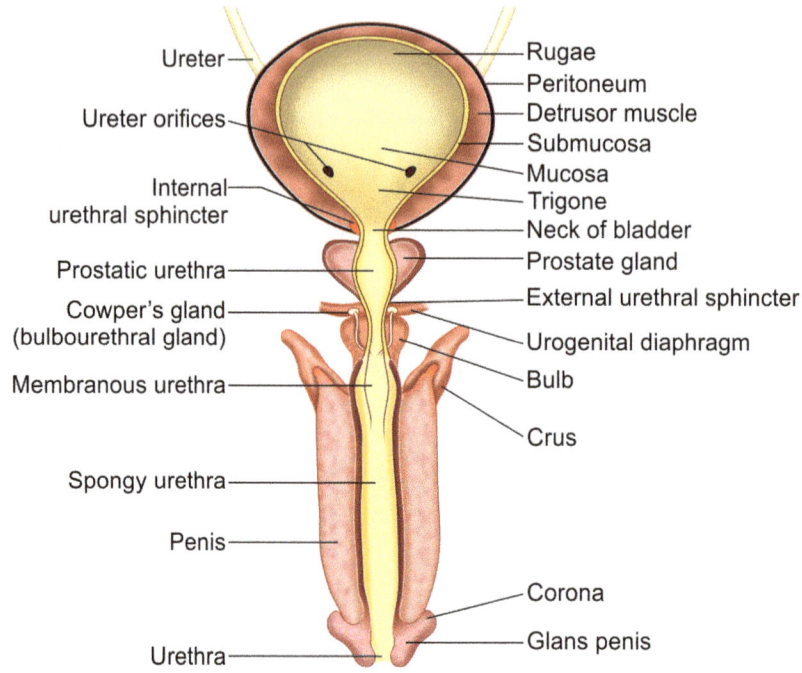

FIGURE 40.1: Urinary bladder and urethra in male.

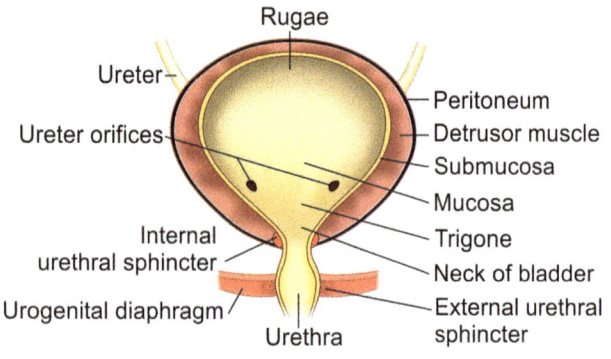

FIGURE 40.2: Urinary bladder and urethra in female.

NERVE SUPPLY TO URINARY BLADDER AND SPHINCTERS

Urinary bladder and the internal sphincter are supplied by sympathetic and parasympathetic divisions of autonomic nervous system whereas, the external sphincter is supplied by the somatic nerve fibers **(Fig. 40.3)**.

SYMPATHETIC NERVE SUPPLY

Sympathetic preganglionic fibers arise from first two lumbar segments (L1 and L2) of spinal cord. After origin, the fibers pass through lateral sympathetic chain without any synapse and terminate in **hypogastric ganglion**.

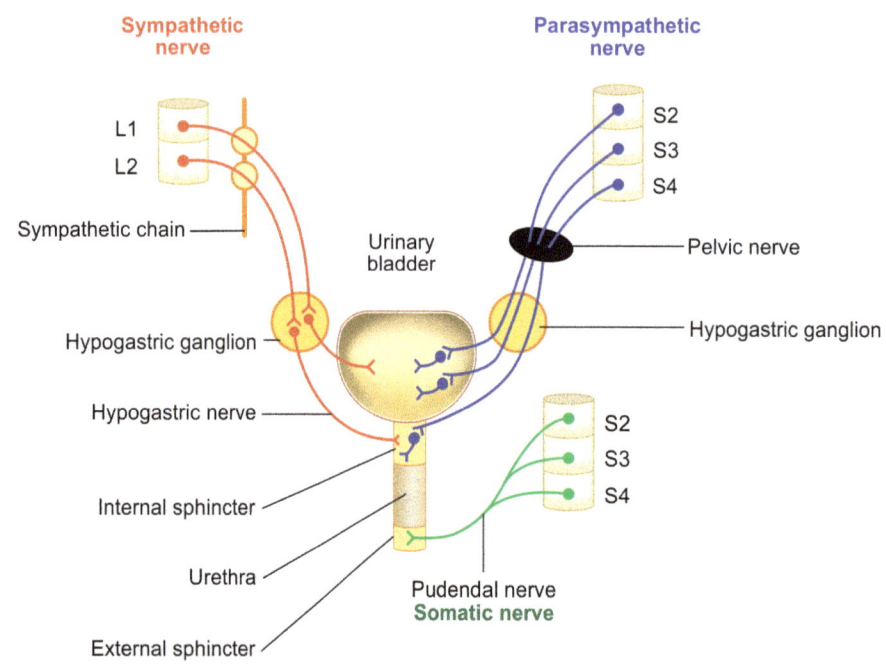

FIGURE 40.3: Nerve supply to urinary bladder and urethra.

TABLE 40.1: Functions of nerves supplying urinary bladder and sphincters.

Nerve	On detrusor muscle	On internal sphincter	On external sphincter	Function
Sympathetic nerve (hypogastric nerve)	Relaxation	Constriction	Not supplied	Filling of urinary bladder
Parasympathetic nerve (pelvic nerve)	Contraction	Relaxation	Not supplied	Emptying of urinary bladder (micturition)
Somatic nerve (pudendal nerve)	Not supplied	Not supplied	Constriction	Voluntary control of micturition

Postganglionic fibers arising from this ganglion form the **hypogastric nerve**, which supplies detrusor muscle and internal sphincter.

Function of Sympathetic Nerve

Sympathetic nerve causes relaxation of detrusor muscle and constriction of the internal sphincter. It results in filling of urinary bladder and so, the sympathetic nerve is called **nerve of filling**.

■ PARASYMPATHETIC NERVE SUPPLY

Preganglionic fibers of parasympathetic nerve form the **pelvic nerve** or **nervous erigens**. Pelvic nerve fibers arise from second to fourth sacral segments (S2, S3 and S4) of spinal cord. These fibers run through **hypogastric ganglion** and synapse with postganglionic neurons situated in close relation to urinary bladder and internal sphincter **(Table 40.1)**.

Function of Parasympathetic Nerve

Pelvic (parasympathetic) nerve causes contraction of detrusor muscle and relaxation of the internal sphincter leading to emptying of urinary bladder **(Table 40.2)**. So, the parasympathetic nerve is called the **nerve of emptying** or **nerve of micturition**.

Pelvic nerve has also the sensory fibers which carry impulses from **stretch receptors** present on the wall of the urinary bladder and urethra to the central nervous system.

■ SOMATIC NERVE SUPPLY

External sphincter is innervated by the somatic nerve called the **pudendal nerve**. It arises from second, third and fourth sacral segments of the spinal cord.

Function of Pudendal Nerve

It maintains the **tonic contraction** of skeletal muscle fibers of external sphincter and keeps the external sphincter constricted always.

During micturition, this nerve is inhibited. It causes relaxation of external sphincter leading to voiding of urine. Thus, the pudendal nerve is responsible for voluntary control of micturition.

■ FILLING OF URINARY BLADDER
■ PROCESS OF FILLING

Urine is continuously formed in nephrons and it is transported drop by drop through the ureters into the urinary bladder. **Peristaltic waves** push the urine from pelvis of ureter into bladder through ureter.

A reasonable volume of urine can be stored in urinary bladder without any discomfort and without much increase in pressure inside the bladder (**intravesical pressure**). It is due to the adaptation of detrusor muscle. Relationship between the volume of urine and pressure in urinary bladder is studied by cystometrogram.

■ CYSTOMETROGRAM

Definition

Cystometry is the technique used to study the relationship between **intravesical pressure** and volume of urine in the bladder.

Cystometrogram is the graphical registration (recording) of pressure changes in urinary bladder in relation to volume of urine collected in it.

In the graph volume of urine is plotted in X-axis and intravesical pressure is plotted in Y-axis **(Fig. 40.4)**.

TABLE 40.2: Urethral sphincters.

Features	Internal urethral sphincter	External urethral sphincter
Situation	Between neck of bladder and upper end of urethra	In urogenital diaphragm
Muscle involved	Made up of smooth muscle fibers: Detrusor muscle	Made up of circular skeletal muscle fibers
Nerve supply	Supplied by autonomic nerves Sympathetic : Hypogastric nerve Parasympathetic : Pelvic nerve	Supplied by somatic nerve: Pudendal nerve

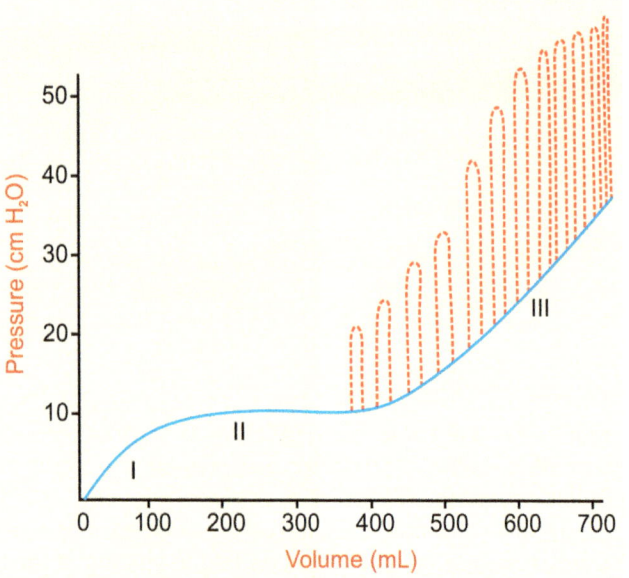

FIGURE 40.4: Cystometrogram.
Dotted lines = Contraction of detrusor muscle.

Description of Cystometrogram

Cystometrogram shows three segments.

Segment I

Initially, when urinary bladder is empty, the intravesical pressure is 0. When about 100 mL of fluid is collected, the pressure rises sharply to about 10 cm H_2O.

Segment II

This segment shows the plateau, i.e. the intravesical pressure remains more or less at 10 cm H_2O (level of segment I) without any change even after introducing 300 mL to 400 mL of fluid. It is because of adaptation of urinary bladder by relaxation.

When about 100 mL of urine is collected, the pressure rises to about 10 cm H_2O and now, the desire for micturition occurs. The desire for micturition is associated with a vague feeling in the perineum. An additional volume of about 200 mL to 300 mL of urine can be collected in bladder without much increase in pressure. However, when total volume rises beyond 400 mL, the pressure rises sharply and the **urge for micturition** starts. Still **voluntary control of micturition** is possible. And, beyond 600 mL to 700 mL of urine, voluntary control starts failing.

Segment III

As pressure increases with collection of 300 mL to 400 mL of fluid, the contraction of detrusor muscle becomes intense, increasing the consciousness and urge for micturition. Still, voluntary control is possible. Voluntary control is possible up to volume of 600 mL to 700 mL at which the pressure rises to about 35 cm H_2O to 40 cm H_2O.

When intravesical pressure rises above 40 cm water, the contraction of detrusor muscle becomes still more intense. And, voluntary control of micturition is not possible. Now, pain sensation develops and micturition should take place.

■ MICTURITION REFLEX

Micturition reflex is the reflex by which micturition occurs. This reflex is elicited by stimulation of **stretch receptors** situated on the wall of urinary bladder and urethra. When about 300 mL to 400 mL of urine is collected in bladder, the pressure inside bladder increases. This stretches the wall of bladder resulting in stimulation of stretch receptors and generation of sensory impulses.

Sensory (afferent) impulses from receptors reach the sacral segments of spinal cord via sensory fibers of pelvic (parasympathetic) nerve. Motor (efferent) impulses produced in spinal cord, travel through motor fibers of pelvic nerve towards bladder and internal sphincter. These motor impulses cause contraction of detrusor muscle and relaxation of internal sphincter so that, urine enters the urethra from bladder **(Fig. 40.5)**.

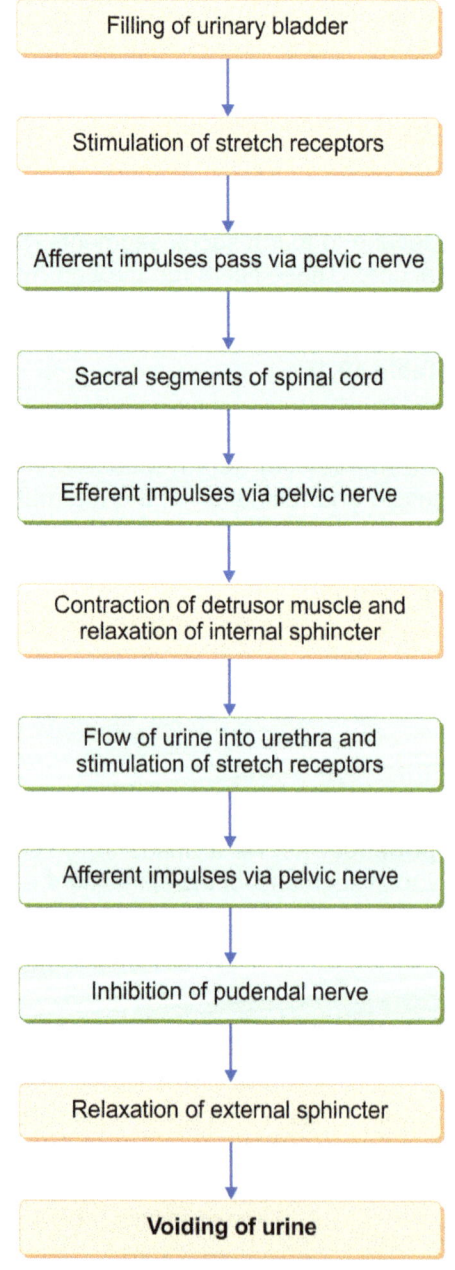

FIGURE 40.5: Micturition reflex.

Once urine enters urethra, stretch receptors in the urethra are stimulated and send afferent impulses to spinal cord via pelvic nerve fibers. These impulses inhibit **pudendal nerve**. So, the external sphincter relaxes and micturition occurs.

During micturition, the flow of urine is facilitated by increase in abdominal pressure due to the voluntary contraction of abdominal muscles.

Higher Centers for Micturition

Spinal centers for micturition are present in sacral and lumbar segments. Spinal centers are regulated by higher centers.

Higher centers are of two types:

1. **Inhibitory centers** which are situated in midbrain and cerebral cortex.
2. **Facilitatory centers** which are situated in pons and cerebral cortex.

■ APPLIED PHYSIOLOGY: ABNORMALITIES OF MICTURITION

■ 1. ATONIC BLADDER: EFFECT OF DESTRUCTION OF SENSORY NERVE FIBERS

Atonic bladder is the urinary bladder with loss of tone in detrusor muscle. It is caused by destruction of sensory (pelvic) nerve fibers of urinary bladder.

Due to destruction of sensory nerve fibers, detrusor muscle loses the tone and becomes flaccid. So, bladder is completely filled with urine without any stretching. Later, overflow occurs in drops as and when urine enters the bladder. It is called **overflow incontinence** or **overflow dribbling**. It occurs in spinal injury and syphilis.

■ 2. AUTOMATIC BLADDER

Automatic bladder is the urinary bladder characterized by **hyperactive micturition reflex** with loss of voluntary control. So, even with small amount of urine collected in the bladder, micturition reflex occurs resulting in emptying of bladder. This occurs in transaction of spinal cord above the sacral segments.

■ 3. NOCTURNAL MICTURITION

Nocturnal micturition is the involuntary voiding of urine during night. It is otherwise known as **enuresis** or **bedwetting**. It occurs due to the absence of voluntary control of micturition. It is a common and normal process in infants and children below 3 years. It is because of incomplete myelination of motor nerve fibers of the bladder. When myelination is complete, voluntary control of micturition develops and bedwetting stops.

Nocturnal micturition occurs after 3 years of age because of neurological disorders such as lumbosacral vertebral defects and impairment of motor area of cerebral cortex.

CHAPTER 41

Skin

CHAPTER OUTLINE

- **STRUCTURE OF SKIN**
  - EPIDERMIS
  - DERMIS
  - APPENDAGES OF SKIN
  - COLOR OF SKIN
- **GLANDS OF SKIN**
  - SEBACEOUS GLANDS
  - SWEAT GLANDS
- **FUNCTIONS OF SKIN**
  - PROTECTIVE FUNCTION
- SENSORY FUNCTION
- STORAGE FUNCTION
- SYNTHETIC FUNCTION
- REGULATION OF BODY TEMPERATURE
- REGULATION OF WATER AND ELECTROLYTE BALANCE
- EXCRETORY FUNCTION
- ABSORPTIVE FUNCTION
- SECRETORY FUNCTION

■ STRUCTURE OF SKIN

Skin forms largest organ of the body. It is not uniformly thick. At some places, it is thick and in some places it is thin. Average thickness of the skin is about 1 mm to 2 mm. Skin is made up of two layers namely, epidermis and dermis.

■ EPIDERMIS

Epidermis is the outer layer of skin. It is formed by stratified epithelium.

Epidermis is formed by five layers of structures:

1. Stratum corneum.
2. Stratum lucidum.
3. Stratum granulosum.
4. Stratum spinosum.
5. Stratum germinativum.

Important feature of epidermis is that, it does not have blood vessels **(Fig. 41.1)**. Nutrition is provided to epidermis by the capillaries of dermis.

■ DERMIS

Dermis is the inner layer of the skin. It is a connective tissue layer made up of dense and stout collagen fibers, fibroblasts and histiocytes.

Dermis is made up of two layers:

1. Superficial papillary layer.
2. Deeper reticular layer.

■ APPENDAGES OF SKIN

Hair follicles with hairs, nails, sweat glands, sebaceous glands and mammary glands are considered as appendages of the skin.

■ COLOR OF SKIN

Color of the skin depends upon **two factors**:

1. *Pigmentation of the Skin*

Cells of the skin contain a brown pigment called melanin. **Melanin** is synthesized by **melanocytes** present mainly in the stratum germinativum and stratum spinosum of epidermis. After synthesis, this pigment spreads to cells of other layers.

Melanin forms the major color determinant of human skin. Skin becomes dark when melanin content increases. It is protein in nature and it is synthesized from the amino acid **tyrosine** via **dihydroxyphenylalanine (DOPA)**.

2. *Hemoglobin in Blood*

Amount and nature of hemoglobin that circulates in the cutaneous blood vessels are also involved in the coloration the skin.

Skin becomes:

i. Pale when hemoglobin content decreases.
ii. Pink when blood rushes to skin due to cutaneous vasodilatation (blushing).

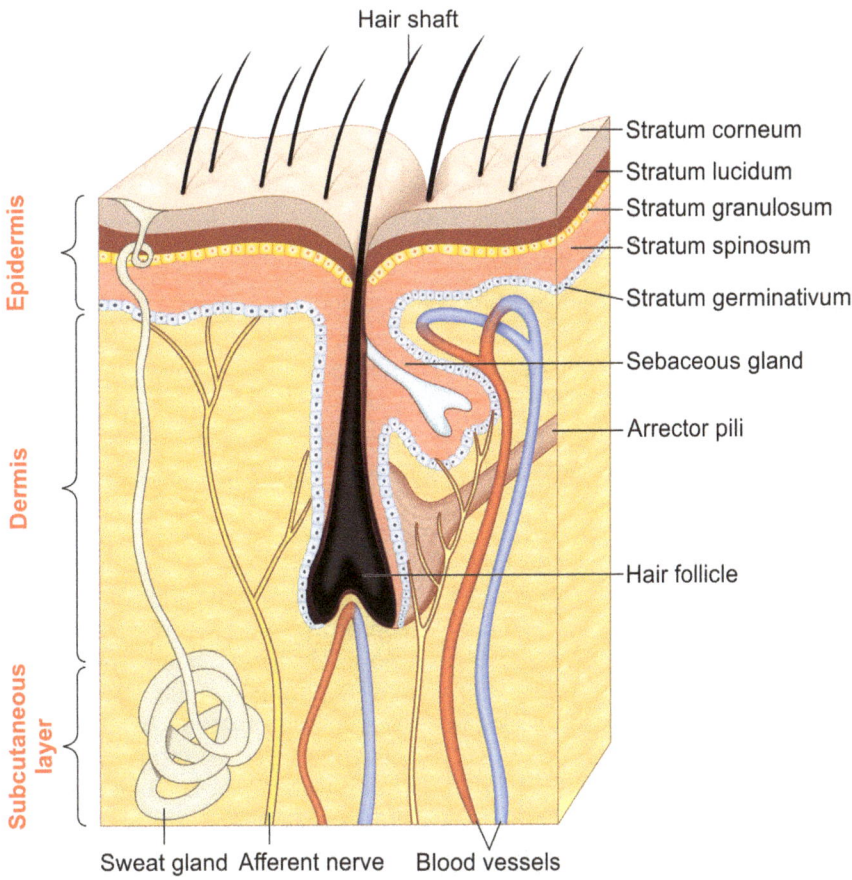

FIGURE 41.1: Structure of skin.
(*Courtesy*: JS Pasricha and Ramji Gupta)

iii. Bluish during cyanosis which is caused by excess amount of reduced hemoglobin.

GLANDS OF SKIN

Skin contains two types of glands, sebaceous glands and the sweat glands.

SEBACEOUS GLANDS

Sebaceous glands are simple or branched alveolar glands situated in the dermis of the skin. These glands are ovoid or spherical in shape and open into the neck of the hair follicle through a duct. In some areas like face, lips, nipple, glans penis and labia minora the sebaceous glands open directly into the exterior.

Sebaceous glands secrete an oily substance called **sebum**.

Composition of Sebum

Sebum contains:

1. Free fatty acids.
2. Triglycerides.
3. Squalene.
4. Sterols.
5. Waxes.
6. Paraffin.

Functions of Sebum

1. Free fatty acid content of the sebum has antibacterial and antifungal actions. Thus, it prevents the infection of skin by bacteria or fungi.
2. Lipid nature of sebum keeps the skin smooth and oily. It protects the skin from unnecessary desquamation and injury caused by dryness.
3. Lipids of the sebum prevent heat loss from the body. It is particularly useful in cold climate.

Activation of Sebaceous Glands at Puberty

Sebaceous glands are inactive till puberty. At the time of puberty these glands are activated by sex hormones in both males and females.

At the time of puberty particularly in males, due to increased secretion of sex hormones especially dehydroepiandrosterone, the sebaceous glands are stimulated suddenly. It leads to development of acne on the face.

Acne

Acne is the localized inflammatory condition of skin characterized by pimples on face, chest and back. It occurs because of over activity of sebaceous glands. **Acne vulgaris** is the common type of acne that is developed

TABLE 41.1: Differences between eccrine and apocrine sweat glands.

Features	Eccrine glands	Apocrine glands
1. Distribution	Throughout the body	Only in limited areas like axilla, pubis, areola and umbilicus
2. Opening	Exterior through sweat pore	Into the hair follicle
3. Period of functioning	Function throughout life	Start functioning only at puberty
4. Secretion	Clear and watery	Thick and milky
5. Regulation of body temperature	Play important role in temperature regulation	Do not play any role in temperature regulation
6. Conditions when secretion increases	During increased temperature and emotional conditions	Only during emotional conditions
7. Control of secretory activity	Under nervous control	Under hormonal control
8. Nerve supply	Sympathetic cholinergic fibers	Sympathetic adrenergic fibers

during adolescence. Acne disappears within few years when the sebaceous glands become adapted to the sex hormones.

■ SWEAT GLANDS

Sweat glands are of two types, eccrine glands and apocrine glands.

Eccrine Glands

Eccrine glands are tubular glands distributed throughout the body **(Table 41.1)**. These glands open out through the sweat pore.

Secretory activity of eccrine glands

Eccrine glands function throughout life since birth. These glands secrete a clear watery sweat. The secretion increases during increase in temperature and emotional conditions.

Eccrine glands play a role in regulating the body temperature by secreting sweat. Sweat contains water, sodium chloride, urea and lactic acid.

Apocrine Glands

Apocrine glands are situated only in certain areas of the body like axilla, pubis, areola and umbilicus. These glands are also tubular in nature but open into the hair follicles.

Secretory activity of apocrine glands

Apocrine sweat glands are nonfunctional till puberty and start functioning only at the time of puberty. In old age, the function of these glands gradually declines.

Secretion of the apocrine glands is thick and milky. At the time of secretion, it is odorless. When microorganisms grow in this secretion, a characteristic odor develops in the regions where apocrine glands are present. Secretion increases in emotional conditions.

Apocrine glands do not play any role in temperature regulation.

Pheromones

Pheromones or **vomeropherins** are substances secreted by apocrine glands. It is observed that the pheromones excreted in axilla of a woman affects the menstrual cycle of her room-mate or another woman living with her. These substances stimulate receptors of vomeronasal receptors. **Vomeronasal receptors** detect the odor of pheromones. Impulses from these receptors are transmitted to hypothalamus, which influences the menstrual cycle via pituitary gonadal axis. Effect of pheromones on the menstrual cycle of other individuals is called **dormitory effect.** Refer Chapter 100 for details of vomeronasal organ and its receptors.

■ FUNCTIONS OF THE SKIN

Primary function of skin is the protection of organs. However, it has many other important functions also.

■ 1. PROTECTIVE FUNCTION

Skin forms covering of all organs of the body and protects these organs from the following **three factors**:

i. Protection from Bacteria and Toxic Substances

Skin covers and protects the organs from having direct contact with external environment. Thus, it prevents the bacterial infection. **Lysozyme** secreted in skin destroys the bacteria. Stratum corneum of epidermis offers resistance against toxic chemicals like acids and alkalis.

ii. Protection from Mechanical Blow

Skin is not tightly placed over the underlying organs or tissues. It is somewhat loose and moves over the underlying subcutaneous tissues. So, the mechanical impact of any blow to skin is not transmitted to underlying tissues.

iii. Protection from Ultraviolet Rays

Skin protects the body from ultraviolet rays of sunlight. Exposure to sunlight increases the production of melanin in skin. Melanin absorbs ultraviolet rays. At the same time, stratum corneum also absorbs the ultraviolet rays.

■ 2. SENSORY FUNCTION

Skin is considered as the largest sense organ in the body. It has many nerve endings, which form the specialized cutaneous receptors (Chapter 79).

These receptors are stimulated by the sensations of touch, pain, pressure or temperature sensation and convey these sensations to the brain via afferent nerves. At the brain level, perception of different sensations occurs.

■ 3. STORAGE FUNCTION

Skin stores fat, water, chloride and sugar. It can also store blood by the dilatation of the cutaneous blood vessels.

■ 4. SYNTHETIC FUNCTION

Vitamin D_3 is synthesized in skin by the action of ultraviolet rays from sunlight on cholesterol (Chapter 46).

■ 5. REGULATION OF BODY TEMPERATURE

Skin plays an important role in the regulation of body temperature. Details are given in Chapter 42.

■ 6. REGULATION OF WATER AND ELECTROLYTE BALANCE

Skin regulates water balance and electrolyte balance by excreting water and salts through sweat.

■ 7. EXCRETORY FUNCTION

Skin excretes small quantities of waste materials like urea, salts and fatty substance.

■ 8. ABSORPTIVE FUNCTION

Skin absorbs the fat-soluble substances and some ointments.

■ 9. SECRETORY FUNCTION

Skin secretes sweat through sweat glands and sebum through sebaceous glands. By secreting sweat, skin regulates body temperature and water balance. Sebum keeps the skin smooth and moist.

Chapter 42

Body Temperature

CHAPTER OUTLINE

- **BODY TEMPERATURE**
  - NORMAL BODY TEMPERATURE
  - TEMPERATURE AT DIFFERENT PARTS OF BODY
- **HEAT BALANCE**
  - HEAT GAIN OR HEAT PRODUCTION IN THE BODY
  - HEAT LOSS FROM THE BODY
- **REGULATION OF BODY TEMPERATURE**
  - ROLE OF HYPOTHALAMUS
  - MECHANISM OF TEMPERATURE REGULATION
- **APPLIED PHYSIOLOGY: THERMOREGULATORY DISORDERS**
  - HYPERTHERMIA: FEVER
  - HYPOTHERMIA

■ BODY TEMPERATURE

Body temperature can be measured by placing the clinical thermometer in different parts of the body such as:

1. Mouth (oral temperature).
2. Axilla (axillary temperature).
3. Rectum (rectal temperature).
4. Over the skin (surface temperature).

■ NORMAL BODY TEMPERATURE

Normal body temperature in human is 37°C (98.6°F) when measured by placing clinical thermometer in the mouth (**oral temperature**). It varies between 35.8°C and 37.3°C (96.4°F and 99.1°F).

■ TEMPERATURE AT DIFFERENT PARTS OF THE BODY

Axillary temperature is 0.3 to 0.6°C (0.5 to 1°F) lower than the oral temperature. And, the **rectal temperature** is 0.3 to 0.6°C (0.5 to 1°F) higher than oral temperature. The **surface temperature** (skin or **superficial temperature**) varies between 29.5°C and 33.9°C (85.1°F and 93°F). Surface temperature is slightly less than oral temperature.

Core Temperature

Core temperature is the average temperature of structures present in deeper part of the body. Core temperature is always more than oral or rectal temperature. Temperature at different parts of the body are given in **Table 42.1**.

■ HEAT BALANCE

Regulation of body temperature depends upon the balance between heat produced in body and heat lost from the body.

■ HEAT GAIN OR HEAT PRODUCTION IN THE BODY

Various mechanisms are involved in production of heat in the body.

1. Metabolic Activities

Major portion of heat produced in the body is due to metabolism of foodstuffs. Liver is the organ in which maximum heat is produced due to metabolic activity.

TABLE 42.1: Temperature at different parts of the body.

Parts	Temperature Fahrenheit	Temperature Celsius
Oral temperature	98.6° (96.4 to 99.1°)	37.0° (35.8 to 37.3°)
Surface temperature	85.1 to 93°	29.5 to 33.9°
Axillary temperature	0.5 to 1° Lower than the oral temperature	0.3 to 0.6°
Rectal temperature	0.5 to 1° Higher than oral temperature	0.3 to 0.6°
Core temperature	100°	37.8°

2. Muscular Activity

Heat is produced in the muscle both at rest and during activities. During rest, heat is produced by muscle tone. About 80% of heat of activity is produced by the activity of skeletal muscles.

3. Role of Hormones

Thyroxine and adrenaline increase the heat production by accelerating metabolic activities.

4. Radiation of Heat from the Environment

Body gains heat by radiation. It occurs when environmental temperature is higher than body temperature.

5. Shivering

Shivering is the shaking of body caused by rapid involuntary contraction or twitching of muscles during exposure to cold. It is a compensatory physiological mechanism in the body, during which enormous heat is produced.

6. Brown Fat Tissue

Brown fat or **brown adipose tissue** is one of the two types of adipose tissues, the other being white adipose tissue. Brown fat produces enormous body heat, particularly in infants.

HEAT LOSS FROM THE BODY

Maximum heat is lost from the body through skin and small amount of heat is lost through respiratory system, kidney and GI tract. When environmental temperature is less than body temperature, heat is lost from the body. Heat loss occurs by the following methods:

1. Conduction

Heat is lost from the surface of the body to other objects such as chair or bed by means of conduction.

2. Radiation

Sixty percent of heat is lost by means of radiation, i.e. transfer of heat by infrared electromagnetic radiation from body to other objects through the surrounding air.

3. Convection

Heat is conducted to the air surrounding the body and then carried away by air currents, i.e. convection.

4. Evaporation: Insensible Perspiration

When body temperature increases sweating occurs. During sweating, water evaporates from sweat and heat is lost from the body. About 22% of heat is lost through evaporation of water.

Perspiration and insensible perspiration

Perspiration means formation of sweat from which water is lost by means of evaporation. Insensible perspiration is the perspiration which occurs before it is being perceived or sensed, i.e. we are not aware of perspiration. In addition to loss of water through sweat, insensible perspiration includes evaporation of water through lungs also. Usually insensible perspiration is about 400 mL/day to 600 mL/day.

REGULATION OF BODY TEMPERATURE

Living organisms are classified into two groups depending upon the maintenance (regulation) of body temperature.

1. **Homeothermic animals** or **warm-blooded animals** are the animals whose body temperature is maintained at a constant level irrespective of the environmental temperature. Birds and mammals including man belong to this category.
2. **Poikilothermic animals** or **cold-blooded animals** are the animals whose body temperature is not constant. It varies according to environmental temperature. Amphibians and reptiles are the poikilothermic animals.

ROLE OF HYPOTHALAMUS

Set Point for Body Temperature

Body temperature is regulated by hypothalamus, which sets the normal range of body temperature. The set point for body temperature under normal physiological conditions is 37°C.

Hypothalamus has **two centers** which regulate the body temperature.

Heat Loss Center

This center is situated in **preoptic nucleus** of anterior hypothalamus. Neurons in preoptic nucleus are heatsensitive nerve cells which are called **thermoreceptors**.

Heat Gain Center

It is otherwise known as heat production center. It is situated in posterior hypothalamic nucleus.

MECHANISM OF TEMPERATURE REGULATION

When Body Temperature Increases

When body temperature increases, blood temperature also increases. When blood with increased temperature passes through hypothalamus, it stimulates the thermoreceptors present in the heat loss center in preoptic nucleus **(Fig. 42.1)**.

Now, the heat loss center brings temperature back to normal by **two mechanisms**:

1. Promotion of heat loss

Heat loss center promotes heat loss from the body by:

i. Increasing the secretion of sweat. When sweat secretion increases, more water is lost from skin along with heat.
ii. Inhibiting the sympathetic centers in posterior hypothalamus. This causes cutaneous vasodilatation. Now, blood flow through skin increases causing excess

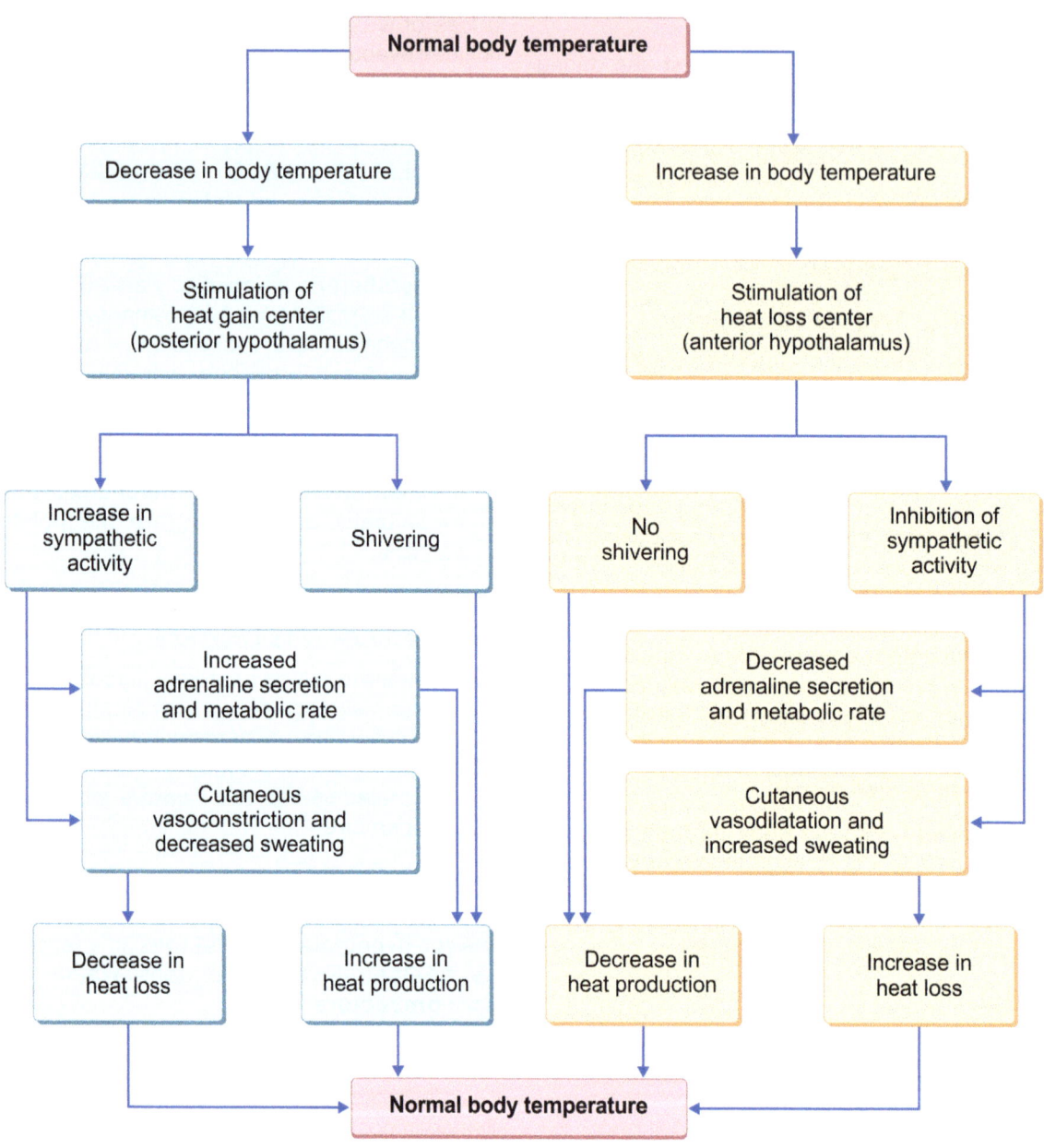

FIGURE 42.1: Regulation of body temperature.

sweating. It increases the heat loss through sweat leading to decrease in body temperature.

2. Prevention of heat production

Heat loss center prevents heat production in the body by inhibiting mechanisms involved in heat production such as shivering and chemical (metabolic) reactions.

When Body Temperature Decreases

When the body temperature decreases it is brought back to normal by **two mechanisms**:

1. Prevention of heat loss

When body temperature decreases, the preoptic thermoreceptors are not activated. So, the posterior hypothalamus is not inhibited. This causes cutaneous vasoconstriction. The blood flow to skin decreases and so the heat loss is prevented.

2. Promotion of heat production

Heat production is promoted by two ways:

i. *Shivering*: Motor center for shivering is situated in posterior hypothalamus. When body temperature is low, this center is activated by heat gain center and, shivering occurs. Enormous heat is produced during shivering due to severe muscular activities.

ii. *Increased metabolic reactions*: Sympathetic centers, which are activated by heat gain center, stimulate secretion of adrenaline and noradrenaline. These hormones, particularly adrenaline increase heat production by accelerating cellular metabolic activities.

Simultaneously, hypothalamus secretes thyrotropin-releasing hormone. It causes release of thyroid stimulating hormone from pituitary. It in turn increases release of thyroxine from thyroid. Thyroxine accelerates the metabolic activities in the body and increases heat production.

The process by which heat is produced in the body by metabolic activities induced by hormones is called **chemical thermogenesis.**

■ APPLIED PHYSIOLOGY: THERMOREGULATORY DISORDERS

■ HYPERTHERMIA: FEVER

Elevation of body temperature above the set point is called hyperthermia, fever or **pyrexia.** Fever itself is not an illness. But it is an important sign of something going wrong in the body. It is the part of body's response to disease.

Fever may be beneficial to body and on many occasions, it plays an important role in helping the body fight diseases, particularly the infections.

Hyperpyrexia

Hyperpyrexia is the rise in body temperature beyond 107.6°F (42°C). Hyperpyrexia results in damage of body tissues. Further increase in temperature becomes life threatening.

Common Causes of Fever

1. Infection by certain substances **(pyrogens)** released from bacteria or parasites.
2. Hyperthyroidism.
3. Brain lesions which involves temperature regulating centers.

■ HYPOTHERMIA

Decrease in body temperature below 95°F (35°C) is called hypothermia. It is considered as the clinical state of subnormal body temperature, when the body fails to produce enough heat to maintain the normal activities. Major setback of this condition is the impairment of metabolic activities of the body. When the temperature drops below 87.8°F (31°C), it becomes fatal. Elderly persons are more susceptible for hypothermia.

MODEL QUESTIONS IN RENAL PHYSIOLOGY AND SKIN

■ LONG QUESTIONS

1. Describe the process of urine formation.
2. What are the different stages of urine formation? Explain glomerular filtration.
3. Give an account of role of renal tubules in the process of urine formation.
4. What is countercurrent mechanism? Describe the anatomical and physiological basis of countercurrent mechanism in kidney.
5. Describe the mechanism involved in concentration of urine.
6. Give an account of micturition.
7. What is normal body temperature? Explain heat balance and regulation of body temperature. Add a note on fever.

■ SHORT QUESTIONS

1. Functions of kidney.
2. Structure of nephron.
3. Juxtaglomerular apparatus.
4. Renin-angiotensin system.
5. Salient features of renal circulation.
6. Glomerular filtration rate.
7. Effective filtration pressure in kidney.
8. Reabsorption of water in renal tubule.
9. Tubular secretion.
10. Countercurrent multiplier/Countercurrent exchanger.
11. Plasma clearance.
12. Nerve supply to urinary bladder and sphincters.
13. Cystometrogram.
14. Micturition reflex.
15. Glands of skin/Sweat glands.
16. Functions of skin.

■ VERY SHORT ANSWER QUESTIONS

1. Renal corpuscle.
2. Differences between two types of nephron.
3. Filtration membrane in glomerulus.
4. GFR.
5. Net filtration pressure.
6. Tubuloglomerular feedback.
7. Selective reabsorption.
8. Define tubular maximum and give example.
9. Define renal threshold and give example.
10. Renal medullary gradient.
11. Role of ADH in concentration of urine.
12. Properties and composition of urine.
13. Urethra in males and females.
14. Atonic bladder/Automatic bladder.
15. Nocturnal enuresis.
16. Apocrine glands/Eccrine glands.
17. Sebaceous glands/Sebum.
18. Temperature at different parts of the body and core temperature.
19. Heat loss center and Heat gain center.
20. Fever/Hypothermia.

SECTION 6 ENDOCRINOLOGY

CHAPTER 43: Overview of Endocrine System

CHAPTER OUTLINE

- **ENDOCRINE SYSTEM**
  - CELL-TO-CELL SIGNALING
  - CHEMICAL MESSENGERS
- **ENDOCRINE GLANDS**
- **CLASSIFICATION OF HORMONES**
- **HORMONAL ACTION**
  - HORMONE RECEPTORS
  - MECHANISM OF HORMONAL ACTION

ENDOCRINE SYSTEM

All physiological activities of the body are regulated by two major controlling systems in the body:

1. Nervous system.
2. Endocrine system.

Both the systems interact with one another and regulate the body functions. This section deals with endocrine system and Section 10 deals with nervous system. Endocrine system functions by secreting some chemical substances called **hormones**.

CELL-TO-CELL SIGNALING

Cell-to-cell signaling is the transfer of information from one cell to another. It is also called **cell signaling** or **intercellular communication**. Cell signaling occurs through chemical messengers.

CHEMICAL MESSENGERS

Most of the chemical messengers are secreted by endocrine glands. Some of them are secreted by nerve endings and the cells of other tissues.

All the chemical messengers carry the message (signal) from **signaling cells (controlling cells)** to **target cells.**

Classification of Chemical Messengers

Chemical messengers are usually classified into two types namely, classical hormones secreted by endocrine glands and local hormones secreted from other tissues.

However, recently chemical messengers are classified into four types:

1. Endocrine messengers.
2. Paracrine messengers.
3. Autocrine messengers.
4. Neurocrine messengers.

1. *Endocrine Messengers*

Endocrine messengers are the classical hormones secreted by endocrine glands. **Classical hormone** is defined as a chemical messenger, synthesized by endocrine gland and transported by blood to the target organs or tissues (site of action).

Examples are growth hormone and insulin.

2. *Paracrine Messengers*

Paracrine messengers are the chemical messengers, which diffuse from control cells to the target cells through interstitial fluid **(Fig. 43.1)**.

Juxtacrine messengers or local hormones

Juxtacrine messengers or **local hormones** are some of the paracrine messengers which directly enter the neighboring target cells through gap junctions.

Examples are prostaglandins and histamine.

3. *Autocrine Messengers*

Autocrine messengers are the chemical messengers that control the source cells which secrete them. So, these messengers are also called **intracellular chemical mediators**.

Examples are leukotrienes.

4. *Neurocrine or Neural Messengers*

Neurocrine or neural messengers are of two types:

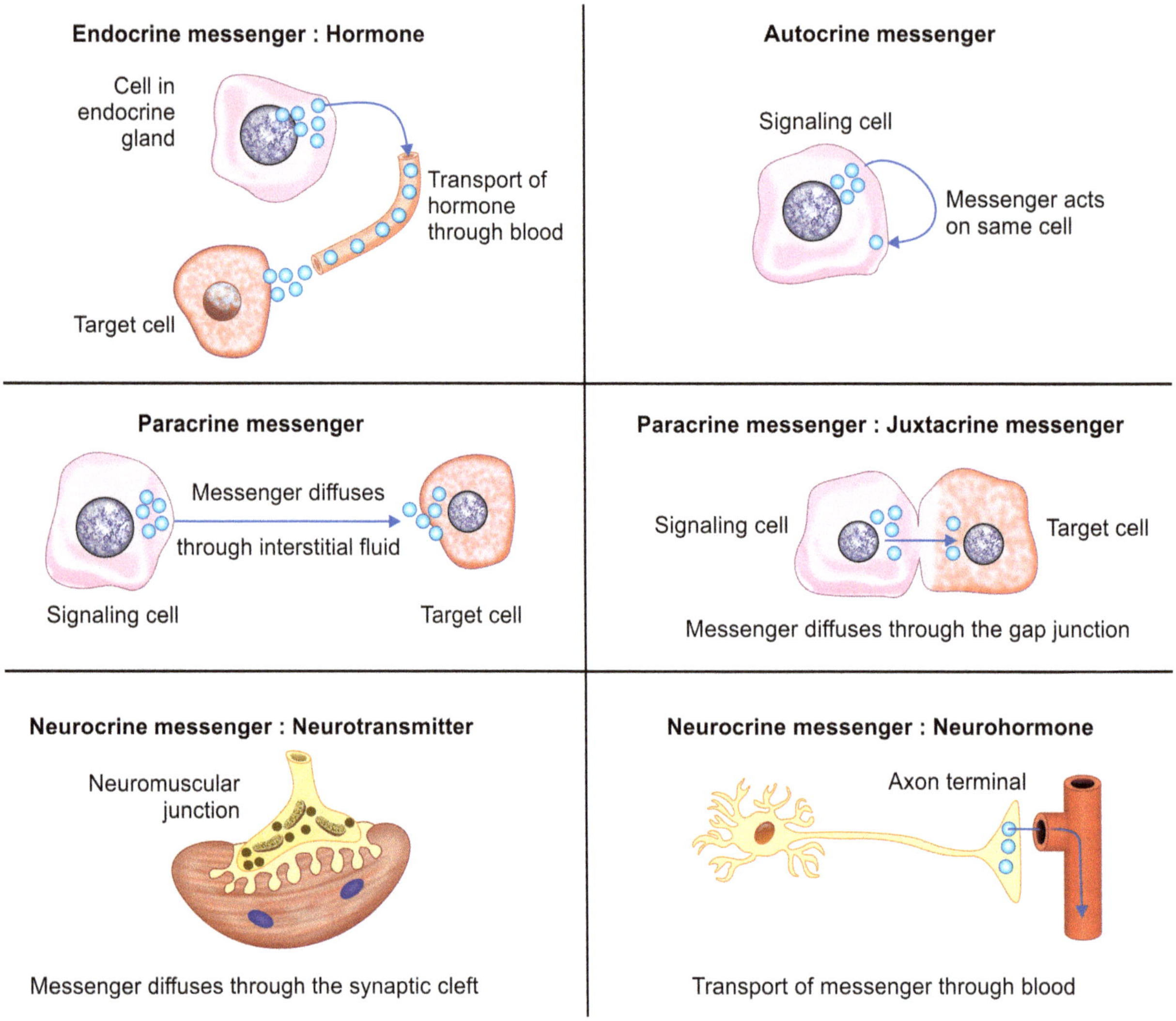

FIGURE 43.1: Chemical messengers.

1. *Neurotransmitter*: Neurotransmitter is the chemical messenger that carries information from a nerve cell to another nerve cell or muscle or another tissue. Examples are acetylcholine and dopamine.
2. *Neurohormone*: Neurohormone is a chemical messenger that is released by the nerve cell directly into the blood and transported to the distant target cells. Example are oxytocin, antidiuretic hormone and hypothalamic releasing hormones.

ENDOCRINE GLANDS

Endocrine glands are the glands which synthesize and release the classical hormones into the blood. Endocrine glands are also called **ductless glands** because the hormones secreted by them are released directly into blood without any duct.

Major endocrine glands are shown in **Figure 43.2**.

Hormones secreted by major endocrine glands are listed in **Table 43.1**.

Hormones secreted by gonads are given in **Table 43.2**.

Hormones secreted by other organs are given in **Table 43.3**.

Local hormones are listed in **Box 43.1**.

CLASSIFICATION OF HORMONES

Based on chemical nature, hormones are classified into three types:

1. Steroid hormones which are synthesized from cholesterol or its derivatives.
2. Protein hormones which are peptides in nature.
3. Hormones derived from amino acid tyrosine.

Classification of hormones depending upon their chemical nature is given in **Table 43.4**.

HORMONAL ACTION

Hormone does not act directly on the cellular structures. It combines with receptors present on the target cells and forms a hormone-receptor complex. This **hormone-receptor complex** induces various changes or reactions in the target cells.

Chapter 43: Overview of Endocrine System

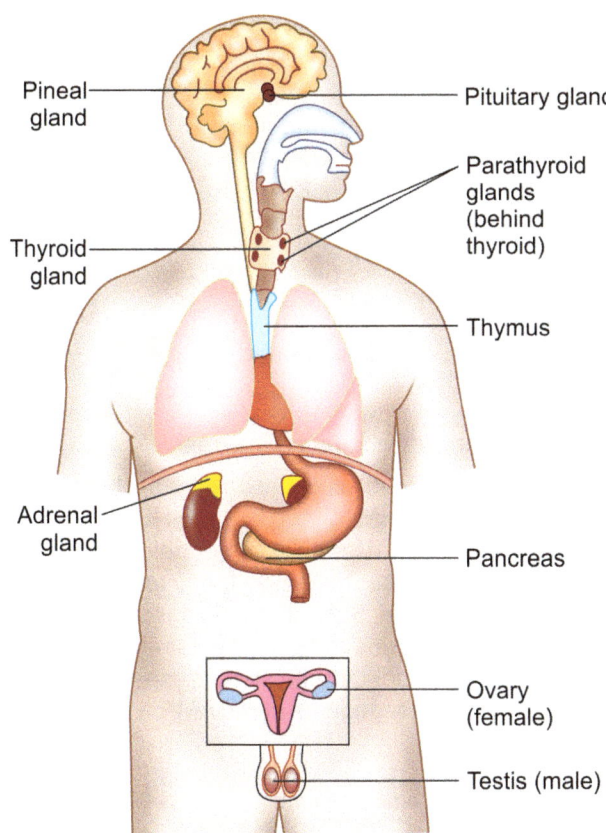

FIGURE 43.2: Diagram showing major endocrine glands.

TABLE 43.2: Hormones secreted by gonads.

Gonad	Hormones
Testis	1. Testosterone 2. Dihydrotestosterone 3. Androstenedion
Ovary	1. Estrogen 2. Progesterone

is specific for one single hormone, i.e. each receptor can combine with only one hormone.

Thus, a hormone can act on a target cell, only if the target cell has the receptor for that particular hormone.

Situation of the Hormone Receptors

Hormone receptors are situated in any of the following parts of a cell:

1. *Cell membrane*: Receptors of protein hormones and adrenal medullary hormones (catecholamines) are situated in the cell membrane **(Fig. 43.3)**.
2. *Cytoplasm*: Receptors of steroid hormones are situated in cytoplasm of the cells.
3. *Nucleus*: Receptors of thyroid hormones are in the nucleus of the cell.

MECHANISM OF HORMONAL ACTION

On the target cell, the hormone-receptor complex acts by **three mechanisms**:

1. By Altering Permeability of Cell Membrane

Neurotransmitter substances in a synapse or neuromuscular junction act by altering the permeability of postsynaptic membrane.

For example, in a **neuromuscular junction**, when an action potential reaches the axon terminal of motor

HORMONE RECEPTORS

Hormone receptors are the large **proteins** present in the target cells to which the hormones bind to execute the hormonal actions.

Each cell has thousands of receptors. Important characteristic feature of the receptors is that each receptor

TABLE 43.1: Hormones secreted by major endocrine glands.

Endocrine gland	Hormones	Endocrine gland	Hormones
Anterior pituitary	1. Growth hormone (GH) 2. Thyroid-stimulating hormone (TSH) 3. Adrenocorticotropic hormone (ACTH) 4. Follicle-stimulating hormone (FSH) 5. Luteinizing hormone (LH) 6. Prolactin	Adrenal cortex	Mineralocorticoids 1. Aldosterone 2. 11-deoxycorticosterone
Posterior pituitary	1. Antidiuretic hormone (ADH) 2. Oxytocin		Glucocorticoids 1. Cortisol 2. Corticosterone
Thyroid gland	1. Thyroxine (T_4) 2. Triiodothyronine (T_3) 3. Calcitonin		Sex hormones 1. Androgens 2. Estrogen 3. Progesterone
Parathyroid gland	1. Parathormone	Adrenal medulla	Catecholamines 1. Adrenaline (epinephrine) 2. Noradrenaline (norepinephrine) 3. Dopamine
Pancreas: Islets of Langerhans	1. Insulin 2. Glucagon 3. Somatostatin 4. Pancreatic polypeptide		

Section 6: Endocrinology

TABLE 43.3: Hormones secreted by other organs.

Organ	Hormones
Pineal gland	1. Melatonin
Thymus	1. Thymosin 2. Thymin
Kidney	1. Erythropoietin 2. Thrombopoietin 3. Renin 4. 1,25-dihydroxycholecalciferol (calcitriol) 5. Prostaglandins
Heart	1. Atrial natriuretic peptide 2. Brain natriuretic peptide 3. C-type natriuretic peptide
Placenta	1. Human chorionic gonadotropin (hCG) 2. Human chorionic somatomammotropin 3. Estrogen 4. Progesterone

BOX 43.1: Local hormones.

1. Prostaglandins
2. Thromboxanes
3. Prostacyclin
4. Leukotrienes
5. Lipoxins
6. Acetylcholine
7. Serotonin
8. Histamine
9. Substance P
10. Heparin
11. Bradykinin
12. Gastrointestinal hormones

nerve, acetylcholine is released from synaptic vesicles. **Acetylcholine** increases permeability of postsynaptic membrane by opening the **ligand-gated sodium channels**. So, sodium ions enter the neuromuscular junction from ECF and cause development of endplate potential.

2. By Activating Intracellular Enzyme

Protein hormones and the catecholamines act by activating the intracellular enzymes.

A hormone which acts on a target cell is called **first messenger** or chemical mediator. It causes formation of a **second messenger**. Second messenger produces the effects of hormone inside the cells. Protein hormones and the catecholamines act through second messenger. Most common second messenger is cyclic AMP.

TABLE 43.4: Classification of hormones depending upon chemical nature.

Chemical nature	Hormones	Source of secretion
Steroids	Aldosterone 11-deoxycorticosterone Cortisol Corticosterone	Adrenal cortex
	Estrogen Progesterone	Ovary Adrenal cortex
	Testosterone Dihydrotestosterone Dehydroepiandrosterone	Testis Adrenal cortex
Proteins	Growth hormone (GH) Thyroid-stimulating hormone (TSH) Adrenocorticotropic hormone (ACTH) Follicle-stimulating hormone (FSH) Luteinizing hormone (LH) Prolactin	Anterior pituitary gland
	Antidiuretic hormone Oxytocin	Posterior pituitary gland
	Insulin Glucagon Somatostatin Pancreatic polypeptide	Pancreas (Islets of Langerhans)
	Human chorionic gonadotropin (hCG) Human chorionic somatomammotropin	Placenta
	Parathormone	Parathyroid gland
	Calcitonin	
Derivatives of tyrosine	Thyroxine (T4) Triiodothyronine (T3)	Thyroid gland
	Adrenaline (epinephrine) Noradrenaline (norepinephrine) Dopamine	Adrenal medulla

Chapter 43: Overview of Endocrine System

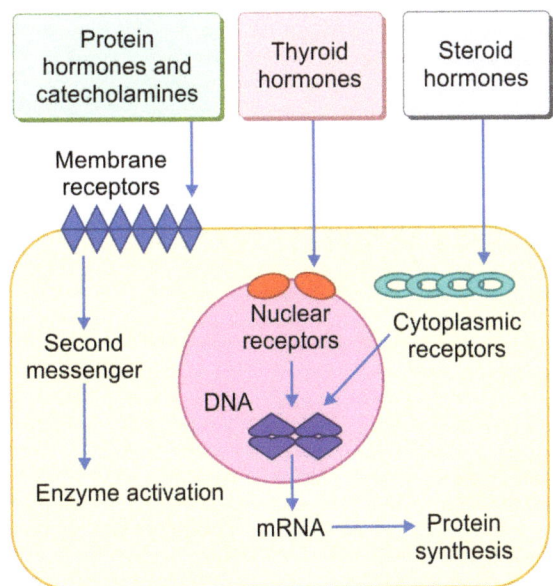

FIGURE 43.3: Situation of hormonal receptors.

Cyclic AMP

Cyclic AMP or cAMP or cyclic adenosine 3'5'-monophosphate acts as second messenger for protein hormones and catecholamines. G proteins or **guanosine nucleotide-binding proteins** are the membrane proteins situated on the inner surface of cell membrane. These proteins are necessary for the formation of cAMP.

Cyclic AMP executes the actions of hormone inside the cell by stimulating the enzymes such as protein kinase A.

3. By Acting on Genes

Thyroid and steroid hormones act by activating the genes of the target cells.

Hormone enters the cell and binds with receptor in cytoplasm (steroid hormone) or in nucleus (thyroid hormone) and forms hormone-receptor complex. This complex binds to DNA and increases transcription of mRNA. The mRNA activates ribosomes. Activated ribosomes produce large quantities of proteins which produce the physiological responses in the target cells

Chapter 44

Pituitary Gland

CHAPTER OUTLINE

- ■ PITUITARY GLAND
  - ■ DIVISIONS
  - ■ REGULATION OF SECRETION
- ■ ANTERIOR PITUITARY OR ADENOHYPOPHYSIS
  - ■ PARTS
  - ■ FUNCTIONAL HISTOLOGY
  - ■ REGULATION
  - ■ HORMONES
  - ■ GROWTH HORMONE
  - ■ OTHER HORMONES
- ■ POSTERIOR PITUITARY OR NEUROHYPOPHYSIS
  - ■ PARTS
  - ■ FUNCTIONAL HISTOLOGY
  - ■ HORMONES
  - ■ ANTIDIURETIC HORMONE
  - ■ OXYTOCIN
- ■ APPLIED PHYSIOLOGY: DISORDERS OF PITUITARY GLAND
  - ■ HYPERACTIVITY OF ANTERIOR PITUITARY
  - ■ HYPOACTIVITY OF ANTERIOR PITUITARY
  - ■ HYPERACTIVITY OF POSTERIOR PITUITARY
  - ■ HYPOACTIVITY OF POSTERIOR PITUITARY
  - ■ HYPOACTIVITY OF ANTERIOR AND POSTERIOR PITUITARY

■ PITUITARY GLAND

Pituitary gland or **hypophysis** is a small gland that lies at the base of brain. It is connected with the hypothalamus by **pituitary stalk** or **hypophyseal stalk**.

■ DIVISIONS OF PITUITARY GLAND

Pituitary gland is divided into two portions:

1. Anterior pituitary or **adenohypophysis**.
2. Posterior pituitary or **neurohypophysis**.

■ REGULATION OF SECRETION OF PITUITARY HORMONES

Hypothalamo-hypophyseal Relationship

Relationship between hypothalamus and pituitary gland is called hypothalamo-hypophyseal relationship. Hormones secreted by hypothalamus are transported to anterior pituitary and posterior pituitary. But the mode of transport of these hormones is different.

Hormones from hypothalamus are transported to anterior pituitary through hypothalamo-hypophyseal portal blood vessels. But, the hormones from hypothalamus to posterior pituitary are transported by nerve fibers of hypothalamo-hypophyseal tract.

■ ANTERIOR PITUITARY

■ PARTS OF ANTERIOR PITUITARY

Anterior pituitary consists of three divisions **(Fig. 44.1)**:

1. Pars distalis.
2. Pars tuberalis.
3. Pars intermedia.

■ FUNCTIONAL HISTOLOGY OF ANTERIOR PITUITARY

Depending upon staining property, the cells of anterior pituitary are classified into two types:

I. **Chromophobe cells** which do not have granules and stain poorly. These cells are not secretory in nature.
II. **Chromophil cells** which contain large granules and are stained darkly. These cells are secretory in nature.

Classification of Chromophil Cells

Chromophil cells are of two types namely, **acidophilic cells** or α-cells and **basophilic cells** or β-cells.

Depending upon the **secretory function**, chromophil cells are classified into five types:

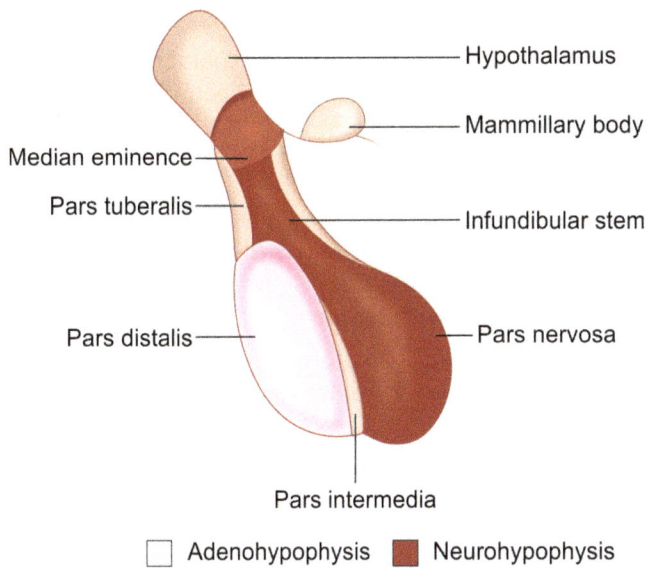

FIGURE 44.1: Parts of pituitary gland.

i. **Somatotrophs** which secrete growth hormone.
ii. **Corticotrophs** which secrete adrenocorticotropic hormone.
iii. **Thyrotrophs** which secrete thyroid stimulating hormone.
iv. **Gonadotrophs** which secrete follicle stimulating hormone and luteinizing hormone.
v. **Lactotrophs** which secrete prolactin.

Somatotrophs and lactotrophs are acidophilic cells, whereas others are basophilic cells.

■ REGULATION OF SECRETION OF ANTERIOR PITUITARY HORMONES

Secretion of anterior pituitary hormones is regulated by hypothalamus. Hypothalamus secretes some releasing and inhibitory hormones (factors) which are transported from hypothalamus to anterior pituitary through hypothalamo-hypophyseal portal vessels.

Releasing and Inhibitory Hormones Secreted by Hypothalamus

1. Growth hormone-releasing hormone (GHRH): Stimulates the release of GH.
2. Growth hormone-releasing polypeptide (GHRP): Stimulates the release of GHRH and GH.
3. Growth hormone-inhibitory hormone (GHIH) or somatostatin: Inhibits GH release.
4. Thyrotropin-releasing hormone (TRH): Stimulates the release of TSH.
5. Corticotropin-releasing hormone (CRH): Stimulates the release of ACTH.
6. Gonadotropin-releasing hormone (GnRH): Stimulates the release of the gonadotropins, FSH and LH.
7. Prolactin-inhibitory hormone (PIH): Inhibits prolactin secretion.

■ HORMONES SECRETED BY ANTERIOR PITUITARY

Anterior pituitary is also known as the **master gland** because it regulates many other endocrine glands.

Six hormones are secreted by the anterior pituitary:
1. Growth hormone (GH) or somatotropic hormone (STH).
2. Thyroid-stimulating hormone (TSH) or thyrotropic hormone.
3. Adrenocorticotropic hormone (ACTH).
4. Follicle stimulating hormone (FSH).
5. Luteinizing hormone (LH) in females or interstitial cell stimulating hormone (ICSH) in males.
6. Prolactin.

Recently, the hormone β-lipotropin is found to be secreted by anterior pituitary.

First five hormones of anterior pituitary stimulate the other endocrine glands. Growth hormone also stimulates the secretory activity of liver and other tissues. Therefore, these five hormones are called **tropic hormones**. Prolactin is concerned with milk secretion.

FSH and LH are together called **gonadotropic hormones** or **gonadotropins** because of their action on the gonads.

■ GROWTH HORMONE

Growth hormone (GH) is secreted by **somatotrophs** which are acidophils of anterior pituitary.

GH is a protein having a single chain polypeptide with 191 amino acids. GH is transported in blood by **GH-binding proteins (GHBP)**.

Basal level of GH concentration in blood of the normal adult is up to 300 g/dL.

Actions of Growth Hormone

Growth hormone is responsible for the growth of almost all tissues of the body, which are capable of growing. It increases the size and number of cells by increasing the mitotic division. GH also causes specific differentiation of certain types of cells like bone cells and muscle cells.

GH also acts on the metabolism of all the three major types of foodstuffs in the body. It increases the synthesis of proteins, mobilization of lipids and conservation of carbohydrates.

1. On metabolism

   a. *On protein metabolism*

   GH accelerates synthesis of proteins by:
   i. Increasing amino acid transport through cell membrane.
   ii. Increasing ribonucleic acid (RNA) translation so more proteins are synthesized.
   iii. Increasing transcription of DNA to RNA: RNA, in turn accelerates the synthesis of proteins in the cells.

iv. **Decreasing catabolism of protein:** It helps in the building up of tissues.
v. Promoting **anabolism of proteins** indirectly by causing release of insulin from β-cells of islets in pancreas, which has anabolic effect on proteins.

b. *On fat metabolism*

GH mobilizes fats from adipose tissue. Because of this, the concentration of fatty acids increases in the body fluids. Fatty acids are used for production of energy by the cells. So, proteins are spared.

During the utilization of fatty acids for production of energy, lot of acetoacetic acid is produced by the liver and released into the body fluids leading to **ketosis**. Sometimes excess mobilization of fat from the adipose tissue causes accumulation of fat in liver, resulting in **fatty liver**.

c. *On carbohydrate metabolism*

Major action of GH on carbohydrates is the conservation of glucose.

Effects of GH on the carbohydrate metabolism are:
i. Decrease in peripheral utilization of glucose for the production of energy.
ii. Increase in deposition of glycogen in the cells. Since, glucose is not utilized for energy production by the cells, it is converted into glycogen which is deposited in the cells.
iii. Decrease in uptake of glucose by the cells. As the deposition of glycogen increases, cells become saturated with glycogen. Because of this, no more glucose can enter the cells. So, the blood glucose level increases.

Diabetogenic effect of GH

Hypersecretion of GH increases blood glucose level enormously. Increased blood sugar stimulates the β-cells in the islets of Langerhans in pancreas continuously and increases insulin secretion. In addition to this, the GH also stimulates the β-cells of islets in pancreas directly and causes secretion of insulin. Because of excess stimulation, the β-cells are burnt out at one stage. This causes deficiency of insulin, which leads to true diabetes mellitus or **full-blown diabetes mellitus**. This is called the **diabetogenic effect of GH**.

2. On bones

In embryonic stage, GH is responsible for the differentiation and development of bone cells. In later stages, GH increases growth of the skeleton. It increases both length as well as thickness of the bones.

GH increases length of the bones until epiphysis fuses with shaft of bone. Usually fusion occurs at puberty. After **epiphyseal fusion**, length of the bones cannot be increased. However, GH stimulates the osteoblasts strongly. So, the bone continues to grow in thickness throughout life.

Mode of Action of GH on Bones and Metabolism

GH acts on bones, growth and protein metabolism through a substance called somatomedin, which is secreted by liver. GH stimulates the liver to secrete somatomedin.

Somatomedin

Somatomedin is a polypeptide. It is of two types:
1. **Insulin like growth factor-I (IGF-I)**, which is also called **somatomedin C**.
2. **Insulin like growth factor-II**.

Among the two somatomedins, somatomedin C (IGF-I) is responsible for the action of bones on bones and metabolism.

Regulation of GH Secretion

Secretion of GH is regulated by hypothalamus and feedback control.

Role of hypothalamus in the secretion of GH

Hypothalamus regulates GH secretion by releasing three hormones:
1. **Growth hormone releasing hormone (GHRH)** that increases secretion of GH by stimulating the somatotrophs of anterior pituitary.
2. **Growth hormone releasing polypeptide (GHRP)** that promotes release of GHRH from hypothalamus and GH from pituitary.
3. **Growth hormone inhibitory hormone (GHIH)** or **somatostatin** which inhibits secretion of GH.

These three hormones are transported from hypothalamus to anterior pituitary by hypothalamo-hypophyseal portal blood vessels. Hypothalamus is in turn influenced by many factors which cause increase or decrease in GH secretion.

Factors which increase the GH secretion are hypoglycemia, fasting, starvation, exercise, stress and trauma.

Factors which decrease the GH secretion are hyperglycemia and increase in free fatty acids in blood.

Feedback control

GH secretion is under negative feedback control (Chapter 4). Hypothalamus releases GHRH and GHRP, which in turn promote the release of GH from anterior pituitary. GH acts on various tissues. It also activates the liver cells to secrete somatomedin C (IGF-I).

Now, the somatomedin C acts in three ways:
i. It increases release of GHIH from hypothalamus. GHIH in turn inhibits release of GH from pituitary.
ii. Somatomedin also inhibits release of GHRP from hypothalamus.
iii. It acts on pituitary directly and inhibits the secretion of GH **(Fig. 44.2)**.

GH inhibits its own secretion by stimulating the release of GHIH from hypothalamus. This type of feedback is called

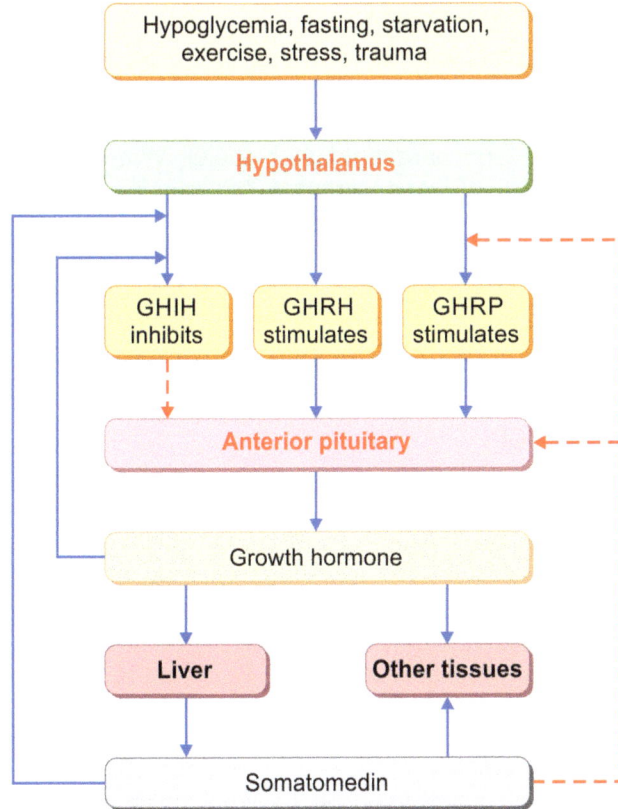

FIGURE 44.2: Regulation of GH secretion.
GHIH = Growth hormone-inhibitory hormone, GHRH = Growth hormone-releasing hormone, GHRP = Growth hormone-releasing polypeptide. Growth hormone and somatomedin stimulate hypothalamus to release GHIH. Somatomedin inhibits anterior pituitary directly. Solid blue line = Stimulation/Secretion, Dashed red line = Inhibition

short-loop feedback control. Similarly, GHRH inhibits its own release by short-loop feedback control.

Whenever, blood level of GH decreases, GHRH is secreted from the hypothalamus. It in turn causes secretion of GH from pituitary.

OTHER HORMONES OF ANTERIOR PITUITARY

Thyroid-stimulating Hormone (TSH)

TSH is necessary for growth and secretory activity of the thyroid gland. Refer Chapter 45 for details of TSH.

Adrenocorticotropic Hormone (ACTH)

ACTH is necessary for structural integrity and the secretory activity of adrenal cortex. Refer Chapter 45 for details of ACTH.

Follicle-stimulating Hormone (FSH)

Actions in males

In males, FSH acts along with testosterone and accelerates the process of spermiogenesis.

Actions in females

1. It is responsible for the development of Graafian follicle from primordial follicle.
2. It stimulates the theca cells of Graafian follicle and causes secretion of estrogen. Refer Chapter 52 for details.
3. Promotes aromatase activity in granulosa cells resulting in conversion of androgens into estrogen.

Luteinizing Hormone (LH)

Actions in males

In males, LH is known as **interstitial cell stimulating hormone (ICSH)** because it stimulates the interstitial cells of Leydig in testes. This hormone is essential for the secretion of testosterone from Leydig cells.

Actions in females

1. LH causes maturation of vesicular follicle into Graafian follicle along with follicle stimulating hormone.
2. It induces synthesis of androgens from theca cells of growing follicle.
3. It is responsible for ovulation.
4. It is necessary for the formation of corpus luteum.
5. It activates the secretory functions of corpus luteum.

Prolactin

Prolactin is necessary for the final preparation of mammary glands for production and secretion of milk.

β-lipotropin

It mobilizes fat from adipose tissue and promotes lipolysis.

POSTERIOR PITUITARY

PARTS OF POSTERIOR PITUITARY

Posterior pituitary consists of three divisions:

1. Pars nervosa or infundibular process.
2. Nural stalk or infundibular stem.
3. Median eminence.

Pars tuberalis of anterior pituitary and the neural stalk of posterior pituitary together form the **hypophyseal stalk**.

FUNCTIONAL HISTOLOGY OF POSTERIOR PITUITARY

Posterior pituitary is made up of nerve cells called **pituicytes** and unmyelinated nerve fibers. Pituicytes act as supporting cells and do not secrete any hormone. Posterior pituitary also has numerous blood vessels, hyaline bodies, neuroglial cells and mast cells.

HORMONES OF POSTERIOR PITUITARY

Posterior pituitary hormones are:

1. Antidiuretic hormone (ADH) or vasopressin.
2. Oxytocin.

Source of Secretion of Posterior Pituitary Hormones

Actually, the posterior pituitary does not secrete any hormone. ADH and oxytocin are synthesized in the hypothalamus. From hypothalamus, these two hormones are transported to the posterior pituitary through the nerve fibers of **hypothalamo-hypophyseal tract (Fig. 44.3)**, by means of axonic flow.

In the posterior pituitary, these hormones are stored at the nerve endings. Whenever, the impulses from hypothalamus reach the posterior pituitary, these hormones are released from the nerve endings into the circulation. Hence, these two hormones are called **neurohormones.**

■ ANTIDIURETIC HORMONE

ADH is secreted mainly by **supraoptic nucleus** of hypothalamus and in small quantity by paraventricular nucleus. From here, this hormone is transported to the posterior pituitary through the nerve fibers of hypothalamo-hypophyseal tract by means of **axonic flow (Fig. 44.3)**.

Antidiuretic hormone is a polypeptide, containing 9 amino acids.

Actions of ADH

Major function of ADH is **retention of water** by acting on kidneys. It increases **facultative reabsorption of water** from distal convoluted tubule and collecting duct in the kidneys (Chapter 36).

ADH increases water reabsorption in the tubular epithelial membrane by regulating water channel proteins called **aquaporins** through **V2 receptors** (Chapter 36).

Vasopressor Action

In large amount, ADH shows vasoconstrictor action in all parts of the body. Due to vasoconstriction, the blood pressure increases. ADH acts on blood vessels through **V1A receptors**.

Regulation of Secretion

Secretion of ADH depends upon volume of body fluid and osmolarity of the body fluids.

Potent stimulants for ADH secretion are:
1. Decrease in ECF volume.
2. Increase in osmolar concentration in ECF.

Role of osmoreceptors

Osmoreceptors are the receptors, which give response to change in osmolar concentration of the blood. Osmoreceptors are situated in the hypothalamus near supraoptic and paraventricular nuclei. When osmolar concentration of blood increases, the osmoreceptors are activated. In turn, the osmoreceptors stimulate supraoptic and paraventricular nuclei. These two nuclei send motor impulses to posterior pituitary through the nerve fibers and cause release of ADH. ADH causes reabsorption of water from the renal tubules. This increases volume of ECF and restores the normal osmolarity.

■ OXYTOCIN

Oxytocin is secreted mainly by the **paraventricular nucleus** and a small quantity is secreted by the supraoptic nucleus in the hypothalamus. And it is transported from hypothalamus to posterior pituitary through the nerve fibers of hypothalamo-hypophyseal tract. In the posterior pituitary, oxytocin is stored in nerve endings of hypothalamohypophyseal tract. When suitable stimuli reach the posterior pituitary from hypothalamus, oxytocin is released into the blood. Oxytocin is secreted in both males and females.

Oxytocin is a polypeptide, having 9 amino acids.

Actions in Females

In females, oxytocin acts on mammary glands and uterus.

Action of oxytocin on mammary glands

It causes ejection of milk from the mammary glands. The process by which milk is ejected from the alveoli of mammary glands is called milk ejection reflex or **milk let-down reflex**.

Milk ejection reflex

Plenty of **touch receptors** are present on the mammary glands, particularly around nipple. When the infant suckles mother's nipple, touch receptors are stimulated and impulses are discharged. Impulses from here are carried by the somatic afferent nerve fibers and reach the paraventricular and supraoptic nuclei of hypothalamus.

Now, hypothalamus in turn, sends impulses to the posterior pituitary through hypothalamohypophyseal tract and cause release of oxytocin into the blood. When the hormone reaches mammary gland, it causes contraction of **myoepithelial cells** resulting in ejection of milk from mammary glands **(Fig. 44.4)**.

As this reflex is initiated by nervous factors and completed by the hormonal action, it is called a **neuroendocrine reflex**. During this reflex, large amount of oxytocin is released by **positive feedback mechanism**.

Action of oxytocin on uterus

Oxytocin acts on pregnant uterus and nonpregnant uterus.

Action on pregnant uterus

On pregnant uterus, at the time of labor, oxytocin causes **contraction of uterus** and helps in **expulsion of fetus**.

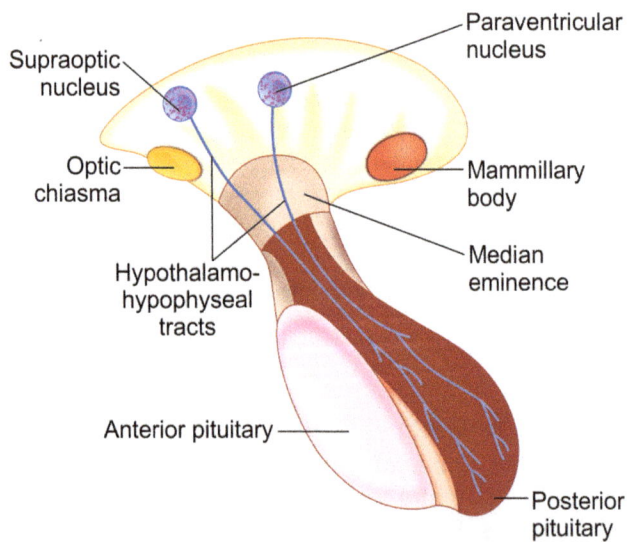

FIGURE 44.3: Hypothalamo-hypophyseal tracts.

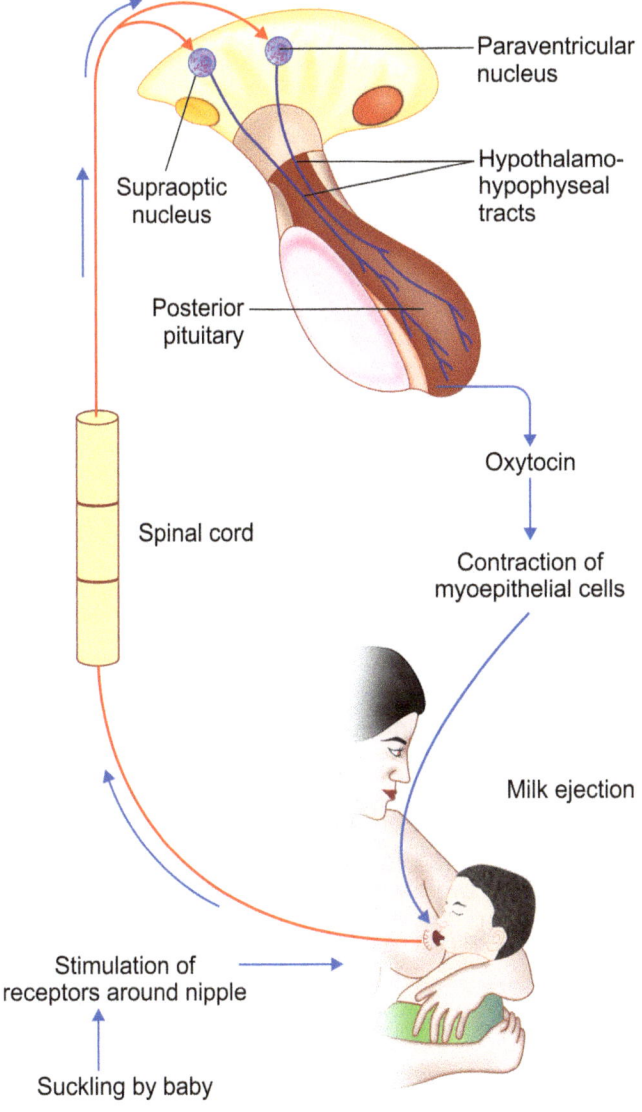

FIGURE 44.4: Milk ejection reflex.

During **labor**, oxytocin induces contraction of uterus, which in turn causes release of more amount of oxytocin.

Action on non-pregnant uterus

On non-pregnant uterus oxytocin facilitates the transport of sperms through female genital tract up to fallopian tube by producing the uterine contraction during sexual intercourse.

During the sexual intercourse, the receptors in the vagina are stimulated. Vaginal receptors generate the impulses, which are transmitted by somatic afferent nerves to the paraventricular and supraoptic nuclei of hypothalamus. When, these two nuclei are stimulated, oxytocin is released and transported by blood. While reaching the female genital tract, the hormone causes antiperistaltic contractions of uterus towards the fallopian tube. It is also a **neuroendocrine reflex.**

Action in Males

In males, release of oxytocin increases during ejaculation. It facilitates release of sperm into urethra by causing contraction of smooth muscle fibers in reproductive tract particularly vas deferens.

Mode of Action of Oxytocin

Oxytocin acts on mammary glands and uterus by activating G protein-coupled **oxytocin receptor**.

■ APPLIED PHYSIOLOGY: DISORDERS OF PITUITARY GLAND

Disorders of pituitary gland are given in **Table 44.1**.

■ HYPERACTIVITY OF ANTERIOR PITUITARY

1. Gigantism

Gigantism is a pituitary disorder characterized by excess growth of the body. The affected subjects look like **giants** with average height of about 7 to 8 feet.

Causes of gigantism

Gigantism is due to hypersecretion of GH in childhood or preadult life **before fusion of epiphysis** of bone with shaft. It occurs due to **pituitary tumors**.

Signs and symptoms of gigantism

i. Because of over growth, the person has a **huge stature** with a height of more than 7 or 8 feet. Limbs are disproportionately long.
ii. Giants are hyperglycemic and they develop glycosuria and **pituitary diabetes**.
iii. Pituitary tumor itself causes constant headache.
iv. Pituitary tumor also causes **visual disturbances** such as bitemporal hemianopia (Chapter 95).

2. Acromegaly

Acromegaly is the pituitary disorder characterized by enlargement, thickening and broadening of bones, particularly in the extremities of the body.

TABLE 44.1: Disorders of pituitary gland.

Parts involved	Hyperactivity	Hypoactivity
Anterior pituitary	Gigantism Acromegaly Acromegalic gigantism Cushing's disease	Dwarfism Acromicria Simmonds' diseases
Posterior pituitary	Syndrome of inappropriate hypersecretion of ADH (SIADH)	Diabetes insipidus
Anterior and posterior pituitary	–	Dystrophia adiposogenitalis Panhypopituitarism

Causes of acromagaly

Acromegaly is due to hypersecretion of GH in adults **after fusion of epiphysis** with shaft of the bone. Hypersecretion of GH is due to adenomatous tumor of anterior pituitary involving the acidophil cells.

Signs and symptoms of acromegaly

i. Striking facial features such as protrusion of supraorbital ridges, broadening of nose, thickening of lips, thickening and wrinkles formation on forehead, and **prognathism** (protrusion of lower jaw) are developed.
Face with these features is called **acromegalic face** or **gorilla face (Fig. 44.5)**.
ii. Hands and feet are enlarged **(Fig. 44.6)** with **kyphosis** (bowing of spine).
iii. Scalp is thickened and thrown into folds or wrinkles like **bulldog scalp**. There is general overgrowth of body hair.
iv. Visceral organs such as lungs, heart, liver and spleen are enlarged.
v. Thyroid gland, parathyroid glands and the adrenal glands show hyperactivity.
vi. Hyperglycemia and glucosuria occur resulting in **diabetes mellitus**.
vii. Hypertension.
viii. Headache.
ix. Visual disturbance (bitemporal hemianopia) is developed.

3. Acromegalic Gigantism

It is a rare disorder with symptoms of both gigantism and acromegaly. Hypersecretion of GH in children, before the fusion of epiphysis with shaft of the bones causes

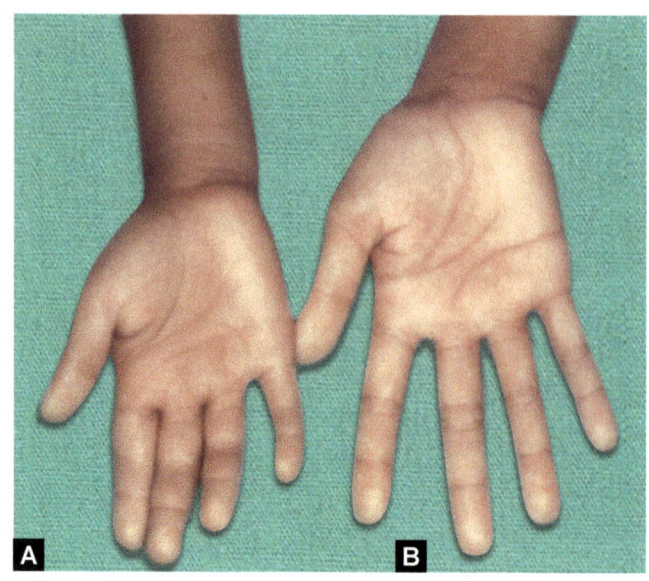

FIGURE 44.6: A. Normal hand. **B.** Acromegalic hand.
(*Courtesy*: Prof Mafauzy Mohamed)

gigantism. And, if hypersecretion of GH is continued even after the fusion of epiphysis, the symptoms of acromegaly also appear.

4. Cushing's Disease

It is also a rare disorder characterized by obesity. Details of this disorder are given in Chapter 48.

HYPOACTIVITY OF ANTERIOR PITUITARY

1. Dwarfism

It is a pituitary disorder in children characterized by stunted growth.

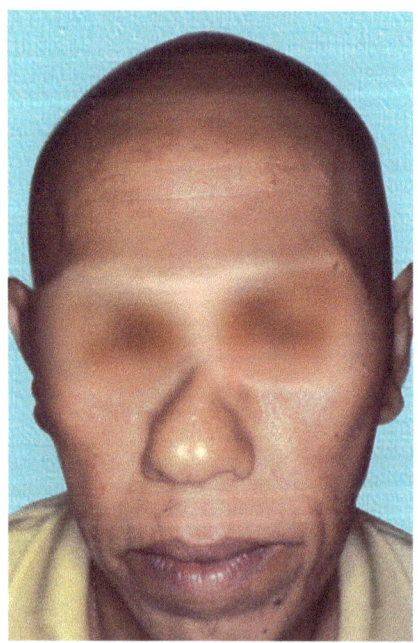

Gorilla face: Protrusion of supraorbital ridges broad nose, thickened lips and protrusion of lower jaw

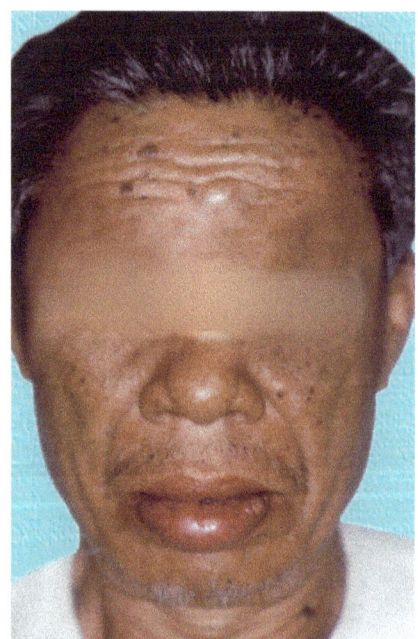

Wrinkled forehead, with other features of acromegalic face

FIGURE 44.5: Acromegaly. (*Courtesy:* Prof Mafauzy Mohamed)

Causes of dwarfism

Hyposecretion of GH in infancy or early childhood causes dwarfism. Hyposecretion of GH occurs in deficiency of GHRH, deficiency of somatomedin C atrophy or degeneration of acidophilic cells in the anterior pituitary and pituitary tumor.

Dwarfism also occurs in **panhypopituitarism.** In this condition, there is reduction in the secretion of all the hormones of anterior pituitary gland.

Signs and symptoms of dwarfism

i. Primary symptom of hypopituitarism in children is the **stunted skeletal growth**. Maximum height of anterior pituitary dwarf at the adult age is only about 3 feet.
ii. But proportions of different parts of the body are almost normal. Only, head becomes slightly larger in relation to the body.
iii. Pituitary dwarfs do not show any deformity and their mental activity is normal with no mental retardation.
iv. Reproductive function is not affected, if there is only GH deficiency. However, in panhypopituitarism, dwarfs do not obtain puberty due to deficiency of gonadotropic hormones.

Other types of dwarfism

Other types of dwarfism are given in **Box 44.1**.

2. *Acromicria*

It is a rare pituitary disorder in adults characterized by atrophy of the extremities of the body.

BOX 44.1: Different types of dwarfism.

Pituitary dwarfism
Caused by hyposecretion of GH in infancy or early childhood
Laron dwarfism
Laron dwarfism or Laron syndrome is due to mutations in genes of GH receptor
Psychosocial dwarfism
Psychosocial or stress dwarfism is a pituitary disorder that occurs due deficiency of GH caused by exposure of the child to extreme emotional deprivation or stress
Dwarfism in dystrophia adiposogenitalis
Dystrophia adiposogenitalis or Fröhlich syndrome is a pituitary disorder caused by hypoactivity of both anterior and posterior pituitary. It results in dwarfism if it affects children
Dwarfism in panhypopituitarism
Panhypopituitarism (pituitary disorder caused by hyposecretion of all hormones of anterior pituitary) results in dwarfism if it affects children
Cretinism
Cretinism is the hypothyroid condition characterized by stunted growth (Chapter 45)

Causes of acromicria

Hyposecretion of GH in adults causes acromicria.

Signs and symptoms of acromicria

i. Atrophy and thinning of extremities of body, (hands and feet) are the major symptoms in acromicria.
ii. Acromicria is mostly associated with hypothyroidism and hyposecretion of adrenocortical hormones.
iii. Affected person becomes lethargic and obese.
iv. Sexual functions are lost.

3. *Simmonds' Disease*

Simmond's disease or **pituitary cachexia** is a rare pituitary disease. This disease occurs mostly in **panhypopituitarism.**

Symptoms of Simmond's disease

i. A major feature of Simmond's disease is the rapidly developing **senile decay**. Thus, a 30 years old person looks like a 60 years old person.
ii. There is loss of hair over the body and loss of teeth.
iii. Skin over face becomes dry and wrinkled. So, there is shrunken appearance of facial features. It is the most common feature of this disease.

■ **HYPERACTIVITY OF POSTERIOR PITUITARY**

Syndrome of Inappropriate Hypersecretion of Antidiuretic Hormone (SIADH)

SIADH is the disease characterized by loss of sodium through urine due to hypersecretion of ADH. SIADH occurs due to cerebral tumors, lung tumors and lung cancers because the tumor cells and cancer cells secrete ADH.

Signs and Symptoms of SIADH

1. Loss of appetite.
2. Weight loss.
3. Nausea and vomiting.
4. Headache.
5. Muscle weakness, spasm and cramps.
6. Fatigue.
7. Restlessness and irritability.

In severe conditions, the patients die because of convulsions and coma.

■ **HYPOACTIVITY OF POSTERIOR PITUITARY**

Diabetes Insipidus

Diabetes insipidus is a posterior pituitary disorder characterized by excess excretion of water through urine.

Causes of Diabetes Insipidus

This disorder develops due to the deficiency ADH which occurs in the following conditions:

1. Lesion (injury) or degeneration of supraoptic and paraventricular nuclei of hypothalamus and hypothalamohypophyseal tract.
2. Atrophy of posterior pituitary.
3. Inability of renal tubules to give response to ADH. Such condition is called **nephrogenic diabetic insipidus**.

Signs and Symptoms Diabetes Insipidus

1. *Polyuria:* Polyuria is the increased urinary output with frequent voiding. It is due to water diuresis. Daily output of urine varies between 4 and 12 liters.
2. *Polydipsia:* Polydipsia is intake of excess water. It is due to stimulation of thirst center in hypothalamus.
3. *Dehydration:* In some cases, thirst center in the hypothalamus is also affected by lesion. Water intake decreases in these patients and, the loss of water through urine is not compensated. So, dehydration develops which may lead to death.

■ HYPOACTIVITY OF ANTERIOR AND POSTERIOR PITUITARY

Dystrophia Adiposogenitalis

Dystrophia adiposogenitalis is a disease characterized by obesity and hypogonadism affecting mainly the adolescent boys. It is also called **Fröhlich's syndrome** or hypothalamic eunuchism.

It is due to hypoactivity of both anterior pituitary and posterior pituitary and disease in hypothalamic regions concerned with food intake and gonadal development.

Symptoms of Dystrophia Adiposogenitalis

1. **Obesity** is the common feature of this disorder. It is due to abnormal stimulation of feeding center resulting in overeating.
2. **Sexual infantilism** (failure to develop secondary sexual characters) or **eunuchism**.
3. **Dwarfism** occurs if the disease starts in growing age. In children, it is called infantile or prepubertal type of Fröhlich's syndrome.

This disease develops in adults also. When it occurs in adults, it is called adult type of Fröhlich's syndrome. In adults, the major symptoms are obesity and atrophy of sex organs.

Chapter 45

Thyroid Gland

CHAPTER OUTLINE

- MORPHOLOGY OF THYROID GLAND
- FUNCTIONAL HISTOLOGY
- HORMONES
- SYNTHESIS OF THYROID HORMONES
- STORAGE OF THYROID HORMONES
- RELEASE OF THYROID HORMONES
- TRANSPORT OF THYROID HORMONES IN THE BLOOD
- FUNCTIONS OF THYROID HORMONES
- MODE OF ACTION OF THYROID HORMONES
- REGULATION OF SECRETION OF THYROID HORMONES
- APPLIED PHYSIOLOGY: DISORDERS OF THYROID GLAND
- THYROID FUNCTION TESTS

■ MORPHOLOGY OF THYROID GLAND

Thyroid is an endocrine gland situated at the root of neck on either side of trachea. It has two lobes, which are connected in the middle by an isthmus (Fig. 45.1). It weighs about 20 to 40 g in adults.

■ FUNCTIONAL HISTOLOGY OF THYROID GLAND

Thyroid gland is composed of large number of closed follicles called **thyroid follicles**. Each follicle is formed by cuboidal epithelial cells namely the **follicular cells** around the follicular cavity (Fig. 45.2). **Follicular cavity** is filled with a colloidal substance known as **thyroglobulin** which is secreted by the follicular cells. Follicular cells secrete tetraiodothyronine (T_4) or thyroxine and triiodothyronine (T_3). In between the follicles, are the **parafollicular cells** or **clear cells** or **C cells**, which secrete calcitonin.

■ HORMONES OF THYROID GLAND

Thyroid gland secretes three hormones:

1. **Tetraiodothyronine (T_4)** or **thyroxine**.
2. **Triiodothyronine (T_3)**.
3. **Calcitonin**.

T_4 is forms about 90% of the total secretion, whereas, T_3 is only 9 to 10%. But the potency of T_3 is four times more than that of T_4. Calcitonin is described in Chapter 46.

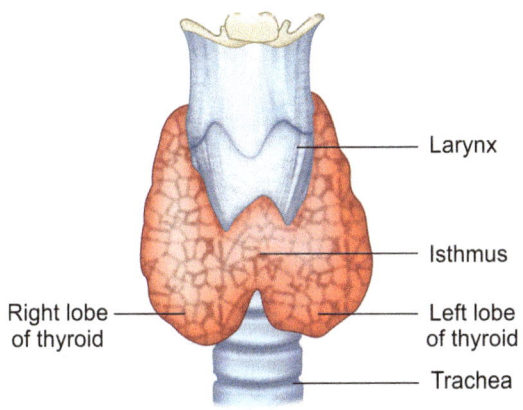

FIGURE 45.1: Thyroid gland.

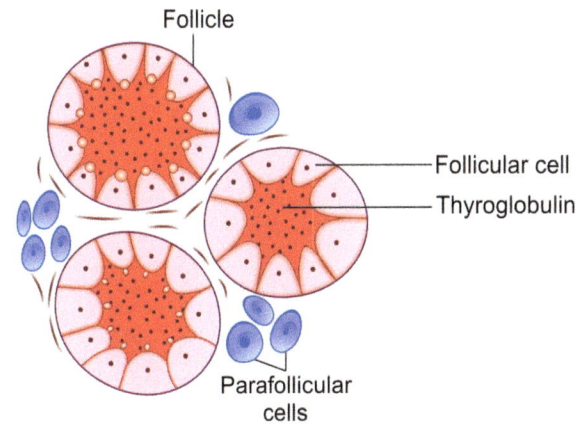

FIGURE 45.2: Histology of thyroid gland.

SYNTHESIS OF THYROID HORMONES

Synthesis of thyroid hormones takes place in thyroglobulin present in follicular cavity. **Iodine** and **tyrosine** are essential for the formation of thyroid hormones. Iodine which is consumed through diet is converted into **iodide** and absorbed from GI tract. Tyrosine is also consumed through diet and is absorbed from the GI.

STAGES OF SYNTHESIS OF THYROID HORMONES

Synthesis of thyroid hormones takes place in **five stages**:

1. Thyroglobulin Synthesis

Endoplasmic reticulum and Golgi apparatus in the follicular cells of thyroid gland synthesize and secrete thyroglobulin continuously. Each thyroglobulin molecule contains 140 tyrosine molecules. After synthesis, the thyroglobulin is stored in the follicle.

2. Iodide Trapping or Iodide Pump

Iodide is transported actively from the blood into follicular cell by a process called iodide trapping. From here, iodide is transported into the follicular cavity.

3. Oxidation of the Iodide

Iodide is oxidized to elementary iodine inside follicular cells in the presence of **thyroid peroxidase**.

4. Iodination of Tyrosine

Iodine is released from follicular cells into the follicular cavity where it binds with thyroglobulin. This process is called **organification of thyroglobulin**. In the thyroglobulin, iodine combines with tyrosine which is already present there by the enzyme **iodinase**. Combination of iodine with tyrosine is known as **iodination (Fig. 45.3)**.

Iodination of tyrosine occurs in several stages. Tyrosine is iodized first into **monoiodotyrosine (MIT)** and later into **diiodotyrosine (DIT)**. MIT and DIT are called the **iodotyrosine residues**.

5. Coupling Reactions

Iodotyrosine residues get coupled with one another through coupling reactions. Coupling occurs in different configurations to give rise to different thyroid hormones.

Coupling reactions are:

i. One molecule of DIT and one molecule of MIT combine to form triiodothyronine (T_3).
ii. Sometimes one molecule of MIT and one molecule of DIT combine to produce another form of T_3 called reverse T_3 or rT_3. **Reverse T_3** is only 1% of thyroid output.
iii. Two molecules of DIT combine to form tetraiodothyronine (T_4) which is thyroxine:

Tyrosine + I = Monoiodotyrosine (MIT)
MIT + I   = Diiodotyrosine (DIT)
DIT + MIT = Triiodothyronine (T_3)
MIT + DIT = Reverse T_3
DIT + DIT = Tetraiodothyronine or thyroxine (T_4)

STORAGE OF THYROID HORMONES

After synthesis, thyroid hormones remain in the form of vesicles within thyroglobulin. In combination with thyroglobulin, thyroid hormones can be stored for several months.

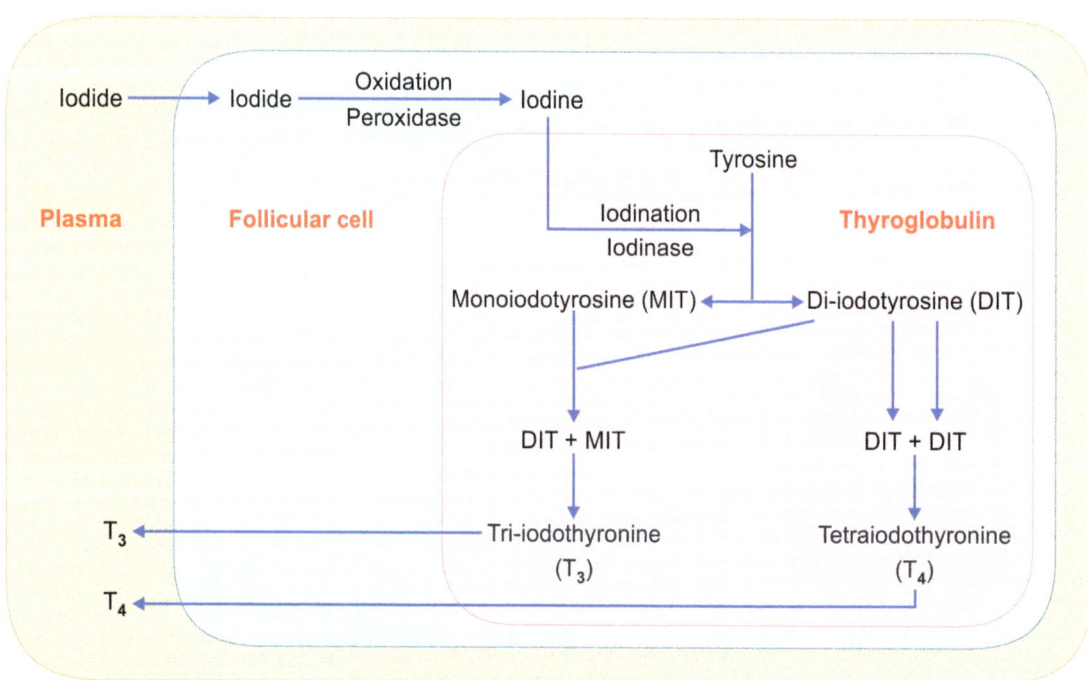

FIGURE 45.3: Synthesis of thyroid hormones.

RELEASE OF THYROID HORMONES FROM THE THYROID GLAND

Hormones are first cleaved from thyroglobulin and then released into the blood.

Only T_3 and T_4 are released into the blood. A small amount of reverse T_3 is also formed. But reverse T_3 is biologically inactive. The MIT and DIT are not released into blood.

TRANSPORT OF THYROID HORMONES IN THE BLOOD

Thyroid hormones are transported in the blood in combination with three types of plasma proteins, **thyroxine-binding globulin (TBG)**, **thyroxine-binding prealbumin (TBPA)** and albumin.

Normal Plasma Level of Thyroid Hormones

Total T_3 = 0.12 µg/dL.
Total T_4 = 8 µg/dL.

FUNCTIONS OF THYROID HORMONES

Thyroid hormones have two major functions viz stimulation of overall metabolic rate in the body and stimulation of growth in children. Actions of thyroid hormones are detailed below.

1. ON BASAL METABOLIC RATE

Basal metabolic rate is defined as the energy (number of calories) required for body functions at rest. Thyroxine increases the basal metabolic rate (BMR) by increasing the oxygen consumption of the tissues. Action that increases the BMR is called **calorigenic action**.

2. ON PROTEIN METABOLISM

Thyroid hormones increase synthesis of proteins. Thyroxine accelerates protein synthesis by the following ways:

i. By increasing translation of RNA in the cells.
ii. By increasing transcription of DNA to RNA.
iii. By increasing activity of mitochondria.
iv. By increasing activity of cellular enzymes.

Though thyroxine increases protein synthesis, it also causes catabolism of proteins.

3. ON CARBOHYDRATE METABOLISM

Thyroxine stimulates almost all processes involved in the metabolism of carbohydrate.
Thyroxine:
i. Increases absorption of glucose from GI tract.
ii. Enhances glucose uptake by the cells, by accelerating transport of glucose through cell membrane.
iii. Accelerates breakdown of glycogen into glucose.
iv. Stimulates gluconeogenesis.

4. ON FAT METABOLISM

Thyroxine decreases the fat storage by mobilizing it from adipose tissues and fat depots. Mobilized fat is converted into free fatty acid and transported by blood. Thus, thyroxine increases the free fatty acid level in blood.

5. ON PLASMA AND LIVER FATS

Thyroxine decreases the cholesterol, phospholipids and triglyceride levels in the plasma. Thyroxine also increases deposition of fats in the liver resulting in **fatty liver**.

6. ON VITAMIN METABOLISM

Thyroxine increases the formation of many enzymes by utilizing vitamins. Hence, vitamin deficiency is possible during hypersecretion of thyroxine.

7. ON BODY TEMPERATURE

Thyroid hormone increases the heat production in the body by accelerating various cellular metabolic processes and increasing BMR.

8. ON GROWTH

Thyroid hormones have general and specific effects on growth. Increase in thyroxine secretion accelerates the growth of the body, especially in growing children. Lack of thyroxine arrests the growth. At the same time, thyroxine causes early closure of epiphysis. So, the height of the individual may be slightly less in hypothyroidism.

Thyroxine is more important to promote growth and development of brain during fetal life and first few years of postnatal life. Deficiency of thyroid hormones during this period leads to **mental retardation**.

9. EFFECT ON BODY WEIGHT

Thyroxine is essential for maintaining body weight. Increase in thyroxine secretion decreases the body weight and fat storage. Decrease in thyroxine secretion increases the body weight because of fat deposition.

10. EFFECT ON BLOOD

Thyroxine increases production of RBCs. It is one of the important general factors necessary for erythropoiesis. Thus, thyroxine increases erythropoietic activity and blood volume.

11. ON CARDIOVASCULAR SYSTEM

Thyroxine increases overall activity of cardiovascular system.

i. On Heart

Thyroxine acts directly on heart and increases rate and force of contraction.

ii. On Blood Vessels

Thyroxine causes vasodilatation by increasing the metabolic activity. During metabolic activity, production of metabolites is increased. These metabolites cause vasodilatation and increase the blood flow.

iii. On Arterial Blood Pressure

Thyroxine increases systolic blood pressure by increasing rate and force of contraction of the heart, blood volume and cardiac output. At the same time, it decreases diastolic pressure by its vasodilator effect. So only the pulse pressure increases and the mean pressure is not altered.

■ 12. EFFECT ON RESPIRATION

Thyroxine increases the rate and force of respiration indirectly. Increased metabolic rate (caused by thyroxine) increases the demand for oxygen and formation of excess carbon dioxide. These two factors stimulate the respiratory centers to increase the rate and force of respiration.

■ 13. ON GASTROINTESTINAL TRACT

Generally, thyroxine increases the appetite and food intake. It also increases the secretions and movements of GI tract.

■ 14. ON CENTRAL NERVOUS SYSTEM

Thyroxine is very essential for the development and maintenance of normal functioning of the central nervous system.

i. On Development of Central Nervous System

Thyroxine is very important to promote growth and development of the brain during fetal life and during the first few years of postnatal life. Thyroid deficiency in infants results in mental retardation.

ii. On Normal Function of Central Nervous System

Thyroxine is a stimulating factor for the brain. So, normal functioning of brain needs the presence of thyroxine. Thyroxine also increases the blood flow to brain.

■ 15. ON SKELETAL MUSCLE

Thyroxine is essential for the normal activity of the skeletal muscles. Slight increase in thyroxine level makes the muscles to work with more vigor. But, hypersecretion of thyroxine causes weakness of the muscles due to the catabolism of proteins.

■ 16. ON SLEEP

Normal thyroxine level is essential to maintain normal sleep. Hypersecretion of thyroxine causes excessive stimulation of the muscles and central nervous system. So, the person feels tired, exhausted, and feels like sleeping. But the person cannot sleep because of the stimulatory effect of thyroxine on neurons. On the other hand, hyposecretion of thyroxine causes **somnolence** (sleepiness).

■ 17. ON SEXUAL FUNCTION

Normal thyroxine level is essential for normal sexual function. In men, hypothyroidism leads to complete loss of **libido** (sexual drive), and hyperthyroidism leads to **impotence**.

In women, hypothyroidism causes **menorrhagia** and **polymenorrhea** (Chapter 53). In some women, it causes irregular menstruation and occasionally **amenorrhea**. Hyperthyroidism in women leads to **oligomenorrhea** and sometimes **amenorrhea** (Chapter 53).

■ 18. ON OTHER ENDOCRINE GLANDS

Because of its metabolic effects, thyroxine increases the demand for secretion of other endocrine glands.

■ MODE OF ACTION OF THYROID HORMONES

Thyroid hormones act by activating the genes.

■ REGULATION OF SECRETION OF THYROID HORMONES

The secretion of thyroid hormones is controlled by anterior pituitary and hypothalamus through feedback mechanism **(Fig. 45.4)**.

■ ROLE OF PITUITARY GLAND

Thyroid-stimulating Hormone

Thyroid-stimulating hormone (TSH) secreted by anterior pituitary is the major factor regulating the synthesis and release of thyroid hormones.

TSH is a peptide hormone with one α-chain and one β-chain. Normal plasma level of TSH is approximately 2 U/mL.

Actions of TSH

TSH accelerates thyroxine synthesis by the following ways:

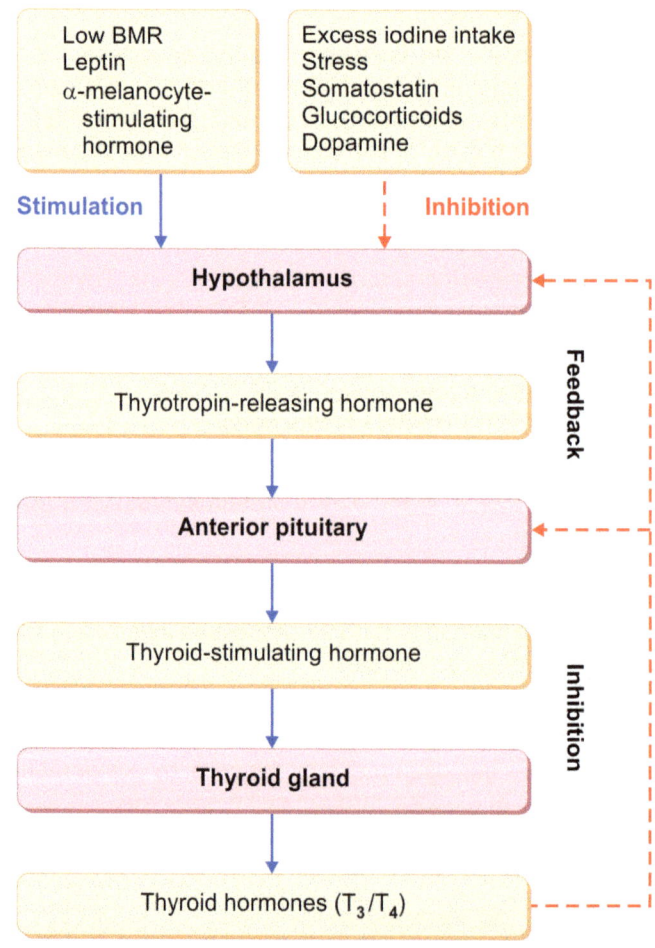

FIGURE 45.4: Regulation of secretion of thyroid hormones.

1. Increases number of follicular cells of thyroid.
2. Accelerates development of thyroid follicles by converting cuboidal cells in thyroid gland into columnar cells.
3. Increases the size and secretory activity of follicular cells.
4. Activates iodide pump and iodide trapping in follicular cells.
5. Increases thyroglobulin secretion into follicles.
6. Increases iodination of tyrosine and coupling to form the hormones.
7. Increases proteolysis of the thyroglobulin, and release of hormones.

Mode of Action of TSH

TSH acts through cyclic AMP mechanism.

ROLE OF HYPOTHALAMUS

Hypothalamus regulates thyroid secretion by inducing release of TSH by thyrotropin-releasing hormone (TRH). From hypothalamus, TRH is transported through hypothalamo-hypophyseal portal vessels to the anterior pituitary. After reaching the pituitary gland, the TRH causes the release of TSH.

FEEDBACK CONTROL

Thyroid hormones regulate their own secretion through negative feedback control by inhibiting the release of TRH from hypothalamus and TSH from anterior pituitary **(Fig. 45.4)**.

ROLE OF IODIDE

Iodide is an important factor regulating the synthesis of thyroid hormones. When the dietary level of iodine is moderate, blood level of thyroid hormones is normal. However, when iodine intake is high, the enzymes necessary for synthesis of thyroid hormones are inhibited by iodide itself resulting in suppression of hormone synthesis.

APPLIED PHYSIOLOGY: DISORDERS OF THYROID GLAND

HYPERTHYROIDISM: THYROTOXICOSIS

Hyperthyroidism refers to excess synthesis and release of thyroid hormones by thyroid gland resulting in increased level of hormones in blood.

Thyrotoxicosis is defined as high level of thyroid hormones in blood. It is the condition caused by not only excess secretion by thyroid glands, but also release of stored hormones.

Causes for Hyperthyroidism

Hyperthyroidism is caused by Graves' disease and thyroid adenoma.

i. *Graves' disease*

Graves' disease is an autoimmune disease. Normally, thyroid-stimulating hormone (TSH) combines with surface receptors of thyroid cells and causes the synthesis of thyroid hormones. In Graves' disease the B lymphocytes (plasma cells) produce autoimmune antibodies called **thyroid stimulating hormone receptor antibodies** (TSHRAb). These antibodies act like TSH by binding with membrane receptors of TSH and activating cAMP system of the thyroid follicular cells. This results in hypersecretion of thyroid hormones.

ii. *Thyroid adenoma*

Sometimes, a localized tumor develops in the thyroid tissue. It is known as thyroid adenoma and it secretes large quantities of thyroid hormones.

Signs and Symptoms of Hyperthyroidism

1. **Intolerance to heat** because production of more heat during increased basal metabolic rate caused by hyperthyroidism.
2. Increased sweating due to vasodilatation.
3. Decreased body weight due to fat mobilization.
4. Diarrhea due to increased motility of GI tract.
5. Muscular weakness due to excess protein catabolism.
6. Neuronal disturbances such as nervousness, extreme fatigue, inability to sleep, mild tremor in hands and psychoneurotic symptoms such as hyperexcitability, extreme anxiety or worry.
7. Toxic goiter.
8. Oligomenorrhea or amenorrhea.
9. Exophthalmos.
10. Polycythemia.
11. Tachycardia and atrial fibrillation.
12. Systolic hypertension.
13. Cardiac failure.

Exophthalmos

Protrusion of eyeballs is called exophthalmos. Exophthalmos in hyperthyroidism is due to the edematous swelling of the retro-orbital tissues and degenerative changes in the extraocular muscles.

Effect of exophthalmos on vision

Severe exophthalmic conditions lead to blindness because of two reasons:
1. Protrusion of the eyeball stretches and damages the optic nerve resulting in blindness.
2. Due to the protrusion of eyeballs, eyelids cannot be closed completely while blinking or during sleep. So, the constant exposure of eyeball to atmosphere causes dryness of the cornea leading to irritation and infection. It finally results in ulceration of the cornea leading to blindness.

HYPOTHYROIDISM

Decreased secretion of thyroid hormones is called hypothyroidism. Hypothyroidism leads to myxedema in adults and cretinism in children.

Myxedema

It is the hypothyroidism in adults characterized by generalized edematous appearance.

Causes for myxedema

1. Diseases of thyroid gland.
2. Genetic disorder.
3. Iodine deficiency.
4. Deficiency of thyroid-stimulating hormone or thyrotropin-releasing hormone.
5. Autoimmune disease called Hashimoto's thyroiditis.

Signs and symptoms of myxedema

1. Edematous appearance throughout the body.
2. Swelling of the face.
3. Bagginess under the eyes.
4. Nonpitting type of edema, i.e. when pressed, it does not make pits and the edema is hard.
5. **Atherosclerosis**: It is the hardening of the walls of arteries because of accumulation of fat. It occurs in myxedema because of increased plasma level of cholesterol which leads to deposition of cholesterol on walls of the arteries. Atherosclerosis produces **arteriosclerosis** which means thickening and stiffening of arterial wall. Arteriosclerosis causes hypertension.

Other general features of hypothyroidism in adults are:

1. Anemia.
2. Fatigue and muscular sluggishness.
3. Extreme somnolence with sleeping up to 14 to 16 hours per day.
4. Menorrhagia and polymenorrhea.
5. Decreased cardiovascular functions such as reduction in rate and force of contraction of the heart, cardiac output and blood volume.
6. Increase in body weight.
7. Constipation.
8. Mental sluggishness.
9. Depressed hair growth.
10. Scaliness of the skin.
11. **Frog-like husky voice**.
12. **Intolerance to cold**.

Cretinism

Cretinism is the hypothyroidism in children characterized by stunted growth.

Causes for cretinism

Cretinism occurs due to congenital absence of thyroid gland, genetic disorder or lack of iodine in the diet.

Features of cretinism

1. A newborn baby with thyroid deficiency may appear normal at the time of birth because thyroxine might have been supplied from mother. But a few weeks after birth, the baby starts developing the signs like sluggish movements and croaking sound while crying. Unless treated immediately, the baby will be mentally retarded permanently.
2. Skeletal growth is more affected than the soft tissues. So, there is **stunted growth.** Abdominal bloating is common in cretins **(Fig. 45.5)**. Tongue becomes so big, that it hangs down with dripping of saliva. The big

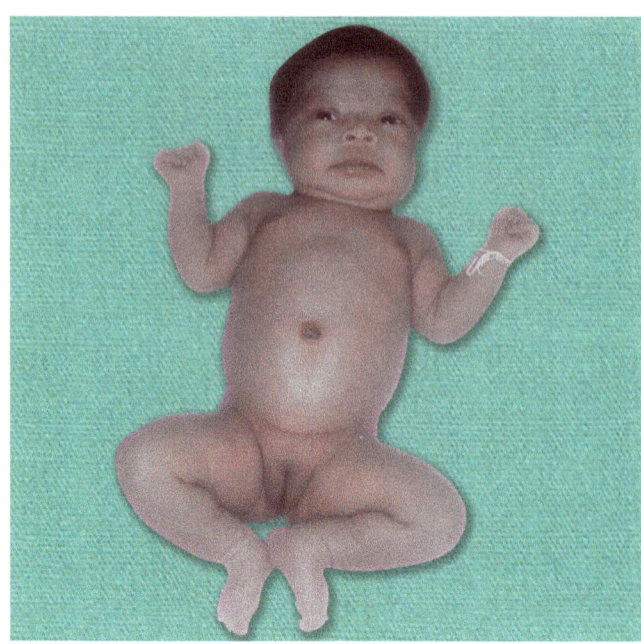

FIGURE 45.5: Cretinism (3-month-old baby).
(Courtesy: Prof Mafauzy Mohamed)

tongue obstructs swallowing and breathing. Tongue produces characteristic **guttural breathing** that may sometimes choke the baby.

■ GOITER

Goiter means enlargement of the thyroid gland. It occurs both in hyperthyroidism and hypothyroidism.

Goiter in Hyperthyroidism: Toxic Goiter

Toxic goiter is the enlargement of thyroid gland with increased secretion of thyroid hormones caused by thyroid tumor.

Goiter in Hypothyroidism: Nontoxic Goiter

Nontoxic goiter is the enlargement of thyroid gland without increase in hormone secretion. It is also called **hypothyroid goiter (Fig. 45.6)**. It is of two types:

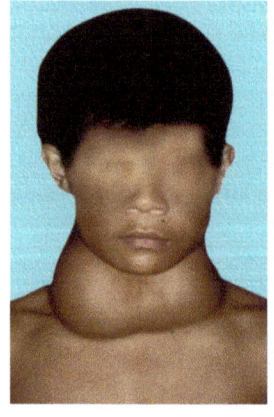 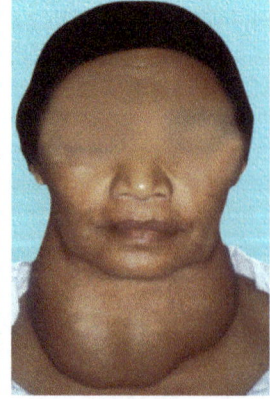

FIGURE 45.6: Nontoxic goiter.
(Courtesy: Prof Mafauzy Mohamed)

1. *Endemic colloid goiter*

It is the nontoxic goiter caused by iodine deficiency. It is also called **iodine deficiency goiter**. Iodine deficiency occurs when intake is less than 50 μg/day.

2. *Idiopathic nontoxic goiter*

It is the goiter due to unknown cause. Enlargement of thyroid gland occurs even without iodine deficiency. The exact cause is not known.

■ TREATMENT FOR THYROID DISORDERS

■ TREATMENT FOR HYPERTHYROIDISM

Hyperthyroidism is treated by two methods:

1. By antithyroid substances such as **thiocyanate**, **thioureylenes** and high concentration of inorganic iodides.
2. By surgical removal.

■ TREATMENT FOR HYPOTHYROIDISM

Only treatment for hypothyroidism is the administration of thyroid extract or ingestion of pure thyroxine in the form of tablets, orally.

■ THYROID FUNCTION TESTS

Functional status of thyroid gland is assessed by the following tests:

1. Measurement of concentration of T_3 and T_4 in plasma.
2. Measurement of measurement of TRH and TSH in plasma.
3. Measurement of basal metabolic rate.

Chapter 46: Parathyroid Glands and Physiology of Bone

CHAPTER OUTLINE

- MORPHOLOGY OF PARATHYROID GLANDS
- PARATHORMONE
- APPLIED PHYSIOLOGY: DISORDERS OF PARATHYROID GLANDS
- CALCITONIN
- CALCIUM METABOLISM
- PHOSPHATE METABOLISM
- PHYSIOLOGY OF BONE

■ MORPHOLOGY OF PARATHYROID GLANDS

There are four parathyroid glands located immediately behind thyroid gland at the upper and lower poles **(Fig. 46.1)**. Parathyroid glands are very small in size measuring about 6 mm long, 3 mm wide and 2 mm thick with dark brown color.

■ FUNCTIONAL HISTOLOGY OF PARATHYROID GLANDS

Each parathyroid gland is made up of **chief cells** and **oxyphil cells**. Chief cells secrete parathormone but, function of the oxyphil cell is not known. It is believed that oxyphil cells are the degenerated chief cells.

■ PARATHORMONE

Parathormone secreted by parathyroid gland is essential for the maintenance of **blood calcium level**.

■ SOURCE, CHEMISTRY AND PLASMA LELVEL

Parathormone (PTH) is secreted by the chief cells of the parathyroid glands. It is protein in nature having 84 amino acids. Normal plasma level of PTH is about 1.5 to 5.5 ng/dL.

■ ACTIONS OF PARATHORMONE

Parathormone maintains the blood calcium level and blood phosphate level.

Action of PTH on Blood Calcium Level

Primary action of PTH is to maintain the blood calcium level within the critical range of 9 to 11 mg/dL. Blood calcium level has to be maintained critically because, it is very important for many activities in the body.

PTH maintains the blood calcium level by acting on bones, kidneys and GI tract.

1. **Effect on bone**
    i. Parathormone increases **osteoclastic activity** (resorption of calcium from the bones) by acting on **osteoclasts** of the bone. Parathormone also stimulates the proliferation of osteoclasts.
    ii. PTH increases the permeability of membranes of osteoblasts for calcium ions. So, calcium ions move from these bone cells into the blood.

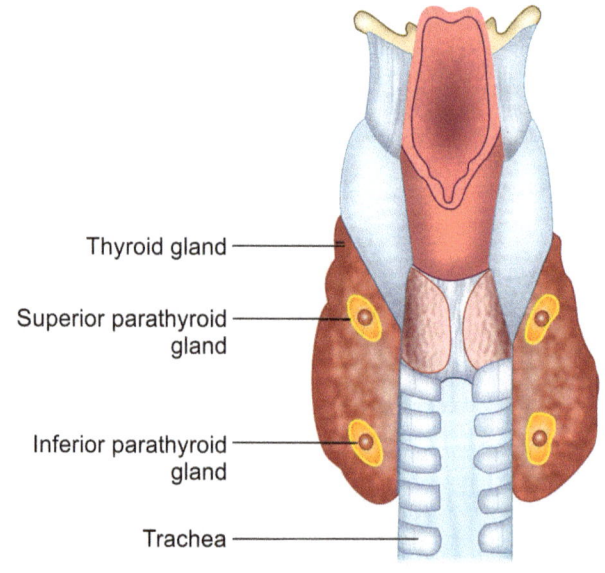

FIGURE 46.1: Parathyroid glands on the posterior surface of thyroid gland.

iii. PTH stimulates osteoclasts and causes release of proteolytic enzymes and some acids such as citric acid and lactic acid. All these substances digest or dissolve the organic matrix of bone, releasing calcium ions into plasma.

2. Effect on kidneys

Parathormone increases reabsorption of calcium from distal convoluted tubule and proximal part of collecting duct into the plasma. It also increases the formation of **1,25-dihydroxycholecalciferol** (activated form of vitamin D) from **25-hydroxycholecalciferol** in kidneys. **Activated vitamin D** is necessary for absorption of calcium form GI tract.

3. Effect on gastrointestinal tract

PTH increases **absorption of calcium** from GI tract by increasing the formation of 1,25-dihydroxycholecalciferol in kidneys.

Role of PTH on activation of vitamin D

Vitamin D is in different forms. But, the most important one is **vitamin D_3** or **cholecalciferol**. Vitamin D_3 is synthesized in the skin from **7-dehydrocholesterol** by the action of ultraviolet rays from sunlight. It is also obtained from dietary sources.

Action of PTH on Blood Phosphate Level

PTH decreases blood level of phosphate by increasing its urinary excretion. It also acts on bone and GI tract.

1. Effect on bone

Along with calcium resorption, PTH also increases phosphate absorption from the bones.

2. Effect on kidneys: Phosphaturic action

Phosphaturic action is excretion of phosphate through urine. PTH inhibits reabsorption of phosphate from renal tubules so that excretion of phosphate through urine increases.

3. Effect on gastrointestinal tract

PTH increases the formation of 1,25-dihydroxy-cholecalciferol in kidneys. This vitamin in turn increases the absorption of phosphate along with calcium from GI tract.

■ **MODE OF ACTION OF PARATHORMONE**

On the target cells, PTH binds with **parathormone receptor** which is coupled to G protein and forms hormone-receptor complex. Hormone-receptor complex causes formation of cAMP, which acts as a second messenger for the hormone.

■ **REGULATION OF PARATHORMONE SECRETION**

Blood level of calcium is the main factor that regulates the secretion of PTH. Blood phosphate level also influences PTH secretion.

Role of Blood Level of Calcium

PTH secretion is **inversely proportional** to blood calcium level. Increase in blood calcium level decreases PTH secretion.

Role of Blood Level of Phosphate

PTH secretion is **directly proportional** to blood phosphate level. Whenever the blood level of phosphate increases, it combines with ionized calcium to form of calcium hydrogen phosphate. This decreases ionized calcium level in blood which stimulates PTH secretion.

■ **APPLIED PHYSIOLOGY: DISORDERS OF PARATHYROID GLANDS**

■ **HYPOPARATHYROIDISM: HYPOCALCEMIA**

Hypoparathyroidism leads to hypocalcemia (decrease in blood calcium level).

Causes for Hypoparathyroidism

1. Surgical removal of parathyroid glands (**parathyroidectomy**).
2. Removal of parathyroid glands during surgical removal of thyroid gland (**thyroidectomy**).
3. Autoimmune disease.
4. Deficiency of receptors for PTH in the target cells. In this, the PTH secretion is normal or increased but the hormone cannot act on the target cells. This condition is called **pseudohypoparathyroidism**.

Hypocalcemia

Hypoparathyroidism causes hypocalcemia by decreasing the resorption of calcium from bones. Hypocalcemia causes neuromuscular hyperexcitability resulting in hypocalcemic tetany.

Hypocalcemic Tetany

Tetany is an abnormal condition characterized by painful muscular spasm (involuntary contraction of muscle or group of muscles) particularly in feet and hand. It is because of hyperexcitability of nerves and skeletal muscles due to calcium deficiency.

Tetany occurs when blood calcium level falls below 6 mg/dL from its normal value of 9.4 mg/dL. It becomes **fatal** when the calcium level falls below 4 mg/dL.

Signs and symptoms of hypocalcemic tetany

1. *Hyperreflexia and convulsions*

Increased neural excitability results in hyperreflexia (overactive reflex actions) and convulsive muscular contractions.

2. *Carpopedal spasm*

Carpopedal spasm is the **spasm** (violent and painful muscular contraction) in hand and feet that occurs due to hypocalcemia. During carpopedal spasm, hand shows a peculiar attitude with flexion at wrist joint and

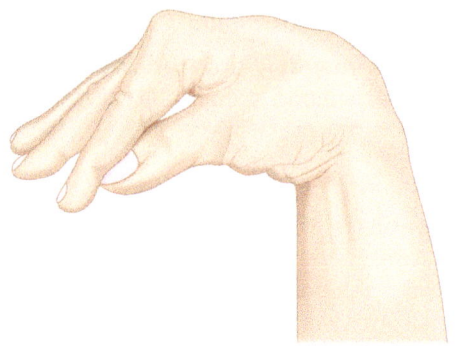

FIGURE 46.2: Carpopedal spasm.

metacarpophalangeal joints, adduction of the thumb, and extension of interphalangeal joints **(Fig. 46.2)**.

3. *Laryngeal stridor*

Stridor means noisy breathing. **Laryngeal stridor** means a loud crowing sound during inspiration which occurs mainly due to **laryngospasm** (involuntary contraction of laryngeal muscles). Laryngeal stridor is a common feature of hypocalcemic tetany.

4. *Cardiovascular changes*

Dilatation of the heart, arrhythmias (irregular heartbeat) hypotension and heart failure.

Latent Tetany or Subclinical Tetany

Latent or subclinical tetany is the neuromuscular hyperexcitability due to hypocalcemia that develops before the onset of tetany. It is characterized by general weakness and cramps in feet and hand. Hyperexcitability in these patients is detected by some signs, which do not appear in normal persons.

1. *Trousseau's sign*

It is the spasm of hand that is developed after 3 minutes of arresting the blood flow to lower arm and hand. Blood flow to lower arm and hand is arrested by inflating blood pressure cuff 20 mm Hg above the patient's systolic pressure.

2. *Chvostek's sign*

Chvostek's sign is the twitch of facial muscles caused by a gentle tap over the facial nerve in front of ear. It is due to the hyperirritability of facial nerve.

3. *Erb's sign*

Hyperexcitability of the skeletal muscles even to a mild electrical stimulus is called Erb's sign. It is also called **Erb-Westphal sign**.

HYPERPARATHYROIDISM: HYPERCALCEMIA

Hyperparathyroidism results in hypercalcemia (increase in blood calcium level).

Causes of Hyperparathyroidism

Causes of hyperparathyroidism are tumor in parathyroid glands and **hyperplasia** (abnormal increase in the number of cells) of parathyroid glands.

Hypercalcemia

Hypercalcemia is the increase in plasma calcium level. It occurs in hyperparathyroidism because of increased resorption of calcium from bones.

Common signs and symptoms of hypercalcemia.

1. Depression of the nervous system.
2. Sluggishness of reflex activities.
3. Lack of appetite.
4. Constipation.
5. Bone diseases.
6. Formation of **calcium-phosphate crystals**. The calcium-phosphate crystals may be deposited in kidneys, thyroid gland, lungs, gastric mucosa and arteries resulting in dysfunction of these organs. **Renal stones** are formed when it is deposited in kidney.

Depressive effects of hypercalcemia are noticed when the blood calcium level increases to 12 mg/dL. The condition becomes severe with 15 mg/dL and it becomes lethal when blood calcium level reaches 17 mg/dL.

PARATHYROID FUNCTION TESTS

Functions of parathyroid glands are assessed by the following tests:

1. Measurement of blood calcium level.
2. Chvostek's sign and Trousseau's sign for hypoparathyroidism.

CALCITONIN

SOURCE, CHEMISTRY AND PLASMA LEVEL OF CALCITONIN

Calcitonin is secreted by the **parafollicular cells** or **clear cells** (**C cells**) situated amongst the follicles in thyroid gland. It is a polypeptide chain with 32 amino acids. Its molecular weight is about 3,400. Plasma level of calcitonin it 1 to 2 ng/dL.

ACTIONS OF CALCITONIN

1. *Action of Calcitonin on Blood Calcium Level*

Calcitonin decreases the blood calcium level and thereby counteracts parathormone. Calcitonin decreases blood calcium level by acting on bones, kidneys and intestine.

i. *Effect on bones*

Calcitonin stimulates **osteoblastic activity** and facilitates the deposition of calcium on bones. At the same time, it suppresses the activity of osteoclasts and inhibits the resorption of calcium from bones. It inhibits even the development of new osteoclasts in bones.

ii. *Effect on kidney*

Calcitonin increases the excretion of calcium through urine, by inhibiting the reabsorption of calcium from the renal tubules.

iii. *Effect on intestine*

It prevents the absorption of calcium from intestine into the blood.

2. Action of Calcitonin on Blood Phosphate Level

With respect to calcium, calcitonin is an antagonist to PTH. But it has similar actions of PTH with respect to phosphate. Calcitonin decreases blood level of phosphate by acting on bones and kidneys.

i. Effect on bones

Calcitonin inhibits the resorption of phosphate from bone and stimulates deposition of phosphate on bones.

ii. Effect on kidney

Calcitonin increases the excretion of phosphate through urine, by inhibiting the reabsorption of calcium from the renal tubules.

■ REGULATION OF CALCITONIN SECRETION

High calcium content in plasma stimulates the calcitonin secretion through a **calcium receptor** in parafollicular cells. Gastrin also is known to stimulate release of calcitonin.

■ CALCIUM METABOLISM
■ IMPORTANCE OF CALCIUM

Calcium is very essential for many activities in the body such as:

1. Bone and teeth formation.
2. Neuronal activity.
3. Activity of all types of muscles.
4. Secretory activity of the glands.
5. Cell division and growth.
6. Coagulation of blood.

■ NORMAL VALUE OF CALCIUM LEVEL

In a normal young healthy adult, there is about 1,100 g of calcium in the body. Normal **blood calcium level** ranges between 9 and 11 mg/dL.

■ SOURCE OF CALCIUM

1. Dietary Source

Calcium is available in several foodstuffs such as milk, cheese, vegetables, meat, egg, grains, sugar, coffee, tea, chocolate, etc.

2. From Bones

Besides dietary calcium, blood also gets calcium from bone by resorption.

■ DAILY REQUIREMENTS OF CALCIUM

Amount of calcium required daily by a normal adult is 1,000 mg.

■ ABSORPTION AND EXCRETION OF CALCIUM

Absorption of Calcium

Calcium taken through dietary sources is absorbed from duodenum. **Vitamin D** is essential for the absorption of calcium from GI tract.

Excretion of Calcium

About 1,000 mg of calcium is excreted daily. Out of this 900 mg is excreted through feces and 100 mg through urine.

■ REGULATION OF BLOOD CALCIUM LEVEL

Blood calcium level is regulated by hormones.

1. Role of Parathormone

Parathormone increases the blood calcium level by bone resorption.

2. Role of 1,25-dihydroxycholecalciferol: Calcitriol

It is the activated form of vitamin D and it increases the blood calcium level by increasing the calcium absorption from small intestine.

3. Role of Calcitonin

It is a calcium lowering hormone. It reduces the blood calcium level mainly by decreasing bone resorption.

4. Role of Growth Hormone

Growth hormone increases the blood calcium level by increasing the intestinal calcium absorption.

5. Role of Glucocorticoids

Glucocorticoids (cortisol) decrease blood calcium by inhibiting intestinal absorption and increasing the renal excretion of calcium.

■ PHOSPHATE METABOLISM

Phosphorus (P) is an essential mineral that is required by every cell in the body for normal function. Phosphorus is present in many food substances, such as peas, dried beans, nuts, milk, cheese and butter. **Inorganic phosphorus (Pi)** is in the form of the **phosphate** (PO_4). Majority of the phosphorus in the body is found as phosphate.

■ IMPORTANCE OF PHOSPHATE

1. Phosphate is an important component of many organic substances such as, ATP, DNA, RNA and many intermediates of metabolic pathways.
2. Along with calcium it forms an important constituent of bone and teeth.
3. It forms a buffer in the maintenance of acid base balance.

■ NORMAL VALUE OF PHOSPHATE LEVEL

Total amount of phosphate in the body is 500 to 800 g. Though it is present in every cell of the body, 85 to 90% of body's phosphate is found in the bones and teeth. Normal plasma level of phosphate is 4 mg/dL.

■ REGULATION OF PHOSPHATE LEVEL

Phosphate level is regulated by hormones.

1. Role of Parathormone

Parathormone decreases the plasma level of phosphate by causing urinary excretion of phosphate.

2. Role of Calcitonin

Calcitonin also decreases the plasma level of phosphate by inhibiting bone resorption and stimulating urinary excretion.

3. Role of 1,25-dihydroxycholecalciferol: Calcitriol

This hormone increases absorption of phosphate from small intestine.

4. Role of Growth Hormones

Growth hormone increases the blood phosphate level by increasing the intestinal phosphate absorption.

5. Role of Glucocorticoids

Glucocorticoids (cortisol) decrease blood phosphate by inhibiting intestinal absorption and increasing the renal excretion of phosphate.

PHYSIOLOGY OF BONE

Bone or **osseous tissue** is a specialized rigid connective tissue that forms the skeleton.

FUNCTIONS OF BONE

1. Protective function

Bone protects soft tissues and vital organs of the body.

2. Mechanical function

It supports the body and brings out various movements of the body.

3. Metabolic function

It is responsible for metabolism and homeostasis of calcium and phosphate in the body.

4. Hematopoietic function

Red bone marrow in the bones is the site of production of blood cells.

CLASSIFICATION OF BONE

Bones are classified into five types depending upon the size and shape:

1. Long bones   : Bones of the limbs.
2. Short bones   : Bones in the wrist and ankle.
3. Flat bones   : Skull bones, mandible, scapula, etc.
4. Irregular bones : Vertebra.
5. Sesamoid bones   : Patella.

PARTS OF BONE

Long bones are formed by a cylindrical tube of bone tissue, which has three portions:

1. **Diaphysis**: Midportion or midshaft.
2. **Epiphysis**: Wider extremity or the head on either end.
3. **Metaphysis**: Portion between the diaphysis and epiphysis (Fig. 46.3).

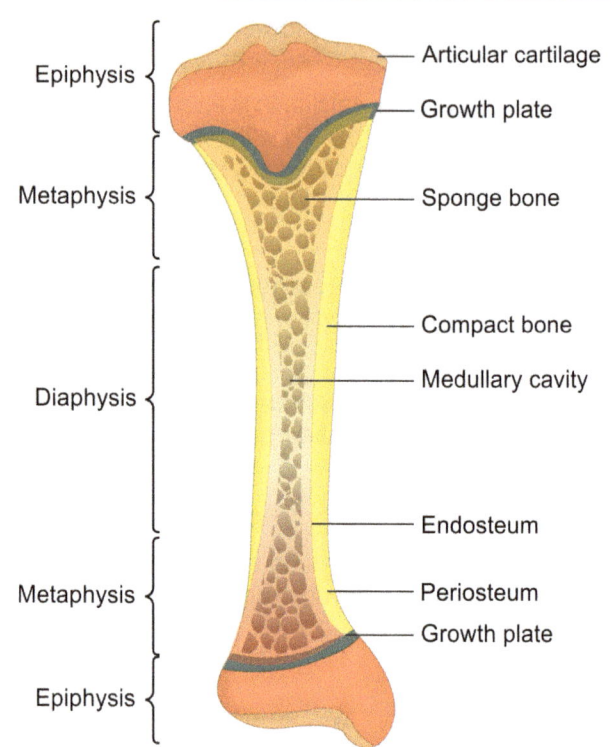

FIGURE 46.3: Parts of long bone.

In growing age, a layer of cartilage called **epiphyseal cartilage** or **epiphyseal plate** or **growth plate** is present in between epiphysis and metaphysis. Epiphyseal plate is responsible for the longitudinal growth of the bones.

STRUCTURE OF BONE

Bone is covered by an outer white fibrous connective layer called **periosteum** and an inner dense fibrous membrane called **endosteum**. Tendons from the muscles are attached to **periosteum**. Heads (epiphysis) of bone are covered by a **hyaline cartilage**. It forms the synovial joint with adjoining bones.

Bones have two layers of structures, outer compact bone and inner spongy bone.

TYPES OF CELLS IN BONE

Bone has three major types of cells:

1. Osteoblasts

Osteoblasts are the bone cells that are concerned with bone formation. Osteoblasts arise from the giant multinucleated primitive cells called the **osteoprogenitor cells**.

Functions of osteoblasts

Osteoblasts:

i. Are responsible for the synthesis of bone matrix.
ii. Are rich in alkaline phosphatase, which is necessary for **calcification** (deposition of calcium in the bone matrix).
iii. Synthesize of the proteins called **matrix Gla-protein** and **osteopontin**, which are involved in the calcification.

Chapter 46: Parathyroid Glands and Physiology of Bone

Fate of osteoblasts

After taking part in bone formation, the osteoblasts differentiate into osteocytes, which are trapped inside lacunae of calcified bone.

2. Osteocytes

Osteocytes are the cells concerned with maintenance of bone. Osteocytes are derived from the matured osteoblasts.

Functions of osteocytes

Osteocytes help to maintain the bone as living tissue because of their metabolic activity.

3. Osteoclasts

Osteoclasts are the bone cells that are concerned with bone resorption. Osteoclasts are the giant phagocytic multinucleated cells found in the lacunae of bone matrix. These bone cells are derived from hematopoietic stem cells via monocytes (CFU-M).

Functions of osteoclasts

Osteoclasts are responsible for bone resorption during bone remodeling. Osteoclasts are also involved in synthesis and release of **lysosomal enzymes** necessary for bone resorption.

■ BONE REMODELING

Bone remodeling is a dynamic lifelong process in which old bone is resorbed and new bone is formed. Usually, it takes place in groups of bone cells called the **basic multicellular units (BMU)**. Entire process of remodeling extends for about 100 days in compact bone and about 200 days in spongy bone.

Bone remodeling includes two processes:

1. *Bone resorption:* **Osteoclastic activity** (destruction of entire bone matrix and removal of calcium). Osteoclasts are responsible for this.
2. *Bone formation:* **Osteoblastic activity** (development and mineralization of new matrix). Osteoblasts are responsible for this.

Significance of Bone Remodeling

In children:
1. Thickness of bone increases.
2. Bone obtains strength.
3. Shape of bone is realtered in relation to growth of the body.

In adults:
1. Maintenance of toughness of bone.
2. Mechanical integrity of skeleton throughout life.
3. Calcium homeostasis.

■ APPLIED PHYSIOLOGY: DISEASES OF BONE

1. Osteoporosis

Osteoporosis is a bone disease characterized by the loss of bone matrix and minerals. It occurs due to excess bone resorption and decreased bone formation. Osteoporosis is common in women after 60 years.

Features of osteoporosis

Because of loss of bone matrix and minerals bone becomes weak and fragile with **high risk of fracture**. Commonly affected bones are vertebrae and hip.

2. Rickets

Rickets is the bone disease in children characterized by inadequate mineralization of bone matrix. It occurs due to vitamin D deficiency.

Features of rickets

i. Collapse of chest wall: Due to the flattening of sides of thorax with projecting sternum called **pigeon chest**, **chicken chest** or **pectus carinatum**.
ii. **Rachitic rosary**: A visible swelling where the ribs join their cartilages.
iii. **Kyphosis**: Excess curvature of upper backbone with convexity backward (forward bending or forward curvature).
iv. **Lordosis**: Excess forward curvature of backbone in lumbar region.
v. **Scoliosis**: Lateral curvature of spine.
vii. Bowing of hands and legs.

3. Osteomalacia

Rickets in adults is called osteomalacia or **adult rickets**. It occurs because of deficiency of vitamin D. It also occurs due to prolonged damage of kidney (**renal rickets**).

Features of osteomalacia

i. Vague pain.
ii. Tenderness in bones and muscles.
iii. **Myopathy** leading to **waddling gait** (**gait** means the manner of walking). In waddling gait, the feet are wide apart and walk resembles that of a duck.

Chapter 47: Endocrine Functions of Pancreas

CHAPTER OUTLINE
- ISLETS OF LANGERHANS
- INSULIN
- GLUCAGON
- SOMATOSTATIN
- PANCREATIC POLYPEPTIDE
- REGULATION OF BLOOD SUGAR LEVEL
- APPLIED PHYSIOLOGY: DISORDERS OF PANCREAS

■ ISLETS OF LANGERHANS

Endocrine function of pancreas is performed by the islets of Langerhans **(Fig. 47.1)**. Human pancreas contains about 1 to 2 million islets.

Islets of Langerhans consist of four types of cells:

1. A cells or α-cells which secrete glucagon.
2. B cells or β-cells which secrete insulin.
3. D cells or γ-cells which secrete somatostatin.
4. F cells or PP cells which secrete pancreatic polypeptide.

■ INSULIN

SOURCE, CHEMISTRY AND BLOOD LEVEL OF INSULIN

Insulin is secreted by B cells or the **β-cells** in islets of Langerhans of pancreas.

Insulin is a polypeptide with 51 amino acids. It has two amino acid chains called α and β-chains which are linked by **disulfide bridges**.

Basal level of insulin in plasma is 10 µU/mL.

ACTIONS OF INSULIN

Insulin is the important hormone that is concerned with regulation of carbohydrate metabolism and blood sugar level. It is also concerned with metabolism of proteins and fats.

1. Action on Carbohydrate Metabolism

Insulin is the only **antidiabetic hormone** secreted in the body, i.e. it is the only hormone in body that reduces blood sugar level. Insulin reduces the blood sugar level by its following actions on carbohydrate metabolism.

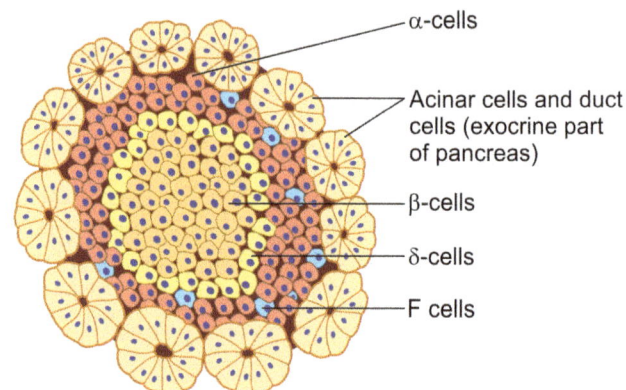

FIGURE 47.1: Islets of Langerhans.

i. By facilitating transport and uptake of glucose by the cells

Insulin facilitates transport of glucose from the blood into cells by increasing the permeability of cell membrane to glucose. Insulin stimulates the rapid uptake of glucose by all the tissues particularly liver, muscle and adipose tissues. Insulin also increases the number of glucose transporters called **GLUT4** in cell membrane.

ii. By increasing peripheral utilization of glucose

Insulin promotes the peripheral utilization of glucose. In the presence of insulin, glucose which enters the cell is oxidized immediately.

iii. By increasing storage of glucose: Glycogenesis

Insulin promotes the rapid conversion of glucose into glycogen (glycogenesis), which is stored in muscle and liver. Insulin activates the enzymes, which are necessary for glycogenesis. In liver, when glycogen content increases beyond its storing capacity, insulin causes conversion of glucose into fatty acids.

iv. *By inhibiting of glycogenolysis*

Insulin inhibits glycogenolysis (breakdown of glycogen into glucose) in muscle and liver.

v. *By inhibiting of gluconeogenesis*

Insulin inhibits gluconeogenesis (formation of glucose) from proteins.

2. Action on Protein Metabolism

Insulin facilitates the synthesis and storage of proteins, and inhibits the cellular utilization of proteins by:

i. Facilitating the transport of amino acids into cell from blood.
ii. Accelerating the synthesis of proteins.
iii. Preventing catabolism.
iv. Preventing conversion of proteins into glucose.

Thus, insulin is responsible for **protein conservation** (protein sparing effect) and synthesis and storage (**anabolic effect**) of proteins in the body.

3. Action on Fat Metabolism

Insulin stimulates the synthesis of fat. It also increases the storage of fat in the adipose tissue. Actions of insulin on fat metabolism are:

i. Insulin promotes the transport of excess glucose into cells, particularly the liver cells. This glucose is utilized for the synthesis of fatty acids and triglycerides.
ii. Insulin facilitates transport of fatty acids into adipose tissue.
iii. It promotes the storage of fat in adipose tissue.

4. Action on Growth

Along with growth hormone, insulin promotes growth of body by its **anabolic action**. It enhances the transport of amino acids into the cell and synthesis of proteins in the cells. It also has the **protein sparing effect**, i.e. it causes conservation of proteins by increasing the glucose utilization by the tissues.

MODE OF ACTION OF ACTION OF INSULIN

On the target cells, insulin binds with **insulin receptor** and forms insulin-receptor complex. This complex executes the action by activating intracellular enzyme system. Insulin receptor is a glycoprotein and it is present in almost all the cells of body. Insulin receptor is formed by four glycoprotein subunits (two α-subunits and two β-subunits).

REGULATION OF SECRETION OF INSULIN

Insulin secretion is mainly regulated by blood glucose level. In addition, other factors like amino acids, lipid derivatives, gastrointestinal and endocrine hormones, and autonomic nerve fibers also stimulate insulin secretion.

1. Role of Blood Glucose Level

When blood glucose level is normal (80 to 100 mg/dL), the rate of insulin secretion is low (up to 10 µU/minute). When blood glucose level increases between 100 and 120 mg/dL, the rate of insulin secretion rises rapidly to 100 µU/minute. When the blood glucose level rises above 200 mg/dL, the rate of insulin secretion also rises very rapidly up to 400 µU/minute.

2. Role of Proteins

Excess amino acids in blood also stimulate insulin secretion.

3. Role of Lipid Derivatives

The **β-keto acids** such as **acetoacetate** also stimulate insulin secretion.

4. Role of Gastrointestinal Hormones

Insulin secretion is increased by some of the gastrointestinal hormones such as gastrin, secretin, cholecystokinin and gastric inhibitory peptide (GIP).

5. Role of Endocrine Hormones

Diabetogenic hormones such as glucagon, growth hormone and cortisol increase the blood sugar level which, in turn stimulate insulin secretion indirectly. Prolonged hypersecretion of these hormones causes exhaustion of β-cells resulting in diabetes mellitus.

6. Role of Autonomic Nerves

Stimulation of parasympathetic nerve to the pancreas (right vagus) increases insulin secretion.

GLUCAGON

SOURCE AND CHEMISTRY OF GLUCAGON

Glucagon is secreted from A cells or **α-cells** in the islets of Langerhans of pancreas. It is also secreted from A cells of stomach and L cells of intestine. Glucagon is a polypeptide with 29 amino acids.

ACTIONS OF GLUCAGON

Actions of glucagon are **antagonistic to insulin** actions. It increases the blood sugar level and peripheral utilization of lipids, and facilitates the conversion of proteins into glucose.

1. Action on Carbohydrate Metabolism

Glucagon increases the blood glucose level by increasing **glycogenolysis** and **gluconeogenesis** in liver and releasing glucose into the blood.

2. Action on Protein Metabolism

Glucagon increases transport of amino acids into liver cells. The amino acids are utilized for gluconeogenesis.

3. Action on Fat Metabolism

Glucagon shows lipolytic and ketogenic actions. It increases lipolysis by increasing the release of free fatty acids from adipose tissue and making them available for peripheral utilization. **Lipolytic activity** of glucagon, in turn promotes **ketogenesis** (formation of ketone bodies) in liver.

4. Other Actions of Glucagon

Glucagon:
i. Inhibits secretion of gastric juice.
ii. Increases secretion of bile from liver.

MODE OF ACTION OF GLUCAGON

On target cells glucagon causes formation of cyclic AMP which brings out the actions of glucagon.

REGULATION OF SECRETION OF GLUCAGON

Secretion of glucagon is controlled mainly by blood glucose and amino acid levels in the blood.

1. Role of Blood Glucose Level

When blood glucose level decreases below 80 mg/dL of blood, α-cells of islets of Langerhans are stimulated and more glucagon is released. Glucagon in turn increases the blood glucose level. On the other hand, when blood sugar level increases, α-cells are inhibited and the secretion of glucagon decreases.

2. Role of Amino Acid Level in Blood

Increase in amino acid level in blood stimulates the secretion of glucagon. Glucagon, in turn converts the amino acids into glucose.

3. Role of Other Factors

Factors which increase glucagon secretion are exercise, stress, gastrin, cholecystokinin and cortisol.

Factors which inhibit glucagon secretion are somatostatin, insulin, free fatty acids and ketones.

SOMATOSTATIN

SOURCE AND CHEMISTRY OF SOMATOSTATIN

Somatostatin is secreted from **D cells (δ-cells)** in islets of Langerhans of pancreas, hypothalamus and D cells in stomach and upper part of small intestine. Somatostatin is a polypeptide.

ACTIONS OF SOMATOSTATIN

1. Somatostatin acts within islets of Langerhans, and inhibits α and β-cells, i.e. it inhibits the secretion of both glucagon and insulin.
2. It decreases the motility of stomach, duodenum and gallbladder.
3. Somatostatin reduces the secretion of gastrointestinal hormones gastrin, CCK, GIP and VIP.
4. Hypothalamic somatostatin inhibits secretion of GH and TSH from anterior pituitary. That is why, it is also called growth hormone inhibitory hormone (GHIH).

MODE OF ACTION OF SOMATOSTATIN

Somatostatin brings out its actions through cAMP.

REGULATION OF SECRETION OF SOMATOSTATIN

Pancreatic Somatostatin

Secretion of pancreatic somatostatin is stimulated by glucose, amino acids and CCK. Tumor of D cells in islets of Langerhans causes hypersecretion of somatostatin. It leads to hyperglycemia and other symptoms of diabetes mellitus.

Gastrointestinal Tract Somatostatin

Secretion of somatostatin in GI tract is increased by the presence of chyme-containing glucose and proteins in stomach and small intestine.

PANCREATIC POLYPEPTIDE

SOURCE AND CHEMISTRY OF PANCREATIC POLYPEPTIDE

Pancreatic polypeptide is secreted by **F cells** or **PP cells** in the islets of Langerhans of pancreas. It is also found in small intestine. It is a polypeptide with 36 amino acids.

ACTIONS OF PANCREATIC POLYPEPTIDE

Exact physiological action of pancreatic polypeptide is not known. It is believed to increase the secretion of glucagon from α-cells in islets of Langerhans.

MODE OF ACTION OF PANCREATIC POLYPEPTIDE

Pancreatic polypeptide brings out its actions through cAMP.

REGULATION OF SECRETION OF PANCREATIC POLYPEPTIDE

Secretion of pancreatic polypeptide is stimulated by the presence of chyme-containing more proteins in small intestine.

REGULATION OF BLOOD SUGAR LEVEL (BLOOD GLUCOSE LEVEL)

NORMAL BLOOD SUGAR LEVEL

In normal persons, blood sugar level is controlled within a narrow range. In early morning after overnight fasting, the **fasting blood sugar** level is low ranging between 70 and 110 mg/dL of blood. Between 1st and 2nd hour after meals, **postprandial blood sugar level** rises from 100 to 140 mg/dL. Sugar level in the blood is brought back to normal at the end of 2nd hour after the meals.

Blood sugar-regulating mechanism is operated through liver and muscle by the influence of pancreatic hormones insulin and glucagon. Many other hormones are also involved in the regulation of blood sugar level.

Among all the hormones, insulin is the only hormone that reduces blood sugar level and it is called antidiabetogenic hormone. Hormones, which increase blood sugar level, are called diabetogenic hormones or **antiinsulin hormones**.

Necessity of Regulation of Blood Glucose Level

Regulation of blood sugar (glucose) level is very essential, because glucose is the only nutrient that is utilized for energy by many tissues such as brain tissues, retina and germinal epithelium of the gonads.

ROLE OF LIVER IN THE MAINTENANCE OF BLOOD SUGAR LEVEL

Liver serves as an important **glucose buffer system**. When blood sugar level increases after a meal, the excess glucose is converted into glycogen and stored in liver. Afterwards, when blood sugar level falls, the glycogen in liver is converted into glucose and released into the blood. Storage of glycogen and release of glucose from liver are mainly regulated by insulin and glucagon.

ROLE OF INSULIN IN THE MAINTENANCE OF BLOOD SUGAR LEVEL

Insulin decreases blood sugar level and it is the only antidiabetic hormone available in the body. Refer the actions on insulin on carbohydrate metabolism in this Chapter.

ROLE OF GLUCAGON IN THE MAINTENANCE OF BLOOD SUGAR LEVEL

Glucagon increases the blood sugar level. Refer actions of glucagon on carbohydrate metabolism in this Chapter.

ROLE OF OTHER HORMONES IN THE MAINTENANCE OF BLOOD SUGAR LEVEL

Other hormones which increase the blood sugar level are:

1. Growth hormone (Chapter 44).
2. Thyroxine (Chapter 45).
3. Cortisol (Chapter 48).
4. Adrenaline (Chapter 49).

Thus, liver helps to maintain the blood sugar level by storing glycogen, when blood glucose level is high after meals; and by releasing glucose, when blood sugar level is low after 2 to 3 hours of food intake. Insulin helps to control blood sugar level, especially after meals. Glucagon and other hormones help to maintain the blood sugar level by raising it in between the meals.

APPLIED PHYSIOLOGY: DISORDERS OF PANCREAS

HYPOACTIVITY: DIABETES MELLITUS

Diabetes mellitus is a metabolic disorder characterized by high blood sugar (glucose) level associated with other manifestations. In most of the cases, the diabetes mellitus develops due to the **deficiency of insulin**.

Classification of Diabetes Mellitus

Diabetes mellitus is of two types, type I and type II. Differences between the two types are given in **Table 47.1**.

Type I Diabetes Mellitus

Type I diabetes mellitus is due to the deficiency of **insulin**. So, it is also called **insulin dependent diabetes mellitus (IDDM)**. Type I diabetes mellitus may occur at any age of life. But it usually occurs before 40 years of age. When it occurs at infancy (due to congenital disorder) or in childhood, it is called **juvenile diabetes**.

Causes of type I diabetes mellitus

1. Degeneration of β-cells in the islets of Langerhans of pancreas.
2. Destruction of β-cells by viral infection.
3. Congenital disorder of β-cells.
4. Destruction of β-cells during autoimmune diseases.

TABLE 47.1: Differences between type I and type II diabetes mellitus.

Features	Type I (IDDM)	Type II (NIDDM)
Age of onset	Usually before 40 years	Usually after 40 years
Major cause	Lack of insulin	Lack of insulin receptor
Insulin deficiency	Yes	Partial deficiency
Immune destruction of β-cells	Yes	No
Involvement of other endocrine disorders	No	Yes
Hereditary cause	Yes	May or may not be
Need for insulin	Always	Not in initial stage May require in later stage
Insulin resistance	No	Yes
Control by oral hypoglycemic agents	No	Yes
Symptoms appear	Rapidly	Slowly
Body weight	Usually thin	Usually overweight
Stress-induced obesity	No	Yes
Ketosis	Yes	May or may not be

Type II Diabetes Mellitus

It is due to the absence or deficiency of **insulin receptors**. It usually occurs after 40 years; hence, it is called maturity onset diabetes mellitus. This type of diabetes mellitus is also called **non-insulin dependent diabetes mellitus (NIDDM)**.

Causes for type II diabetes mellitus

In this type of diabetes, structure and function of β-cells and blood level of insulin are normal. But insulin receptors may be less, absent or abnormal, resulting in insulin resistance.

Common causes of insulin resistance are:

1. Genetic disorders (significant factors causing type II diabetes mellitus).
2. Lifestyle changes such as bad eating habits and physical inactivity, leading to obesity.
3. Stress.

Diabetes Mellitus Associated with other Endocrine Disorders

Diabetes is very common in some of the endocrine disorders such as gigantism, acromegaly and Cushing's syndrome. This type of diabetes mellitus is called **secondary diabetes**.

Signs and Symptoms of Diabetes Mellitus

1. Glucosuria

Loss of glucose in urine is known as glucosuria. Normally glucose does not appear in urine. When glucose level rises above 180 mg/dL in blood, glucose appears in urine. It is the **renal threshold** level for glucose.

2. Osmotic diuresis

Diuresis due to osmotic effects is called **osmotic diuresis**. Excess glucose in the renal tubules develops osmotic effect which decreases the reabsorption of water from renal tubules resulting in diuresis. It leads to polyuria and polydipsia.

3. Polyuria

Excess urine formation with increase in frequency of voiding urine is called polyuria. It is due to the osmotic diuresis caused by increase in blood sugar level.

4. Polydipsia

Polydipsia is the increase in water intake. Excess loss of water decreases water content and increases salt content in the body. This stimulates the thirst center in hypothalamus. Thirst center in turn induces water intake.

5. Polyphagia

Polyphagia means the intake of excess food. It is very common in diabetes mellitus.

6. Asthenia

Asthenia is the loss of strength. Body becomes very weak. There is loss of energy. Asthenia occurs because of **protein depletion** caused by lack of insulin.

7. Acidosis

During insulin deficiency since glucose cannot be utilized by the peripheral tissues large amount of fat is broken down to release energy. It causes the formation of **excess ketoacids** leading to **acidosis**.

8. Acetone breathing

In cases of severe ketoacidosis, acetone is expired in the expiratory air, giving the characteristic **acetone breath odor** or **fruity breath odor**. It is a life-threatening condition of severe diabetes.

9. Kussmaul breathing

Kussmaul breathing is the increase in rate and depth of respiration caused by severe acidosis.

10. Circulatory shock

Osmotic diuresis leads to dehydration, which causes circulatory shock. It occurs only in severe diabetes.

11. Coma

Coma occurs in severe cases of diabetes mellitus. Increase in blood sugar level develops hyperosmolarity of plasma which also leads to coma. It is called **hyperosmolar coma**.

Complications of Diabetes Mellitus

Prolonged hyperglycemia in diabetes mellitus causes dysfunction and injury of many tissues resulting in some complications such as:

1. Cardiovascular complications such as **hypertension** and **myocardial infarction**.
2. Degenerative changes in retina called **diabetic retinopathy**.
3. Degenerative changes in kidney known as **diabetic nephropathy**.
4. Degeneration of autonomic and peripheral nerves called **diabetic neuropathy**.

Diagnostic Tests for Diabetes Mellitus

Diagnosis of diabetes mellitus includes the determination of:

1. Fasting blood sugar.
2. Postprandial blood sugar.
3. Glucose tolerance test (GTT).
4. Hemoglobin A1c (HbA1c) or glycosylated (glycated) hemoglobin test.

    Determination of HbA1c is commonly done to monitor the glycemic control of the persons already diagnosed with diabetes mellitus.

■ HYPERACTIVITY: HYPERINSULINISM

Hyperinsulinism is the hypersecretion of insulin.

Cause of Hyperinsulinism

Hyperinsulinism occurs due to the tumor of β-cells in the islets of Langerhans.

Signs and Symptoms of Hyperinsulinism

1. Hypoglycemia

Blood sugar level falls below 50 mg/dL.

2. Manifestations of central nervous system

Manifestations of central nervous system occur when the blood sugar level decreases. All the manifestations are together called **neuroglycopenic symptoms** which include nervousness, tremor all over the body and sweating. If not treated immediately, it leads to clonic convulsions and unconsciousness. Slowly, the convulsions cease and coma occurs due to damage of neurons.

Chapter 48: Adrenal Cortex

CHAPTER OUTLINE

- IMPORTANCE OF ADRENAL GLANDS
- FUNCTIONAL ANATOMY OF ADRENAL GLANDS
- FUNCTIONAL HISTOLOGY OF ADRENAL CORTEX
- HORMONES SECRETED BY ADRENAL CORTEX
- MINERALOCORTICOIDS
- GLUCOCORTICOIDS
- ADRENAL SEX HORMONES
- APPLIED PHYSIOLOGY: DISORDERS OF ADRENAL COTEX

IMPORTANCE OF ADRENAL GLANDS

Adrenal glands are called the **life-saving glands.** It is because the absence of adrenocortical hormones causes death within a week and absence of adrenomedullary hormones, drastically decreases the resistance to mental and physical stress.

FUNCTIONAL ANATOMY OF ADRENAL GLANDS

There are two adrenal glands. Each gland is situated on the upper pole of each kidney. Because of their situation, adrenal glands are called **suprarenal glands**.

Adrenal gland (Fig. 48.1) is made of two distinct parts:

1. *Adrenal cortex*: Outer portion, constituting 80% of the gland.
2. *Adrenal medulla*: Central portion, constituting 20% of the gland.

Each part of the gland is different from other one in development, structure and functions.

FUNCTIONAL HISTOLOGY OF ADRENAL CORTEX

Adrenal cortex is formed by three distinct layers of structures:

1. **Zona glomerulosa** or outer layer.
2. **Zona fasciculata** or middle layer.
3. **Zona reticularis** or inner layer.

HORMONES SECRETED BY ADRENAL CORTEX

Hormones secreted by adrenal cortex are collectively known as **adrenocortical hormones** or **corticosteroids**.

Based on their functions, the corticosteroids are classified into three groups:

I. Mineralocorticoids.
II. Glucocorticoids.
III. Sex hormones.

MINERALOCORTICOIDS

Mineralocorticoids are the corticosteroids which act on minerals (electrolytes), particularly sodium and potassium. Mineralocorticoids are secreted by zona glomerulosa of adrenal cortex **(Table 48.1)**.

Mineralocorticoids are aldosterone and 11-deoxycorticosterone. Mineralocorticoids are C_{21} steroids having 21 carbon atoms. Plasma level of aldosterone and 11-deoxycorticosterone is 0.006 µg/dL.

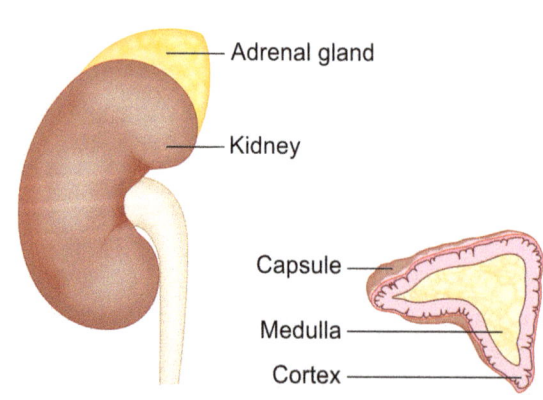

FIGURE 48.1: Adrenal gland.

TABLE 48.1: Hormones secreted by different layers of adrenal cortex.

Layer	Hormones
Zona glomerulosa	Mineralocorticoids
Zona fasciculata	Glucocorticoids Small quantity of sex hormones
Zona reticularis	Sex hormones Small quantity of glucocorticoids

FUNCTIONS OF MINERALOCORTICOIDS

Ninety percent of mineralocorticoid activity is provided by **aldosterone**.

Life-saving Hormone

Aldosterone is **life-saving hormone**, because the absence of this hormone causes death within a week.

Actions of aldosterone are explained below.

1. Action on Sodium Ions

Aldosterone helps in the conservation of sodium in the body. Aldosterone increases reabsorption of sodium from distal convoluted tubule and collecting duct in the kidney. It also increases sodium absorption from the intestine, sweat glands and salivary glands.

2. Action on Extracellular Fluid Volume

When sodium ions are reabsorbed from the renal tubules, almost an equal amount of water is also reabsorbed. So, the net result is increase in ECF volume.

3. Action on Blood Pressure

Increase in ECF volume and blood volume finally leads to increase in blood pressure.

Aldosterone escape or escape phenomenon

Aldosterone escape means escape of the kidney from **salt-retaining effect** of excess of aldosterone as in the case of primary hyperaldosteronism. When aldosterone level increases, there is excess retention of sodium and water. This increases the ECF volume and blood pressure.

Aldosterone-induced high blood pressure decreases the ECF volume through two types of reactions:

i. It stimulates secretion of **atrial natriuretic peptide (ANP)** from atrial muscles of the heart. ANP causes excretion of sodium in spite of increase in aldosterone secretion.
ii. It causes **pressure diuresis** (excretion of excess salt and water by high blood pressure) through urine. This decreases the salt and water content in ECF in spite of hypersecretion of aldosterone.

Significance of aldosterone escape

Because of aldosterone escape, edema does not occur in primary hyperaldosteronism.

4. Action on Potassium Ions

Aldosterone increases the potassium excretion through renal tubules.

5. Action on Hydrogen Ion Concentration

Aldosterone induces excretion of hydrogen ions by increasing tubular secretion of hydrogen ions. This is essential to maintain acid-base balance in the body.

MODE OF ACTION OF MINERALOCORTICOIDS

Mineralocorticoids act through the messenger RNA mechanism.

REGULATION OF SECRETION OF MINERALOCORTICOIDS

Aldosterone secretion is regulated by four important factors **(Fig. 48.2)**. Factors stimulating secretion of aldosterone are given below in the order of their potency:

1. Increase in potassium ion concentration in ECF.
2. Decrease in sodium ion concentration in ECF.
3. Decrease in ECF volume.
4. Adrenocorticotropic hormone.

Increase in the concentration of potassium ions is the most effective stimulant for aldosterone secretion. It acts directly on the zona glomerulosa and increases the secretion of aldosterone. Decrease in sodium ion concentration and ECF volume stimulates aldosterone secretion through renin-angiotensin mechanism.

Adrenocorticotropic hormone mainly stimulates the secretion of glucocorticoids. It has only a mild stimulating effect on aldosterone secretion.

GLUCOCORTICOIDS

Glucocorticoids are the corticosteroids which act mainly on glucose metabolism. Glucocorticoids are secreted mainly by zona fasciculata of adrenal cortex. A small quantity of glucocorticoids is also secreted by zona reticularis.

Glucocorticoids are cortisol, corticosterone and cortisone. Glucocorticoids are C_{21} steroids having 21 carbon atoms. Plasma level of cortisol is 13.9 μg/dL and that of corticosterone is 0.4 μg/dL.

FUNCTIONS OF GLUCOCORTICOIDS

Cortisol is more potent and it has 95% of glucocorticoid activity.

Life-protecting Hormone

Cortisol is a life protecting hormone, because it helps to withstand the stress and trauma in life.

Actions of glucocorticoids are explained below.

1. Action on Carbohydrate Metabolism

Glucocorticoids increase the blood glucose level by two ways:

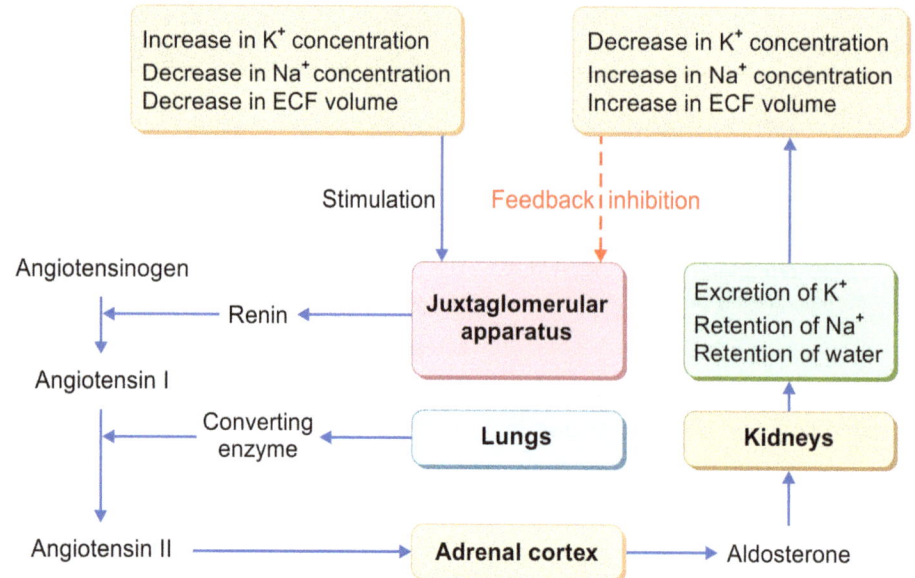

FIGURE 48.2: Regulation of aldosterone secretion.

i. By promoting gluconeogenesis in liver from amino acids.
ii. By inhibiting glucose uptake and utilization by peripheral cells.

2. Action on Protein Metabolism

Glucocorticoids promote catabolism of proteins by the following methods:

i. Glucocorticoids decrease the protein in body cells, except liver cells by accelerating protein catabolism and release of amino acids from the tissues.
ii. Glucocorticoids increase the transport of amino acids into hepatic cells. In hepatic cells, the amino acids are used for synthesis of proteins, plasma proteins and for gluconeogenesis.

Thus, glucocorticoids cause mobilization of proteins from tissues other than liver.

3. Action on Fat Metabolism

Glucocorticoids cause mobilization and redistribution of fats. Actions on fats are:

i. Mobilization of fatty acids from adipose tissue.
ii. Increasing the concentration of fatty acids in blood.
iii. Increasing the utilization of fat for energy.
  By increasing the utilization of fats for energy release, glucocorticoids cause the formation of a large amount of ketone bodies. It is called **ketogenic effect** of glucocorticoids.

4. Action on Water Metabolism

Glucocorticoids are involved in the maintenance of water balance by accelerating excretion of water.

5. Action on Mineral Metabolism

Glucocorticoids enhance the retention of sodium and to lesser extent, increase the excretion of potassium. Glucocorticoids decrease blood calcium by inhibiting absorption of calcium from intestine and increasing the excretion of calcium through urine.

6. Action on Bone

Glucocorticoids stimulate **osteoclastic activity** (bone resorption) and inhibit **osteoblastic activity** (bone formation and mineralization).

7. Action on Muscles

Glucocorticoids cause catabolism of proteins from muscle.

8. Action Blood Cells

Glucocorticoids decrease eosinophil count by increasing the destruction of eosinophils in reticuloendothelial cells. These hormones also decrease the number of basophils and lymphocytes, and increase the number of circulating neutrophils, RBCs and platelets.

9. Action on Vascular Response

Presence of glucocorticoids is essential for the constrictor action of catecholamines (adrenaline and noradrenaline). In adrenal insufficiency, the blood vessels fail to respond to adrenaline and noradrenaline leading to vascular collapse.

10. Action on Central Nervous System

Glucocorticoids are essential for normal functioning of nervous system. Insufficiency of these hormones causes personality changes like irritability and lack of concentration.

11. Permissive Action of Glucocorticoids

Permissive action of glucocorticoids is the execution of actions of some hormones only in the presence of glucocorticoids. Examples are calorigenic effects, lipolytic effects, pressor effects and bronchodilator effect of catecholamines.

12. Action on Resistance to Stress

Exposure to any type of stress, either physical or mental, increases the secretion of adrenocorticotropic hormone (ACTH). ACTH in turn increases glucocorticoid secretion. Increase in glucocorticoid level is very essential for survival, as it offers high resistance to body against stress.

13. Anti-inflammatory Effects

Inflammation is defined as a localized protective response induced by injury or destruction of tissues. When tissue is injured by mechanical or chemical factors, some substances are released from the affected area, which produce series of changes in the affected area.

Glucocorticoids prevent the inflammatory changes in injured or infected tissues. In addition to preventing inflammatory reactions, if inflammation has already started, the glucocorticoids cause an early resolution of inflammation and rapid healing.

14. Antiallergic Actions

Corticosteroids prevent the various reactions in allergic conditions as in the case of inflammation.

15. Immunosuppressive Action

Glucocorticoids suppress the immune system of body by decreasing the number of circulating T lymphocytes and proliferation of T lymphocytes in lymphoid tissues.

■ MODE OF ACTION OF GLUCOCORTICOIDS

Glucocorticoids act through the messenger RNA mechanism.

■ REGULATION OF SECRETION OF GLUCOCORTICOIDS

Glucocorticoid secretion is regulated by anterior pituitary and hypothalamus.

Role of Anterior Pituitary: ACTH

Anterior pituitary controls the activities of adrenal cortex by secreting ACTH. ACTH is secreted by the basophilic chromophilic cells of anterior pituitary. It is a single chained polypeptide with 39 amino acids. Its concentration in plasma is 3 ng/dL.

ACTH is mainly concerned with regulation of cortisol secretion. It plays only a minor role in the regulation of mineralocorticoid secretion.

Actions of ACTH

ACTH is necessary for structural integrity and the secretory activity of adrenal cortex. It has other functions also.

Actions of ACTH on adrenal cortex

1. Maintenance of structural integrity, and vascularization of zona fasciculata and zona reticularis of adrenal cortex.
2. Acceleration of synthesis of glucocorticoids by converting cholesterol into pregnenolone, which is the precursor of glucocorticoids.
3. Release of glucocorticoids.

Other (nonadrenal) actions of ACTH

1. Mobilization of fats from tissues.
2. Melanocyte stimulating effect: Because of structural similarity with **melanocyte stimulating hormone**, ACTH shows melanocyte stimulating effect. It causes darkening of skin by acting on melanophores which are the cutaneous pigment cells containing melanin.

Mode of Action of ACTH

ACTH acts by the formation of cyclic AMP.

Role of Hypothalamus

Hypothalamus also regulates cortisol secretion by controlling the ACTH secretion through corticotropin releasing factor (CRF) or corticotropin releasing hormone. CRF stimulates the corticotrophs of anterior pituitary and causes synthesis and release of ACTH.

Feedback Control

Cortisol regulates its own secretion through negative feedback control by inhibiting the release of CRF from hypothalamus and ACTH from anterior pituitary **(Fig. 48.3)**.

■ ADRENAL SEX HORMONES

Adrenal sex hormones are secreted mainly by zona reticularis. Zona fasciculata secretes small quantities of sex hormones. Adrenal cortex secretes mainly **androgens** (male sex hormones). But small quantities of estrogen and progesterone are also secreted by adrenal cortex.

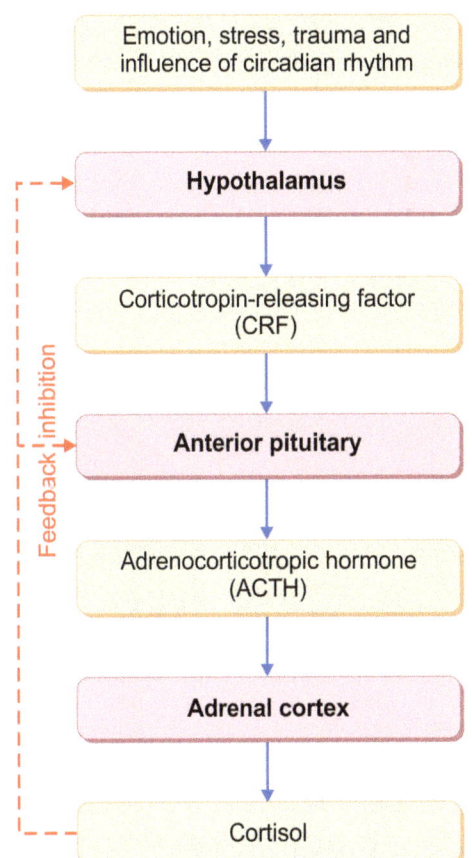

FIGURE 48.3: Regulation of cortisol secretion.

Androgens secreted by adrenal cortex are dehydroepiandrosterone, androstenedione and testosterone. Dehydroepiandrosterone is the most active adrenal androgen.

Androgens, are responsible for masculine features of the body (Chapter 51). But in normal conditions, the adrenal androgens have insignificant physiological effects, because of the low amount of secretion both in males and females.

■ APPLIED PHYSIOLOGY: DISORDERS OF ADRENAL CORTEX

■ HYPERACTIVITY OF ADRENAL CORTEX

Hypersecretion of adrenocortical hormones leads to:
1. Cushing's syndrome.
2. Hyperaldosteronism.
3. Adrenogenital syndrome.

■ 1. CUSHING'S SYNDROME

Cushing's syndrome is a disorder characterized by obesity **(Fig. 48.4)**.

Causes of Cushing's Syndrome

Cushing's syndrome is due to the hypersecretion of glucocorticoids, particularly cortisol. It may be either due to pituitary origin or adrenal origin. If it is due to pituitary origin, it is known as **Cushing's disease**. If it is due to adrenal origin, it is called **Cushing's syndrome**. Generally, these two terms are used interchangeably.

Cushing's disease by pituitary origin is due to increased secretion of ACTH. ACTH causes hyperplasia of adrenal cortex leading to hypersecretion of cortisol. Cushing's syndrome by adrenal origin is due to hypersecretion of cortisol by tumor or carcinoma in zona fasciculata of adrenal cortex.

Signs and Symptoms of Cushing's Syndrome

Signs and symptoms developed during Cushing's syndrome are listed in **Box 48.1**.

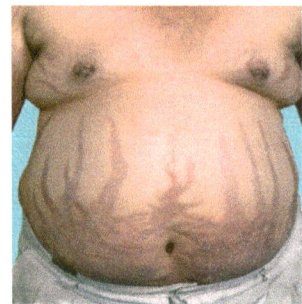
Pot belly with purple striae

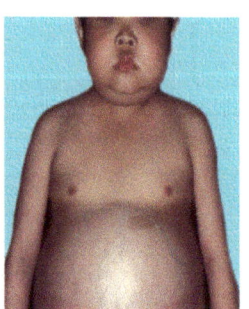
Fat deposition in upper abdomen, thorax and face (moon face) with thin hands

FIGURE 48.4: Cushing's syndrome.
(*Courtesy:* Prof Mafauzy Mohamed)

BOX 48.1: Signs and symptoms of Cushing's syndrome.

1. Abnormal features due to disproportionate distribution of fat
a. Moon face: Edematous facial appearance due to accumulation of fat and retention of water and salt
b. Torso: Fat accumulation in the chest and abdomen. Torso means trunk.
c. Buffalo hump: Fat deposit on the back of neck and shoulder
d. Pot belly: Fat accumulation in upper abdomen
2. Purple striae
Reddish purple stripes on abdomen due to:
a. Stretching of abdominal wall by excess subcutaneous fat
b. Rupture of subdermal tissues due to stretching
c. Deficiency of collagen fibers due to protein depletion
3. Thinning of extremities
Due to protein depletion
4. Thinning of skin and subcutaneous tissue
Due to protein depletion
5. Acanthosis
Skin disease characterized by dark patches in axilla, neck and groin
6. Pigmentation of skin
Due to melanocyte-stimulating effect of ACTH
7. Facial plethora
Redness of face
8. Hirsutism
Heavy growth of hair on body and face
9. Weakening of muscles
Because of protein depletion
10. Susceptibility of bone for fracture
Due to bone resorption and osteoporosis
11. Hyperglycemia and glucosuria
Due to gluconeogenesis and inhibition of peripheral utilization of glucose
In severe conditions adrenal diabetes develops
12. Hypertension
Caused by mineralocorticoid effects of glucocorticoids: Retention of sodium and water resulting in increase in ECF volume and blood volume
13. Susceptibility for infection
Due to immunosuppression
14. Poor wound healing
Prevention of wound healing due to hypersecretion of cortisol

Tests for Cushing's Syndrome

i. Observation of external features.
ii. Determination of blood sugar and cortisol levels.
iii. Analysis of urine for 17-hydroxysteroids.

2. HYPERALDOSTERONISM

Increased secretion of aldosterone is called hyperaldosteronism.

Types and Causes of Hyperaldosteronism

Depending upon the causes, hyperaldosteronism is classified into two types:

i. **Primary hyperaldosteronism** or **Conn's syndrome** occurs due to tumor in zona glomerulosa of adrenal cortex. In primary hyperaldosteronism, edema does not occur because of escape phenomenon (see above).
ii. **Secondary hyperaldosteronism** which occurs due to extra adrenal causes such as congestive cardiac failure toxemia of pregnancy and cirrhosis of liver.

Signs and Symptoms of Hyperaldosteronism

i. Increase in ECF volume and blood volume resulting in hypertension.
ii. Severe depletion of potassium causes renal damage. And kidneys fail to produce concentrated urine. This leads to polyuria and polydipsia.
iii. Muscular weakness due to potassium depletion.
iv. Metabolic alkalosis.

3. ADRENOGENITAL SYNDROME

Adrenogenital syndrome is a group of diseases caused by secretion of abnormal quantities of adrenal androgens.

Causes of Adrenogenital Syndrome

It is due to the tumor of zona reticularis in adrenal cortex.

Symptoms of Adrenogenital Syndrome

Adrenogenital syndrome is characterized by the tendency for the development of secondary sexual character of opposite sex.

In females, increased secretion of androgens causes development of male secondary sexual characters. The condition is called adrenal **virilism**. In males, the tumor of estrogen-secreting cells produces more than normal quantity of estrogens resulting in symptoms such as **feminization**, **gynecomastia** (enlargement of breast) and **atrophy of testes**.

HYPOACTIVITY OF ADRENAL CORTEX

Hyposecretion of adrenocortical hormones leads to the following conditions:
1. Addison's disease or chronic adrenal insufficiency.
2. Congenital adrenal hyperplasia.

1. ADDISON'S DISEASE OR CHRONIC ADRENAL INSUFFICIENCY

Addison's disease is an endocrine disorder caused by failure of adrenal cortex to secrete corticosteroids (**Box 48.2**).

Addison's disease is classified into three types:
i. Primary Addison's disease that occurs due to adrenal cause.

BOX 48.2: Disorders of adrenal cortex.

During hyperactivity
1. Cushing's syndrome
2. Hyperaldosteronism
3. Adrenogenital syndrome

During hypoactivity
1. Addison's disease
2. Congenital adrenal hyperplasia In boys: Macrogenitosomia praecox In girls: Virilism or pseudohermaphroditism

ii. Secondary Addison's disease which is due to failure of anterior pituitary to secrete ACTH.
iii. Tertiary Addison's disease which is due to failure of hypothalamus to secrete CRF.

Causes for Primary Addison's Disease

i. Atrophy or destruction of adrenal cortex.
ii. Malignancy of adrenal cortex.
iii. Congenital failure to secrete cortisol.

Signs and symptoms

Common signs and symptom are:
i. Pigmentation of skin and mucous membrane.
ii. Muscular weakness.
iii. Dehydration with loss of sodium.
iv. Hypotension.
v. Decrease in size of the heart.
vi. Hypoglycemia.
vii. Nausea, vomiting and diarrhea.
viii. Loss of body weight.
ix. Susceptibility to any type of infection.
x. Inability to withstand any stress resulting in Addisonian crisis (see below).

Addisonian Crisis or Adrenal Crisis or Acute Adrenal Insufficiency

It is a common symptom of Addison's disease characterized by sudden collapse associated with an increase in need for large quantities of glucocorticoids. The condition becomes fatal, if not treated in time.

2. CONGENITAL ADRENAL HYPERPLASIA

It is a congenital disorder characterized by increase in size of adrenal cortex resulting in hypersecretion of adrenal androgens.

Causes of Congenital Adrenal Hyperplasia

Even though the size of the gland increases, cortisol secretion decreases. It is because of congenital deficiency of enzymes necessary for the synthesis of cortisol called 21-hydroxylases.

Lack of this enzyme reduces the synthesis of cortisol. It in turn, increases the secretion of ACTH from pituitary by feedback mechanism. ACTH stimulates the adrenal cortex causing hyperplasia. Cortisol cannot be synthesized because of lack of 21-hydroxylase. Therefore, the secretion of androgens increases. It results in sexual abnormalities.

Symptoms of Congenital Adrenal Hyperplasia

Characteristic features of adrenal hyperplasia are virilism and excess body growth.

In boys

Adrenal hyperplasia produces a condition known as **macrogenitosomia praecox (Fig. 48.5)**.

Features of this condition are:
 i. Precocious body growth, causing stocky appearance called **infant Hercules**.
 ii. Precocious sexual development with enlarged penis even at age of 4 years.

In girls

In girls, adrenal hyperplasia produces **masculinization**. It is otherwise called **virilism**. In some cases of genetic disorders, the female child is born with external genitalia of male type. This condition is called **pseudohermaphroditism**.

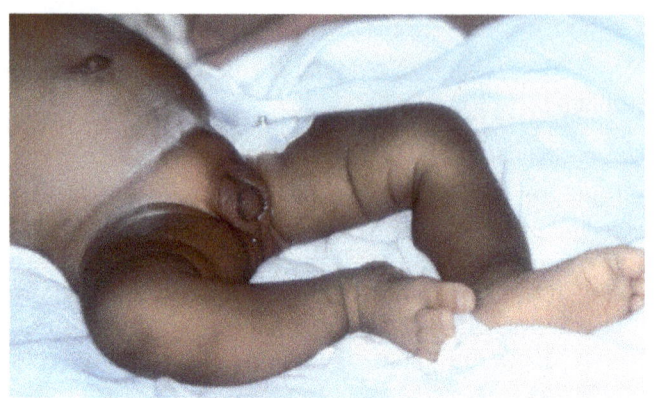

FIGURE 48.5: Congenital adrenal hyperplasia (macrogenitosomia praecox).
(*Courtesy:* Prof Mafauzy Mohamed)

Chapter 49: Adrenal Medulla

CHAPTER OUTLINE

- FUNCTIONAL HISTOLOGY OF ADRENAL MEDULLA
- HORMONES SECRETED BY ADRENAL MEDULLA
- SYNTHESIS OF CATECHOLAMINES
- ACTIONS OF ADRENALINE AND NORADRENALINE
- REGULATION OF SECRETION OF ADRENALINE AND NORADRENALINE
- DOPAMINE
- APPLIED PHYSIOLOGY: PHEOCHROMOCYTOMA

FUNCTIONAL HISTOLOGY OF ADRENAL MEDULLA

Medulla is the inner part of adrenal gland and it forms 20% of mass of adrenal gland. Adrenal medulla is made up of interlacing cords of cells known as **chromaffin cells** or **pheochrome cells**.

Chromaffin cells present adrenal medulla are of two types, adrenaline secreting cells (90%) and noradrenaline secreting cells (10%).

HORMONES SECRETED BY ADRENAL MEDULLA

Adrenal medullary hormones are the amines derived from catechol and so these hormones are called catecholamines.

Catecholamines secreted by adrenal medulla are:

1. Adrenaline or epinephrine.
2. Noradrenaline or norepinephrine.
3. Dopamine.

Plasma level of catecholamines

1. Adrenaline   : 3   µg/dL
2. Noradrenaline : 30   µg/dL
3. Dopamine   : 3.5 µg/dL

SYNTHESIS OF CATECHOLAMINES

Catecholamines are synthesized from amino acid **tyrosine** in the chromaffin cells of adrenal medulla. First dopamine is synthesized. Then noradrenaline is derived from dopamine. And finally, adrenaline is derived from noradrenaline.

ACTIONS OF ADRENALINE AND NORADRENALINE

Adrenaline and noradrenaline stimulate the nervous system. Adrenaline has significant effects on metabolic functions and both adrenaline and noradrenaline have significant effects on cardiovascular system.

MODE OF ACTION OF ADRENALINE AND NORADRENALINE: ADRENERGIC RECEPTORS

Actions of adrenaline and noradrenaline are executed by binding with receptors called adrenergic receptors which are present in the target organs.

Adrenergic receptors are of two types:

1. **Alpha-adrenergic receptors,** which are subdivided into alpha-1 and alpha-2 receptors.
2. **Beta-adrenergic receptors,** which are subdivided into beta-1 and beta-2 receptors.

ACTIONS OF ADRENALINE AND NORADRENALINE

Actions of adrenaline and noradrenaline on various target organs depend upon the type of receptors present in cells of the organs. Adrenaline acts through both alpha and beta receptors equally. Noradrenaline acts mainly through alpha receptors and occasionally through beta receptors.

1. Actions on Metabolism

Adrenaline influences the metabolic functions more than noradrenaline:

  i. *General metabolism:* Adrenaline increases oxygen consumption and carbon dioxide removal. It increases basal metabolic rate. So, it is said to be a **calorigenic hormone**.
  ii. *Carbohydrate metabolism:* Adrenaline increases the blood glucose level by increasing the glycogenolysis in liver and muscle.
  iii. *Fat metabolism:* Adrenaline causes mobilization of free fatty acids from adipose tissues. Catecholamines need the presence of glucocorticoids for this action.

2. Action on Blood

Adrenaline decreases blood coagulation time. It increases RBC count in blood by contracting smooth muscles of splenic capsule and releasing RBCs from spleen into circulation.

3. Action on Heart

Adrenaline has stronger effects on heart than noradrenaline. It increases overall activity of the heart, i.e.:

  i. Heart rate (chronotropic effect).
  ii. Force of contraction (inotropic effect).
  iii. Excitability of heart muscle (bathmotropic effect).
  iv. Conductivity in heart muscle (dromotropic effect).

4. Action on Blood Vessels

Noradrenaline has strong effects on blood vessels. It causes constriction of all blood vessels throughout the body. So, it is called '**General vasoconstrictor**'. Vasoconstrictor effect of noradrenaline increases total peripheral resistance.

Adrenaline also causes constriction of blood vessels. However, it causes dilatation of blood vessels in skeletal muscle, liver and heart through receptors. So, the total peripheral resistance is decreased by adrenaline.

5. Action on Blood Pressure

Adrenaline increases systolic blood pressure by increasing the force of contraction of the heart and cardiac output. But it decreases diastolic blood pressure by reducing the total peripheral resistance.

Noradrenaline increases diastolic pressure due to general vasoconstrictor effect by increasing the total peripheral resistance. It also increases the systolic blood pressure to a slight extent by its actions on heart. Action of catecholamines on blood pressure needs the presence of glucocorticoids.

6. Action on Respiration

Adrenaline increases rate and force of respiration. Adrenaline injection produces apnea, which is known as **adrenaline apnea**. It also causes **bronchodilation**.

7. Action on Skin

Adrenaline causes contraction of arrector pili. It also increases the secretion of sweat.

8. Action on Skeletal Muscle

Adrenaline causes severe contraction and quick fatigue of skeletal muscle. It increases glycogenolysis and release of glucose from muscle into blood. It also causes vasodilatation in skeletal muscles.

9. Action on Smooth Muscle

Catecholamines cause contraction of smooth muscles in the following organs:

  i. Splenic capsule.
  ii. Sphincters of GI tract.
  iii. Arrector pili of skin.
  iv. Gallbladder.
  v. Uterus.
  vi. Dilator pupillae of iris.

Catecholamines cause relaxation of smooth muscles in the following organs:

  i. Nonsphincteric part of GI tract (esophagus, stomach and intestine).
  ii. Bronchioles.
  iii. Urinary bladder.

10. Action on Central Nervous System

Adrenaline increases the activity of brain. Adrenaline secretion increases during **fight or flight reactions** after exposure to stress. It enhances the cortical arousal and other facilitatory functions of central nervous system.

11. Other Actions of Catecholamines

  i. On salivary glands: Cause mild increase in salivary secretion.
  ii. On sweat glands: Increase the secretion of apocrine sweat glands.
  iii. On lacrimal glands: Increase the secretion of tears.
  iv. On ACTH secretion: Adrenaline increases ACTH secretion.
  v. On nerve fibers: Adrenaline accelerates electrical activities in nerve fibers.
  vi. On renin secretion: Increase the secretion of renin from kidney.

■ REGULATION OF SECRETION OF ADRENALINE AND NORADRENALINE

Adrenaline and noradrenaline are secreted from adrenal medulla in small quantities even during rest. During stress conditions, due to sympathoadrenal discharge, a large quantity of catecholamines is secreted. These hormones prepare the body for fight or flight reactions.

Catecholamine secretion increases during exposure to cold and hypoglycemia also.

DOPAMINE

Dopamine is secreted by adrenal medulla. Dopamine is also secreted by **dopaminergic neurons** in some areas of brain particularly, **basal ganglia**. In brain, this hormone acts as a neurotransmitter.

Injected dopamine produces following effects:

1. Vasoconstriction by releasing norepinephrine.
2. Vasodilatation in mesentery.
3. Increase in heart rate.
4. Increase in systolic blood pressure. Dopamine does not affect diastolic blood pressure.

Deficiency of dopamine in basal ganglia produces nervous disorder called Parkinsonism (Chapter 86).

APPLIED PHYSIOLOGY: PHEOCHROMOCYTOMA

Pheochromocytoma is a condition characterized by hypersecretion of catecholamines.

Cause of Pheochromocytoma

Pheochromocytoma is caused by tumor of pheochrome cells in adrenal medulla. It is also caused rarely by tumor of sympathetic ganglia (**extra-adrenal pheochromocytoma**).

Signs and Symptoms of Pheochromocytoma

Characteristic feature of pheochromocytoma is hypertension. This type of hypertension is known as endocrine or **secondary hypertension**.

Other common features of pheochromocytoma:
1. Chest pain.
2. Palpitation and tachycardia.
3. Fever.
4. Headache.
5. Metabolic disorders.
6. Nausea and vomiting.
7. Sweating and flushing.
8. Weight loss.

Chapter 50: Endocrine Functions of Other Organs and Local Hormones

CHAPTER OUTLINE

- **PINEAL GLAND**
  - SITUATION AND STRUCTURE
  - FUNCTIONS
- **THYMUS**
  - SITUATION AND STRUCTURE
  - FUNCTIONS
- **KIDNEYS**
  - ERYTHROPOIETIN
  - THROMBOPOIETIN
  - RENIN
  - 1,25-DIHYDROXYCHOLECALCIFEROL: CALCITRIOL
- **PROSTAGLANDINS**
- **HEART**
  - ATRIAL NATRIURETIC PEPTIDE
  - BRAIN NATRIURETIC PEPTIDE
  - C-TYPE NATRIURETIC PEPTIDE
- **LOCAL HORMONES**
  - LOCAL HORMONES SYNTHESIZED IN TISSUES
  - LOCAL HORMONES SYNTHESIZED IN BLOOD

PINEAL GLAND

SITUATION AND STRUCTURE OF PINEAL GLAND

Pineal gland or **epiphysis of cerebri** is a small cone-shaped gland located in diencephalic area of brain above the hypothalamus. It is about 10 mm long.

Pineal gland has two types of cells, the parenchymal epithelial cells and neuroglial cells. In adults, the pineal gland is **calcified**. But the **parenchymal cells** exist and secrete the hormonal substance.

FUNCTIONS OF PINEAL GLAND

Pineal gland controls the sexual activities in animals. But it plays little role in regulating the sexual functions in human being. Pineal gland secretes a hormonal substance called melatonin.

Melatonin

Melatonin is secreted by parenchymal cells of pineal gland. It is an **indole** (N-acetyl-5-methoxytryptamine).

Actions of Melatonin

Melatonin inhibits the onset of puberty by inhibiting the gonads.

Diurnal variation in melatonin secretion

Melatonin secretion is more in darkness than in daylight. Secretion of melatonin varies according to activities in different periods of the day, i.e. **circadian rhythm**. Hypothalamus is responsible for the circadian fluctuations of melatonin secretion.

THYMUS

SITUATION AND STRUCTURE OF THYMUS

It is situated in front of trachea below the thyroid gland. Thymus is small in newborn infants and gradually enlarges till puberty, and then decreases in size.

Thymus is formed by two **lobes**. Each lobe is divided into many **lobules**. Each lobule has two layers of structures namely outer cortex and inner medulla.

Cortex consists of large number of T lymphocytes and supporting reticular cells. **Medulla** contains large number of reticular cells and a smaller number of T lymphocytes.

FUNCTIONS OF THYMUS

Thymus has lymphoid function and endocrine function. It is responsible for development of immunity in the body. Thymus has two functions:

1. Processing of T Lymphocytes

Lymphocytes, produced in bone marrow, are processed in thymus into T lymphocytes.

2. Endocrine Function of Thymus

Thymus secretes two hormones:

i. Thymosin

Thymosin is a peptide. It accelerates lymphopoiesis and proliferation of T lymphocytes.

ii. Thymin or thymopoietin

It suppresses the neuromuscular activity by inhibiting acetylcholine release.

Hyperactivity of thymus causes **myasthenia gravis**.

KIDNEYS

Kidneys secrete five hormonal substances:

1. Erythropoietin.
2. Thrombopoietin.
3. Renin.
4. 1,25-dihydroxycholecalciferol (calcitriol).
5. Prostaglandins.

Recently, it is discovered that kidney secretes small quantity of C-type natriuretic peptide (see below).

1. ERYTHROPOIETIN

Erythropoietin is secreted by endothelial cells of peritubular capillaries in the kidney. It is a glycoprotein with 165 amino acids. Erythropoietin stimulates the bone marrow and causes erythropoiesis. Details are given in Chapter 8.

2. THROMBOPOIETIN

Thrombopoietin is a glycoprotein. It is secreted by kidneys and liver. It stimulates production of platelets.

3. RENIN

Renin is secreted by granular cells of juxtaglomerular apparatus of the kidney.

Actions of Renin

Renin converts angiotensinogen into angiotensin I which is in turn converted into angiotensin II. Details of renin and angiotensin II are given in Chapter 34.

4. 1,25-DIHYDROXYCHOLECALCIFEROL: CALCITRIOL

In kidney, 1,25-dihydroxycholecalciferol or **calcitriol** or **activated vitamin D** is formed from **cholecalciferol** (vitamin D_3) (Chapter 46).

Action of 1,25-dihydroxycholecalciferol

Activated vitamin D help in maintenance of blood calcium level by accelerating absorption of calcium from intestine into the blood. Details are given in Chapter 46.

5. PROSTAGLANDINS

Prostaglandins PGA_2 and PGE_2 are secreted by juxtaglomerular cells and type I interstitial cells present in medulla of kidney. Prostaglandins decrease the blood pressure by systemic vasodilatation (see below).

HEART

Heart secretes three hormones.

1. ATRIAL NATRIURETIC PEPTIDE

Atrial natriuretic peptide (ANP) is a polypeptide with 28 amino acids. It is secreted by atrial musculature of the heart. It is found in hypothalamus of brain also.

Actions of Atrial Natriuretic Peptide

ANP increases excretion of sodium ions through urine. It is also involved in escape phenomenon. Refer Chapter 48 for details. ANP decreases the blood pressure by vasodilatation and by inhibiting vasoconstrictor effect of angiotensin II and catecholamines.

2. BRAIN NATRIURETIC PEPTIDE

Brain natriuretic peptide (BNP) or **B-type natriuretic peptide**. It is a polypeptide with 32 amino acids. It is secreted by the cardiac muscle and some parts of brain. BNP has same actions of ANP (see above). Its actions on brain are not known.

3. C-TYPE NATRIURETIC PEPTIDE

C-type natriuretic peptide (CNP) is a peptide hormone with 22 amino acid. It is secreted in myocardium, blood vessels, gastrointestinal tract, kidneys and brain. It has similar action of atrial natriuretic peptide.

LOCAL HORMONES

Local hormones are the substances which act on same area of their secretion or in immediate neighborhood.

Local hormones are classified into two types:

I. Hormones synthesized in tissues.
II. Hormones synthesized in blood.

LOCAL HORMONES SYNTHESIZED IN TISSUES

Local hormones synthesized in the tissues are of two types, prostaglandins and its related substances and other local hormones.

Prostaglandins and Its Related Hormones: Eicosanoids

Prostaglandins and other hormones which are derived from arachidonic acid are collectively called **eicosanoids**.

Eicosanoids are five types:

1. Prostaglandins.
2. Thromboxanes.

3. Prostacyclin.
4. Leukotrienes.
5. Lipoxins.

1. Prostaglandins

Prostaglandins were first discovered in human **semen**. But almost all tissues of the body synthesize prostaglandins. Prostaglandins are unsaturated fatty acids with a cyclopentane ring and 20 carbon atoms.

Types of prostaglandins

A variety of prostaglandins are identified. Active forms of prostaglandins are PGA_2, PGD_2, PGE_2, and PGF_2.

Actions of prostaglandins

i. *Action on blood:* Prostaglandins accelerate the capacity of RBCs to pass through minute blood vessels.
ii. *Action on blood vessels:* PGE_2 causes **vasodilatation**.
iii. *Action on GI tract:* Prostaglandins reduce gastric secretion.
iv. *Action on respiratory system:* PGE_2 causes **bronchodilatation**.
v. *Action on lipids:* Prostaglandins inhibit the release of free fatty acids from adipose tissue.
vi. *Action on nervous system:* Prostaglandins control or alter the actions of neurotransmitters.
vii. *Action on kidney:* Prostaglandins stimulate juxtaglomerular apparatus and enhance the secretion of renin.
viii. *Action on reproduction:*
   a. Prostaglandins cause degeneration of corpus luteum **(luteolysis)**.
   b. Prostaglandins increase the receptive capacity of cervical mucosa for sperms.
   c. Prostaglandins cause **reverse peristaltic movement** of uterus and fallopian tubes during coitus. This in turn, increases the velocity of sperm transport in female genital tract.
   d. Prostaglandins (PGE_2) facilitate **labor** by increasing the force of uterine contractions.

2. Thromboxanes

Thromboxanes are derived from **arachidonic acid**.

Thromboxanes are of two types, thromboxane A_2 which is secreted in platelets and thromboxane B_2 the metabolite of thromboxane A_2. Thromboxane A_2 causes vasoconstriction. It accelerates platelets aggregation during **hemostasis**. It also accelerates the clot formation.

3. Prostacyclin

Prostacyclin is also a derivative of arachidonic acid. It is produced in the endothelial cells and smooth muscle cells of blood vessels. Prostacyclin causes vasodilatation and inhibits platelet aggregation.

4. Leukotrienes

Leukotrienes are derived from arachidonic acid via 5-hydroperoxyeicosatetraenoic acid (5-HETE). Leukotrienes are the mediators of allergic responses.

These hormones also promote inflammatory reactions. Release of leukotrienes increases when some allergic agents combine with antibodies like IgE.

Leukotrienes cause bronchiolar constriction, arteriolar constriction, vascular permeability and attraction of neutrophils and eosinophils towards the site of inflammation.

5. Lipoxins

Lipoxins are also derived from arachidonic acid via 15-hydroperoxyeicosatetraenoic acid (15-HETE). Lipoxins are of two types namely, Lipoxin A and Lipoxin B.

Lipoxin A causes dilation of minute blood vessels. Both the types inhibit the cytotoxic effects of killer T cells.

■ OTHER LOCAL HORMONES SYNTHESIZED IN TISSUES

In addition to prostaglandins and related hormonal substances, tissues secrete some more hormones which are given listed below:

1. Acetylcholine

Acetylcholine is the **cholinergic neurotransmitter**. It is the transmitter substance at neuromuscular junction. It is also secreted by other nerve endings and other cells.

Source of secretion of acetylcholine

i. Presynaptic terminals.
ii. Preganglionic parasympathetic nerve.
iii. Postganglionic parasympathetic nerve.
iv. Preganglionic sympathetic nerve.
v. Postganglionic sympathetic cholinergic nerves, such as nerves supplying eccrine sweat glands and sympathetic vasodilator nerves in skeletal muscle.
vi. Nerves in amacrine cells of retina.
vii. Mast cell.
viii. Gastric mucosa.
ix. Lungs.
x. Many regions of brain.

Actions of acetylcholine

Acetylcholine:
i. Is an **excitatory neurotransmitter**.
ii. Produces excitatory function of synapse by opening the sodium channels.
iii. Activates smooth muscles in GI tract and urinary tract.
vi. Activates skeletal muscles.
v. Inhibits cardiac function.
vi. Causes dilatation of blood vessels.

Destruction of acetylcholine

Acetylcholine is very quick in action. Immediately after executing the action, it is destroyed by acetylcholinesterase. This enzyme is present in basal lamina of the synaptic cleft.

2. Serotonin

Serotonin or as 5-hydroxytryptamine is secreted in CNS, retina, GI tract lungs and platelets.

Actions of serotonin

i. Serotonin is an **inhibitory neurotransmitter**.
ii. It inhibits impulses of pain sensation in posterior gray horn of spinal cord.
iii. It causes mood depression and induces sleep (Chapter 89).
iv. It also causes vasoconstriction.

3. Histamine

Histamine is secreted in nerve endings of hypothalamus, limbic cortex and other parts of cerebral cortex, spinal cord and gastrointestinal tract. Histamine is also released from tissues during allergic condition, inflammation or damage.

Actions of histamine

i. It is an **excitatory neurotransmitter**.
ii. Histamine released from tissues causes vasodilatation and enhances the capillary permeability for fluid and plasma proteins from blood into the affected tissues. So, the accumulation of fluid with proteins develops local edema.
iii. In GI tract, histamine increases the motility.

4. Substance P

Substance P is secreted in nerve endings (first order neurons of pain pathway) in spinal cord and in retina.

It is also secreted in GI tract.

Actions of substance P

Substance P is the neurotransmitter for pain sensation. is also the neurotransmitter substance in GI tract. In GI tract, it increases the mixing and propulsive movements of small intestine.

5. Heparin

Heparin is secreted by mast cells and basophils.

Actions of heparin

Heparin is a naturally produced anticoagulant. Refer Chapter 15 for other details.

6. Leptin

Leptin is a protein hormone with 167 amino acids and it is secreted by adipocytes in adipose tissues.

Actions of leptin

Leptin controls **food intake** and **adipose tissue**. It acts on hypothalamus and inhibits the feeding center resulting in stoppage of food intake (Chapter 84). Thus, leptin is responsible for control of food intake and body weight.

7. Gastrointestinal Hormones

i. Gastrin (Chapter 27).
ii. Secretin (Chapter 28).
iii. Cholecystokinin (Chapter 28).
iv. Gastric inhibitory peptide (GIP) (Chapter 27).
v. Vasoactive intestinal polypeptide (VIP) (Chapter 27).
vi. Pancreatic polypeptide (Chapter 28).
vii. Somatostatin (Chapter 28).
viii. Peptide YY (Chapter 28).

■ LOCAL HORMONES SYNTHESIZED IN BLOOD

Local hormones produced in the blood are:

1. Serotonin.
2. Angiotensinogen.
3. Kinins.

Serotonin is described above. Angiotensinogen is explained in Chapter 34.

Kinins are protein hormones circulating in blood. Kinins dilate blood vessels and decreases the blood pressure and increase blood flow throughout the body. Kinins also increase permeability of capillaries during inflammatory conditions resulting in edema in the affected area.

MODEL QUESTIONS IN ENDOCRINOLOGY

■ LONG QUESTIONS

1. Enumerate the hormones secreted by pituitary gland. Describe actions and regulation of secretion of growth hormone. Write in brief about effects of hypersecretion of anterior pituitary gland.
2. Describe the synthesis, storage, release, transport, functions and regulation of secretion of thyroid hormones.
3. Explain the functions and regulation of secretion of parathormone. Add a note on the disorders of parathormone secretion.
4. List the hormones secreted by pancreas. Explain functions and regulation of secretion of insulin.
5. Describe in detail the regulation of blood sugar level.
6. Classify the hormones secreted by adrenal cortex. Explain actions and regulation of secretion of cortisol.
7. Enumerate the corticosteroids. Describe actions and regulation of secretion of aldosterone.
8. What are catecholamines? Explain the synthesis, metabolism, actions and regulation of secretion of catecholamines.

■ SHORT QUESTIONS

1. Growth hormone.
2. Thyroid stimulating hormone.
3. Adrenocorticotropic hormone.
4. Oxytocin.
5. Antidiuretic hormone.
6. Milk ejection/neuroendocrine reflex.
7. Gigantism.
8. Dwarfism.
9. Disorders of posterior pituitary gland.
10. Thyroxine.
11. Hyperthyroidism/hypothyroidism.
12. Goiter.
13. Cretinism.
14. Myxedema.
15. Parathormone.
16. Tetany.
17. Hypercalcemia/hypocalcemia.
18. Insulin.
19. Glucagon.
20. Diabetes mellitus.
21. Hyperinsulinism.
22. Cortisol.
23. Aldosterone.
24. Cushing's syndrome or disease.
25. Hyperaldosteronism.
26. Adrenogenital syndrome.
27. Addison's disease.
28. Actions of catecholamines.
29. Prostaglandins.
30. Acetylcholine.

■ VERY SHORT ANSWER QUESTIONS

1. Any hormone.
2. Any endocrine disorder.
3. Cell-to-cell signaling.
4. Define classical hormone, neurotransmitter and neurohormone. Give examples.
5. Classify classical hormone.
6. Hormonal receptors.
7. Cyclic AMP.
8. Hypothalamo-hypophyseal relationship.
9. Parts and cell types in anterior pituitary. Name the hormone secreted by each cell type.
10. Feedback control of regulation GH secretion.
11. Diabetogenic effect of growth hormone.
12. Role of osmoreceptors in regulations of ADH secretion.
13. Acromegaly/acromegalic gigantism.
14. Acromicria.
15. Simmond's disease.
16. Fröhlich's syndrome.
17. Diabetes insipidus.
18. Thyroglobuilin.
19. Exophthalmos.
20. Carpopedal spasm.
21. Trousseau's sign and Chvostek's sign.
22. Importance of calcium.
23. Effect of parathormone and calcitonin on blood calcium level.
24. Osteoporosis.
25. Rickets.
26. Cells of islets of Langerhans and their secretions.
27. Somatostatin.
28. Pancreatic polypeptide.
29. Complications of prolonged diabetes mellitus.
30. Aldosterone escape.
31. Action of ACTH on adrenal cortex.
32. Adrenal androgens.
33. Dopamine.
34. Pheochromocytoma.
35. Functions of pineal gland.
36. Functions of thymus.
37. Endocrine function of heart.
38. Serotonin.
39. Histamine.
40. Substance P.

SECTION 7 REPRODUCTIVE SYSTEM

CHAPTER 51

Male Reproductive System

CHAPTER OUTLINE

- REPRODUCTIVE SYSTEM
- MALE REPRODUCTIVE ORGANS
- FUNCTIONAL ANATOMY OF TESTES
- ACCESSORY SEX ORGANS IN MALES
- FUNCTIONS OF TESTIS
- GAMETOGENIC FUNCTIONS OF TESTIS: SPERMATOGENESIS
- ENDOCRINE FUNCTIONS OF TESTIS
- SEMEN
- MALE CLIMACTERIC
- APPLIED PHYSIOLOGY

■ REPRODUCTIVE SYSTEM

Reproductive system ensures the continuation of species. **Gonads** are the primary reproductive organs which produce the gametes. Gametes are the sperms and ova. Sperms are produced in males by a pair of testes. And, ova are produced in females by a pair of ovaries.

Normally, most of the animals including humans are either definite males or definite females. However, in some organisms like earthworms and snails, both sexes may be present in the same organism and this condition is known as **hermaphroditism**.

In humans and most of the higher animals, reproduction occurs sexually, i.e. by mating. However, there are some species like insects which can produce offspring without mating.

■ MALE REPRODUCTIVE ORGANS

Male reproductive organs include **primary sex organs** and **accessory sex organs**. Testes are the primary sex organs or gonads in males.

Accessory sex organs in males are seminal vesicles, prostate gland, urethra and penis. See below for details of accessory sex organs in males.

■ FUNCTIONAL ANATOMY OF TESTES

There are two testes in almost all the species (singular = **testis**). Testes are ovoid or walnut-shaped bodies located in the sac-like structure called **scrotum** (Fig. 51.1).

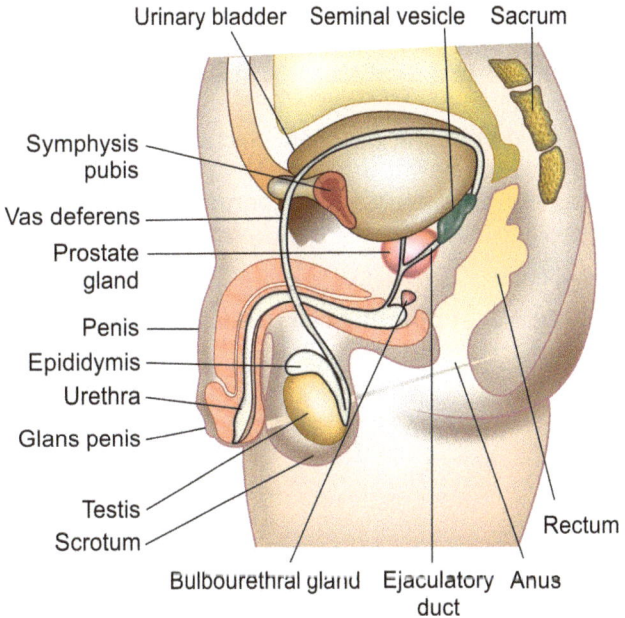

FIGURE 51.1: Male reproductive system and other organs of pelvis.

■ COVERINGS OF TESTIS

Each testis is enclosed by three coverings:

1. *Tunica vasculosa*: Tunica vasculosa is the innermost covering of testis. It is made up of connective tissue. And it is rich in blood vessels.
2. *Tunica albuginea*: This is the middle covering and it is a dense fibrous capsule.

3. *Tunica vaginalis*: Tunica vaginalis is the outermost covering formed by visceral and parietal layers.

■ PARENCHYMA OF TESTIS

Lobules of Testis

Tunica albuginea on the posterior surface of testis is thickened to form **mediastinum testis**. From this, a **septula testis** radiates into testis and bind with tunica albuginea at various points. Because of this, testis is divided into a number of **pyramidal lobules (Fig. 51.2)**.

Each testis has about 200 to 300 lobules. Each lobule contains 1 to 4 coiled tubules known as the seminiferous tubules.

Seminiferous Tubules

Seminiferous tubules are thread-like convoluted tubular structures in which the spermatozoa or sperms are produced. There are about 400 to 600 seminiferous tubules in each testis. Length of each seminiferous tubule is between 30 cm and 70 cm. Its diameter is between 150 μ and 300 μ.

Epithelium of seminiferous tubules consists of two types of cells, namely, spermatogenic cells or germ cells and Sertoli cells or supporting cells.

Spermatogenic cells

Spermatogenic cells or **germ cells** present in seminiferous tubules are the precursor cells of spermatozoa. These cells lie in between Sertoli cells. Spermatogenic cells are attached to Sertoli cells by means of cytoplasmic connection.

In children, spermatogenic cells are in the primitive stage called **spermatogonia**. With onset of puberty, spermatogonia develop into sperms through different stages.

Sertoli cells

Sertoli cells or **supporting cells** are large and tall irregular columnar cells.

Functions of Sertoli cells

Sertoli cells:
1. Support and nourish the spermatogenic cells till spermatozoa are released from them.
2. Secretes the enzyme **aromatase** which converts androgens into estrogen.
3. Secrete **androgen-binding protein (ABP)** which is essential for testosterone activity particularly in spermatogenesis.
4. Secrete **estrogen-binding protein (EBP)**.
5. Secrete **inhibin** which inhibits the release of follicle stimulating hormone (FSH) from anterior pituitary.
6. Secrete **activin** which increases FSH release.
7. Secrete **Müllerian regression factor (MRF)** in fetal testes. MRF is also called **Müllerian inhibiting substance (MIS)**. MRF is responsible for the regression of Müllerian duct during sex differentiation in fetus (see below).
8. Tight junctions between Sertoli cells form blood-testis barrier.

Blood-Testis Barrier

Blood-testis barrier is a mechanical barrier that separates blood from seminiferous tubules of the testes. It is formed by **tight junctions** between the adjacent Sertoli cells near the basal membrane of seminiferous tubule.

Blood-testis barrier protects the seminiferous tubules and spermatogenic cells by preventing the entry of toxic substances from blood into testis. At the same time, it permits nutritive and other essential substances necessary for spermatogenic cells.

Rete Testis, Vas Efferens, Epididymis and Vas Deferens

Each seminiferous lobule opens into a network of thin walled channels called the rete testis. From rete testis, 8 to 15 tubules called vas efferens arise. Vas efferens join together and form the **head of epididymis** and then converge to form **duct of epididymis**.

Duct of epididymis is an enormously convoluted tubule with a length of about 4 meters. It begins at head, where it receives vas efferens. At the caudal pole of testis, epididymis turns sharply upon itself and continues as vas deferens without any definite demarcation.

Interstitial Cells of Leydig

Interstitial cells of Leydig are the hormone secreting cells in testes. These cells are situated in between the seminiferous tubules.

■ ACCESSORY SEX ORGANS IN MALES
■ SEMINAL VESICLES

Seminal vesicles are paired glands situated in lower abdomen on either side of the prostate gland behind urinary bladder. Each seminal vesicle is a hollow sac of irregular shape. It is lined by complexly folded mucous membrane which secretes seminal fluid.

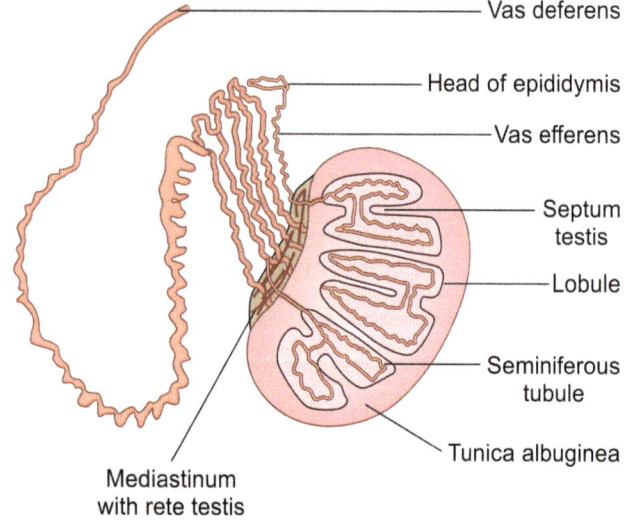

FIGURE 51.2: Structure of testis.

Seminal Fluid

Seminal fluid from each seminal vesicle is added to semen in the **ejaculatory duct** through **ampulla of vas deferens**. Ejaculatory duct opens into urethra.

Seminal fluid is mucoid and viscous in nature. It is neutral or slightly alkaline in reaction. It adds to the bulk of semen as it forms 60% of total semen. Seminal vesicles secrete several important substances. Refer Figure 51.5 for the products secreted by seminal vesicles.

Functions of Seminal Fluid

1. Nutrition to sperms

Fructose and other nutritive substances present in seminal fluid are utilized by sperms after being ejaculated into female genital tract.

2. Clotting of semen

As soon as semen is ejaculated it is clotted because of conversion of **fibrinogen** of seminal fluid into **fibrin**. Clotting of semen is essential for holding the sperms in uterine cervix.

3. On fertilization

Prostaglandin of seminal fluid enhances fertilization of ovum by the following processes:

i. Increasing the receptive capacity of cervical mucosa for sperms.
ii. Causing **reverse peristalsis** in uterus and fallopian tubes. This, in turn, facilitates the transport of sperms through female genital tract during coitus.

PROSTATE GLAND

Prostate gland weighs about 40 g. It is formed by 20 to 30 separate secretory glands, which open separately into the urethra. Prostate secretes prostatic fluid.

Prostatic Fluid

Prostatic fluid is a thin, milky and alkaline fluid. It forms 30% of total semen. Refer Figure 51.5 for the products secreted by prostate gland.

Functions of Prostatic Fluid

1. Maintenance of sperm motility

Prostatic fluid provides optimum pH for the motility of sperms. Sperms are nonmotile at a pH of less than 6.0. Vaginal secretions in females are highly acidic with a pH of 3.5 to 4.0.

Prostatic secretion neutralizes the acidity and maintains a pH of 6.0 to 6.5. At this pH, the sperms become motile and the chances of fertilization are enhanced.

2. Clotting of semen

Clotting enzymes present in prostatic fluid convert fibrinogen (from seminal vesicles) into clot.

3. Lysis of clot

The clot is dissolved by fibrinolysin of the prostatic fluid so that, the sperms become motile.

URETHRA

Male urethra is about 20 cm long. After origin from bladder it traverses the prostate gland, which lies below the bladder and then runs through the penis. Ejaculatory duct opens into urethra. Other details of urethra are given in Chapter 40.

Internal urethra passes through penis as **external urethra**. Urethra contains mucus glands throughout its length, which are called **glands of Littre**. Bilateral **bulbo-urethral glands** also open into the urethra.

PENIS

Penis is the male genital organ. Urethra passes through penis and opens to the exterior. Penis is formed by three erectile tissue masses, i.e. a paired **corpora cavernosa** and an unpaired **corpus spongiosum**. Corpus spongiosum surrounds the urethra and terminates distally to form **glans penis**.

FUNCTIONS OF TESTIS

Testis performs two functions:

1. Gametogenic function by which gametes are produced in gonads.
2. Endocrine function by which male sex hormones are secreted.

GAMETOGENIC FUNCTIONS OF TESTIS: SPERMATOGENESIS

Spermatogenesis is the process by which male gametes called **spermatozoa** (sperms) are formed from spermatogonia (primitive spermatogenic cells) in the testis **(Fig. 51.3)**. It takes 74 days for the formation of sperm from a spermatogonia.

STAGES OF SPERMATOGENESIS

Spermatogenesis occurs in four stages:

1. Stage of Proliferation

Each spermatogonium contains diploid number (23 pairs) of chromosomes. One member of each pair is derived from mother and the other one from father. The 23 pairs include 22 pairs of autosomal chromosomes and one pair of sex chromosomes. Sex chromosomes are one X chromosome and one Y chromosome.

During the proliferative stage, **spermatogonia** divide by mitosis without any change in chromosomal number. In man, there are usually seven generations of spermatogonia. Spermatogonia migrate along with Sertoli cells towards the lumen of seminiferous tubule.

Last generation of spermatogonia enters the stage of growth as **primary spermatocyte**.

2. Stage of Growth

Primary spermatocyte grows into a large cell in this stage. And there is no other change in spermatocyte during this stage.

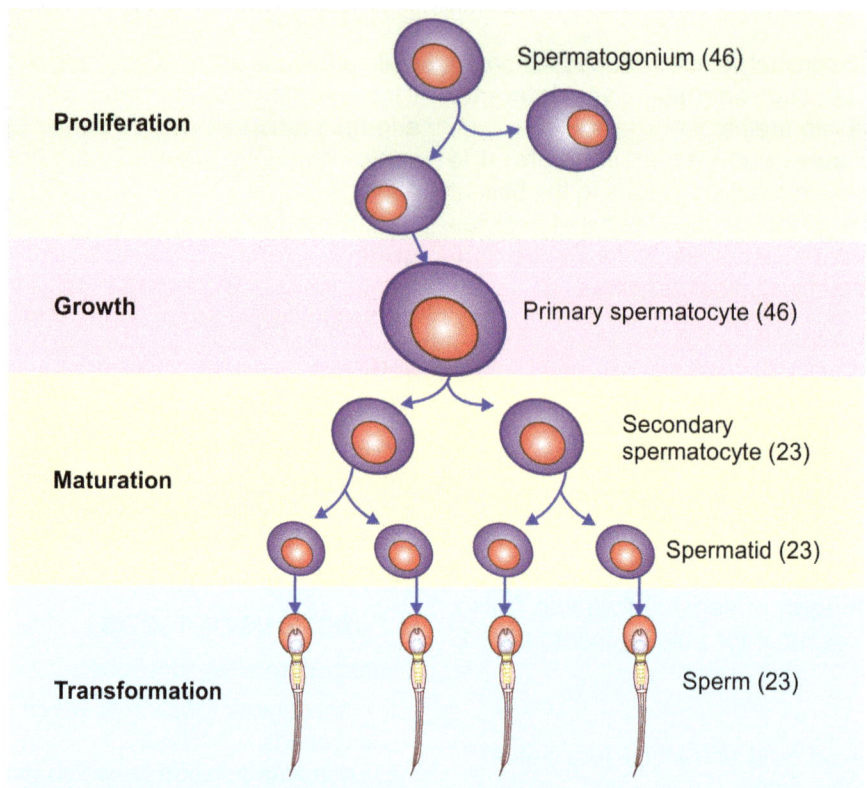

FIGURE 51.3: Spermatogenesis. Number in parenthesis indicates chromosomal number.

3. Stage of Maturation

After reaching the full size, each primary spermatocyte quickly undergoes meiotic or maturation division, which occurs in two phases. In the first phase each primary spermatocyte divides into two **secondary spermatocytes**. Each secondary spermatocyte receives only haploid or half the number of chromosomes. Total of 23 chromosomes include 22 autosomes and one X or Y chromosome.

During the second phase, each secondary spermatocyte undergoes second meiotic division resulting in two smaller cells called **spermatids**. Each spermatid has haploid number of chromosomes.

4. Stage of Transformation

Spermatids are transformed into **matured spermatozoa** (sperms). Transformation occurs in two stages.

i. Spermiogenesis

Spermiogeneis is the process by which spermatids become matured spermatozoa.

Changes taking place during spermiogenesis are:

a. Condensation of nuclear material.
b. Formation of acrosome, mitochondrial spiral filament and tail structures.
c. Removal of unwanted quantity of cytoplasm.

ii. Spermiation

Spermiation is the process by which the matured sperms are released from Sertoli cells into the lumen of seminiferous tubules. Structure of sperm is explained later in this chapter.

ROLE OF SERTOLI CELLS IN SPERMATOGENESIS

Sertoli cells influence spermatogenesis by many ways (see above).

ROLE OF HORMONES IN SPERMATOGENESIS

Spermatogenesis is influenced by many hormones which act either directly or indirectly.

Hormones necessary for spermatogenesis are:

1. Follicle Stimulating Hormone

FSH is responsible for the initiation of spermatogenesis. It binds with Sertoli cells and spermatogonia and induces the proliferation of spermatogonia **(Table 51.1)**.

2. Luteinizing Hormone

In males this hormone is called **interstitial cell stimulating hormone**. It is essential for the secretion of testosterone from Leydig cells.

3. Growth Hormone

Growth hormone is essential for the general metabolic processes in testis. It is also necessary for proliferation of spermatogonia.

4. Testosterone

Testosterone is responsible for sequence of later stages in spermatogenesis. It is also responsible for maintenance of spermatogenesis.

TABLE 51.1: Hormones necessary for spermatogenesis.

Stage of spermatogenesis	Hormones necessary
Stage of proliferation	• Follicle-stimulating hormone • Growth hormone
Stage of growth	• Testosterone • Growth hormone
Stage of maturation	• Testosterone • Growth hormone
Stage of transformation	• Testosterone • Estrogen

5. Estrogen

Estrogen is formed from testosterone in Sertoli cells. It is necessary for spermiogenesis.

6. Inhibin

Inhibin is a peptide hormone and serves as a transforming growth factor. It is secreted by Sertoli cells. In females, it is secreted by granulosa cells of ovarian follicles. Its secretion is stimulated by FSH. Inhibin inhibits FSH secretion through feedback mechanism leading to decrease in the pace of spermatogenesis.

7. Activin

It is also a peptide hormone secreted in gonads by Sertoli cells and Leydig cells. Activin has opposite actions of inhibin. It increases secretion of FSH and accelerates spermatogenesis.

■ OTHER FACTORS AFFECTING SPERMATOGENESIS

1. Increase in the body temperature prevents spermatogenesis. It occurs in cryptorchidism (see below). Normally, temperature in the scrotum is about 2°C less than the body temperature. But in cryptorchidism the testes are in the abdomen where the temperature is always higher than that of scrotum. Increase in temperature stops spermatogenesis.
2. Infectious diseases such as mumps cause degeneration of seminiferous tubules and absence of spermatogenesis.

■ ENDOCRINE FUNCTIONS OF TESTIS

Testis secretes **male sex hormones** which are collectively called the **androgens**. Androgens secreted by testis are testosterone, dihydrotestosterone and androstenedione. Androgens are secreted in large quantities by interstitial cells of Leydig in testes and in small quantity by zona reticularis in adrenal cortex.

Androgens are steroid hormones synthesized from cholesterol or acetate. Testosterone is a C19 steroid. The plasma level of testosterone in an adult male varies between 300 ng/dL and 700 ng/dL. In adult female the testosterone level is 30 mg/dL to 60 mg/dL.

■ TESTOSTERONE SECRETION IN DIFFERENT PERIODS OF LIFE

Testosterone is secreted in fetus by **genital ridge**. In childhood, no testosterone is secreted until 10 to 12 years of age. Afterwards, testosterone secretion starts and, it increases rapidly at the onset of puberty and lasts through most of the remaining part of life. Testosterone secretion starts decreasing after 40 years and becomes almost zero by the age of 90 years.

■ FUNCTIONS OF TESTOSTERONE IN FETAL LIFE

Fetal testes begin to secrete testosterone at about 2nd to 4th month of fetal life. Testosterone performs **three functions** in fetus:

1. Sex Differentiation in Fetus

Testosterone is responsible for the sex differentiation of fetus.

Fetus has two genital ducts:

  i. **Müllerian duct** which gives rise to female accessory sex organs such as vagina, uterus and fallopian tube.
  ii. **Wolffian duct** which gives rise to male accessory sex organs such as epididymis, vas deferens and seminal vesicles.

If testosterone is secreted from the **genital ridge** of the fetus at about 7th week of intrauterine life, the Müllerian duct system disappears and male sex organs develop from Wolffian duct. In addition to testosterone, **Müllerian regression factor (MRF)** secreted by Sertoli cells is also responsible for regression of Müllerian duct.

In the absence of testosterone, Wolffian duct regresses and female sex organs develop from Müllerian duct.

2. Development of Accessory Sex Organs and External Genitalia

Testosterone is also essential for the growth of the external genitalia viz. penis and scrotum and other accessory sex organs namely genital ducts, seminal vesicles and prostate.

3. Descent of Testes

Testes which are developed in the abdominal cavity are pushed down into the scrotum through inguinal canal just before birth. The process by which testes enter the scrotum is called the descent of testes. Testosterone is necessary for descent of testes.

Cryptorchidism

Cryptorchidism is a congenital disorder characterized by the failure of one or both testes to descent from abdomen into scrotum. In such case, the testes are called **undescended testes**.

FUNCTIONS OF TESTOSTERONE IN ADULT LIFE

1. Effect on Sex Organs

Testosterone increases the size of penis, scrotum and the testes after puberty. All these organs are enlarged many folds between the onset of puberty and the age of 20 years, under the influence of testosterone. Testosterone is also necessary for spermatogenesis.

2. Effect on Basal Metabolic Rate

At the time of puberty and earlier part of adult life, testosterone increases the basal metabolic rate to about 5 to 10% by its anabolic effects on protein metabolism.

3. Effect on Electrolyte and Water Balance

Testosterone increases the sodium reabsorption from renal tubules along with water. It leads to increase in ECF volume.

4. Effect on Blood

Testosterone has got **erythropoietic action**. So, after puberty, testosterone causes mild increase in RBC count. It also increases blood volume by increasing the water retention and ECF volume.

5. Effect on Secondary Sexual Characters

Secondary sexual characters are the physical and behavioral characteristics that distinguish the male from female. These characters appear at the time of puberty. Testosterone is responsible for the development of secondary sexual characters in males. Secondary sexual characters in males are given below.

i. Effect on muscular growth

Testosterone increases the muscle mass due to its anabolic effects on proteins. It accelerates transport of amino acids into the muscle cells, synthesis of proteins and storage of proteins in the muscles.

ii. Effect on bone growth

After puberty, testosterone increases the thickness of bones by increasing the matrix content and calcium deposition.

In addition to increase in the size and strength of bones, testosterone also causes early **fusion of epiphyses** of long bones with shaft. So, if testes are removed before puberty, the fusion of epiphyses is delayed and the height of the person increases.

iii. Effect on shoulder and rib cage

Testosterone causes broadening of shoulder bones and rib cage.

iv. Effect on pelvic bones

Testosterone has a specific effect on pelvis which results in:

  a. Lengthening of pelvis.
  b. Funnel-like shape of pelvis.
  c. Narrowing of pelvic outlet.

Thus, pelvis in males is different from that of females, which is broad and round or oval in shape.

v. Effect on skin

Testosterone increases the thickness of skin and ruggedness of subcutaneous tissue by increasing the deposition of proteins in skin. It also increases the quantity of **melanin pigment**, which is responsible for deepening of the skin color.

Testosterone enhances the secretory activity of **sebaceous glands**. So, at the time of puberty, when body is exposed to sudden increase in testosterone secretion, the excess secretion of sebum leads to development of **acne** on the face. After few years, the skin gets adapted to testosterone secretion and, the acne disappears.

vi. Effect on hair distribution

Testosterone causes male type of hair distribution on the body, i.e. hair growth over the pubis, along linea alba up to umbilicus, on face, on chest and other parts of the body such as back and limbs. In males, the pubic hair has the base of the triangle downwards whereas in females it is upwards. Testosterone decreases the hair growth on head and may cause baldness if there is genetic background.

vii. Effect on voice

At the time of adolescence, boys have a cracking voice. It is because of testosterone effect which causes:

  a. Hypertrophy of laryngeal muscles.
  b. Enlargement of larynx and lengthening.
  c. Thickening of vocal cords.

Later, the **cracking voice** changes gradually into a typical adult male voice.

MODE OF ACTION OF TESTOSTERONE

Testosterone acts via genes.

REGULATION OF TESTOSTERONE SECRETION

In Fetus

During fetal life, the testosterone secretion from testis is stimulated by human chorionic gonadotropin (hCG).

In Adults

Interstitial cell stimulating hormone (ICSH) or luteinizing hormone (LH) stimulates the Leydig cells and the quantity of testosterone secreted is directly proportional to the amount of ICSH available.

Secretion of LH from anterior pituitary gland is stimulated by gonadotropin releasing hormone (GnRH) or luteinizing hormone releasing hormone (LHRH) from hypothalamus.

Feedback Control

Testosterone regulates its own secretion by **negative feedback** mechanism. It acts on hypothalamus and inhibits the secretion of LHRH. When LHRH secretion is inhibited, LH is not released from anterior pituitary resulting in stoppage of testosterone secretion from testes. On the other hand, when testosterone production is low, lack of inhibition of hypothalamus leads to secretion of testosterone through LHRH and LH **(Fig. 51.4)**.

■ SEMEN

Semen is a white or gray fluid that contains spermatozoa (sperms). It is the collection of fluids from testes, seminal vesicles, prostate gland and bulbourethral glands. Semen is discharged during sexual act and the process of discharge of semen is called **ejaculation.**

Testes contribute sperms. Prostate secretion gives milky appearance to semen. And, the secretions from seminal vesicles and bulbourethral glands provide mucoid consistency to semen.

At the time of ejaculation, human semen is liquid in nature. After some time, the **fibrinogen** secreted from seminal vesicle is converted into a weak **coagulum** by the clotting enzymes secreted from prostate gland. The coagulum is liquefied after about 30 minutes, as it is lysed by **fibrinolysin**. Fibrinolysin is the activated form of **profibrinolysin** produced in prostate gland.

When semen is ejaculated, the sperms are **nonmotile** due to the viscosity of coagulum. When the coagulum dissolves, the sperms become **motile**.

■ PROPERTIES OF SEMEN

Specific gravity : 1.028
Volume : 2 to 6 mL per ejaculation
Reaction : It is alkaline with a pH of 7.5. Alkalinity is due to the secretions from prostate gland

■ COMPOSITION OF SEMEN

Semen contains 10% sperms and 90% of fluid part which is called **seminal plasma**. The seminal plasma contains the products from seminal vesicle and prostate gland **(Fig. 51.5)**. It also has small amount of secretions from the mucus glands, particularly the bulbourethral glands.

■ SPERM

Sperm or spermatozoon (pleural = spermatozoa) is the male reproductive cell, developed in the testis. The matured sperm is 60 μ long.

Sperm Count

Total count of sperm is about 100 to 150 million/mL of semen. Sterility occurs when the sperm count falls below 20 million/mL.

Survival Time of Sperm

Though the sperms can be stored in male genital tract for longer periods, after ejaculation the survival time is only about 24 to 48 hours at a temperature equivalent to body temperature.

Motility of Sperm

Rate of motility of sperm in female genital tract is about 3 mm/min. Sperms reach the fallopian tube in about 30 to 60 minutes after sexual intercourse. Uterine contractions during sexual act facilitate the movement of sperms.

Structure of Sperm

Each sperm consists **four parts**:

1. Head

Head of sperm is oval in shape (in front view), with a length of 3 to 5 μ and width of up to 3 μ. Anterior portion of head is thin **(Fig. 51.6)**.

Head is formed by thin cytoplasm with a condensed nucleus and it is covered by a thin cell membrane. Anterior two-thirds of the head appear like a thick cap and it is called **acrosome**. Acrosome develops from Golgi apparatus and it is made up of mucopolysaccharide and acid phosphatase. It also contains **hyaluronidase** and **proteolytic enzymes** which are essential for the sperm to fertilize the ovum.

2. Neck

Head is connected to the body by a short neck. Anterior end of the neck is formed by thick disk-shaped **anterior end knob**, which is also called proximal centriole. Posterior end of neck is formed by another similar structure known as **posterior end knob**. It gives rise to the **axial filament** of body.

Often, the neck and body of sperm are together called **midpiece**.

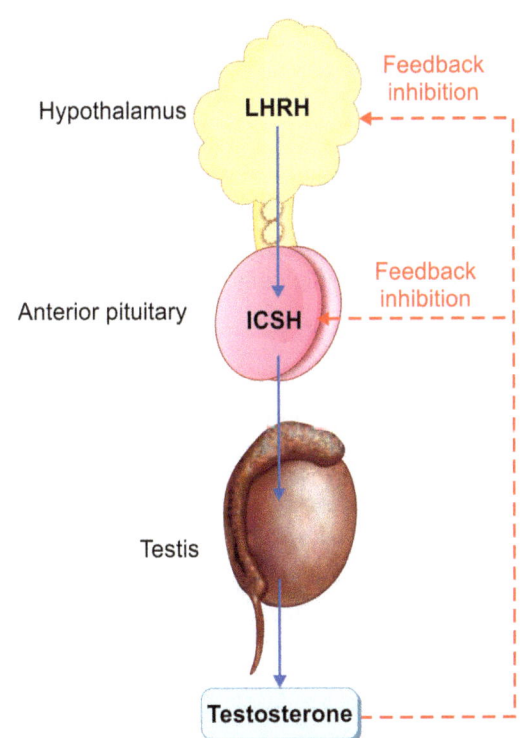

FIGURE 51.4: Regulation of testosterone secretion.
LHRH = Luteinizing hormone-releasing hormone,
ICSH = Interstitial cell stimulating hormone

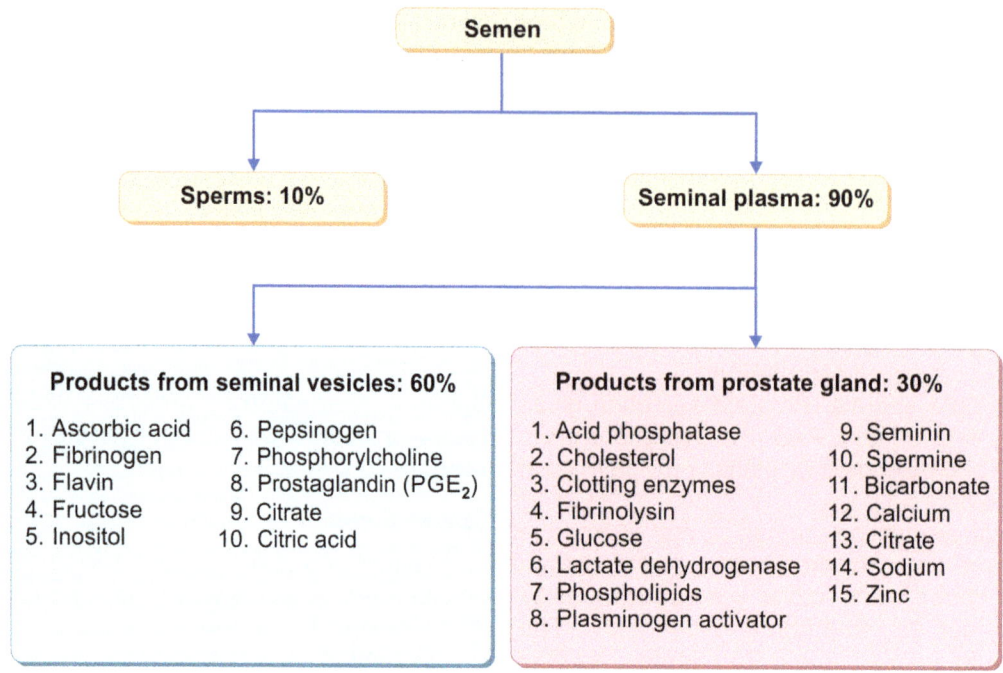

FIGURE 51.5: Composition of semen.

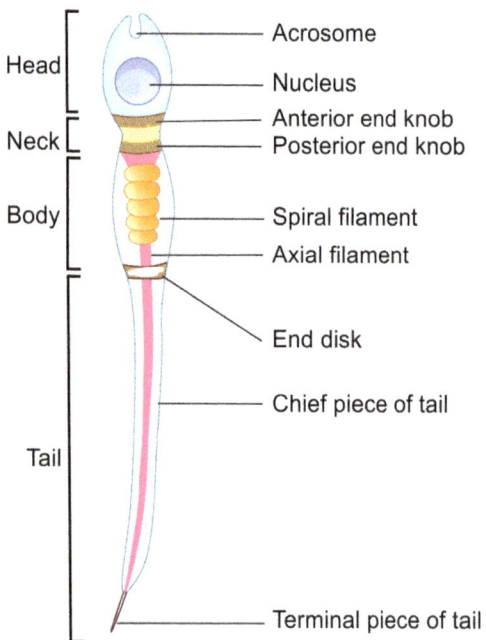

FIGURE 51.6: Human sperm.

3. Body

It is cylindrical with a length of 5 to 9 μ and the thickness of 1 μ. Body of the sperm consists of a central core called axial filament covered by thin cytoplasmic capsule.

Axial filament starts from posterior end knob of the neck. It passes through the body and a perforated disk called end disk or end ring centriole. Finally, axial filament reaches the tail as **axial thread**.

In the body, axial filament is surrounded by a closely wound **spiral filament** consisting of mitochondria.

4. Tail

Tail of the sperm consists of two segments:
  i. **Chief or main piece** of tail which is enclosed by cytoplasmic capsule and has an axial thread. It is 40 to 50 μ long.
 ii. **Terminal or end piece** of tail that has only the axial filament.

■ MALE CLIMACTERIC

Male andropause or climacteric is the condition in men characterized by emotional and physical changes in the body due to low androgen level with aging. It is also called **viropause**. After the age of 50, testosterone secretion starts declining because of decrease in number and secretory activity of Leydig cells.

■ APPLIED PHYSIOLOGY

■ EFFECTS OF EXTIRPATION OF TESTES

Removal of tests is called **castration**. Effects of castration depend upon the age when testes are removed.

1. Effects of Extirpation of Testes before Puberty: Eunuchism

If a boy loses the testes before puberty, he continues to have **infantile sexual characters** throughout life. This condition is called eunuchism.

Sex organs do not increase in size and the male secondary sexual characters do not develop. Voice remains like that of a child.

There is abnormal deposition of fat on buttocks, hip, pubis and breast, resembling the feminine distribution.

2. Effects of Extirpation of Testes Immediately after Puberty

If testes are removed after puberty, some of the male secondary sexual characters revert to those of a child and other masculine characters are retained.

Functions of sex organs are suppressed. Seminal vesicles and prostate undergo atrophy. Penis remains smaller. There may be loss of sexual desire and sexual activities.

3. Effect of Extirpation of Testes in Adults

Removal of testis in adults does not cause loss of secondary sexual characters. But accessory sex organs start degenerating. Sexual desire is not totally lost. Erection occurs but ejaculation is rare because of degeneration of accessory sex organs and lack of sperms.

■ HYPERGONADISM IN MALES

Hypergonadism is the condition characterized by hypersecretion of sex hormones from gonads.

Cause of Hypergonadism

Hypergonadism in males is mainly due to the tumor of Leydig cells. It is common in prepubertal boys who develop precocious pseudopuberty.

Symptoms of Hypergonadism

There is rapid growth of musculature and bones. But, height of the person is less because of early closure of epiphysis. There is excess development of sex organs and secondary sexual characters.

Tumors also secrete estrogenic hormones which cause **gynecomastia** (enlargement of breasts).

■ HYPOGONADISM IN MALES

Hypogonadism is a condition characterized by reduction in the functional activity of gonads.

Causes of Hypogonadism

Common causes for hypogonadism in males are:

1. Congenital nonfunctioning of testes or under developed testes.
2. Cryptorchidism associated with partial or total degeneration of testes.
3. Castration.
4. Absence of androgen receptors in testes.

Signs and Symptoms of Hypogonadism

Clinical picture of male hypogonadism depends upon whether the testicular deficiency develops before or after puberty.

Before puberty

Features of hypogonadism are similar to those developed due to extirpation of testes before puberty, which are described above.

After puberty

Symptoms are similar to those developed due to the removal of testes after puberty (see above).

In adults

Same symptoms, which develop after extirpation of testis, occur in this condition.

Dystrophia adiposogenitalis

It is the disorder characterized by obesity and hypogonadism in adolescent boys. It is also called **Fröhlich's syndrome** or **hypothalamic eunuchism**. Refer Chapter 84 for details.

Chapter 52: Female Reproductive System

CHAPTER OUTLINE

- FEMALE REPRODUCTIVE ORGANS
- FUNCTIONAL ANATOMY OF OVARY
- FUNCTIONS OF OVARY
- ACCESSORY SEX ORGANS IN FEMALES
- OVARIAN HORMONES
- SEXUAL LIFE IN FEMALES
- CLIMACTERIC AND MENOPAUSE

FEMALE REPRODUCTIVE ORGANS

Female reproductive system comprises primary sex organs and accessory sex organs (**Figs 52.1** and **52.2**).

Primary sex organs are a pair of **ovaries**, which produce **ova** and secrete female sex hormones. Accessory sex organs are given below.

FUNCTIONAL ANATOMY OF OVARY

Ovaries are flattened ovoid bodies with dimensions of 4 cm in length, 2 cm in width and 1 cm in thickness. On cross section, each ovary shows two zones, medulla and cortex.

MEDULLA

Medulla of ovary or **zona vasculosa** is the inner portion of ovary. It has the stroma of loose connective tissues. It contains blood vessels, lymphatics, nerve fibers and bundles of smooth muscle fibers near the hilum.

CORTEX

Cortex is the outer broader portion of ovary and it has compact cellular layers. Cortex is covered by **germinal epithelium** underneath a fibrous layer known as **tunica albuginea**. Cortex consists of ovarian follicles at different stages, connective tissue and interstitial cells.

When the fetus develops, **primary germ cells** called **oogonia** develop from germinal epithelium. Oogonia give rise to **immature ova** called **primary oocytes**. Primary oocytes move towards the inner substance of cortex. A layer of **granulosa cells** from ovarian stroma surrounds each primary oocyte. Primary oocyte along with granulosa cells is called the **primordial follicle**.

At 7th or 8th month of intrauterine life, about 6 million primordial follicles are found in the ovary. But, at the time of birth, only 1 million primordial follicles are seen in both the ovaries. Remaining follicles degenerate. At the time of puberty, number reduces further to about 3,00,000 to 4,00,000. After menarche, during every menstrual cycle, one of the follicles matures and releases its ovum. Only one ovum is released from any one of the ovaries during each menstrual cycle.

During each cycle, many of the follicles degenerate and become **atretic follicles** which disappear without leaving any scar.

FUNCTIONS OF OVARY

Functions of ovaries are:

1. Secretion of female sex hormones.
2. Oogenesis.
3. Menstrual cycle.

Sex hormones are discussed later in this chapter. Menstrual cycle is explained in the next chapter. Oogenesis is explained below.

OOGENESIS

Oogenesis is the process of origin and development of ovum. It occurs in three stages.

Stages of Oogenesis

1. *Stage of proliferation*

In fetus, cells of germinal epithelium undergo repeated mitotic division to form diploid **oogonia**. All the oogonia are formed during fetal life itself and not after birth.

2. *Stage of growth*

Oogonia give rise to **immature ova** called **primary oocytes**. Each primary oocyte is enclosed in primordial

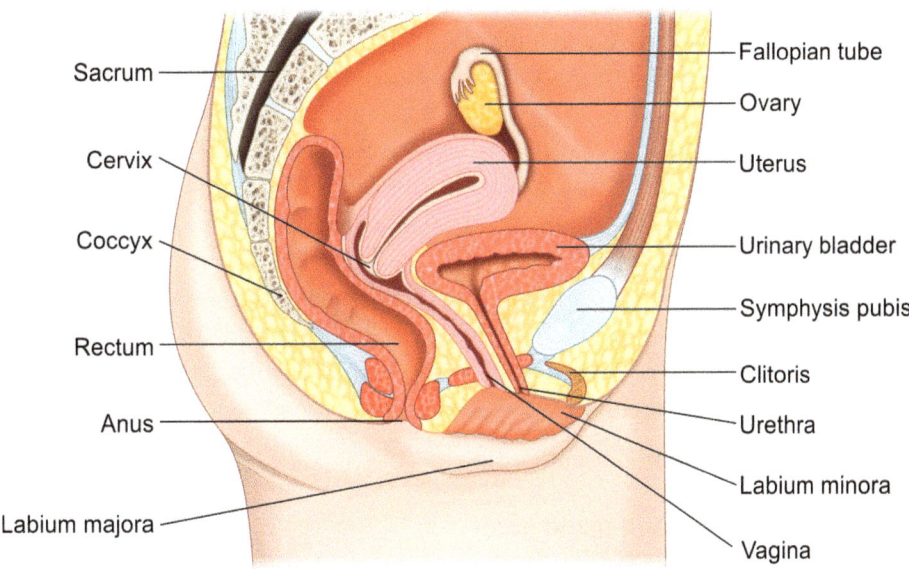

FIGURE 52.1: Female reproductive organs and other organs of pelvis.

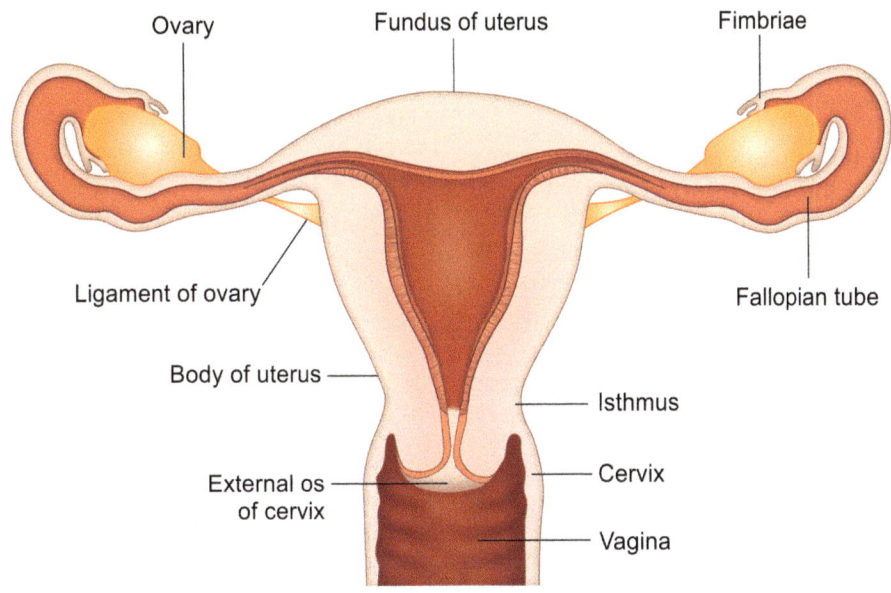

FIGURE 52.2: Female reproductive system.

ovarian follicle (see above). Primary oocyte has diploid number (23 pairs) of chromosomes.

3. Stage of maturation

Just before ovulation, meiotic division takes place. Primary oocyte divides into a **secondary oocyte** and a **first polar body**. First polar body is expelled out. Secondary oocyte contains only 23 chromosomes (haploid). Remaining 23 chromosomes are lost in the expelled first polar body.

After ovulation the secondary oocyte is released into abdominal cavity because of rupture of Graafian follicle (Chapter 53). Then, the secondary oocyte enters fallopian tube through fimbriated end. When fertilization occurs, the secondary oocyte divides into a **matured ovum** and a **second polar body**. Second polar body is expelled. Matured ovum has 23 chromosomes.

■ ACCESSORY SEX ORGANS IN FEMALES

Accessory sex organs in females are:

1. A system of genital ducts that includes fallopian tubes, uterus, cervix and vagina.
2. External genitalia which are labia majora, labia minora and clitoris.

Mammary glands are not the female genital organs but are the important glands of female reproductive system.

■ UTERUS

Uterus is otherwise known as **womb**. It lies in the pelvic cavity, in between the rectum and urinary bladder. Uterus is a hollow muscular organ with a thick wall. It has a central cavity, which opens into **vagina** through **cervix**. On either side at its upper part, the **fallopian tubes** open. Uterus communicates with peritoneal cavity through fallopian tubes. There is a constriction almost at the middle of uterus called **isthmus**.

Divisions of Uterus

Uterus is divided into three portions:

1. Fundus (above entrance of fallopian tubes).
2. Body (between fundus and isthmus).
3. Cervix (below isthmus).

Structure of Uterine Wall

Uterine wall made up of three layers of structures:

1. Outer serous layer or **perimetrium** derived from peritoneum.
2. Middle muscular layer or **myometrium** made up of smooth muscle fibers.
3. Inner mucus layer or **endometrium** made up of ciliated columnar epithelial cells, connective tissue and uterine glands **(Fig. 52.3)**.

■ CERVIX

Cervix is the lower constricted part of uterus. It is divided into two portions:

1. Upper **supravaginal portion** which communicates with body of uterus through **internal os** (orifice) of cervix.
2. Lower **vaginal portion** which communicates with vagina through **external os**.

■ VAGINA

Vagina is a short tubular organ. It is lined by mucous membrane which is formed by stratified epithelial cells.

■ OVARIAN HORMONES

Ovary secretes the female sex hormones estrogen and progesterone. Ovary also secretes few more hormones namely, inhibin, relaxin and small quantities of androgens.

■ ESTROGEN

In a normal nonpregnant female, estrogen is secreted in large quantity by **theca interna** cells of ovarian follicles and in small quantity by **corpus luteum** of the ovaries. A small quantity of estrogen is also secreted by **adrenal cortex**. During pregnancy, a large amount of estrogen is secreted by the **placenta**. Estrogen is a C18 steroid.

Forms of Estrogen

Estrogen is present in three forms in plasma, β-estradiol, estrone and estriol.

Quantity and potency of **β-estradiol** are more than those of estrone and estriol. Plasma level of estrogen in females at normal reproductive age varies during different phases of menstrual cycle. In follicular phase, it is 30 to 200 pg/mL.

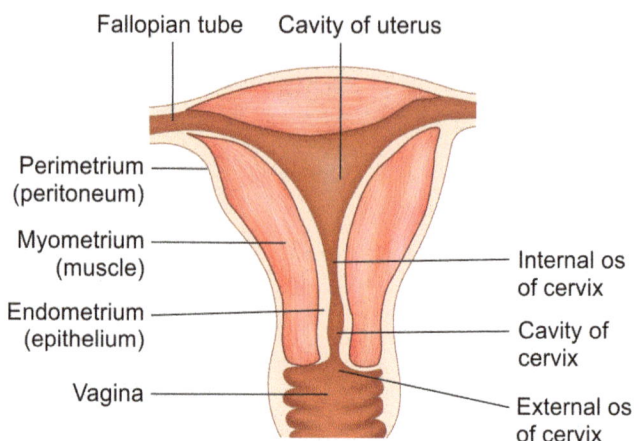

FIGURE 52.3: Section of uterus.

Functions of Estrogen

Major function of the estrogen is to promote cellular proliferation and tissue growth in sex organs and in other tissues related to reproduction. Effects of estrogen are given below.

1. Effect on ovarian follicles

Estrogen promotes the growth of ovarian follicles by increasing the proliferation of the follicular cells. It also increases the secretory activity of theca cells. Refer Chapter 53 for details.

2. Effect on uterus

Estrogen produces the following changes in uterus:

i. Enlargement of uterus by the proliferation of endometrial cells.
ii. Increase in the blood supply to endometrium.
iii. Deposition of glycogen and fats in endometrium.
iv. Proliferation and dilatation of blood vessels of endometrium.
v. Proliferation and dilatation of the endometrial glands.
vi. Increase in the spontaneous activity of the uterine muscles and their sensitivity to oxytocin.
vii. Increase in the contractility of the uterine muscles.

All these changes prepare uterus for pregnancy.

3. Effect on fallopian tubes

Estrogen:
i. Acts on mucosal lining of fallopian tubes and increases the number and size of ciliated epithelial cells lining the fallopian tubes.
ii. Increases the activity of cilia, so that the movement of ovum in fallopian tube is facilitated.
iii. Enhances the proliferation of glandular tissues in fallopian tubes.

All these changes are necessary for fertilization of ovum.

4. Effect on vagina

Estrogen:
i. Changes the vaginal epithelium from cuboidal into stratified type. Stratified epithelium is more resistant to trauma and infection.

ii. Increases the layers of vaginal epithelium by proliferation.
iii. Reduces the pH of vagina making it more acidic.

All these changes are necessary for prevention of vaginal infections.

5. Effect on secondary sexual characters

Estrogen is responsible for the development of secondary sexual characters in females.

Secondary sexual characters in female are:

i. *Hair distribution:* Hair develops in the pubic region and axilla. In females, pubic hair has the base of triangle upwards. Body hair growth is less. Scalp hair grows profusely.
ii. *Skin:* Skin becomes soft and smooth. Vascularity also increases in skin.
iii. *Body shape:* Shoulders become narrow, hip broadens, the thighs converge and the arms diverge. Fat deposition increases in the breasts and buttocks.
iv. *Pelvis:* Estrogen has a specific effect on pelvis which results in:
   a. Broadening of pelvis with increased transverse diameter.
   b. Round or oval-shaped pelvis
   c. Round or oval-shaped pelvic outlet.
   Thus, pelvis in females is different from that of males, which is funnel-like shaped.
v. *Voice:* Larynx remains in prepubertal stage, which produces high-pitch voice.

6. Effect on breast

Estrogen causes:
i. Development of stromal tissues of breasts.
ii. Growth of an extensive ductile system.
iii. Deposition of fat in ductile system.

All these effects prepare the breasts for lactation.

7. Effect on bones

Estrogen increases **osteoblastic activity**. So, at the time of puberty, the growth rate increases enormously. But, at the same time, estrogen causes early **fusion of epiphysis** with the shaft. This effect is much stronger in the females than the similar effect of testosterone in males. As a result, growth of females usually ceases few years earlier than in the males.

In old age, the estrogen is not secreted or it becomes scanty. It leads to **osteoporosis** by which the bones become extremely weak and fragile. And, because of this, the bones are highly susceptible for fractures.

8. Effect on metabolism

i. *On protein metabolism:* Estrogen induces anabolism of proteins by which it increases the total body protein.
ii. *On fat metabolism:* Estrogen causes deposition of fat in the subcutaneous tissues, breasts, buttocks and thighs.

9. Effect on electrolyte balance

Estrogen causes sodium and water retention from the renal tubules. This effect is normally insignificant but in pregnancy, it becomes more significant.

Mode of Action of Estrogen

Estrogen acts through genes.

Regulation of Estrogen Secretion

Secretion of estrogen is regulated by **follicle stimulating hormone (FSH)** released from anterior pituitary. Release of FSH is stimulated by the **gonadotropin releasing hormone (GnRH)** secreted from hypothalamus.

FSH stimulates the secretory activities of theca and granulosa cells. Estrogen inhibits secretion of FSH and GnRH by negative feedback. Inhibin secreted by granulosa cells also decreases estrogen secretion by inhibiting secretion of FSH and GnRH **(Fig. 52.4)**.

■ PROGESTERONE

A small quantity of progesterone is secreted by **theca interna** cells of ovarian follicles during the first half of menstrual cycle, i.e. during follicular stage. But, a large quantity of progesterone is secreted during the latter half of each menstrual cycle, i.e. during secretory phase by the **corpus luteum**. Small amount of progesterone is secreted from **adrenal cortex** also.

During pregnancy, a large amount of progesterone is secreted by **corpus luteum** in the first trimester. In the second trimester corpus luteum degenerates. **Placenta** secretes large quantity of progesterone in second and third trimesters.

Progesterone is a C21 steroid. Plasma level of progesterone in females at normal reproductive age varies during different phases of menstrual cycle. In follicular phase, it is about 0.9 ng/mL (Refer Fig. 53.6).

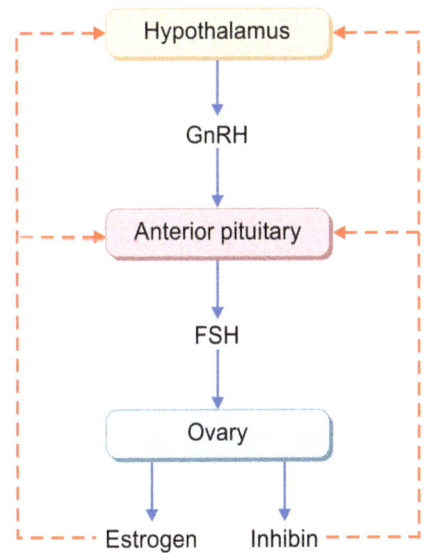

FIGURE 52.4: Regulation of estrogen secretion. Red dashed lines = Inhibition

Functions of Progesterone

Progesterone is concerned mainly with final preparation of the uterus for pregnancy and the breasts for lactation. Effects of progesterone are given below.

1. Effect on fallopian tubes

Progesterone promotes secretory activities of mucosal lining of the fallopian tubes. Secretions of fallopian tubes are necessary for nutrition of the fertilized ovum while it is in fallopian tube before implantation.

2. Effect on uterus

Progesterone promotes secretory activities of uterine endometrium during the secretory phase of the menstrual cycle.

Thus, the uterus is prepared for implantation of fertilized ovum by the following actions of progesterone.

Progesterone:
  i. Increases thickness of endometrium by increasing the number and size of cells.
  ii. Increases size of uterine glands and make them more tortuous.
  iii. Increases secretory activities of uterine glands.
  iv. Increases deposition of lipid and glycogen in endometrium.
  v. Increases the blood supply to endometrium.
  vi. Decreases the frequency of uterine contractions during pregnancy. Because of this, expulsion of implanted ovum is prevented.

3. Effect on cervix

Progesterone increases thickness of cervical mucosa and thereby inhibits transport of sperm into uterus. This effect is utilized in the contraceptive actions of mini pills.

4. Effect on mammary glands

Progesterone promotes development of the lobules and alveoli of mammary glands by proliferating and enlarging the alveolar cells. It also makes the breasts secretory in nature. It makes the breasts to swell by increasing the secretory activity and fluid accumulation in subcutaneous tissue.

5. Thermogenic effect

Progesterone increases the body temperature after ovulation. The mechanism of thermogenic action is not known. It is suggested that progesterone increases the body temperature by acting on hypothalamic centers for temperature regulation.

6. Effect on respiration

During luteal phase of menstrual cycle and during pregnancy, progesterone increases the ventilation via respiratory center. This results in decreased partial pressure of carbon dioxide in the alveoli.

Mode of Action of Progesterone

Like estrogen, progesterone also acts through genes.

Regulation of Secretion of Progesterone

Luteinizing hormone (LH) from anterior pituitary activates the corpus luteum to secrete progesterone. Secretion of LH is influenced by the **gonadotropin releasing hormone (GnRH)** secreted in hypothalamus. Progesterone inhibits release of LH from anterior pituitary by negative feedback.

■ SEXUAL LIFE IN FEMALES

Lifespan of a female is divided into three periods.

■ FIRST PERIOD

First period extends from birth to puberty. During this period, primary and accessory sex organs do not function. These organs remain quiescent. Puberty occurs at the age of 12 to 15 years.

■ SECOND PERIOD

Second period extends from onset of puberty to the onset of menopause. First menstrual cycle is known as **menarche**. Permanent stoppage of the menstrual cycle in old age is called **menopause,** which occurs at the age of about 45 to 50 years. During the period between menarche and menopause, women menstruate and reproduce.

■ THIRD PERIOD

Third period extends after menopause to the rest of the life.

■ CLIMACTERIC AND MENOPAUSE

Climacteric is the period in old age when reproductive system undergoes changes due to the decreased secretion of sex hormones estrogen and progesterone. It occurs at the age of 45 to 55. In females, climacteric is accompanied by menopause.

Menopause is defined as the period characterized by permanent cessation of menstruation. Normally, it occurs at the age of 45 to 55 years.

■ CHANGES DURING MENOPAUSE: POSTMENOPAUSAL SYNDROME

Postmenopausal syndrome is the group of symptoms that appear in women immediately after menopause. It is characterized by certain physical, physiological and psychological changes. Symptoms start appearing soon after the ovaries stop functioning.

Cause for symptoms is the lack of estrogen and progesterone. The symptoms may persist till the body gets acclimatized to absence of estrogen and progesterone. Symptoms do not appear in all women. Some women develop mild symptoms and some women develop severe symptoms. Symptoms last for few months to few years.

Most of the women manage it very well. But, about 15% of the women need treatment. In many cases, **psychotherapy** works very well. If it fails, **hormone replacement therapy** is given.

Chapter 53

Menstrual Cycle

CHAPTER OUTLINE

- **DEFINITION, DURATION AND CHANGES**
  - DEFINITION
  - DURATION OF MENSTRUAL CYCLE
  - CHANGES DURING MENSTRUAL CYCLE
- **OVARIAN CHANGES DURING MENSTRUAL CYCLE**
  - FOLLICULAR PHASE
  - OVULATION
  - LUTEAL PHASE
- **UTERINE CHANGES DURING MENSTRUAL CYCLE**
  - MENSTRUAL PHASE
  - PROLIFERATIVE PHASE
  - SECRETORY PHASE
- **CHANGES IN CERVIX DURING MENSTRUAL CYCLE**
  - PROLIFERATIVE PHASE
  - SECRETORY PHASE
- **CHANGES IN VAGINA DURING MENSTRUAL CYCLE**
  - PROLIFERATIVE PHASE
  - SECRETORY PHASE
- **REGULATION OF MENSTRUAL CYCLE**
  - HORMONES INVOLVED IN REGULATION
- **APPLIED PHYSIOLOGY: MENSTRUAL DISORDERS**
  - MENSTRUAL SYMPTOMS
  - PREMENSTRUAL SYNDROME
  - ABNORMAL MENSTRUATION
  - ANOVULATORY CYCLE

■ DEFINITION, DURATION AND CHANGES

■ DEFINITION

Menstrual cycle is defined as the cyclic events that take place in a rhythmic fashion during the reproductive period of a woman's life. Menstrual cycle starts at the age of 12 to 15 years, which marks the onset of puberty. Commencement of menstrual cycle is called **menarche**. Menstrual cycle ceases at the age of 45 to 50 years. Permanent cessation of menstrual cycle in old age is called **menopause**.

■ DURATION OF MENSTRUAL CYCLE

Duration of menstrual cycle is usually 28 days. But, under physiological conditions, it may vary between 20 and 40 days.

■ CHANGES DURING MENSTRUAL CYCLE

Series of changes occur in ovary and accessory sex organs during each menstrual cycle. All the changes place simultaneously.

Changes taking place during menstrual cycle are:

I. Ovarian changes.
II. Uterine changes.
III. Vaginal changes.
IV. Changes in cervix.

■ OVARIAN CHANGES DURING MENSTRUAL CYCLE

Changes in each during menstrual cycle occur in two phases, follicular phase and luteal phase.

■ FOLLICULAR PHASE

Follicular phase extends from 5th day of cycle until the time of ovulation, which takes place on 14th day. During this phase development of ovarian follicles and maturation of ovum take place.

Ovarian Follicles

Ovarian follicles are glandular structures present in the cortex of ovary. Each follicle consists of an **immature** ovum surrounded by epithelial cells called **granulosa cells**. The follicles gradually grow into a matured follicle through various stages.

Different follicles are:

1. Primordial follicle.
2. Primary follicle.
3. Vesicular follicle.
4. Matured follicle or Graafian follicle.

1. Primordial Follicle

At the time of puberty, both the ovaries contain 3,00,000 to 4,00,000 primordial follicles. Diameter of primordial follicle is about 15 to 20 μ and that of ovum is about 10 μ. Each primordial follicle has an immature ovum which is incompletely surrounded by the **granulosa cells (Fig. 53.1)**. Granulosa cells provide nutrition to ovum during childhood.

Granulosa cells also secrete **oocyte maturation inhibiting factor** which keeps the ovum in the immature stage. All the ova present in ovaries are formed before birth. No new ovum is developed after birth.

During onset of puberty, under the influence of **follicle stimulating hormone (FSH)** and **luteinizing hormone (LH)** the primordial follicles start growing through various stages.

2. Primary Follicle

Primordial follicle becomes the primary follicle, when ovum is completely surrounded by the granulosa cells. During this stage the follicle and ovum inside the follicle increase in size. Diameter of this follicle increases to 30 to 40 μ and that of ovum increases to about 20 μ. Primary follicle is not covered by a definite connective tissue capsule.

Characteristic changes taking place during development of primary follicles are:

i. Proliferation of granulosa cells and increase in size of the follicle.
ii. Increase in size of ovum.
iii. Onset of formation of connective tissue capsule around the follicle.

Primary follicles develop into vesicular follicles.

3. Vesicular Follicle

Under the influence of FSH, about 6 to 12 primary follicles start growing and develop into the vesicular follicles.

During development of vesicular follicles, many changes take place in granulosa cells and ovum. And a covering sheath is formed.

Changes in granulosa cells

i. First, the proliferation of granulosa cells occurs.
ii. A cavity called **follicular cavity** or **antrum** is formed in between the granulosa cells.
iii. Antrum is filled with a serous fluid called the liquor folliculi.
iv. Ovum is pushed to one side and it is surrounded by granulosa cells which forms the **germ hill** or **cumulus oophorus**.
v. Granulosa cells which line the antrum form membrana granulosa.
vi. Cells of germ hill become columnar and form corona radiata.

Changes in ovum

i. First, the ovum increases in size and its diameter increases to 100 to 150 μ.
ii. Nucleus becomes larger and vesicular.
iii. Cytoplasm becomes granular.
iv. Thick membrane is formed around the ovum which is called **zona pellucida**.
v. A narrow cleft called **perivitelline space** appears between ovum and zona pellucida.

Formation of covering sheath

Spindle cells from the stroma of ovarian cortex are modified and form a covering sheath around the follicle. This covering sheath is known as **follicular sheath** or **theca folliculi**.

Theca folliculi divides into two layers:

a. *Theca interna*: Theca interna is the inner vascular layer with loose connective tissue. This layer contains epithelial cells which secrete female sex hormones, especially estrogen. Hormones are released into the fluid of antrum.
b. *Theca externa*: Theca externa is the outer layer of follicular capsule and consists of thickly packed fibers and spindle-shaped cells.

After about 7th day of menstrual cycle, one of the vesicular follicles develops further to form Graafian follicle. Other vesicular follicles degenerate by means of **apoptosis**.

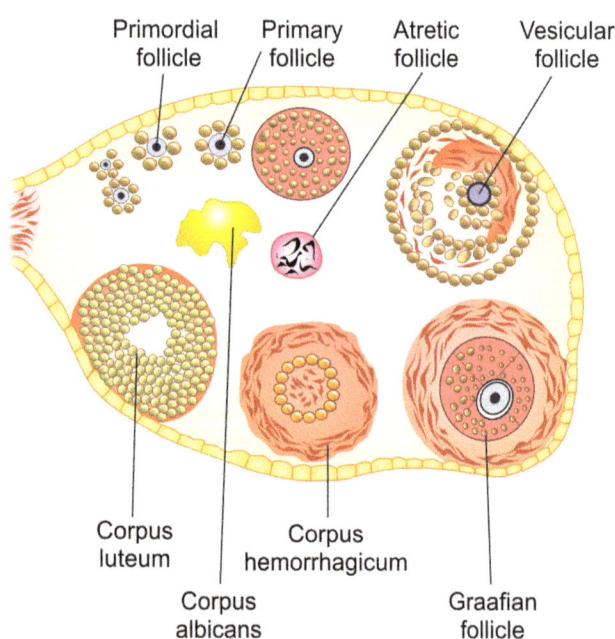

FIGURE 53.1: Ovarian follicles and corpus luteum.

4. Graafian Follicle

Graafian follicle is the matured ovarian follicle with maturing ovum. It is named after the Dutch physician and anatomist **Regnier De Graaf (Fig. 53.2)**. Many changes take place during the development of Graafian follicle:

i. Size of the follicle increases to about 10 to 12 mm.
ii. At one point, follicle encroaches upon tunica albuginea and protrudes upon the surface of ovary. This protrusion is called **stigma**. At the stigma, tunica albuginea becomes thin.
iii. Follicular cavity becomes larger and distended with fluid.
iv. Ovum attains maximum size.
v. Zona pellucida becomes thick.
vi. Corona radiata becomes prominent.
vii. Small spaces filled with fluid appear between the cells of germ hill outside the corona radiata. These spaces weaken the attachment of the ovum to the follicular wall.
viii. Theca interna becomes prominent. Its thickness becomes double with formation of rich capillary network.
ix. On 14th day of menstrual cycle, the Graafian follicle is ready for the process of ovulation.

◼ OVULATION

Ovulation is the process by which Graafian follicle is ruptured with consequent discharge of ovum into abdominal cavity. Ovulation occurs usually on 14th day of menstrual cycle in a normal cycle of 28 days.

The ovum, which is released into abdominal cavity, enters the fallopian tube through fimbriated end of tube. Usually, only one ovum is released from any one of the ovaries. LH is responsible for ovulation. Prior to ovulation, large amount of LH is secreted (**LH surge**) which causes changes in the Graafian follicle leading to ovulation.

LH Surge

LH surge is defined as rapid increase in secretion of luteinizing hormone 24 to 48 hours prior to ovulation.

Stages of Ovulation

1. Rupture of Graafian follicles takes place at the stigma.
2. Follicular fluid oozes out.
3. Germ hillock is freed from wall.
4. Ovum is expelled out into the abdominal cavity along with some amount of fluid and granulosa cells **(Fig 53.3)**.
5. From abdominal cavity, the ovum enters the fallopian tube through the fimbriated end.

Ovum becomes **haploid** before or during ovulation by the formation of polar bodies. After ovulation, the ovum is viable only for 24 to 48 hours. So, it must be fertilized within that time.

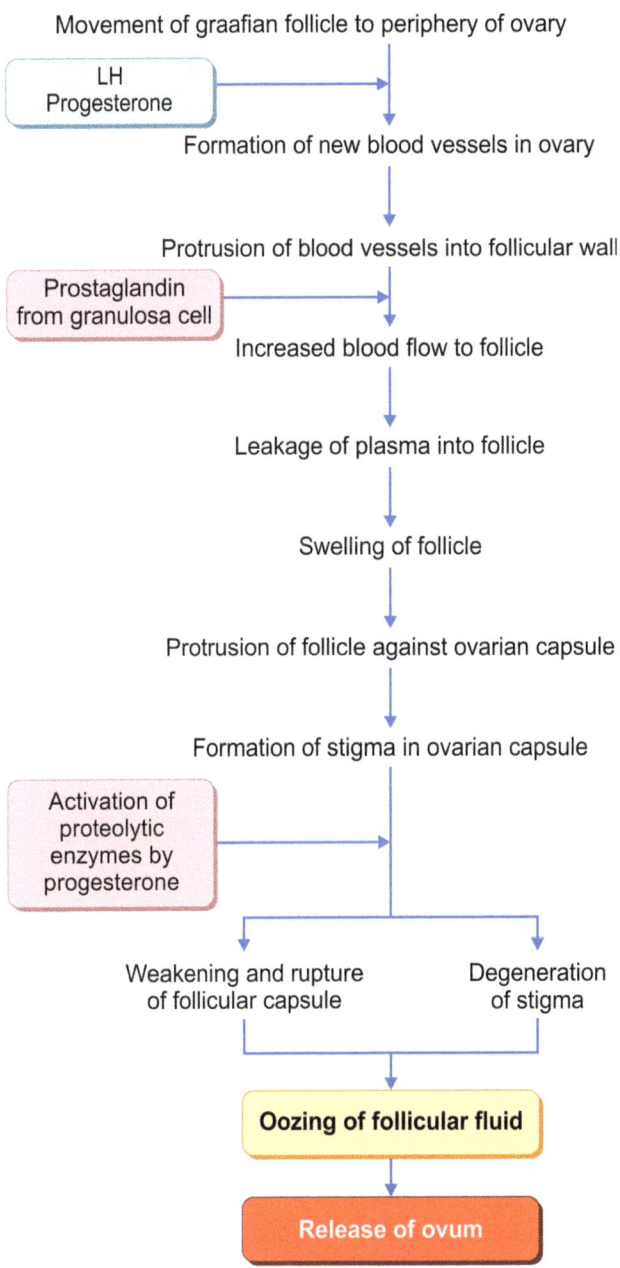

FIGURE 53.3: Process of ovulation.
LH = Luteinizing hormone

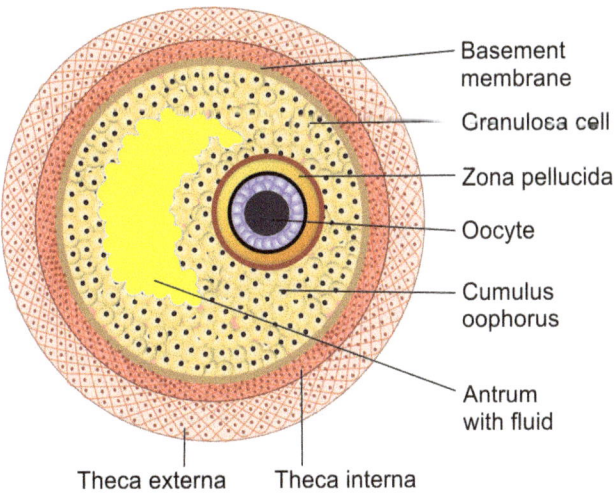

FIGURE 53.2: Graafian follicle.

Fertilized ovum is called **zygote**. Zygote moves from fallopian tube and reaches the uterus on 3rd day after ovulation. It is **implanted** in the uterine wall on 6th or 7th day. If fertilization does not occur, ovum degenerates. Generally, only one ovum is released from one of the ovaries.

Determination of Ovulation Time

Ovulation time can be determined by the following methods:

1. *By determining basal body temperature:* There is a slight fall in the basal temperature just prior to ovulation. And, the temperature increases after ovulation. Alteration in the temperature is very mild and it is about ± 0.3 to 0.5°C.
2. *By determining hormonal excretion in urine:* At the time of ovulation, there is an increase in the urinary excretion of metabolic end products of estrogen and progesterone.
3. *By determination of hormonal level in plasma:* Plasma level of FSH, LH, estrogen and progesterone are altered at the time of ovulation and after ovulation.
4. *Ultrasound scanning:* Process of ovulation is observed by ultrasound scanning.
5. *Cervical mucus pattern:* When the cervical mucus spread on a slide is examined under microscope, it shows a fern pattern. This pattern disappears after ovulation.

Significance of Determining Ovulation Time

Family planning by rhythm method may be well adopted by determination of ovulation time (Chapter 55).

■ LUTEAL PHASE

Luteal phase extends between 15th and 28th day of menstrual cycle. During this phase corpus luteum is developed and hence the name luteal phase **(Fig. 53.4)**.

Corpus Luteum

Corpus luteum is a glandular yellow body developed from the ruptured Graafian follicle after the release of ovum. It is also called **yellow body**.

Development of Corpus Luteum

Soon after the rupture of Graafian follicle and release of ovum, the follicle is filled with blood. Now the follicle is called **corpus hemorrhagicum**. Blood clots slowly and corpus hemorrhagicum is transformed into a corpus luteum.

In the corpus luteum, the granulosa cells and theca interna cells are transformed into **lutein cells** namely granulosa lutein cells and theca lutein cells by accumulation of fine lipid granules and the yellowish pigment granules. These yellowish pigment granules give the characteristic yellow color to corpus luteum.

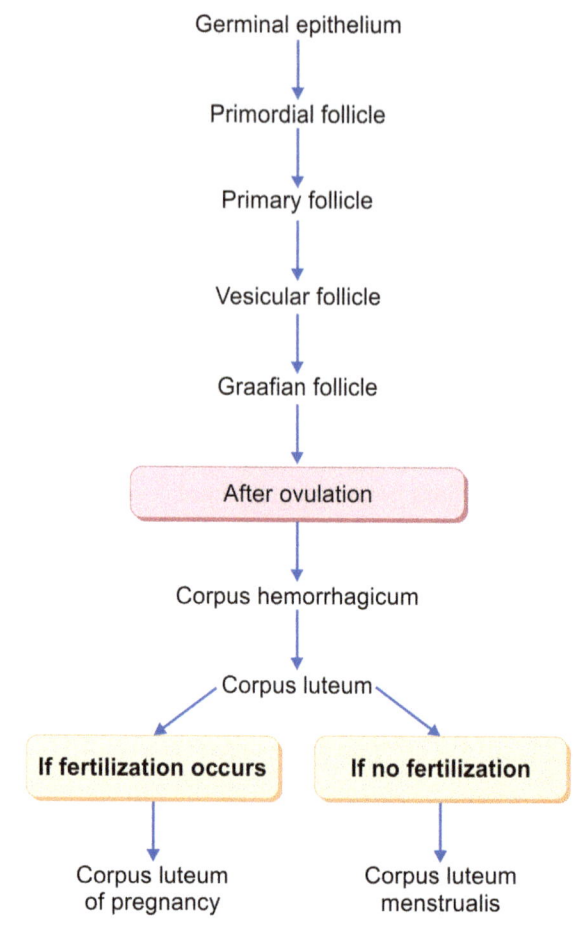

FIGURE 53.4: Schematic diagram showing different ovarian follicles and corpus luteum.

Functions of Corpus Luteum

1. **Secretion of hormones**

Corpus luteum acts as a **temporary endocrine gland**. It secretes large quantity of progesterone and small amount of estrogen. LH influences the secretion of these two hormones.

2. **Maintenance of pregnancy**

If pregnancy occurs, corpus luteum maintains the pregnancy for about 3 months of pregnancy till placenta starts secreting estrogen and progesterone.

Fate of Corpus Luteum

Fate of corpus luteum depends upon whether ovum is fertilized or not.

If the ovum is not fertilized

If fertilization does not take place, corpus luteum reaches the maximum size about 1 week after ovulation. During this period, it secretes large quantity of progesterone with small quantity of estrogen. Then, it degenerates into the **corpus luteum menstrualis**. Afterwards, the corpus luteum menstrualis is transformed into a whitish scar called **corpus albicans**. The process by which corpus luteum undergoes regression is called **luteolysis**.

If ovum is fertilized

If ovum is fertilized and pregnancy occurs, the corpus luteum persists and increases in size. It attains a diameter of 20 to 30 mm and it is transformed into **corpus luteum graviditatis (verum)** or **corpus luteum of pregnancy (Fig. 53.4)**. It remains in the ovary for 3 to 4 months. During this period, it secretes large amount of progesterone with small quantity of estrogen, which are essential for the maintenance of pregnancy. After 3 to 4 months, placenta starts secreting these hormones and corpus luteum degenerates.

■ UTERINE CHANGES DURING MENSTRUAL CYCLE

During each menstrual cycle, along with ovarian changes, uterine changes also occur simultaneously.

Uterine changes in uterus take place in three phases:

1. Menstrual phase.
2. Proliferative phase.
3. Secretory phase.

■ MENSTRUAL PHASE

After ovulation, if pregnancy does not occur, the thickened endometrium is shed or desquamated. This desquamated endometrium is expelled out through vagina along with some blood and tissue fluid. The process of shedding and exit of uterine lining along with blood and fluid is called **menstruation** or **menstrual bleeding**. It lasts for about 4 to 5 days **(Fig. 53.5)**. This period is called menstrual phase or menstrual period. It is also called **menses**, **emmenia** or **catamenia**.

The day when bleeding starts is considered as the 1st day of the menstrual cycle. Two days before onset of bleeding, that is on 26th or 27th day of the previous cycle, there is sudden reduction in the release of estrogen and progesterone from ovary. Decreased level of these two hormones is responsible for menstruation.

Changes in Endometrium during Menstrual Phase

1. Lack of estrogen and progesterone causes sudden involution of endometrium.
2. It leads to reduction in the thickness of endometrium, up to 65% of original thickness.
3. During the next 24 hours, the tortuous blood vessels in the endometrium undergo severe constriction.
4. Vasoconstriction leads to hypoxia, which results in **necrosis** of the endometrium.
5. Necrosis causes rupture of blood vessels and oozing of blood.
6. Outer layer of the **necrotic endometrium** is separated and passes out along with blood.
7. This process is continued for about 24 to 36 hours.
8. Within 48 hours after the reduction in secretion of estrogen and progesterone, superficial layers of endometrium are completely desquamated.
9. Desquamated tissues and the blood in endometrial cavity initiate the contraction of uterus.
10. Uterine contractions expel the blood along with **desquamated uterine tissues** to the exterior through vagina.

During normal menstruation, about 35 mL of blood along with 35 mL of **serous fluid** is expelled. The blood clots as soon as it oozes into the uterine cavity. **Fibrinolysin** causes **lysis of clot** in uterine cavity itself so that, the expelled menstrual fluid does not clot. However, in pathological conditions involving uterus, the lysis of blood clot does not occur. So, the menstrual fluid comes out with blood clot.

Menstruation stops between 3rd and 7th day of menstrual cycle. At the end of menstrual phase, the thickness of endometrium is only about 1 mm. This is followed by proliferative phase.

■ PROLIFERATIVE PHASE

Proliferative phase extends usually from 5th to 14th day of menstruation, i.e. between the day when menstruation stops and the day of ovulation. It corresponds to the follicular phase of ovarian cycle **(Table 53.1)**.

At the end of menstrual phase, only a thin layer (1 mm) of endometrium remains as most of the endometrial stroma is desquamated.

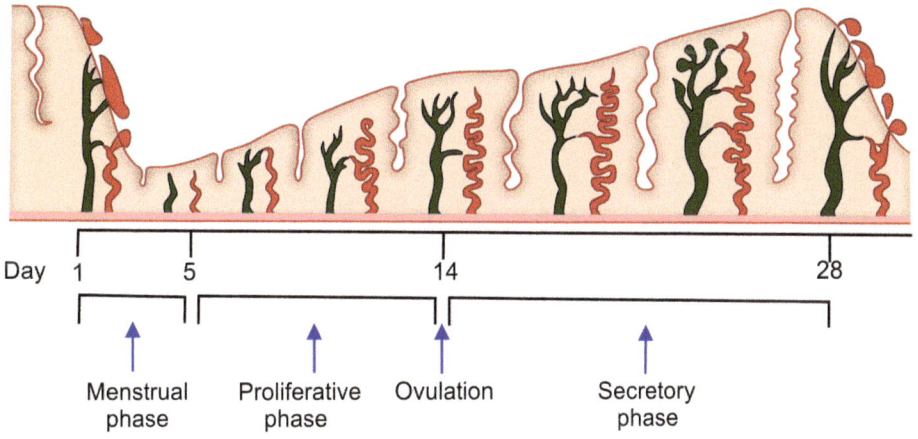

FIGURE 53.5: Uterine changes during menstrual cycle.

TABLE 53.1: Menstrual cycle in nutshell.

Organ changes	Phase and hormones involved	Event	Process
Ovarian changes	Follicular phase (5th to 14th day) FSH, LH and E	Maturation of ovum	Ovarian follicle → Primordial follicle → Primary follicle → Vesicular follicle → Graafian follicle
		Release of ovum (ovulation)	Rupture of Graafian follicle → Release of ovum into abdominal cavity
	Luteal phase (15th to 28th day) FSH, LH, E and P	Formation of corpus luteum	Ruptured Graafian follicle → Corpus hemorrhagicum → Corpus luteum
Uterine changes	Menstrual phase (1st to 5th day) Increased E and P and Lack of FSH and LH	Desquamation and expulsion of endometrium	Involution of endometrium → Vasoconstriction and hypoxia → Rupture of blood vessels → Necrosis of endometrium → Thinning of endometrium to 1 mm → Expulsion of desquamated endometrium
	Proliferative phase (6th to 14th day) E and P	Increase in the thickness of endometrium	Proliferation of endometrial cells → Development of uterine glands and blood vessels → Increase in the thickness of endometrium to 3 to 4 mm
	Secretory phase (15th to 28th day) E and P	Preparation of uterus to receive fertilized ovum	Increase in number and size of blood vessels and uterine glands → Increase in blood supply → Tortuosity of blood vessels and uterine glands → Deposition of lipid and glycogen in endometrium → Increase in thickness of endometrium to 6 mm
Cervical changes	Proliferative phase	Helps in survival and motility of sperm	Mucous membrane becomes thinner and more alkaline
	Secretory phase	Holding the sperms	Mucous membrane becomes thick and adhesive
Vaginal changes	Proliferative phase	Increase in resistance for infection	Cornification of epithelial cells
	Secretory phase		Proliferation of epithelial cells and infiltration with leukocytes

FSH = Follicle stimulating hormone. LH = Luteinizing hormone. E = Estrogen. P = Progesterone

Changes in Endometrium during Proliferative Phase

1. Endometrial cells proliferate rapidly.
2. Epithelium reappears on the surface of endometrium within the first 4 to 7 days.
3. Uterine glands start developing within the endometrial stroma.
4. Blood vessels also appear in the stroma.
5. Proliferation of endometrial cells occurs continuously so that the endometrium reaches the thickness of 3 to 4 mm at the end of proliferative phase.

All these uterine changes during proliferative phase occur because of the influence of estrogen released from ovary. On 14th day, **ovulation** occurs under the influence of LH. This is followed by secretory phase.

SECRETORY PHASE

Secretory phase extends between 15th and 28th day of the menstrual cycle, i.e. between the day of ovulation and the day when menstruation of next cycle commences.

After ovulation, corpus luteum is developed in the ovary. It secretes a large quantity of progesterone along with a small amount of estrogen. Estrogen causes further proliferation of cells in uterus. Because of this, endometrium becomes very thick. Progesterone causes further enlargement of endometrial stroma and further growth of glands.

Under the influence of progesterone, endometrial glands commence their secretory function. Many changes occur in the endometrium before commencement of secretory function.

Changes in Endometrium during Secretory Phase

1. Endometrial glands become more tortuous. Because of increase in size, the glands become tortuous to get accommodated within the endometrium.
2. Cytoplasm of stromal cells increases because of the deposition of glycogen and lipids.
3. Many new blood vessels appear within endometrial stroma. Blood vessels also become tortuous.
4. Blood supply to endometrium increases.
5. Thickness of endometrium increases up to 6 mm.

Actually, secretory phase is the preparatory period during which, uterus is prepared for **implantation** of ovum. At the end of secretory phase, the thickness of endometrium is 5 to 6 mm. All these uterine changes during secretory phase occur due to the influence of estrogen and progesterone. Estrogen is responsible for repair of damaged endometrium and growth of the glands. Progesterone is responsible for further growth of these structures and secretory activities in the endometrium.

If a **fertilized ovum** is implanted during this phase and, if the implanted ovum starts developing into a **fetus**, further changes occur in the uterus for the survival of the developing fetus. If the implanted ovum is unfertilized or if pregnancy does not occur, **menstruation** occurs after this phase and a new cycle begins.

CHANGES IN CERVIX DURING MENSTRUAL CYCLE

Mucous membrane of cervix also shows cyclic changes during different phases of menstrual cycle.

Proliferative Phase

Under the influence of estrogen, during proliferative phase, mucous membrane of cervix becomes thin and **alkaline**. It helps in the survival and motility of spermatozoa.

Secretory Phase

Because of actions of progesterone during secretory phase, the mucous membrane of cervix becomes thick and adhesive.

CHANGES IN VAGINA DURING MENSTRUAL CYCLE

Proliferative Phase

Epithelial cells of vagina are **cornified**. Estrogen released from ovary is responsible for the cornification of vaginal epithelial cells.

Secretory Phase

Vaginal epithelium proliferates due to the actions of progesterone. Vaginal epithelium is **infiltrated with leukocytes**. These two changes increase the resistance for infection.

REGULATION OF MENSTRUAL CYCLE

Menstrual cycle is regulated by hormones of hypothalamic-pituitary-ovarian axis.

HORMONES INVOLVED IN REGULATION

Hormones involved in regulation of menstrual cycle are:
1. Hypothalamic hormone: GnRH.
2. Anterior pituitary hormones: FSH and LH.
3. Ovarian hormones: Estrogen and progesterone.

Hypothalamic Hormone

Gonadotropin releasing hormone (GnRH) from hypothalamus triggers the onset of cyclic changes during menstrual cycle by stimulating secretion of follicle stimulating hormone (FSH) and luteinizing hormone (LH) from anterior pituitary.

Anterior Pituitary Hormones

FSH and LH secreted from anterior pituitary modulate the ovarian and uterine changes by acting directly and/or indirectly via ovarian hormones. FSH stimulates the recruitment and growth of immature ovarian follicles. LH triggers ovulation and sustains corpus luteum.

Secretion of FSH and LH is under the influence of GnRH.

Ovarian Hormones

Estrogen and progesterone which are secreted by follicle and corpus luteum show many activities during menstrual cycle. Ovarian follicle secretes large quantity of estrogen and corpus luteum secretes large quantity of progesterone.

Estrogen secretion reaches the peak twice in each cycle; once during follicular phase just before ovulation and another one during luteal phase **(Fig. 53.6)**. On the other hand, progesterone is virtually absent during follicular phase till prior to ovulation. But it plays a critical role during luteal phase.

Estrogen is responsible for the growth of follicles. Both the steroids act together to produce the changes in uterus, cervix and vagina.

Both the ovarian hormones are under the influence of GnRH which acts via FSH and LH. In addition, the secretion of GnRH, FSH and LH is regulated by ovarian hormones.

■ APPLIED PHYSIOLOGY: MENSTRUAL DISORDERS
■ 1. MENSTRUAL SYMPTOMS

Menstrual symptoms are the unpleasant symptoms with discomfort, which appear in many women during menstruation. These symptoms are due to hormonal withdrawal, leading to cramps in uterine muscle before or during menstruation.

Common menstrual symptoms are abdominal pain, dysmenorrhea (menstrual pain), headache, irritability and depression.

■ 2. PREMENSTRUAL SYNDROME

Premenstrual syndrome (PMS) is the symptom of stress that appears before the onset of menstruation. It is also

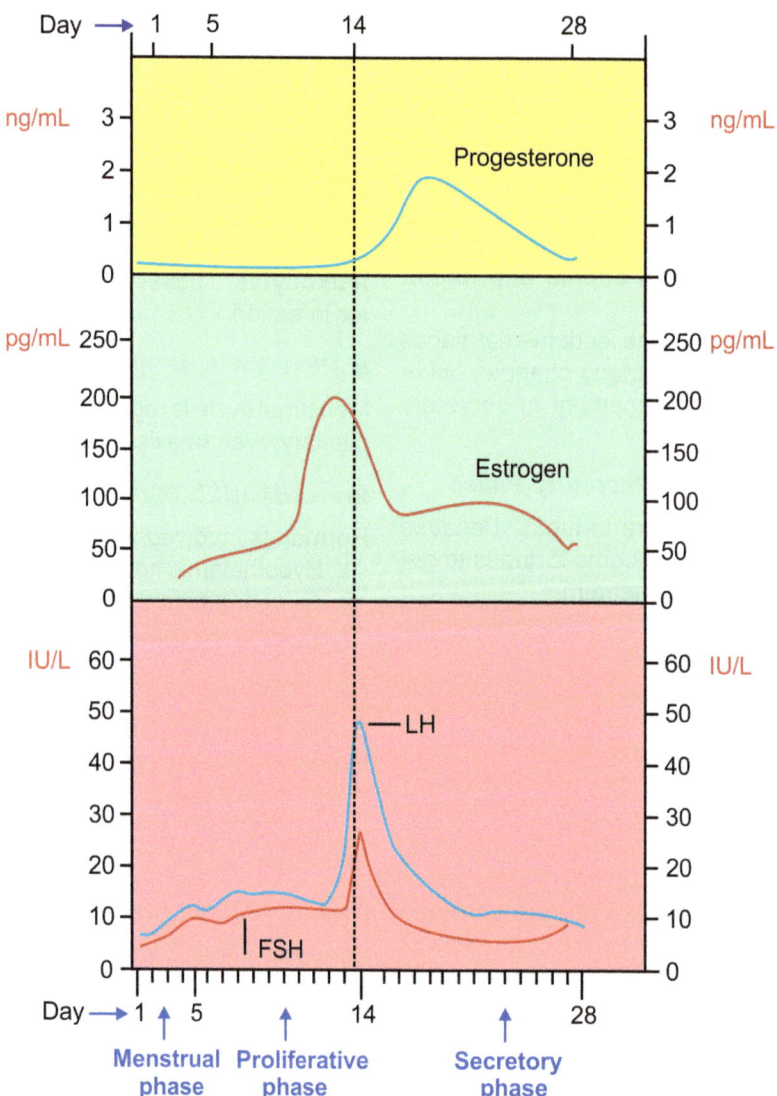

FIGURE 53.6: Hormonal level during menstrual cycle.
LH = Luteinizing hormones, FSH = Follicle-stimulating hormone

TABLE 53.2: Abnormal menstrual cycle.

Abnormality	Feature
1. Amenorrhea	Absence of menstrual bleeding
2. Hypomenorrhea or scanty menstruation	Scanty and light menstrual bleeding
3. Menorrhagia or heavy menstrual bleeding	Heavy and prolonged menstrual bleeding
4. Oligomenorrhea	Less menstrual bleeding with decreased frequency
5. Polymenorrhea	Increased frequency of menstrual bleeding with short menstrual cycle
6. Dysmenorrhea or painful periods or menstrual cramps	Menstruation with pain
7. Metrorrhagia	Abnormal uterine bleeding between menstruations

called premenstrual stress syndrome, premenstrual stress or premenstrual tension. It lasts for about 4 to 5 days prior to menstruation. Symptoms appear due to salt and water retention caused by estrogen.

Common symptoms of this condition are anxiety, emotional instability, headache, depression, constipation, abdominal cramping and bloating (abdominal swelling).

3. ABNORMAL MENSTRUATION

Abnormal types of menstruation are listed in **Table 53.2**.

4. ANOVULATORY CYCLE

Anovulatory cycle is the menstrual cycle in which ovulation does not occur. Menstrual bleeding occurs but the release of ovum does not occur. It is common during puberty and few years before menopause.

When it occurs before menopause, it is called **perimenopause**. If it occurs very often during childbearing years, it leads to infertility.

Chapter 54

Pregnancy, Parturition, Mammary Glands and Lactation

CHAPTER OUTLINE

- DEVELOPMENT OF OVUM
- FERTILIZATION OF THE OVUM
- SEX CHROMOSOMES AND SEX DETERMINATION
- IMPLANTATION AND DEVELOPMENT OF EMBRYO
- PLACENTA
- MATERNAL CHANGES IN PHYSIOLOGICAL SYSTEMS
- GESTATION PERIOD
- PARTURITION
- PREGNANCY TESTS
- MAMMARY GLANDS
- BREAST MILK

DEVELOPMENT OF OVUM

Ovum is released from Graafian follicle of ovary into the abdominal cavity at the time of ovulation. From abdominal cavity, ovum enters fallopian tube through the fimbriated end.

Ovum of matured follicle in the ovary is in **primary oocyte** stage with **diploid number** (23 pairs) of chromosomes. Just before ovulation, meiotic division takes place in the ovum. **Primary oocyte** divides into a **secondary oocyte** and a **first polar body**. First polar body is expelled out. Secondary oocyte contains only 23 chromosomes (haploid). Remaining 23 chromosomes are lost in the expelled first polar body.

Thus, when ovum is released into abdominal cavity during ovulation, it is in the **secondary oocyte stage** with haploid number of chromosomes.

FERTILIZATION OF THE OVUM

Fertilization is the fusion (union) of male and female gametes (sperm and ovum) to form a new offspring.

Ovum is released into abdominal cavity during ovulation. If sexual intercourse occurs at this time and semen is ejaculated in the vagina, sperms travel through vagina and uterus to reach the fallopian tube. Among 200 to 300 million of sperms entering female genital tract, only one succeeds in fertilizing the ovum.

During fertilization, the sperm enters the ovum by penetrating **granulosa cells** present around the ovum. It is facilitated by **hyaluronidase** and **proteolytic enzymes** present in the acrosome of sperm.

SEX CHROMOSOMES AND SEX DETERMINATION

SEX CHROMOSOMES

All the dividing cells in the body have 23 pairs of chromosomes. Among the 23 pairs, 22 pairs are called **somatic chromosomes** or **autosomes**. Remaining one pair of chromosomes is called **sex chromosomes**. Sex chromosomes are X and Y chromosomes.

SEX DETERMINATION

Sex chromosomes are responsible for sex determination. During fertilization of ovum, 23 chromosomes from ovum and 23 chromosomes from the sperm unite together to form the 23 pairs (46) of chromosomes in the fertilized ovum.

Now, sex determination occurs. Ovum contains the X chromosome. Sperm has either X chromosome or Y chromosome. When the ovum is fertilized by a sperm with X chromosome, the child will be female with XX chromosome. And, if the ovum is fertilized by a sperm with Y chromosome, sex of the child will be male with XY chromosome. So, the sex of the child depends upon the male partner.

Role of testosterone in **sex differentiation** is explained in Chapter 51.

IMPLANTATION AND DEVELOPMENT OF EMBRYO

Implantation is the process by which the fertilized ovum implants (fixes itself or gets attached) in the endometrium of uterus. After fertilization, the ovum is known as **zygote**. Zygote takes 3 to 5 days to reach the uterine cavity from fallopian tube. While travelling through fallopian tube, the zygote receives its nutrition from the secretions of fallopian tube.

After reaching uterus, the developing zygote remains freely in uterine cavity for 2 to 4 days before it is implanted. Just before implantation, the zygote develops into **morula**.

Already uterus is prepared by progesterone secreted from the corpus luteum during secretory phase of menstrual cycle. After implantation, morula develops into **embryo**. Placenta develops between morula and endometrium.

■ PLACENTA

Placenta is a temporary membranous vascular organ that develops during pregnancy. It is expelled after child birth. Placenta forms a link between the fetus and mother. It is considered as an **anchor** for the growing fetus. It is not only the physical attachment between fetus and mother but also forms the **physiological connection** between the two.

Placenta is implanted in the wall of uterus. It is formed from both embryonic and maternal tissues. So, it consists of two parts namely **fetal part** and **mother's part**. It is connected to the fetus by **umbilical cord** which contains blood vessels and connective tissue.

Delivery of fetus is followed by the expulsion of placenta. After expulsion of placenta, the umbilical cord is cut. Site of attachment of placenta in the center of anterior abdomen of fetus is called **naval** or **umbilicus**.

■ FUNCTIONS OF PLACENTA

Nutritive Function

Various nutritive substances, electrolytes and hormones necessary for the development of fetus diffuse from the mother's blood into fetal blood through placenta.

Excretory Function

Metabolic end products and other waste products from the fetal body are excreted into the mother's blood through placenta.

Respiratory Function

Fetal lungs are nonfunctioning and placenta forms the respiratory organ for fetus. Oxygen necessary for fetus is received by diffusion from maternal blood through placenta. And carbon dioxide from the fetal blood diffuses into mother's blood through placenta.

Endocrine Function

Placenta secretes **five hormones**:

1. Human chorionic gonadotropin

Human chorionic gonadotropin (hCG) is a glycoprotein.

Actions of hCG

i. On corpus luteum: This hormone is responsible for preservation and the secretory activity of corpus luteum.

ii. On fetal testes: Action of hCG on fetal testes is similar to that of LH in adults. It stimulates the interstitial cells of Leydig and causes secretion of testosterone which is necessary for the development of sex organs in male fetus.

2. Estrogen

Placental estrogen is similar to ovarian estrogen in structure and function.

Actions of placental estrogen

i. On uterus: Estrogen causes enlargement of uterus, so that the growing fetus can be accommodated.
ii. On breasts: Estrogen is responsible for the enlargement of breasts and growth of duct system in breasts.
iii. On pelvis: Estrogen relaxes pelvic ligaments. It facilitates the passage of fetus through birth canal at the time of labor.

3. Progesterone

Placental progesterone is similar to ovarian progesterone in structure and function.

Actions of placental progesterone

i. On uterus: Progesterone accelerates the proliferation and development of decidual cells in the endometrium of uterus. Progesterone inhibits the contraction of muscles in pregnant uterus and prevents expulsion of fetus during pregnancy.
ii. On breasts: Progesterone causes enlargement of breasts and growth of duct system of the breasts.

4. Human chorionic somatomammotropin

Human chorionic somatomammotropin (HCS) is a protein hormone secreted from placenta. It acts on mammary glands and enhance the growth of fetus by influencing the metabolic activities.

5. Relaxin

Relaxin is a polypeptide which is secreted by corpus luteum. It is also secreted in large quantity by placenta and mammary glands at the time of labor.

■ FETOPLACENTAL UNIT

Fetoplacental unit is the interaction between fetus and placenta in the formation of steroid hormones. This type of interaction between fetus and placenta occurs, because some of the enzymes involved in steroid synthesis present in fetus are absent in placenta and, those enzymes which are absent in fetus are present in placenta.

Due to this interaction during synthesis of steroid hormones, fetus and placenta are together called fetoplacental unit.

■ MATERNAL CHANGES IN PHYSIOLOGICAL SYSTEMS DURING PREGNANCY

■ 1. BLOOD

Blood volume increases by about 20% or about 1 L. It is because of increase in plasma volume. This leads to hemodilution. Because of great demand for iron by fetus, the mother usually develops anemia.

2. CARDIOVASCULAR SYSTEM

i. Cardiac Output

Cardiac output increases by about 30% in the first trimester. After the 3rd month, cardiac output starts decreasing and reaches almost the normal level in later stages of pregnancy.

ii. Blood Pressure

Arterial blood pressure remains unchanged during the first trimester. During the second trimester, there is a slight decrease in blood pressure. In third semester blood pressure increases. In some women, hypertension may develop if proper prenatal care is not taken.

Pre-eclampsia or toxemia of pregnancy

Pre-eclampsia or toxemia of pregnancy is the **hypertensive** disorder of pregnancy that occurs in 3 to 4% of the pregnant women. It usually occurs during last trimester of pregnancy.

Eclampsia

Eclampsia is the serious condition of pre-eclampsia characterized by severe **vascular spasm**, dangerous **hypertension** and **convulsions** almost like **seizures**. It occurs just before, during or immediately after delivery. It leads to **death**, if timely treatment is not given.

3. RESPIRATORY SYSTEM

Overall activity of respiratory system increases slightly. Tidal volume, pulmonary ventilation and oxygen utilization are increased.

4. EXCRETORY SYSTEM

Renal blood flow and glomerular filtration rate increase resulting in increase in urine formation. It is because of increase in fluid intake and the increased excretory products from fetus. Urine becomes diluted with the specific gravity of 1,025. In the first trimester, frequency of micturition increases.

5. DIGESTIVE SYSTEM

i. Morning Sickness

Morning sickness is the feeling of sickness during early part of pregnancy. It is characterized by **nausea, vomiting** and tiredness or **giddiness**. Morning sickness starts around 4 to 6 weeks of pregnancy and reaches the peak between 9 and 11 weeks. In most of the women symptoms disappear in 14 to 16 weeks.

Morning sickness is due to high level of **human chorionic gonadotropin (hCG)**.

ii. Other Changes in Digestive System

Indigestion and **hypochlorhydria** (decrease in the amount of hydrochloric acid in gastric juice) and constipation are also common during pregnancy.

6. ENDOCRINE SYSTEM

i. Anterior Pituitary

During pregnancy, size of anterior pituitary increases by about 50%. And secretion of corticotropin, thyrotropin and prolactin increases. However, the secretion of FSH and LH decreases very much. It is because of negative feedback control by estrogen and progesterone which are continuously secreted from corpus luteum initially and placenta later on.

ii. Adrenal Cortex

There is moderate increase in secretion of cortisol and aldosterone. Aldosterone is responsible for the retention of water and sodium.

iii. Thyroid Gland

Size and the secretory activity of thyroid gland increase during pregnancy.

iii. Parathyroid Gland

Parathyroid glands also show an increase in the size and secretory activity.

7. NERVOUS SYSTEM

There is general excitement of nervous system during pregnancy. It leads to the **psychological imbalance,** such as change in the moods, excitement or depression in the early stages of pregnancy. During the later months of pregnancy, the woman becomes very much excited because of anticipation of delivery of the baby, labor pain, etc.

GESTATION PERIOD

Gestation period means the pregnancy period. The average gestation period is about 280 days or 40 weeks from the date of **last menstrual period (LMP)**. Traditionally it is calculated as 10 lunar months. However, in terms of modern calendar, it is calculated as 9 months and 7 days. If the menstrual cycle is normal 28 days cycle, the fertilization of ovum by the sperm occurs on 14th day after last menstrual period.

Thus, the actual duration of human pregnancy is 280 − 14 = 266 days. If the pregnancy ends before 28th week, it is referred as **miscarriage**.

PARTURITION

Parturition is the expulsion or delivery of the fetus from mother's body. It occurs at the end of pregnancy. The process by which **delivery of fetus** occurs is called **labor**. It involves various actions, such as contraction of uterus, dilatation of cervix and opening of vaginal canal.

BRAXTON HICKS CONTRACTIONS

Braxton Hicks contractions are the weak, irregular, short and usually painless uterine contractions which start after 6th week of pregnancy. These contractions are named after the British doctor, who discovered them in 1872. It is suggested that such contractions do not induce cervical dilatation, but may cause softening of cervix. Often called the **practice contractions,** Braxton Hicks contractions help the uterus practice for upcoming labor. Sometimes these contractions cause discomfort.

■ FALSE LABOR CONTRACTIONS

While nearing the time of delivery, Braxton Hicks contractions become intense and are called **false labor contractions**. False labor contractions are believed to help cervical dilatation.

■ STAGES OF PARTURITION

Parturition occurs in three stages.

First Stage

First, strong uterine contractions called **labor contractions** commence. These labor contractions arise from the fundus of uterus and move downwards so that the head of fetus is pushed against the cervix. It results in dilatation of cervix and opening of vaginal canal. This stage extends for a variable period of time.

Second Stage

In this stage, the fetus is delivered out from uterus through cervix and vaginal canal. This stage lasts for about one hour.

Third Stage

During this stage, the **placenta** is detached from decidua and is expelled out from uterus. It occurs within 10 to 15 minutes after the delivery of the child.

■ PREGNANCY TESTS

Pregnancy test is the test used to detect or confirm pregnancy. Pregnancy tests are based on presence of **human chorionic gonadotropin (hCG)** in urine of woman suspected for pregnancy. Both biological and immunological tests are available to determine the presence of hCG in the urine of the pregnant woman. However, biological tests for pregnancy are replaced by immunological tests because of several disadvantages.

■ IMMUNOLOGICAL TESTS

Immunological tests are more accurate and the result is obtained quickly within few minutes. These tests are based on **double antigen-antibody reactions**. Most commonly performed immunological test is known as Gravindex test.

Principle

Principle is to determine the agglutination of sheep RBCs coated with hCG. Latex particles could also be used instead of sheep RBCs.

Requisites

Antiserum from rabbit

Urine from a pregnant woman is collected and hCG is isolated. This hCG is injected into a rabbit.

The rabbit develops antibodies against hCG. This antibody is called **hCG antibody** or **anti-hCG**. Rabbit's blood is obtained and serum is separated. Serum containing hCG antibody is called **rabbit antiserum** or **hCG antiserum**. It is readily available in the market.

Red blood cells from sheep

RBCs are obtained from sheep's blood and are coated with pure hCG obtained from urine of the pregnant women. Nowadays, instead of sheep's RBCs, the rubberized synthetic particles called the **latex particles** are used.

Urine

Fresh urine sample of the woman, who needs to confirm pregnancy, is collected.

Procedure

One drop of hCG antiserum is taken on a glass slide. One drop of urine from the woman who wants to confirm pregnancy is added to this and both are mixed well. If urine contains hCG, all the antibodies of antiserum are used up for agglutination of hCG molecules. The agglutination of hCG molecules by the antiserum is not visible, because it is colorless.

Now, one drop of latex particles is added to this and mixed.

Observation and Result

If the urine contains hCG, it is agglutinated by the antibodies of the antiserum, and all the antibodies are fully used up. No free antibody is available. Later when latex particles are added, these particles are not agglutinated because the free antibody is not available. Thus, the absence of agglutination of latex particles indicates that the woman is pregnant.

If the urine without hCG is mixed with antiserum, the antibodies are freely available. When latex particles are added, the antibodies cause agglutination of these latex particles. Agglutination of latex particles can be seen clearly even with naked eye. Thus, the presence of agglutination of latex particles indicates that the woman is not pregnant **(Fig. 54.1)**.

Nowadays **pregnancy test strip** is used. Advantage of this test strip is, it can be used even in the first few days of conception. Most sensitive test can detect hCG level as low as 20 mIU/mL.

■ MAMMARY GLANDS
■ DEVELOPMENT OF MAMMARY GLANDS

At Birth

At the time of birth, mammary gland is rudimentary and consists of only a tiny nipple and few radiating ducts from it.

At Childhood

Till puberty, there is no difference in the structure of mammary gland between male and female.

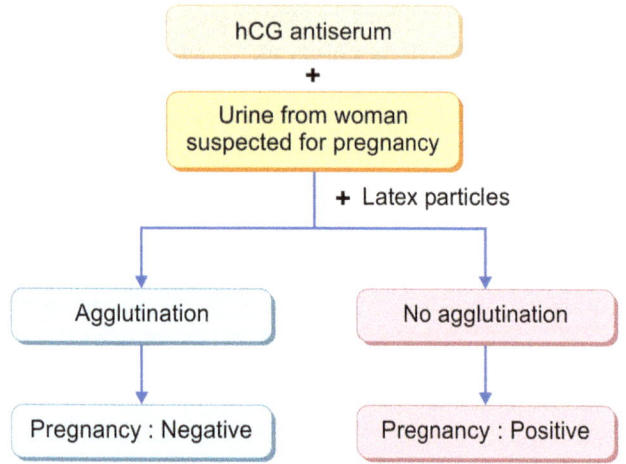

FIGURE 54.1: Immunological test for pregnancy.

At Puberty

At the time of puberty and afterwards there is a vast change in the structure of female mammary gland due to hormonal influence. The beginning of changes in the mammary gland is called **thelarche**. It occurs at the time of puberty, just before **menarche** (Chapter 53). At puberty, there is growth of duct system and formation of glandular tissue. Progressive enlargement occurs, which is also due to the deposition of fat.

During Pregnancy

During pregnancy, the mammary glands enlarge to a great extent accompanied by marked changes in structure. During first half of pregnancy, the duct system develops further with appearance of many new alveoli. No milk is secreted by the gland now.

During the second half, there is enormous growth of glandular tissues and the development is completed for the production of milk just before the end of gestation period.

ROLE OF HORMONES IN GROWTH OF MAMMARY GLANDS

Various hormones are involved in the development and growth of breasts at different stages:

1. Estrogen which causes growth and branching of duct system and accumulation of fat in breasts.
2. Progesterone which stimulates the development of glandular tissues and stroma of mammary glands.
3. Prolactin that is necessary for milk secretion. It also accelerates growth of mammary glands during pregnancy by causing proliferation of epithelial cells of alveoli.
4. Placental hormones namely estrogen and progesterone cause further development of mammary glands during pregnancy by stimulating the proliferation of ducts and glandular cells.
5. Other hormones such as growth hormone, thyroxine, cortisol and relaxin enhance the overall growth and development of mammary glands in all stages.

LACTATION

Lactation means synthesis, secretion and ejection of milk. It involves two processes:

A. Milk secretion.
B. Milk ejection.

A. MILK SECRETION

Milk secretion refers to **synthesis of milk** by alveolar epithelium and its passage through the duct system. This process occurs in two phases:

1. Initiation of milk secretion or lactogenesis.
2. Maintenance of milk secretion or galactopoiesis.

1. Initiation of Milk Secretion or Lactogenesis

Although small amount of milk secretion occurs at later months of pregnancy, a free flow of milk occurs only after the delivery of the child. The milk secreted initially before parturition is called **colostrum**.

Colostrum is lemon yellow in color and it is rich in protein (particularly globulins) and salts. But its sugar content is low. It contains almost all the components of milk except fat.

Role of hormones in lactogenesis

During pregnancy, particularly in later months, large quantity of prolactin is secreted. But the activity of this hormone is suppressed by estrogen and progesterone secreted by placenta. Because of this, lactation is prevented during pregnancy.

Immediately after the delivery of baby and expulsion of placenta, there is sudden loss of estrogen and progesterone. Now, the prolactin is free to exert its action on breasts and to promote lactogenesis.

2. Maintenance of Milk Secretion or Galactopoiesis

Galactopoiesis occurs up to 7 to 9 months after delivery of child provided feeding the baby with mother's milk is continued till then. In fact, the milk production is continued only if feeding the baby is continued.

Role of hormones in galactopoiesis

Galactopoiesis depends upon prolactin secretion. Other hormones like growth hormone, thyroxine and cortisol are essential for continuous supply of glucose, amino acids, fatty acids, calcium and other substances necessary for the milk production **(Fig. 54.2)**.

B. MILK EJECTION

Milk ejection is the discharge of milk from mammary gland. It depends upon suckling exerted by the baby and on contractile mechanism in breast, which expels milk from alveoli into the ducts.

Milk ejection is a reflex phenomenon. It is called milk ejection reflex or milk let down reflex. It is a neuroendocrine reflex.

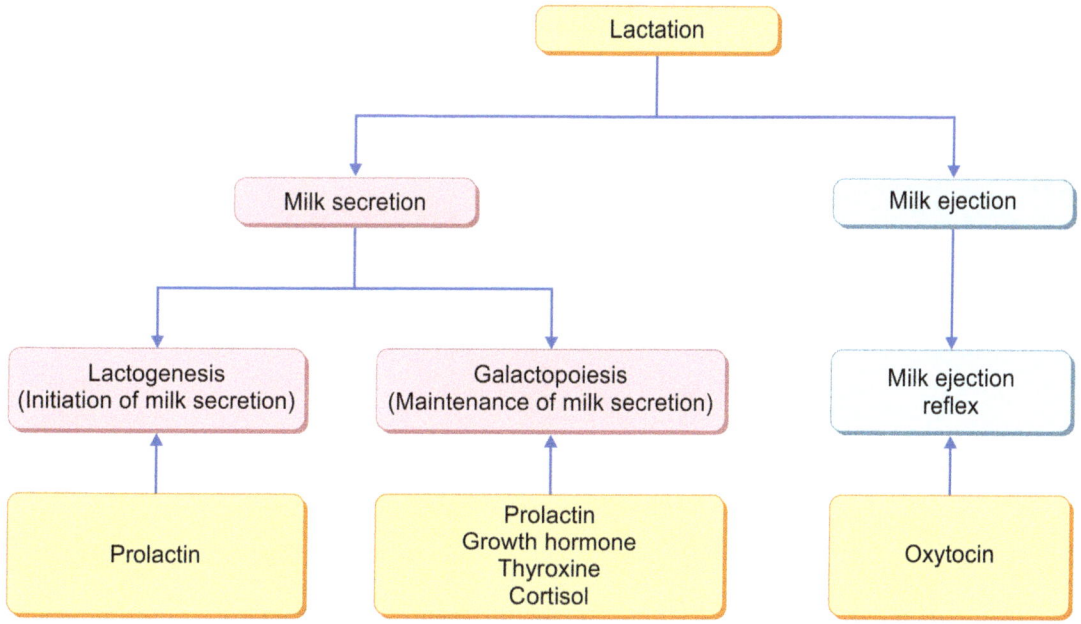

FIGURE 54.2: Process of lactation and role of hormones.

Milk Ejection Reflex

Milk ejection reflex is explained in Chapter 44.

■ BREAST MILK

Breast or human milk forms the primary source of nutrition for infants.

■ COMPOSITION OF MILK

Breast milk contains about 88.5% of water and 11.5% of solids.

Solids include:
1. Nutrients: Lactose, casein, lactalbumin, lactoglobulin, cholesterol and essential fatty acids
2. Minerals: Sodium, calcium, potassium, magnesium, chloride, phosphorous, negligible quantity of iron and copper
3. Vitamins: A, B, C, D, E and K
4. Immunoglobulins: IgA, IgG and IgM
5. Antibacterial agents: Lysozyme and lactoferrin
6. Cells: Neutrophils and other leukocytes, macrophages and stem cells
7. Other substances: Digestive enzymes, hormones, transforming growth factor-β, interleukin-10 and insulin-like growth factor 1.

■ ADVANTAGES OF BREAST MILK

Breast milk is always considered superior to animal milk (cow milk or goat milk) because it consists of sufficient quantity of all the substances necessary for infants such as iron, vitamins and minerals.

Besides nourishment of infant, the breast milk also provides several antibodies which help the infant resist the infection by lethal bacteria. Even some phagocytic cells, such as neutrophils and macrophages are secreted in milk. Phagocytic cells protect the infant by destroying microbes in the infant's body.

CHAPTER 55

Fertility Control

CHAPTER OUTLINE

- **CONTRACEPTIVE METHODS**
- **RHYTHM METHOD**
- **BARRIER METHODS**
  - PHYSICAL BARRIERS
  - CHEMICAL BARRIERS
- **INTRAUTERINE CONTRACEPTIVE DEVICE (IUCD)**
- **HORMONAL CONTRACEPTIVES**
  - ORAL CONTRACEPTIVES
  - HORMONAL IMPLANTS
- **OTHER HORMONAL CONTRACEPTIVES**
- **MEDICAL TERMINATION OF PREGNANCY (MTP): ABORTION**
  - DILATATION AND CURETTAGE (D AND C)
  - VACUUM ASPIRATION
  - ADMINISTRATION OF PROSTAGLANDIN
- **SURGICAL METHOD (STERILIZATION): PERMANENT METHOD**
  - TUBECTOMY
  - VASECTOMY

■ CONTRACEPTIVE METHODS

Contraception means prevention of pregnancy. It is also called **birth control**, **fertility control** or **family planning**.

Contraceptive method or fertility control method is the method or device that is used by a woman to prevent pregnancy. Contraceptive methods may be temporary or permanent. Several methods are available for fertility control. Each method has its own advantages and disadvantages.

■ RHYTHM METHOD

Rhythm method of fertility control is based on the time of ovulation.

■ FERTILE PERIOD

After ovulation, i.e. on the 14th day of menstrual cycle, the ovum is fertilized during its passage through fallopian tubes. Its viability is only for 2 days after ovulation, and should be fertilized within this period.

Sperms survive only for about 24 to 48 hours after ejaculation in the female genital tract. If sexual intercourse occurs during this period, i.e. few days before and few days after ovulation, there is chance of pregnancy. This period is called fertile or dangerous period. Pregnancy can be avoided if there is no sexual intercourse during this period. Prevention of pregnancy by avoiding sexual mating during this period is called rhythm method.

■ INFERTILE OR STERILE OR SAFE PERIOD

Periods when pregnancy does not occur are 4 to 5 days after menstrual bleeding and 5 to 6 days before the onset of next cycle. These periods are together called infertile or sterile or **safe period.**

■ ADVANTAGES AND DISADVANTAGES OF RHYTHM METHOD

It is one of the most successful methods of fertility control, provided the woman knows exact day of ovulation. However, it is not a successful method because of various reasons. Basic knowledge about the menstrual cycle is necessary to determine the day of ovulation. Self restrain is essential to avoid sexual intercourse. Because of these practical difficulties, this method is not popular.

■ BARRIER METHODS

Barriers are used to prevent the entry of sperm into uterine cavity during sexual intercourse. Barriers are of two types namely, physical barriers and chemical barriers.

■ PHYSICAL BARRIERS

Physical barriers are condoms, cervical cap, diaphragm and vaginal sponge.

1. *Condom*

Condom is one of the barriers used for contraception. It is available for both males and females.

Male condom

Condom is the commonly used barrier by men. Male condom is a thin leak-proof and stretchy pouch made of latex or plastic, polyurethane. It is fitted over erectile penis just before intercourse. It does not permit entrance of semen into the female genital tract during coitus.

Female condom

Female condom, also called **internal condom** is a soft pouch made of polyurethane. It is put inside vagina before intercourse, and it forms a barrier to stop sperm to meet the ovum.

Advantages of condoms

1. If used correctly, condoms are most effective contraceptive devices.
2. Condoms are the only contraceptive devices that protect against **sexually transmitted infections (STI)** including infection by **human immunodeficiency virus (HIV)**.
3. Used only at the time of intercourse.

Disadvantages of condoms

1. If not used correctly, condoms particularly in men may tear or slip off.
2. One or both partners may not feel comfortable with condom and may feel interference of condom with sex sensation.

2. Cervical Cap

Cervical cap is the commonly used barrier device in females. It is a small bowl-shaped cup made from latex or silicon. When inserted into the vagina it fits tightly over cervix. Cervical cap is mostly used with spermicidal gel or cream. **Spermicide** is a substance that kills sperms.

Advantages and disadvantages of cervical cap

Cervical cap does not contain hormone but, its disadvantages are more. It is not an effective contraceptive device. Also, it does not protect against STI. Cervical cap is not available easily and it is also little difficult to insert.

3. Diaphragm

Diaphragm is a shallow flexible cup-shaped device made up of soft silicon. It is inserted into vagina to cover the cervix. It is always used with **spermicidal agent**.

Advantages and disadvantages of diaphragm

For many women diaphragm is a safest device but does not protect from the spread of STI. Repeated use of spermicide along with diaphragm may irritate vagina and increase the risk of infection.

4. Vaginal Sponge

Vaginal sponge is a contraceptive sponge that prevents entry of sperm into uterus. It is a small disk-shaped sponge made up of soft polyurethane foam. It also contains spermicide. After insertion into vagina, it covers cervix tightly.

Advantages and disadvantages of vaginal sponge

Sponge is the most effective device when used correctly. However, it does not protect against STI.

■ CHEMICAL BARRIERS

Chemical barriers are the substances which are applied in female genital tract before coitus to destroy the sperms. Destruction of sperms is called spermicidal action. Spermicidal substances are available in the form of foam tablets, jelly, cream and paste which are inserted into vagina deep up to cervix. Common chemical substance present in spermicidal agents is nonoxynol-9. Chemical barriers have not become popular because of so many drawbacks.

Advantages and Disadvantages of Chemical Barriers

Any spermicide is cheap and easy to use. But most of the spermicides cause vaginal irritation. Nonoxynal-9 may be allergic to many women. It also increases the risk of getting infected by HIV.

■ INTRAUTERINE CONTRACEPTIVE DEVICE (IUCD): PREVENTION OF FERTILIZATION AND IMPLANTATION OF OVUM

Intrauterine contraceptive device (IUCD) is a contraceptive device that is inserted into uterus. It prevents fertilization and the implantation of ovum. IUCD is a small device made from metal, polyurethane or other polymers.

■ TYPES OF IUCD

Three types of IUCD are available which are given below.

1. Nonmedicated IUCD

Nonmedicated IUCD is the **first generation** IUCD which is made from plastic. It is available in different shapes.

Common one is the **Lippes loop** which is "S" shaped. It is made up of polyethylene. Nonmedicated IUCD works by changing intrauterine environment which becomes spermicidal. This device causes a mild and sterile inflammatory reaction in uterine wall which is enough for spermicidal action.

Lippes loop is outdated now because of availability of new generations of IUCDs.

2. Copper IUCD

Copper IUCD or the **second generation** of IUCD is made from plastic and copper is added to it. Among the different varieties of copper bearing IUCDs, **Copper T** has become more popular. It is a T-shaped device made up of polyethylene frame. Copper-bearing IUCD also works like nonmedicated IUCD. In addition, it releases free copper and copper salts which cause mild changes in endometrial secretions and increase viscosity of cervical mucus to prevent entry of sperm into cervix.

3. Hormone-Releasing IUCD

Hormone-releasing IUCD is the **third generation** of IUCD. It releases hormone slowly into uterus after insertion. Most common one is called **progestasert**. It is filled with progesterone and it has a permeable polymer membrane to release the hormone.

Progestasert prevents **implantation of ovum** by maintaining high level of progesterone in endometrium. In addition, it also increases viscosity of cervical mucus to prevent sperm entry. When the hormone is exhausted, the device must be replaced **(Table 55.1)**.

■ DISADVANTAGES OF IUCD

IUCD has some disadvantages. It has the tendency to:
1. Cause heavy bleeding in some women.
2. Promote infection.
3. Come out of uterus accidentally.
4. Copper-bearing IUCD cannot be used for long time because release of copper ions is affected after some period due to deposition of materials like minerals. So, the device needs to be replaced periodically.
5. Same with hormone-releasing IUCD also. When the hormone is exhausted, the device must be replaced.

■ HORMONAL CONTRACEPTIVES

Hormonal contraceptives prevent pregnancy by inhibiting maturation of follicles and ovulation. This leads to alteration of normal menstrual cycle. Menstrual cycle becomes the **anovulatory cycle**. Some chemical contraceptives prevent entry of sperm into cervix by increasing the viscosity of cervical mucus. Some contraceptives prevent implantation of fertilized ovum.

Hormonal contraceptives are of different types namely, oral contraceptives, hormonal implants, injectable contraceptives, vaginal ring, contraceptive patch and hormonal IUCD.

■ ORAL CONTRACEPTIVES

Oral contraceptives are the drugs taken by mouth (pills) to prevent pregnancy. These pills prevent pregnancy by inhibiting maturation of follicles and ovulation. This leads to alteration of normal menstrual cycle. The menstrual cycle becomes the anovulatory cycle.

This method of fertility control is called **pill method** and pills are called **contraceptive pills** or birth control pills. These pills contain synthetic estrogen and synthetic progesterone.

Contraceptive pills are of four types:
1. Classical or combined pills.
2. Sequential pills.
3. Minipills or micropills.
4. Postcoital or emergency contraceptive pills.

1. Classical or Combined Pills

Classical or combined pills contain a moderate dose of synthetic estrogen like ethinyl estradiol or mestranol and a mild dose of synthetic progesterone like norethindrone or norgestrel.

These pills are taken daily from 5th to 25th day of menstrual cycle. Withdrawal of the pills after 25th day causes menstrual bleeding. Intake of pills is resumed again after 5th day of the next cycle.

Mechanism of action of classical pills

During continuous intake of the pills, there is relatively large amount of estrogen and progesterone in the blood. It suppresses the release of gonadotropins, FSH and LH from pituitary by means of feedback mechanism. Lack of FSH and LH prevents the maturation of follicle, and ovulation. In addition, progesterone increases the thickness of mucosa in cervix, which is not favorable for transport of sperm. When the pills are withdrawn after 21 days, the menstrual flow starts.

2. Sequential Pills

Sequential pills contain a high dose of estrogen along with moderate dose of progesterone. These pills are taken in two courses:

i. Daily for 15 days from 5th to 20th day of the menstrual cycle.
ii. Then during the last 5 days, i.e. 23rd to 28th day. Sequential pills also prevent ovulation.

3. Minipills of Micropills

Minipills contain a low dose of only progesterone and are taken throughout the menstrual cycle. It prevents pregnancy without affecting ovulation. Progesterone increases the thickness of cervical mucosa, so that the transport of sperms is inhibited. It also prevents implantation of ovum.

4. Postcoital Pills or Emergency Contraceptive Pills

Postcoital pills or **emergency contraceptive pills** are taken to prevent pregnancy after unprotected sex. These pills contain either **levonorgestrel** (synthetic progesterone) or **ethinyl estradiol** (synthetic estrogen).

Disadvantages of Oral Contraceptives

About 40% of women who use contraceptive pills may have minor transient side effects. However, long-term use of oral contraceptives causes some serious side effects such as hypertension, heart attack, stroke and cancer.

■ HORMONAL IMPLANTS OR LONG-TERM CONTRACEPTIVES

To avoid taking pills daily, the long-term contraceptives are used. These contraceptives are in the form of implants containing mainly progesterone. The implants which are inserted beneath skin release the drug slowly and prevent fertility for 4 to 5 years. Though it seems to be effective, it may produce amenorrhea.

■ OTHER HORMONAL CONTRACEPTIVES

Other hormonal contraceptive devices include:
1. Injectables which may be progesterone only injectable or combination injectable.

TABLE 55.1: Contraceptive methods.

Gender	Name of the method	Devices/Techniques	Mechanism of action
Both genders	Rhythm method	Knowledge and cooperation between the couple	By avoiding coitus during fertile period Fertile Period: Few days before and few days after ovulation Safe period: 5 to 6 days after menstrual bleeding and 5 to 6 days before onset of next cycle
Females	Physical barriers	1. Condom 2. Cervical cap 3. Diaphragm 4. Vaginal sponge	Cover the cervix and prevents entry of sperm into uterus
	Chemical methods	1. Foam tablets 2. Jelly 3. Cream 4. Paste	Inserted into vagina just before coitus Kills the sperms
	Intrauterine contraceptive devices (IUCD)	1. Non-medicated: Lippes loop 2. Copper-bearing: Copper T 3. Hormone-releasing: Progestasert	Inserted high in the uterus Prevent fertilization: 1. By reducing chances of sperm survival and entry of sperm into uterus 2. By impeding the movement of ovum into uterus
	Hormonal contraceptives	1. Oral contraceptives: Combination pills, sequential pills and mini pills 2. Hormonal implants 3. Others	Inhibit maturation of ovarian follicles and ovulation
	Medical termination of pregnancy (MTP)	Dilatation and curettage (D and C)	Dilatation of cervix and removal of implanted zygote
		Vacuum aspiration	Removal of implanted zygote by vacuum aspiration
		Prostaglandin administration	Expulsion of implanted zygote by inducing uterine contractions
	Surgical method	Tubectomy	Fallopian tubes are cut and the cut ends are ligated Prevents the entry of fertilized zygote into uterus for implantation
Males	Physical barrier	Male condom	Covers the penis and prevents entry of sperms into vagina
	Surgical method	Vasectomy	Vas deferens are cut and the cut ends are ligated Prevents the entry of sperms into the ejaculatory duct

2. Vaginal ring which contains progesterone.
3. Contraceptive patch containing hormone which is applied to skin over abdomen, buttock, lateral aspect of upper arm and upper torso.
4. Hormone-bearing IUCD which is already described.

MEDICAL TERMINATION OF PREGNANCY (MTP): ABORTION

Abortion is done during first few months of pregnancy. This method is called medical termination of pregnancy (MTP). There are three ways of doing MTP.

1. DILATATION AND CURETTAGE (D AND C)

In this method, the cervix is dilated and the implanted ovum or zygote is removed.

2. VACUUM ASPIRATION

The implanted ovum is removed by vacuum aspiration method. This is done up to 12 weeks of pregnancy.

3. ADMINISTRATION OF PROSTAGLANDIN

Administration of prostaglandin like PGE_2 and PGF_2 intravaginally increases uterine contractions resulting in abortion.

SURGICAL METHOD (STERILIZATION): PERMANENT METHOD

Permanent sterility is obtained by surgical methods. It is also called **sterilization**.

IN FEMALES: TUBECTOMY

In tubectomy, fallopian tubes are cut and both the cut ends are ligated. It prevents entry of ovum into uterus. This operation done through vaginal orifice in the postpartum period. During other periods, it is done by abdominal incision. Tubectomy is done quickly (in few minutes) by using a laparoscope.

Though tubectomy causes permanent sterility, if necessary, **recanalization** of fallopian tube can be done using plastic tube by another surgical procedure.

IN MALES: VASECTOMY

In vasectomy, vas deferens is cut and the cut ends are ligated. So, the sperms cannot enter the ejaculatory duct and semen is devoid of sperms. It is done by surgical procedure with local anesthesia. If necessary, the **recanalization** of vas deferens can be done with plastic tube.

MODEL QUESTIONS IN REPRODUCTIVE SYSTEM

■ LONG QUESTIONS

1. Describe the functions of testis and regulation of testicular functions.
2. Describe the actions and regulation of secretion of testosterone.
3. What are the female sex hormones? Explain their actions.
4. What is menstrual cycle? Explain the ovarian changes taking place during menstrual cycle.
5. Describe the uterine changes during menstrual cycle.

■ SHORT QUESTIONS

1. Spermatogenesis.
2. Testosterone.
3. Cryptorchidism.
4. Secondary sexual characters in males.
5. Semen.
6. Effects of removal of testes.
7. Estrogen.
8. Progesterone.
9. Follicle stimulating hormone.
10. Luteinizing hormone.
11. Gonadotropins.
12. Secondary sexual characters in females.
13. Ovarian follicles.
14. Ovulation.
15. Corpus luteum.
16. Functions of placenta.
17. Pregnancy tests.
18. Milk ejection reflex.
19. Safe period/Rhythm method.
20. Oral contraceptives.
21. MTP.
22. Tubectomy.
23. Condoms.
24. IUCD.
25. Vasectomy.

■ VERY SHORT ANSWER QUESTIONS

1. Prostate gland
2. Sertoli cells.
3. Sex differentiation in fetus/Müllerian and Wolffian ducts.
4. Descend of testes and cryptorchidism.
5. Regulation of testosterone secretion.
7. Properties and composition of semen.
8. Structure of sperm.
9. Hypergonadism in males.
10. Hypogonadism in males.
11. Graafian follicle.
12. Corpus luteum.
13. LH surge.
14. Changes in cervix during menstrual cycle.
15. Changes in vagina during menstrual cycle.
16. Abnormal menstruation.
17. Anovulatory cycle.
18. Hormonal regulation of ovulation.
19. Menopause.
20. Fertilization of ovum.
21. Sex chromosome and sex determination.
22. Braxton Hicks contractions.
23. Stages of parturition.
24. Endocrine function of placenta.
25. Human chorionic gonadotropin.
26. Human chorionic somatomammotropin.
27. Breast milk.
28. Rhythm method of fertility control.
29. Medical termination of pregnancy.
30. Surgical method of fertility control/Sterilization.

Section 8: Cardiovascular System

Chapter 56: Overview of Cardiovascular System

CHAPTER OUTLINE

- **CARDIOVASCULAR SYSTEM**
- **HEART**
  - RIGHT SIDE
  - LEFT SIDE
  - SEPTA
  - LAYERS OF WALL
  - VALVES
- **ACTIONS OF HEART**
  - CHRONOTROPIC ACTION
  - INOTROPIC ACTION
  - DROMOTROPIC ACTION
  - BATHMOTROPIC ACTION
  - LUSITROPIC ACTION
- **BLOOD VESSELS**
- **ARTERIAL SYSTEM**
- **VENOUS SYSTEM**
- **DIVISION OF CIRCULATION**

CARDIOVASCULAR SYSTEM

Cardiovascular system is made up of heart and blood vessels. Heart pumps the blood into blood vessels. Blood vessels circulate the blood throughout body and transport nutrients and oxygen to the tissues and remove carbon dioxide and waste products from the tissues.

HEART

Heart is a muscular organ that pumps blood throughout the circulatory system. It situated in between the two lungs in mediastinum. It is made up of four chambers, viz. two atria and two ventricles. Musculature is more and thick in the ventricles than in the atria. Force of contraction of the heart depends upon the thickness of muscular wall of heart chambers.

RIGHT SIDE OF HEART

Right side of the heart has two chambers, upper **right atrium** and lower **right ventricle**. Right atrium is a thin walled and low-pressure chamber. It has got the **pacemaker** known as **sinoatrial node** that produces cardiac impulses and atrioventricular node that conducts the impulses to the ventricles.

Right atrium receives venous (deoxygenated) blood via two large veins:

1. **Superior vena cava** that returns venous blood from the head, neck and upper limbs.
2. **Inferior vena cava** that returns venous blood from lower parts of the body (Fig. 56.1).

Right atrium communicates with the right ventricle through **tricuspid valve**. Venous blood from right atrium enters the right ventricle through this valve.

From right ventricle, **pulmonary artery** arises. This artery carries venous blood from right ventricle to the lungs. In the lungs, deoxygenated blood is oxygenated.

LEFT SIDE OF HEART

Left side of the heart has two chambers, upper **left atrium** and lower **left ventricle**. Left atrium is a thin walled and low-pressure chamber. It receives oxygenated blood from the lungs through **pulmonary veins**. This is the only exception in the body where an artery carries venous blood and vein carries the arterial blood.

Blood from left atrium enters the left ventricle through the **bicuspid valve** (mitral valve). Wall of the left ventricle is very thick. Left ventricle pumps the arterial blood to different parts of the body through systemic aorta.

SEPTA OF HEART

Right and left atria of heart are separated from one another by **interatrial septum**. The ventricles are separated from one another by **interventricular septum**.

LAYERS OF WALL OF HEART

Heart is made up of three layers of tissues:

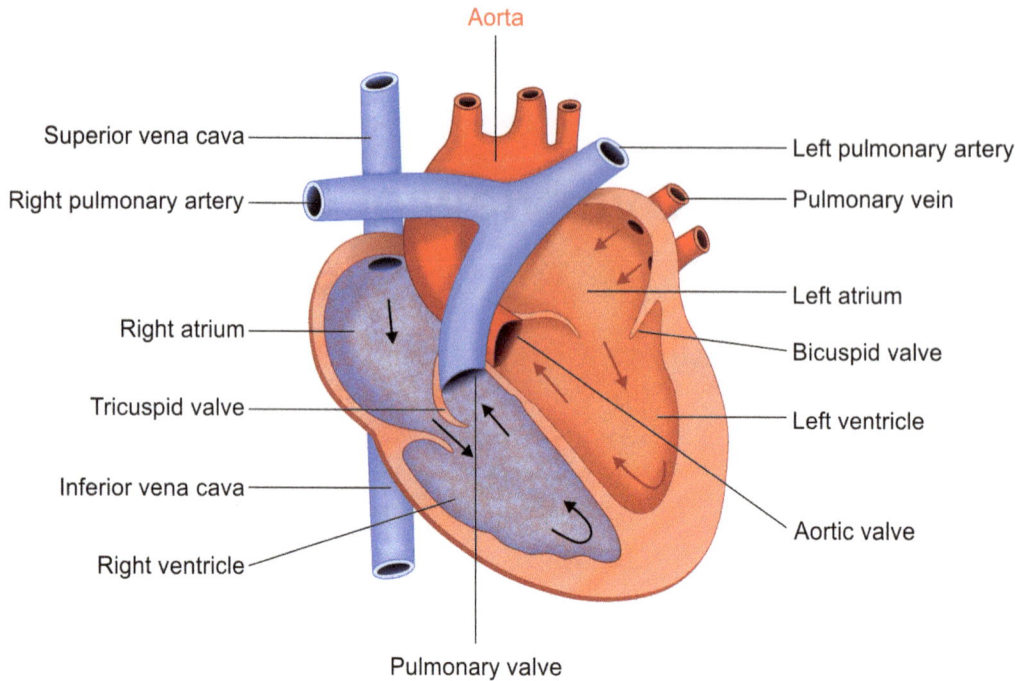

FIGURE 56.1: Section of the heart.

1. Outer pericardium.
2. Middle myocardium.
3. Inner endocardium.

1. Pericardium

Pericardium is the outer covering of heart. It is made up of two layers:

i. Outer **parietal pericardium** which forms a strong protective sac around the heart.
ii. Inner **visceral pericardium** or **epicardium** that covers myocardium.

Layers of pericardium are separated by a space called **pericardial space** or **pericardial cavity** which contains a thin film of fluid.

2. Myocardium

Myocardium is the middle layer of wall of the heart and it is formed by cardiac muscle fibers. Refer Chapter 19 for features of cardiac muscles.

Myocardium is formed by three types of cardiac muscle fibers:

i. Muscle fibers which form contractile unit of heart.
ii. Muscle fibers which form pacemaker.
iii. Muscle fibers which form the conductive system.

i. Muscle fibers which form contractile unit of heart

Cardiac muscle fibers are **striated** and **involuntary** and **branched**. Cardiac muscle fiber is covered by sarcolemma. It has a centrally placed nucleus. Myofibrils are embedded in the sarcoplasm. Sarcomere of the cardiac muscle has all the contractile proteins namely, actin, myosin, troponin and tropomyosin. Cardiac muscles also have sarcotubular system like that of skeletal muscle.

Intercalated disk

Intercalated disk is a tough double membranous structure situated between branches of neighboring cardiac muscle fibers. It is formed by fusion of the membrane of the cardiac muscle branches (Fig. 56.2).

Syncytium

Structure of the cardiac muscle is considered as a syncytium. Syncytium means the tissue in which there is cytoplasmic continuity between the adjacent cells.

However, in cardiac muscle, there is no continuity of the cytoplasm and the muscle fibers are separated from each other by cell membrane. But at the sides, membranes of adjacent muscle fibers fuse together to form gap junctions. Gap junctions facilitate rapid conduction of electrical activity from one fiber to another. This makes the cardiac muscle fibers act like a single unit called physiological syncytium.

Syncytium in human heart has two portions, atrial syncytium and ventricular syncytium which are connected by atrioventricular ring.

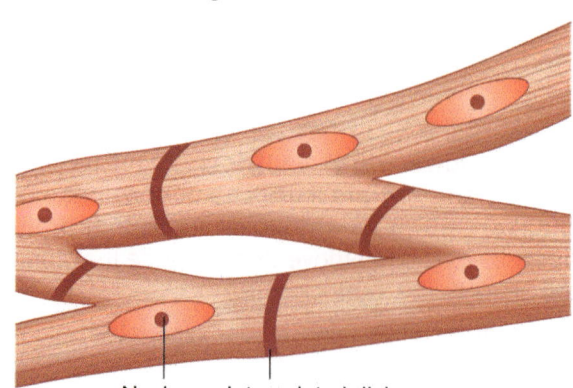

FIGURE 56.2: Cardiac muscle fibers.

ii. Muscle fibers which form pacemaker

Some of the muscle fibers of heart are modified into a specialized structure known as pacemaker.

Pacemaker

Pacemaker is a structure in heart that generates the impulses for heartbeat. It is formed by the **pacemaker cells** called **P cells**. Sinoatrial (SA) node forms the pacemaker in human heart. Details of pacemaker are given in next chapter.

iii. Muscle fibers which form conductive system

Conductive system of the heart is formed by modified cardiac muscle fibers. Impulses from SA node is transmitted to the atria directly. However, the impulses are transmitted to ventricles, through various components of conducting system which are given in the next chapter.

3. Endocardium

Endocardium is the inner most layer of heart wall. It is formed by single layer of endothelial cells lining the inner surface of the heart. Endocardium continues as endothelium of the blood vessels.

VALVES OF THE HEART

Human heart has four valves. Two of the valves are in between atria and the ventricles called atrioventricular valves. Other two valves are semilunar valves which are placed at the opening of blood vessels arising from the ventricles, i.e. systemic aorta and pulmonary artery. Valves of the heart permit flow of blood through the heart in only one direction.

Atrioventricular Valves

Left atrioventricular valve is otherwise known as **mitral valve** or **bicuspid valve**. It is formed by two valvular cusps or flaps **(Fig. 56.3)**. Right atrioventricular valve is known as **tricuspid valve** and it is formed by three cusps.

Brim of the atrioventricular valves is attached to the atrioventricular ring, which is the fibrous connection between the atria and ventricles. Cusps of the valves are attached to **papillary muscles** by means of **chordae tendineae**.

Semilunar Valves

Semilunar valves are present at the openings of systemic aorta and pulmonary artery and are known as aortic valve and pulmonary valve respectively. Because of the half-moon shape, these two valves are called semilunar valves. Semilunar valves are made up of three flaps.

ACTIONS OF HEART

Actions of heart are classified into five types:

1. CHRONOTROPIC ACTION

Chronotropic action is the frequency of heartbeat or heart rate. It is of two types:

i. Tachycardia or increase in heart rate.
ii. Bradycardia or decrease in heart rate.

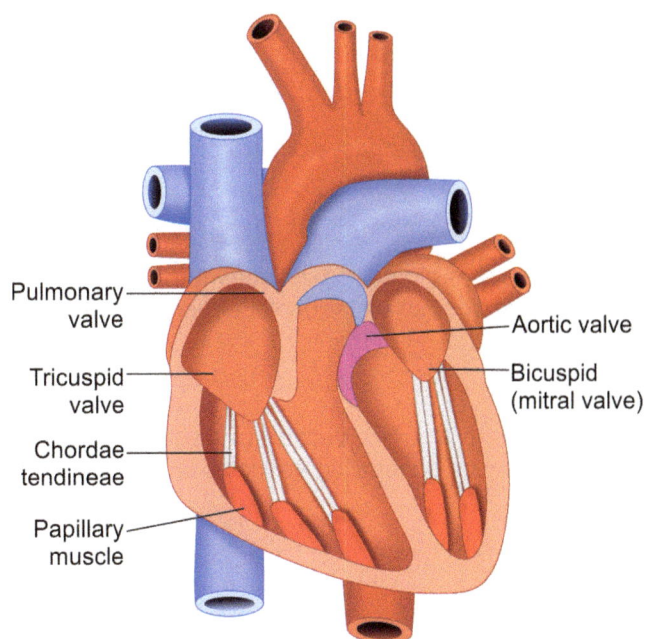

FIGURE 56.3: Valves of the heart.

2. INOTROPIC ACTION

Inotropic action is the force of contraction of heart. It is of two types:

i. Positive inotropic action or increase in force of contraction.
ii. Negative inotropic action or decrease in force of contraction.

3. DROMOTROPIC ACTION

Dromotropic action is the conduction of impulse through heart. It is of two types:

i. Positive dromotropic action or increase in velocity of conduction.
ii. Negative dromotropic action or decrease in velocity of conduction.

4. BATHMOTROPIC ACTION

Bathmotropic action is the excitability of cardiac muscle. It is also of two types:

i. Positive bathmotropic action or increase in excitability of cardiac muscle.
ii. Negative bathmotropic action or the decrease in excitability of cardiac muscle.

5. LUSITROPIC ACTION

Lusitropic action is the ability of cardiac muscle to relax after contraction. It is also of two types:

i. Positive lusitropic action or increase in relaxation of cardiac muscle.
ii. Negative lusitropic action or decrease in relaxation of cardiac muscle **(Table 56.1)**.

Regulation of Actions of Heart

All the actions of heart are continuously regulated. All the actions are altered by nervous stimulation, hormones or hormonal substances of the body and drugs used to treat cardiovascular diseases.

BLOOD VESSELS

Vessels of the circulatory system are divided into arterial system and venous system.

VESSELS OF ARTERIAL AND VENOUS SYSTEMS

Arterial system of circulation includes the aorta, arteries and arterioles. Venous system includes venules, veins and venae cavae.

CAPILLARIES

Capillaries form the link between arterial system and venous system by connecting arterioles and venules (see below).

END ARTERY OR FUNCTIONAL TERMINAL ARTERY

End artery or functional terminal artery is the artery that does not join with other vessel and it is the only vessel supplying oxygenated blood to an organ or a part of the body.

Examples of end artery are arteries in spleen and kidney.

ANASTOMOSIS

Anastomosis means connection between two tubular structures. In cardiovascular system, anastomosis refers to connection between two vessels such as one artery and one vein.

TABLE 56.1: Actions of heart.

Action	Definition
Chronotropic action	Frequency of heartbeat
Inotropic action	Force of contraction of heart
Dromotropic action	Conduction of impulse through heart
Bathmotropic action	Excitability of cardiac muscle
Lusitropic action	Relaxation of cardiac muscle

COLLATERAL CIRCULATION

Collateral circulation is the alternate circulation of blood maintained to a tissue or an organ through network of minute blood vessels that become enlarged and anastomose with adjacent vessels. This happens when the major blood vessel of that tissue or organ is obstructed.

ARTERIAL SYSTEM

Arterial system comprises the aorta, arteries and arterioles. The walls of aorta and arteries are formed by three layers:

1. Outer **tunica adventitia**, which is made up of connective tissue layer
2. Middle **tunica media**, which is formed by smooth muscles.
3. Inner **tunica intima**, which is made up of endothelium.

Branches of arteries become narrower and while reaching the periphery small arteries are continued as terminal arterioles. Arterioles are continued as capillaries which are small, thin walled vessels. Capillaries are functionally very important, because the exchange of

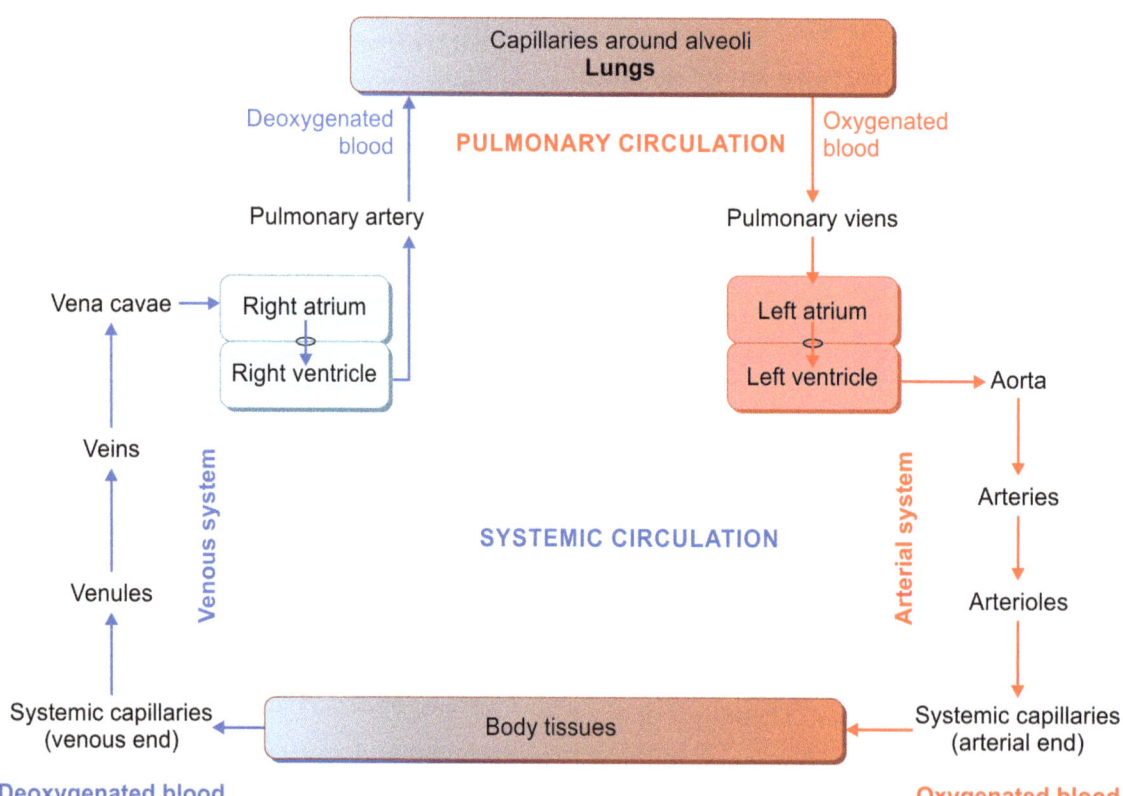

FIGURE 56.4: Schematic diagram showing systemic and pulmonary circulation.

materials between blood and the tissues occurs through these vessels.

VENOUS SYSTEM

From the capillaries, venous system starts and it includes venules, veins and venae cavae. Capillaries end in the venules. The venules are smaller vessels with thin muscular wall than the arterioles. Venules are continued as veins, which form superior and inferior venae cavae which enter the right atrium.

DIVISION OF CIRCULATION

Blood flows through two divisions of circulatory system:

1. Systemic circulation.
2. Pulmonary circulation.

SYSTEMIC CIRCULATION

It is otherwise known as **greater circulation (Fig. 56.4)**. Blood which is pumped from left ventricle passes through a series of blood vessels of arterial system and reaches the tissues. Exchange of various substances between blood and the tissues takes place in the capillaries. After the exchange of substances in capillaries, blood enters the venous system and returns to right atrium and then passes to right ventricles.

PULMONARY CIRCULATION

It is otherwise called **lesser circulation**. Blood is pumped from right ventricle to lungs through pulmonary artery. The exchange of gases occurs between blood and alveoli of the lungs through pulmonary capillary membrane. Oxygenated blood returns to left atrium through the pulmonary veins.

Thus, the left side of heart contains oxygenated or arterial blood and right side of the heart contains venous blood.

Chapter 57

Properties of Cardiac Muscle

CHAPTER OUTLINE

- **EXCITABILITY**
  - **DEFINITION**
  - **ELECTRICAL POTENTIALS IN CARDIAC MUSCLE**
  - **IONIC BASIS OF ACTION POTENTIAL**
  - **SPREAD OF ACTION POTENTIAL THROUGH CARDIAC MUSCLE**
- **RHYTHMICITY**
  - **DEFINITION**
  - **PACEMAKER**
  - **ELECTRICAL POTENTIAL IN SA NODE**
- **CONDUCTIVITY**
  - **CONDUCTIVE SYSTEM IN HUMAN HEART**
  - **VELOCITY OF IMPULSE AT DIFFERENT PARTS OF CONDUCTIVE SYSTEM**
- **CONTRACTILITY**
  - **ALL-OR-NONE LAW**
  - **STAIRCASE PHENOMENON**
  - **SUMMATION OF SUBLIMINAL STIMULI**
  - **REFRACTORY PERIOD**

■ EXCITABILITY

■ DEFINITION

Excitability is defined as the ability of a living tissue to give response to a stimulus. In all tissues, initial response to a stimulus is the electrical activity in the form of action potential. It is followed by mechanical activity in the form of contraction, secretion, etc.

■ ELECTRICAL POTENTIALS IN CARDIAC MUSCLE

Basics of electrical potentials in the muscle are explained in Chapter 22. Resting membrane potential in single cardiac muscle fiber is – 85 to – 95 mV.

Action Potential in Cardiac Muscle

Action potential occurs in **four phases**:

i. Initial Depolarization

Initial depolarization is very rapid and it lasts for about 2 msec. Amplitude of the depolarization is about + 20 mV **(Fig. 57.1)**.

ii. Initial Repolarization

Immediately after depolarization, there is an initial rapid repolarization for a short period of about 2 msec. End of this rapid repolarization is represented by a **notch**.

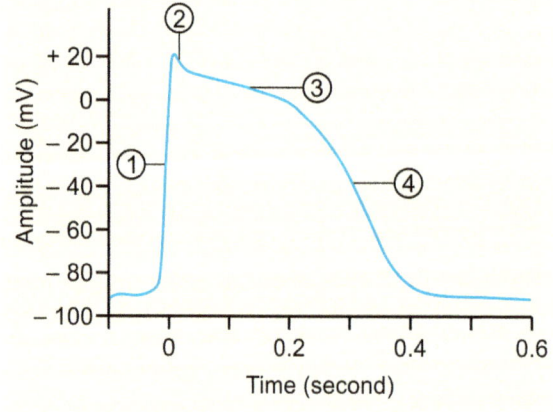

FIGURE 57.1: Action potential in ventricular muscle.
1 = Depolarization, 2 = Initial rapid repolarization,
3 = Plateau, 4 = Final repolarization.

iii. Plateau: Final Depolarization

Afterwards, the muscle fiber remains in depolarized state for some time before further repolarization. It forms the plateau (stable period) in action potential curve. This plateau lasts for about 200 msec (0.2 second) in atrial muscle fibers and for about 300 msec (0.3 second) in ventricular muscle fibers. Due to the long plateau in action potential, the contraction time is longer in cardiac muscle.

Chapter 57: Properties of Cardiac Muscle

iv. Final Repolarization

Final repolarization occurs after the plateau. It is a slow process and it lasts for about 50 to 80 msec (0.05 to 0.08 second) before the re-establishment of resting membrane potential.

■ IONIC BASIS OF ACTION POTENTIAL

1. Initial depolarization is due to opening of fast sodium channels and the **rapid influx of sodium ions**.
2. Initial repolarization is due to the transient (short duration) opening of potassium channels and **efflux of potassium ions** in a small quantity from the muscle fiber. Simultaneously, the fast sodium channels close suddenly and slow sodium channels open resulting in **slow influx of sodium ions** in a low quantity.
3. Plateau (final depolarization) is because of the opening of calcium channels which are kept opened for a longer period. This causes **influx of calcium ions** in large numbers. Entry of both calcium and sodium ions is responsible for prolonged depolarization, i.e. plateau.
4. Final repolarization is due to increase in **efflux of potassium ions**.

■ SPREAD OF ACTION POTENTIAL THROUGH CARDIAC MUSCLE

Action potential spreads through the cardiac muscle very rapidly. It is because of the presence of gap junctions between cardiac muscle fibers. Action potential is transmitted from atria to ventricles through the fibers of specialized conductive system, which is explained later in this chapter.

■ RHYTHMICITY

■ DEFINITION

Rhythmicity or **autorhythmicity** or **self-excitation** is the ability of a tissue to produce its own impulses regularly. This property is present in all the tissues of heart.

However, heart has a specialized excitatory structure called pacemaker which discharges the impulses rapidly. From this, the impulses spread to other parts through the specialized conductive system.

■ PACEMAKER

Pacemaker is defined as the part of heart from which the impulses for heartbeat are produced normally. In mammalian heart, the pacemaker is sinoatrial node (SA node).

SA Node

SA node is a small strip of **modified cardiac muscle** situated in the superior part of lateral wall of right atrium. This node is formed by **pacemaker cells** called **P cells**. Fibers of SA node is continuous with atrial muscle fibers, so that the impulses from SA node spread rapidly through atria.

Other parts of heart like AV node, atria and ventricle also can produce the impulses and function as pacemaker.

Still SA node is called the pacemaker because the rate of production of impulse (rhythmicity) is more in SA node than in other parts. It is about 70 to 80/min.

Spread of Impulses from SA Node

Heart has got a specialized conductive system by which, the impulses from SA node spread to other parts of the heart (see below).

Rate of Generation of Impulses by Different Parts of Human Heart

Rate of generation of impulses by different parts of heart is given in **Table 57.1**.

■ ELECTRICAL POTENTIAL IN SA NODE

Electrical potential in SA node is different from that of other cardiac muscle fibers. In SA node, each impulse triggers the next impulse. It is mainly due to the unstable resting membrane potential.

Resting membrane potential in SA node cells exists only for a very short duration and it has a negativity of – 55 to – 60 mV. It is different from the negativity of – 85 to – 95 mV in other cardiac muscle fibers.

Action Potential in SA Node

Action potential in SA node has **three phases**:

Phase 1: Pacemaker potential

Pacemaker potential in SA node is also called **spontaneous depolarization** or **pacemaker current**. During this phase the spontaneous depolarization starts very slowly and reaches the threshold level of – 40 mV very slowly.

Phase 2: Rapid depolarization

Pacemaker potential triggers the rapid depolarization. Depolarization reaches the voltage of + 5 mV.

Phase 3: Rapid repolarization

Rapid depolarization is followed by rapid repolarization. Repolarization reaches a voltage of – 55 to – 60 mV resulting in **hyperpolarization** and ends in resting membrane potential **(Fig. 57.2)**.

Once again, the cycle is repeated with spontaneous depolarization.

TABLE 57.1: Rate of generation of impulses by different parts of human heart.

Part of the heart	Rate of generation of impulses (per minute)
1. SA node	70 to 89
2. AV node	40 to 60
3. Atrial muscle	40 to 60
4. Purkinje fibers	35 to 40
5. Ventricular muscle	20 to 40

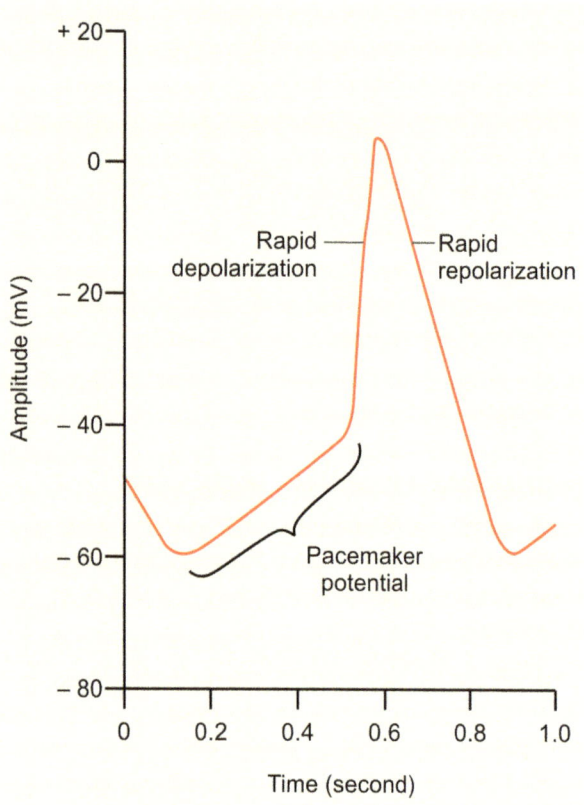

FIGURE 57.2: Action potential in SA node.

CONDUCTIVITY

Heart has a specialized conductive system through which the impulses from SA node are transmitted to all other parts of the heart **(Fig. 57.3)**.

CONDUCTIVE SYSTEM IN HUMAN HEART

Conductive system of the heart is formed by the **modified cardiac muscle fibers**. Conductive tissues of the heart are also called the **junctional tissues**.

Components of Conductive System in Heart

1. AV node.
2. Bundle of His.
3. Right and left bundle branches.
4. Purkinje fibers.

SA node is situated in right atrium (see above). AV node is situated in right posterior portion of intra-atrial septum. The impulses from SA node are conducted throughout right and left atria. These impulses also reach the AV node via some specialized fibers called **intermodal fibers**.

From AV node, the **bundle of His** arises. It divides into right and left **bundle branches** which run on either side of the interventricular septum. From each branch of bundle of His, many **Purkinje fibers** arise and spread all over the ventricular myocardium.

VELOCITY OF IMPULSES AT DIFFERENT PARTS OF THE CONDUCTIVE SYSTEM

Velocity of electrical impulse through different parts of conductive system is given in **Table 57.2**. Velocity is maximum at Purkinje fibers and minimum at AV node. So, when electrical impulse travels from SA node to AV node it is slowed down for a very short period before traveling down through bundle of His. This delay is called **AV nodal delay.**

CONTRACTILITY

Contractility is ability of the tissue to shorten in length (contraction) when stimulated. Various factors affect the

TABLE 57.2: Velocity of impulse through conductive system of heart.

Part of conductive system	Velocity (M/sec)
1. Atrial muscle	0.3
2. Internodal fibers	1.0
3. AV node	0.05
4. Bundle of His	0.12
5. Purkinje fibers	4.0
6. Ventricular muscle	0.5

Velocity of impulse is maximum at Purkinje fibers and minimum at AV node.

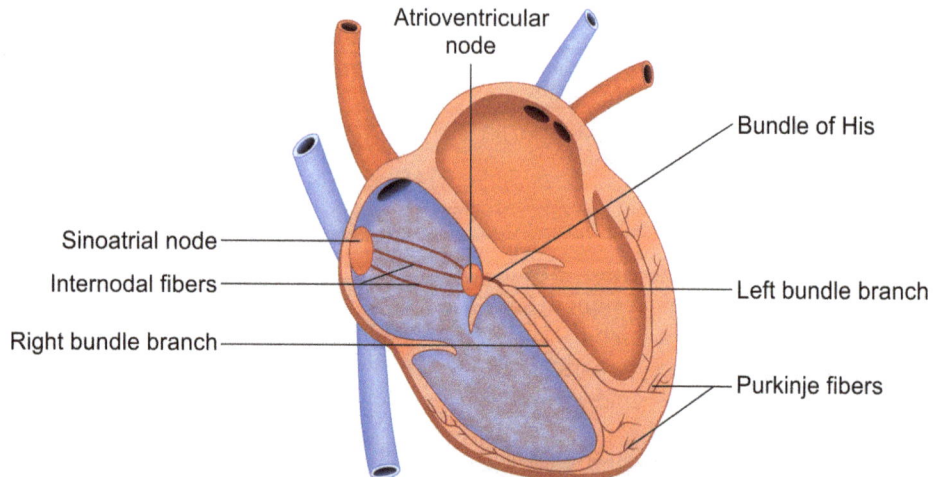

FIGURE 57.3: Sinoatrial node and conductive system of the heart.

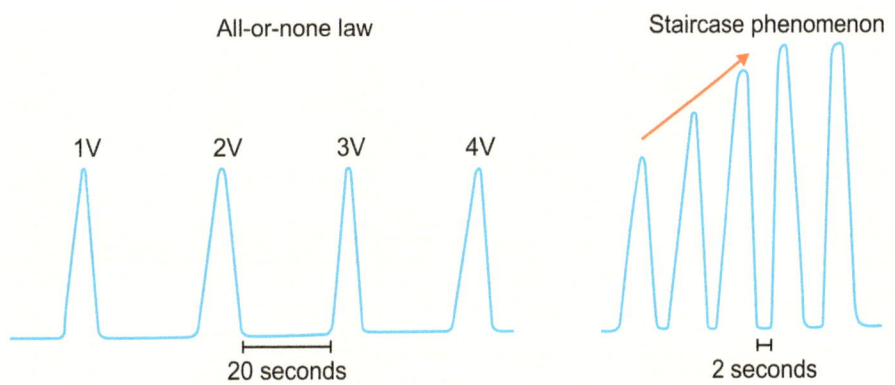

FIGURE 57.4: All-or-none law and staircase phenomenon in cardiac muscle.

contractile properties of the cardiac muscle. Contractile properties are explained below.

ALL-OR-NONE LAW

According to all-or-none law, when a stimulus is applied, whatever may be the strength, the whole cardiac muscle gives maximum response or it does not give any response at all. Below the threshold level, i.e. if strength of stimulus is not adequate, the muscle does not give response.

Cause for All-or-none Law

All-or-none law is applicable to whole cardiac muscle. It is because of **cardiac syncytium**. In skeletal muscle, all-or-none law is applicable only to a single muscle fiber.

STAIRCASE PHENOMENON

When the ventricle is stimulated successively (at a short interval of 2 seconds) without changing the strength, the force of contraction increases gradually for the first few contractions, and then it remains same. Gradual increase in the force of contraction is called staircase phenomenon.

Cause for Staircase Phenomenon

Staircase phenomenon occurs because of the beneficial effect which facilitates the force of successive contraction. So, there is a gradual increase in force of contraction (Fig. 57.4).

SUMMATION OF SUBLIMINAL STIMULI

When a stimulus with a subliminal strength is applied, the heart does not show any response. When few stimuli with same subliminal strength are applied in succession, the heart shows response by contraction. It is due to summation of the stimuli.

REFRACTORY PERIOD

Refractory period is the period in which the muscle does not show any response to a stimulus.

Refractory period is of two types:

1. Absolute refractory period.
2. Relative refractory period.

Absolute Refractory Period

Absolute refractory period is the period during which the muscle does not show any response at all, whatever may be the strength of stimulus. It is because, the depolarization occurs during this period. So, a second depolarization is not possible.

Relative Refractory Period

Relative refractory period is the period during which the muscle shows response if strength of stimulus is increased to maximum. It is the stage at which the muscle is in repolarizing state.

Refractory Period in Cardiac Muscle

Cardiac muscle has a **long refractory period** compared to that of skeletal muscle. Absolute refractory period extends throughout the contraction period of cardiac muscle. It is for 0.27 second and relative refractory period extends during first half of relaxation period which is about 0.26 second. So, the total refractory period is 0.53 second.

Significance of Long Refractory Period In Cardiac Muscle

Long refractory period in cardiac muscle has three advantages:

1. Summation of contractions does not occur.
2. Fatigue does not occur.
3. Tetanus does not occur.

Chapter 58: Cardiac Cycle

CHAPTER OUTLINE

- **DEFINITION AND EVENTS**
- **SUBDIVISIONS AND DURATION**
  - ATRIAL EVENTS
  - VENTRICULAR EVENTS
- **DESCRIPTION OF ATRIAL EVENTS**
  - ATRIAL SYSTOLE
  - ATRIAL DIASTOLE
- **DESCRIPTION OF VENTRICULAR EVENTS**
  - ISOMETRIC CONTRACTION PERIOD
  - EJECTION PERIOD
  - PROTODIASTOLE
  - ISOMETRIC RELAXATION PERIOD
  - RAPID FILLING PHASE
- SLOW FILLING PHASE
- LAST RAPID FILLING PHASE
- **PRESSURE CHANGES DURING CARDIAC CYCLE**
  - INTRA-ATRIAL PRESSURE CHANGES
  - INTRAVENTRICULAR PRESSURE CHANGES
  - AORTIC PRESSURE CHANGES
- **VENTRICULAR VOLUME CHANGES DURING CARDIAC CYCLE**
  - SIGNIFICANCE
  - VOLUME OF BLOOD IN RIGHT AND LEFT VENTRICLES

■ DEFINITION AND EVENTS OF CARDIAC CYCLE

Cardiac cycle is defined as the sequence of coordinated events in the heart which are repeated during every heartbeat in a cyclic manner. Each heartbeat consists of two major periods called **systole** and **diastole**. Systole is the contraction of the cardiac muscle and diastole is the relaxation of cardiac muscle.

Events of cardiac cycle are classified into two divisions:

1. Atrial events which constitute atrial systole and atrial diastole.
2. Ventricular events which constitute ventricular systole and ventricular diastole.

■ SUBDIVISIONS AND DURATION OF EVENTS OF CARDIAC CYCLE

When the heart beats at the normal rate of 72/minute, the duration of each cardiac cycle is about 0.8 second.

■ ATRIAL EVENTS

1. Atrial systole : 0.11 (0.1) second.
2. Atrial diastole : 0.69 (0.7) second.

■ VENTRICULAR EVENTS

Ventricular events are divided into two divisions:

1. Ventricular systole : 0.27 (0.3) second
2. Ventricular diastole : 0.53 (0.5) second

In clinical practice, the term 'systole' refers to ventricular systole and 'diastole' refers to ventricular diastole. Ventricular systole is divided into two subdivisions and ventricular diastole is divided into five subdivisions. Subdivisions of systole and diastole are given in **Box 58.1**.

BOX 58.1: Subdivisions of ventricular events.

Ventricular systole (0.27 sec)	
1. Isometric contraction	0.05 sec
2. Ejection period	0.22 sec
Ventricular diastole (0.53 sec)	
1. Protodiastole	0.04 sec
2. Isometric relaxation	0.08 sec
3. Rapid filling	0.11 sec
4. Slow filling	0.19 sec
5. Last rapid filling (atrial systole)	0.11 sec

Among the atrial events, atrial systole occurs during last phase of ventricular diastole. So, it is also called **last rapid period**. Atrial diastole is not considered as a separate phase, since it coincides with the whole of ventricular systole and earlier part of ventricular diastole.

■ DESCRIPTION OF ATRIAL EVENTS OF CARDIAC CYCLE

For the sake of better understanding, the description of events of cardiac cycle is commenced with atrial systole.

■ ATRIAL SYSTOLE

Atrial systole is also known as **second** or **last rapid filling phase** or **presystole**. It is considered as the last phase of ventricular diastole. Its duration is 0.11 second. During this period, only a small amount, i.e. 10% of blood is forced from atria into ventricles **(Fig. 58.1)**.

Pressure and Volume Changes

During atrial systole, the intra-atrial pressure increases. Intraventricular pressure and ventricular volume also increase, but slightly.

Fourth Heart Sound

Contraction of atrial musculature causes the production of fourth heart sound during this phase.

■ ATRIAL DIASTOLE

After atrial systole, the atrial diastole starts. Atrial diastole lasts for about 0.7 second (accurate duration is 0.69 second).

■ DESCRIPTION OF VENTRICULAR EVENTS OF CARDIAC CYCLE

■ ISOMETRIC CONTRACTION PERIOD

Isometric contraction is the type of muscular contraction characterized by increase in tension without any change in the length of muscle fibers. Isometric contraction of ventricular muscle is also called **isovolumetric contraction**.

Isometric contraction period in cardiac cycle is the first phase of ventricular systole. It lasts for 0.05 second **(Table 58.1)**. Immediately after atrial systole, the atrioventricular valves are closed due to increase in ventricular pressure. Semilunar valves are already closed. Now, the ventricles contract as closed cavities in such a way that, there is no change in the volume of ventricular chambers or in length of muscle fibers. Only, the tension increases in ventricular musculature.

Because of increased tension in ventricular musculature during isometric contraction, the pressure increases sharply inside ventricles.

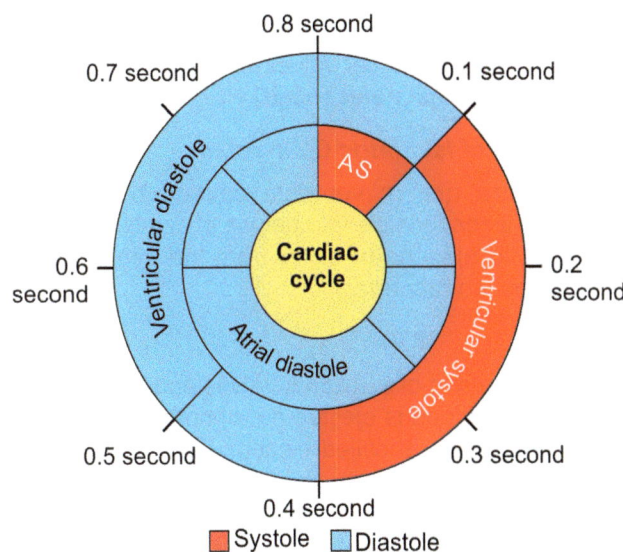

FIGURE 58.1: Atrial and ventricular events of cardiac cycle. AS = Atrial systole.

TABLE 58.1: Atrial and ventricular events of cardiac cycle.

Events	Duration of events (second)	Divisions	Duration of divisions (second)	Subdivisions	Duration of subdivisions (second)	Primary action
Atrial events	0.8	Atrial systole	0.11	–	–	Ventricular filling
		Atrial diastole	0.69	–	–	Atrial filling
Ventricular events	0.8	Ventricular systole	0.27	Isovolumetric contraction period	0.05	Steep increase in pressure
				Rapid ejection period	0.13	Pumping of blood into systemic and pulmonary blood vessels
				Slow ejection period	0.09	
		Ventricular diastole	0.53	Protodiastole	0.04	Beginning of diastole
				Isovolumetric relaxation period	0.08	Rapid fall in pressure
				First rapid filling phase	0.11	Filling of ventricles
				Slow filling phase	0.19	
				Last rapid filling phase	0.11	

Note: Most of the atrial events and ventricular events overlap.

First Heart Sound

Closure of atrioventricular valves at the beginning of this phase produces first heart sound.

Significance of Isometric Contraction

The pressure rise in ventricle caused by isometric contraction is responsible for opening of semilunar valves. This leads to ejection of blood from the ventricles into aorta and pulmonary artery.

■ EJECTION PERIOD

Due to the opening of semilunar valves and contraction of ventricles, the blood is ejected out of both the ventricles. Hence, this period is called ejection period. Duration of this period is 0.22 second.

Ejection period is of two stages:

i. First stage is called **rapid ejection period**. Immediately after the opening of semilunar valves, a large amount of blood is rapidly ejected from both the ventricles. It lasts for 0.13 second.
ii. Second stage is called **slow ejection period**. During this stage, the blood is ejected slowly with much less force. Duration of this period is 0.09 second.

End-systolic Volume

Ventricles are not emptied at the end of ejection period and some amount of blood remains in each ventricle. Amount of blood remaining in ventricles at the end of ejection period (i.e. at the end of systole) is called end-systolic volume. It is 60 to 80 mL per ventricle.

Ejection Fraction

Ejection fraction means the fraction (or portion) of end-diastolic volume (see below) that is ejected out by each ventricle per beat. From 130 to 150 mL of end-diastolic volume, 70 mL is ejected out by each ventricle (stroke volume). Normal ejection fraction is 60 to 65%.

■ PROTODIASTOLE

This is the first stage of ventricular diastole hence the name protodiastole. Duration of this period is 0.04 second. During this period, the pressure in ventricles drops due to ejection of blood. At the end of this period, intraventricular pressure becomes less than the pressure in aorta and pulmonary artery. This causes closure of semilunar valves. Atrioventricular valves are already closed (see above).

No other change occurs in the heart during this period. Thus, protodiastole indicates only the end of systole and beginning of diastole.

Second Heart Sound

Closure of semilunar valves during this phase produces second heart sound.

■ ISOMETRIC RELAXATION PERIOD

Isometric relaxation is the type of muscular relaxation characterized by decrease in tension but, without any change in the length of muscle fibers. Isometric relaxation of ventricular muscle is also called **isovolumetric relaxation**.

During isometric relaxation period, once again all the valves of the heart are closed. Now, both the ventricles relax as closed cavities, without any change in volume or length of the muscle fiber. But intraventricular pressure decreases during this period. Duration of isometric relaxation period is 0.08 second.

Significance of Isometric Relaxation

During isometric relaxation period, the ventricular pressure decreases greatly. When the ventricular pressure becomes less than pressure in atria, the atrioventricular valves open. Thus, the fall in pressure in the ventricles, caused by isometric relaxation is responsible for the opening of atrioventricular valves, resulting in filling of ventricles.

■ RAPID FILLING

When AV valves are opened, there is a sudden rush of blood from atria into ventricles. So, this period is called the **first rapid filling period**. Filling during this period occurs without atrial systole. About 70% of filling takes place during this phase which lasts for 0.11 second.

Third Heart Sound

Rushing of blood into ventricles during this phase produces third heart sound **(Fig. 58.2)**.

■ SLOW FILLING

After a sudden rush of blood, the ventricular filling becomes slow. Now, it is called the slow filling. It is also called **diastasis**. Filling during this phase also occurs without atrial systole. About 20% of filling occurs in this phase. Duration of slow filling phase is 0.19 second.

■ LAST RAPID FILLING

Filling becomes once again rapid because of atrial systole. After slow filling period, the atria contract and push a small amount of blood into the ventricles. About 10% of ventricular filling takes place during this period. Flow of additional amount of blood into ventricle due to atrial systole is called **atrial kick.**

End-diastolic Volume

End-diastolic volume is the amount of blood remaining in each ventricle at the end of diastole. It is about 130 mL to 150 mL per ventricle.

■ PRESSURE CHANGES DURING CARDIAC CYCLE

■ INTRA-ATRIAL PRESSURE CHANGES DURING CARDIAC CYCLE

Significance of Intra-atrial Pressure

Pressure in the atria is called the intra-atrial pressure. Intra-atrial pressure is responsible for opening of the atrioventricular valves and ventricular filling. It is also the main factor for the development of venous pulse.

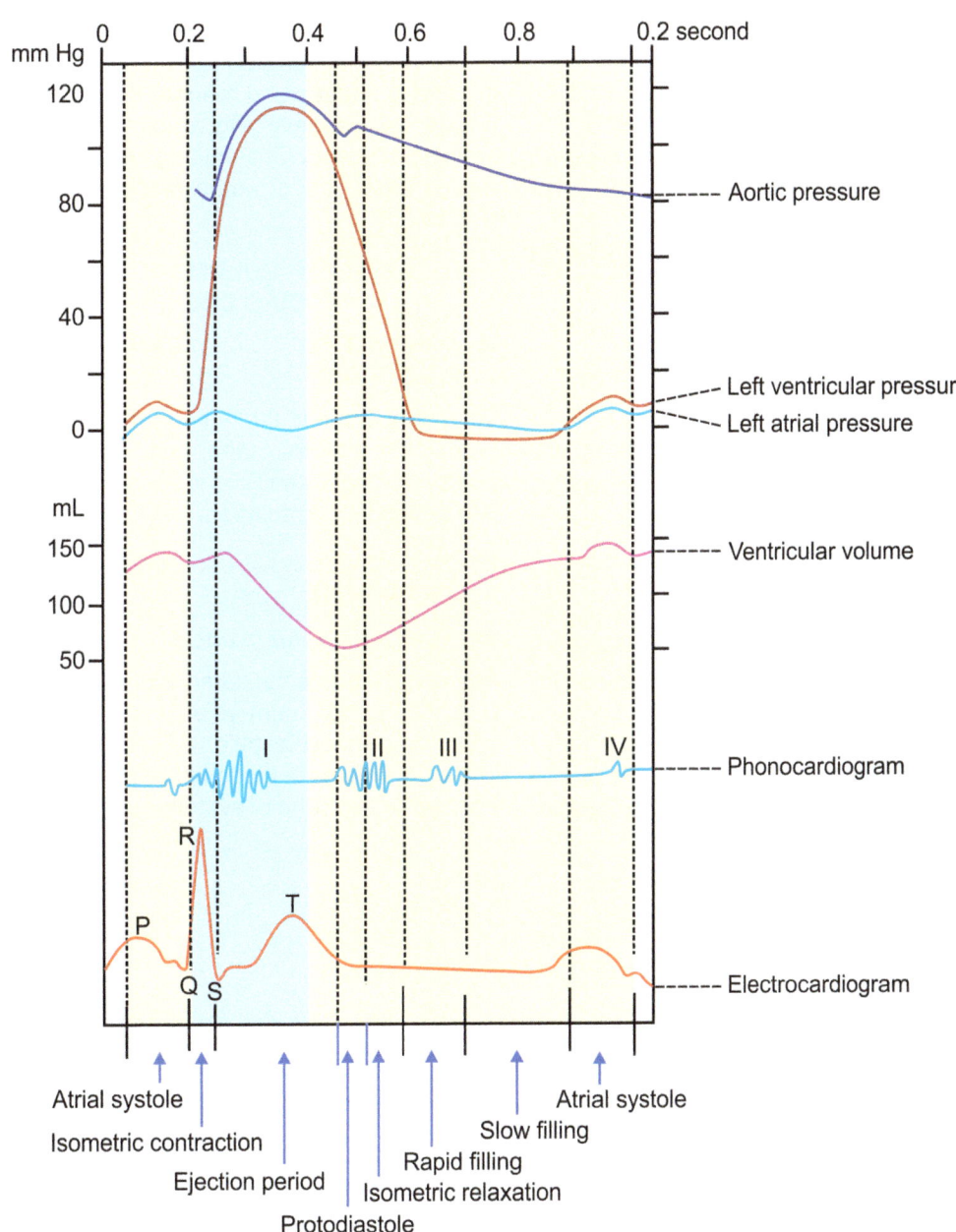

FIGURE 58.2: Comprehensive diagram (Wiggers diagram) ECG, phonocardiogram, pressure changes and volume changes during cardiac cycle.

Pressure Changes during Cardiac Cycle

During atrial diastole, the pressure in atrial falls down and reaches 0 mm Hg because of relaxation. During atrial systole pressure rises sharply up to 5 mm Hg in right atrium and 7 mm Hg in left atrium.

Maximum and minimum pressures in the left and right atria are given in **Table 58.2**.

■ INTRAVENTRICULAR PRESSURE CHANGES DURING CARDIAC CYCLE

Significance of Intraventricular Pressure

Intraventricular pressure is the pressure developed inside the ventricles of heart. It is essential for the circulation of

TABLE 58.2: Pressure changes during cardiac cycle.

Area	Maximum Pressure	Minimum pressure
Left atrium	7 to 8 mm Hg	0 to 2 mm Hg
Right atrium	5 to 6 mm Hg	0 to 2 mm Hg
Left ventricle	120 mm Hg	5 mm Hg
Right ventricle	25 mm Hg	2 to 3 mm Hg
Systemic aorta	120 mm Hg	80 mm Hg
Pulmonary artery	25 mm Hg	7 to 8 mm Hg

blood, because the flow of blood through systemic and pulmonary circulation depends upon pressure at which the blood is pumped out of ventricles.

Pressure Changes during Cardiac Cycle

Pressure in ventricles reach maximum during ejection period and reaches minimum during final phase of ventricular diastole.

Maximum and minimum pressures in the left and right ventricles are given in **Table 58.2**.

■ AORTIC PRESSURE CHANGES DURING CARDIAC CYCLE

Significance Aortic Pressure

Aortic pressure is the pressure developed in the aorta. It is necessary to maintain the blood flow through the circulatory system.

Pressure Changes during Cardiac Cycle

Pressure in systemic aorta is always higher than that of pulmonary artery. It is because of the higher pressure in left ventricle than in the right ventricle. Maximum and minimum pressures in aorta are given in **Table 58.2**.

Minimum pressure in systemic aorta is much greater than the minimum pressure in the left ventricle. It is due to the presence of elastic tissues in the aorta, which enable the aorta to recoil and maintain the minimum pressure at a higher level.

During ejection period of cardiac cycle, the pressure in aorta increases and reaches the peak. During diastole, it reduces gradually and reaches the minimum level. At the time of closure of semilunar valves, an incisura occurs due to back flow of some blood towards the ventricles **(Fig. 58.2)**.

■ VENTRICULAR VOLUME CHANGES DURING CARDIAC CYCLE

■ SIGNIFICANCE OF VOLUME OF BLOOD IN VENTRICLES

Volume of blood in the left ventricle is an important factor to maintain cardiac output and blood circulation. Volume of blood in right ventricle is responsible for flow of blood into pulmonary circulation.

■ VOLUME OF BLOOD IN RIGHT AND LEFT VENTRICLES

End-diastolic Volume and End-systolic Volume

Amount of blood is the same in both right and left ventricles **(Fig. 58.2)**. Maximum volume of blood in each ventricle after filling (end-diastolic volume) is 130 mL to 150 mL. Minimum volume of blood left in the ventricles at the end of ejection period (end of systolic volume) is 60 mL to 80 mL.

Chapter 59: Heart Sounds and Cardiac Murmur

CHAPTER OUTLINE

- **PRODUCTION OF HEART SOUNDS**
  - DIFFERENT HEART SOUNDS
  - IMPORTANCE OF HEART SOUNDS
- **DESCRIPTION OF HEART SOUNDS**
  - FIRST HEART SOUNDS
  - SECOND HEART SOUNDS
  - THIRD HEART SOUNDS
  - FOURTH HEART SOUNDS
- **METHODS OF STUDY OF HEART SOUNDS**
  - BY STETHOSCOPE
  - BY MICROPHONE
  - BY PHONOCARDIOGRAM
- **CARDIAC MURMUR**

PRODUCTION OF HEART SOUNDS

Heart sounds are the sounds produced by mechanical activities of the heart during each cardiac cycle. Heart sounds are produced by flow of blood through chambers of the heart. Contraction of cardiac muscle and closure of valves of the heart.

Heart sounds are heard by placing the ear over the chest or by using a stethoscope or microphone. These sounds are also recorded graphically.

DIFFERENT HEART SOUNDS

Four heart sounds are produced during each cardiac cycle. First and second heart sounds are called **classical heart sounds**. These sounds are more prominent and resemble the spoken words '**LUB**' (or LUBB) and '**DUB**' (or DUP) respectively. These two heart sounds are heard by using the stethoscope.

IMPORTANCE OF HEART SOUNDS

Evaluation of heart sounds has important diagnostic value in clinical practice because alteration in heart sounds indicates the cardiac diseases involving valves of the heart.

DESCRIPTION OF HEART SOUNDS

FIRST HEART SOUND

First heart sound is heard during **isometric contraction** period and earlier part of **ejection period (Table 59.1)**.

Causes of First Heart Sound

Major cause for first heart sound is the sudden and synchronous (simultaneous) closure of **atrioventricular valves**. In addition to this, ejection of blood from ventricles into aorta and pulmonary artery and contraction of cardiac muscles also contribute in the production of the first heart sound.

Characteristics of First Heart Sound

First heart sound is a long, soft and low-pitched sound. It resembles the spoken word '**LUBB**' (or LUB). Duration of this sound is 0.10 to 0.17 second. Its frequency is 25 to 45 cycles/second.

SECOND HEART SOUND

Second heart sound is produced at the end of **protodiastolic period**.

Cause for Second Heart Sound

Second heart sound is produced due to the sudden and synchronous closure of **semilunar valves**.

Characteristics for Second Heart Sound

Second heart sound is a short, sharp and high-pitched sound. It resembles the spoken word '**DUBB**' (or DUP). Duration of the second heart sound is 0.10 to 0.14 second. Its frequency is 50 cycles/second.

THIRD HEART SOUND

Third heart sound is a low-pitched sound that is produced during **rapid filling period** of the cardiac cycle. Usually, the third heart sound is **inaudible** by stethoscope and it can be heard only by using microphone.

TABLE 59.1: Heart sounds.

Features	First heart sound	Second heart sound	Third heart Sound	Fourth heart sound
Cause	Closure of atrioventricular valves	Closure of semilunar Valves	Rushing of blood into ventricle	Contraction of atrial musculature
Occurs during	Isometric contraction period and part of ejection period	Protodiastole and part of isometric relaxation period	Rapid filling phase	Atrial systole
Characteristics	Long, soft and low pitched Resembles the word 'LUBB'	Short, sharp and high pitched Resembles the word 'DUP'	Low pitched	Inaudible sound
Duration (second)	0.10 to 0.17	0.10 to 0.14	0.07 to 0.10	0.02 to 0.04
Frequency (cycles per sec)	25 to 45	50	1 to 6	1 to 4

Cause for Third Heart Sound

Third heart sound is produced by the **rushing of blood** into ventricles during rapid filling phase.

Characteristics of Third Heart Sound

Third heart sound is a short and low-pitched sound. Duration of this sound is 0.07 to 0.10 second. Its frequency is 1 to 6 cycles/second.

Conditions When Third Heart Sound Becomes Audible by Stethoscope

Third heart sound can be heard by stethoscope in children and athletes. Pathological conditions when third heart sound becomes loud and audible by stethoscope are aortic regurgitation, cardiac failure and cardiomyopathy with dilated ventricles.

When third heart sound is heard by stethoscope the condition is called **triple heart sound**. Third heart sound is usually heard best with the bell of stethoscope placed at the apex beat area when the patient is in left lateral decubitus (lying on left side) position.

■ FOURTH HEART SOUND

Normally, the fourth heart sound is an **inaudible** sound. It becomes audible only in pathological conditions. It is studied only by graphical recording, i.e. by **phonocardiography**. This sound is produced during **atrial systole** (late diastole) and it is considered as the physiologic atrial sound. It is also called **atrial gallop** or **presystolic gallop**.

Cause for Fourth Heart Sound

Fourth heart sound is produced by contraction of atrial musculature during atrial systole.

Characteristics of Fourth Heart Sound

Fourth heart sound is a short and low-pitched sound. Duration of this sound is 0.02 to 0.04 second, and its frequency is 1 to 4 cycles/second.

Conditions When Fourth Heart Sound Becomes Audible

Forth heart sound becomes audible by stethoscope when the ventricles become stiff. Ventricular stiffness occurs in conditions like ventricular hypertrophy, longstanding hypertension and aortic stenosis. To overcome the ventricular stiffness, atria contract forcefully producing audible fourth heart sound.

When fourth heart sound is heard by stethoscope the condition is called **triple heart sound** (see below). It is usually heard best with the bell of stethoscope placed at the apex beat area when the patient is in supine or left semilateral position.

■ METHODS OF STUDY OF HEART SOUNDS

Heart sounds are studied by **three methods:**

■ BY USING STETHOSCOPE: AUSCULTATION AREAS

First and second heart sounds are heard on the auscultation areas by using the stethoscope. Chest piece of the stethoscope is placed over 4 areas on the chest, which are called auscultation areas.

Auscultation areas

1. *Mitral area (bicuspid area)*

Mitral area is in the left 5th intercostal space half inch medial to midclavicular line. Sound produced by the closure of mitral valve (first heart sound) is transmitted well into this area. It is also called apex beat area because apex beat is felt in this area.

Apex beat is the thrust (pushing forcefully) of the apex of ventricles, against chest wall during systole.

2. *Tricuspid area*

Tricuspid area is on the left border of lower end of sternum **(Fig. 59.1)**. Sound produced by the closure of tricuspid valve (first heart sound) is transmitted well into this area.

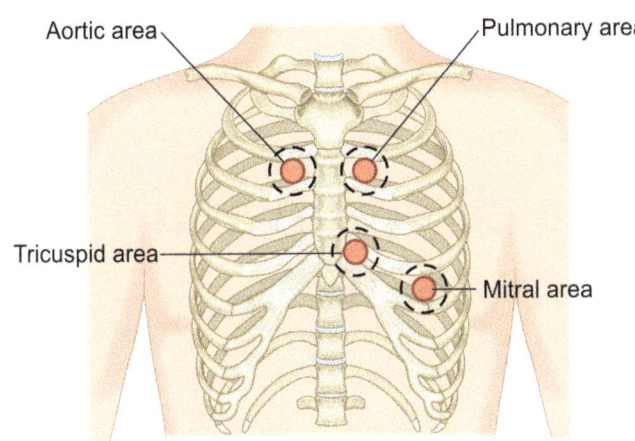

FIGURE 59.1: Auscultatory areas.

3. Pulmonary area

Pulmonary area is on the left 2nd intercostal space, close to sternum. Sound produced by the closure of pulmonary valve (second heart sound) is heard well on this area.

4. Aortic area

Aortic area is over the right 2nd intercostal space, close to sternum. On this area, the sound produced by closure of aortic valve (second heart sound) is heard well.

First heart sound is best heard in mitral and tricuspid areas. However, it is heard in other areas also but the intensity is less. Similarly, the second heart sound is best heard in pulmonary and aortic areas. It is also heard in other areas with less intensity.

■ BY MICROPHONE

A highly sensitive microphone is placed over the chest. Heart sounds are amplified by means of an amplifier and heard by using a loudspeaker. First, second and third heart sounds are heard by this method.

■ BY PHONOCARDIOGRAM

Phonocardiography is the technique used to record the heart sounds. Phonocardiogram is the graphical record of heart sounds. It is done by placing an electronic sound transducer over the chest. This transducer is connected to a recording device like polygraph. All the four heart sounds can be recorded in phonocardiogram. It helps to analyze the frequency of the sound waves **(Fig. 58.2)**.

■ CARDIAC MURMUR

Cardiac murmur is the abnormal or unusual heart sound heard by stethoscope along with normal heart sounds. Cardiac murmur is also called **abnormal heart sound** or **cardiac bruit**.

Abnormal sound is produced because of change in the pattern of blood flow. Normally, blood flows in stream line through the heart and the blood vessels. However, during the abnormal conditions like valvular diseases, the blood flow becomes turbulent. This produces the cardiac murmur.

Cardiac murmur is heard by placing the chest piece of the stethoscope over the auscultatory areas. Murmur due to disease of a particular valve is heard well over the auscultatory area of that valve. Sometimes, the murmur is felt by palpation as 'thrills'. In some patients, the murmur is heard without any aid even at a distance of few feet away from the patient.

Valvular diseases are of two types:

1. **Stenosis** or narrowing of heart valve: Blood flows rapidly with turbulence through narrow orifice of the valve resulting in murmur.
2. **Incompetence** or weakening of heart valve: When the valve becomes weak, it cannot close properly. It causes back flow of blood resulting in turbulence. This disease is also called regurgitation or valvular insufficiency.

Classification of Murmur

Cardiac murmur is classified into three types:

1. **Systolic murmur** produced during systole of the heart.
2. **Diastolic murmur** produced during diastole of the heart.
3. **Continuous murmur** produced continuously (heard in conditions such as **patent ductus arteriosus**).

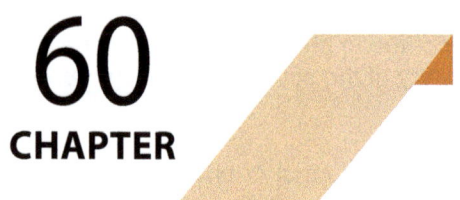

Chapter 60: Electrocardiogram and Arrhythmia

CHAPTER OUTLINE

- **DEFINITIONS AND USES OF ECG**
- **ELECTROCARDIOGRAPHIC GRID**
  - DURATION
  - AMPLITUDE
  - SPEED OF THE PAPER
- **ECG LEADS**
  - BIPOLAR LIMB LEADS
  - UNIPOLAR LEADS
- **WAVES OF NORMAL ECG**
  - 'P' WAVE
  - 'QRS' COMPLEX
  - 'T' WAVE
- **'U' WAVE**
- **INTERVALS AND SEGMENTS OF ECG**
  - 'P-R' INTERVAL
  - 'Q-T' INTERVAL
  - 'S-T' SEGMENT
  - 'R-R' INTERVAL
- **ARRHYTHMIA**
  - DEFINITION AND CLASSIFICATION
  - NORMOTOPIC ARRHYTHMIA
  - ECTOPIC ARRHYTHMIA
  - ABNORMAL PACEMAKER
  - ARTIFICIAL PACEMAKER

DEFINITIONS AND USES OF ECG

Electrocardiography

Electrocardiography is a **technique** by which electrical activities of the heart are studied.

Electrocardiograph

Electrocardiograph is the **instrument** (ECG machine) by which the electrical activities of heart are recorded.

Electrocardiogram (ECG)

Electrocardiogram is the record or **graphical registration** of electrical activities of the heart, which occur prior to the onset of mechanical activities. It is the **summed electrical activity** of all the cardiac muscle fibers recorded from the surface of the body.

Uses of ECG

ECG is useful in determining heart rate and heart rhythm. ECG is also useful in diagnosing the following conditions:

1. Myocardial ischemia.
2. Heart attack.
3. Coronary artery disease.
4. Hypertrophy of heart chambers.

ELECTROCARDIOGRAPHIC GRID

Electrocardiograph or ECG machine amplifies the electrical signals produced from the heart and records these signals on a moving ECG paper.

ECG grid means to markings (lines) on ECG paper. ECG paper has horizontal and vertical lines at regular intervals of 1 mm. Every 5th line (5 mm) is thickened.

DURATION

Time duration of different ECG waves is plotted horizontally on X-axis.

1 mm = 0.04 second
5 mm = 0.20 second.

AMPLITUDE

Amplitude of ECG waves is plotted vertically on Y-axis.

1 mm = 0.1 mV
5 mm = 0.5 mV.

SPEED OF THE PAPER

Movement of paper through the machine can be adjusted in two speeds, 25 mm/sec and 50 mm/sec. Usually, the speed of the paper during recording is fixed at 25 mm/sec. If the heart rate is very high, speed of the paper is changed to 50 mm/sec.

ECG LEADS

ECG is recorded by placing series of **electrodes** on the surface of the body. These electrodes are called ECG leads and are connected to the ECG machine.

Electrodes are fixed on the limbs. Usually right arm, left arm and left leg are chosen. Heart is said to be in the center of an imaginary equilateral triangle drawn by connecting the roots of these three limbs. This triangle is called **Einthoven's triangle**. Electrical potential generated from the heart appears simultaneously on the roots of these three limbs.

ECG is recorded in 12 leads **(Table 60.1)** which are classified into two categories, bipolar leads and unipolar leads.

1. BIPOLAR LIMB LEADS

Bipolar limb leads are otherwise known as **standard limb leads**. Two limbs are connected to obtain these leads and both the electrodes are **active recording electrodes**, i.e. one electrode is positive and the other one is negative **(Fig. 60.1)**.

Standard limb leads are of three types:

1. Lead I: By connecting **right arm and left arm**.
2. Lead II: By connecting **right arm and left leg**.
3. Lead III: By connecting **left arm and left leg**.

2. UNIPOLAR LEADS

Here, one electrode is active electrode and the other one is an indifferent electrode. Active electrode is positive and the indifferent electrode is serving as a composite negative electrode.

Unipolar leads are of two types, unipolar limb leads and unipolar chest leads.

i. Unipolar Limb Leads

Unipolar limb leads are also called **augmented limb leads**. **Active electrode** is connected to one of the limbs. **Indifferent electrode** is obtained by connecting the other two limbs through a resistance.

Unipolar limb leads are of three types:

1. aVR lead: Active electrode is from **right arm**.
2. aVL lead: Active electrode is from **left arm**.
3. aVF lead: Active electrode is from **left leg** (foot).

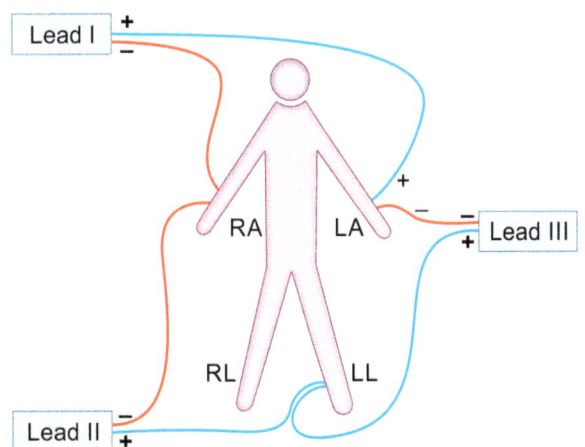

FIGURE 60.1: Position of electrodes for standard limb leads. RA = Right arm, LA = Left arm, LL = Left leg, RL = Right leg (ground electrode)

ii. Unipolar Chest Leads

Indifferent electrode is obtained by connecting the three limbs, left arm, left leg and right arm through a resistance of 5,000 ohms. **Active electrode** is called **chest electrode.** It is placed on six points over the chest **(Fig. 60.2)**. V indicates **vector**, which shows the direction of flow of current.

Position of chest leads

V_1: Over 4th intercostal space near right sternal margin.
V_2: Over 4th intercostal space near left sternal margin.
V_3: In between V_2 and V_4.
V_4: Over left 5th intercostal space on the midclavicular line.
V_5: Over left 5th intercostal space on the anterior axillary line.
V_6: Over left 5th intercostal space on the midaxillary line.

Ground or Earth Electrode

While recording ECG in each lead, a ground or earth electrode is connected to **right leg** of the subject. Ground electrode prevents any artifact arising from machine.

WAVES OF NORMAL ELECTROCARDIOGRAM

A normal ECG consists of waves, complexes, intervals and segments. Waves of ECG recorded by limb lead II are considered as the typical waves.

TABLE 60.1: Twelve leads of ECG.

Bipolar limb leads	Unipolar leads	
	Unipolar limb leads	Unipolar Chest leads
1. Limb lead I	4. aVR lead	7. V_1
2. Limb lead II	5. aVL lead	8. V_2
3. Limb lead III	6. aVF lead	9. V_3
		10. V_4
		11. V_5
		12. V_6

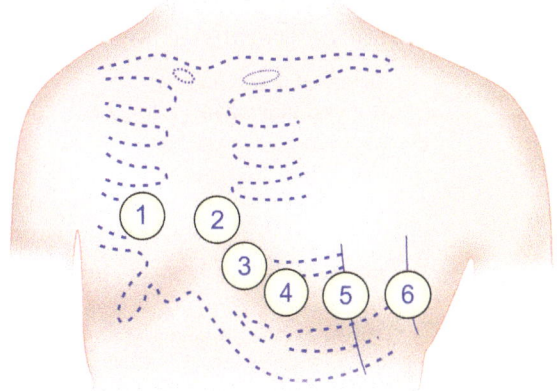

FIGURE 60.2: Position of electrodes for chest leads (V_1 to V_6).

Normal electrocardiogram has the following waves namely P, Q, R, S and T **(Table 60.2, Figs 60.3 and 60.4)**. Einthoven had named the waves of ECG starting from the middle of the English alphabets (P) instead of starting from the beginning (A).

Major complexes in ECG are:

1. 'P' wave, the atrial complex.
2. 'QRS' complex, the initial ventricular complex.
3. 'T' wave, the final ventricular complex.
4. 'QRST', the ventricular complex.

■ 'P' WAVE

It is a positive wave and the first wave in ECG. It is also called **atrial complex**. Its duration is 0.1 second and its amplitude is 0.1 to 0.12.

Cause of 'P' Wave

'P' wave is a positive wave produced due to the **depolarization** of atrial musculature. Atrial repolarization is not recorded as a separate wave in ECG because it merges with ventricular depolarization (QRS complex).

■ 'QRS' COMPLEX

It is also called the **initial ventricular complex**. 'Q' wave is a small negative wave. It is continued as the tall 'R' wave, which is a positive wave. 'R' wave is followed by a small negative wave, the 'S' wave. Its duration is 0.08 to 0.10 second.

Amplitude of 'QRS' complex:

'Q' wave : 0.1 to 0.2 mV
'R' wave : 1 mV
'S' wave : 0.4 mV

'QRS' complex is due to **depolarization** of ventricular musculature. 'Q' wave is due to the depolarization of basal portion of interventricular septum. 'R' wave is due to the depolarization of apical portion of interventricular septum and apical portion of ventricular muscle. And, 'S' wave is due to the depolarization of basal portion of ventricular muscle near the atrioventricular ring.

■ 'T' WAVE

It is the **final ventricular complex** and is a positive wave. Duration of 'T' wave is 0.2 second and its amplitude is 0.3 mV. 'T' wave is due to the **repolarization** of ventricular musculature.

■ 'U' WAVE

'U' wave is not always seen. It is also an insignificant wave in ECG. It is due to repolarization of **papillary muscle** and **Purkinje fibers**.

■ INTERVALS AND SEGMENTS OF ECG

■ 'P-R' INTERVAL

It is the interval between onset of 'P' wave and the onset of 'Q' wave.

'P-R' interval signifies the atrial depolarization and conduction of impulses through AV node. It shows the duration of conduction of the impulses from SA node to ventricles through atrial muscle and AV node.

Normal duration is 0.18 second and varies between 0.12 and 0.2 second. If it is more than 0.2 second, that signifies the delay in conduction of impulse from SA node to ventricles. Usually, the delay occurs in AV node. So, it is called the **AV nodal delay**.

■ 'Q-T' INTERVAL

It is the interval between the onset of 'Q' wave and the end of 'T' wave.

'Q-T' interval indicates the ventricular depolarization and ventricular repolarization, i.e. it signifies the electrical activity in ventricles.

Normal duration of this interval is between 0.4 and 0.42 second.

■ 'S-T' SEGMENT

Time interval between the end of 'S' wave and onset of 'T' wave is called 'S-T' segment. It is an **isoelectric period.** Its normal duration of 0.08 second.

TABLE 60.2: Waves of normal ECG.

Wave/Segment	From – To	Cause	Duration (second)	Amplitude (mV)
P wave	–	Atrial depolarization	0.1	0.1 to 0.12
QRS complex	Onset of Q wave to the end of S wave	Ventricular depolarization	0.08 to 0.10	Q = 0.1 to 0.2 R = 1 S = 0.4
T wave	–	Ventricular repolarization	0.2	0.3
U wave	–	Repolarization of papillary muscle or Purkinje fibers	0.16 to 0.2	0.1 to 0.2
P-R interval	Onset of P wave to onset of Q wave	Atrial depolarization and conduction through AV node	0.18 (0.12 to 0.2)	–
Q-T interval	Onset of Q wave and end of T wave	Ventricular depolarization and ventricular repolarization	0.4 to 0.42	–
S-T segment	End of S wave and onset of T wave	Isoelectric	0.08	–

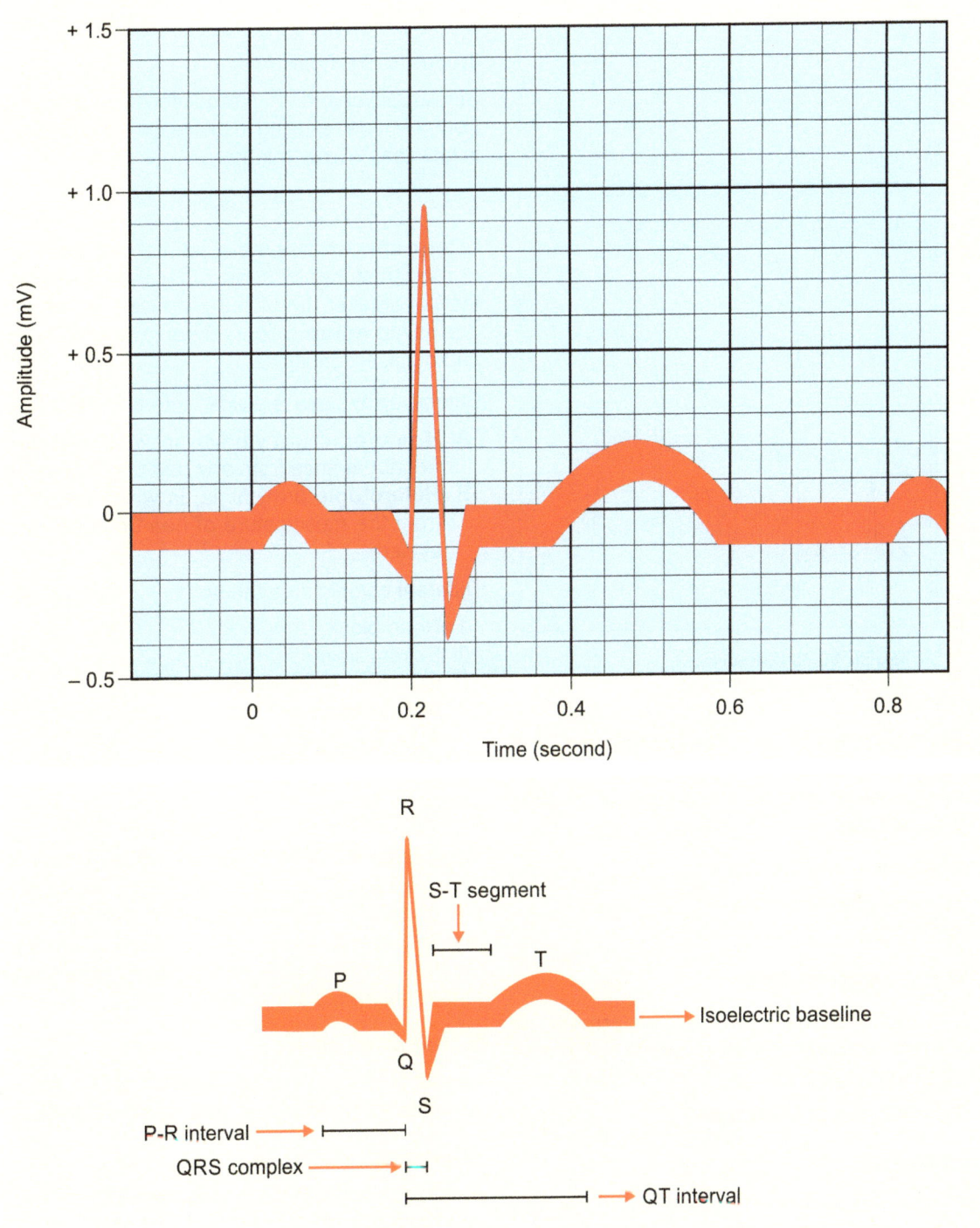

FIGURE 60.3: Waves of normal ECG.

J Point

J point is the point in ECG from where 'S-T' segment starts. It is the junction between QRS complex and 'S-T' segment.

■ 'R-R' INTERVAL

'R-R' interval is the time interval between two consecutive 'R' waves. 'R-R' interval signifies the duration of one cardiac cycle. Normal duration of 'R-R' interval is 0.8 second.

'R-R' interval signifies the duration of one **cardiac cycle**. Measurement of 'R-R' interval helps to calculate heart rate.

■ ARRHYTHMIA

■ DEFINITION AND CLASSIFICATION

Arrhythmia refers to **irregular heartbeat** or disturbance in the rhythm of heart. In arrhythmia, heartbeat may be fast or slow or there may be an extra beat or a missed beat. In

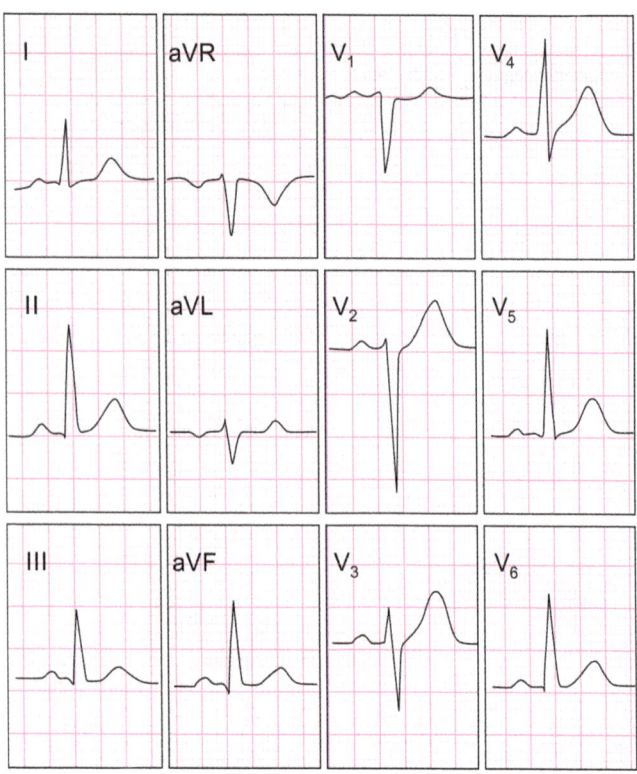

FIGURE 60.4: 12-lead ECG.
(*Courtesy:* Dr Atul Ruthra)

arrhythmia, SA node may or may not be the pacemaker. If SA node is not the pacemaker, any other part of the heart such as atrial muscle, AV node and ventricular muscle becomes the pacemaker.

Arrhythmia is classified into two types:

I. Normotopic arrhythmia.
II. Ectopic arrhythmia.

■ NORMOTOPIC ARRHYTHMIA

Normotopic arrhythmia is the irregular heartbeat, in which SA node is the pacemaker. Normotopic arrhythmia occurs in both physiological and pathological conditions.

Normotopic arrhythmia is of three types:

1. Sinus Arrhythmia

Sinus arrhythmia is a normal rhythmical increase and decrease in heart rate, in relation to respiration. It is also called **respiratory sinus arrhythmia** (RSA). Normal sinus rhythm means the normal heartbeat with SA node as the pacemaker. Normal heart rate is 72 per minute. However, under physiological conditions, in a normal healthy person, heart rate varies according to the phases of respiratory cycle. Heart rate increases during inspiration and decreases during expiration.

2. Sinus Tachycardia

Sinus tachycardia is the increase in discharge of impulses from SA node, resulting in increase in heart rate. Discharge of impulses from SA node is very rapid and the heart rate increases up to 100 per minute and sometimes up to 150 per minute.

3. Sinus Bradycardia

Sinus bradycardia is the reduction in discharge of impulses from SA node resulting in decrease in heart rate. Heart rate is less than 60 per minute.

■ ECTOPIC ARRHYTHMIA

Ectopic arrhythmia is the abnormal heartbeat, in which one of the structures of heart other than SA node becomes the pacemaker. Impulses produced by these structures are called **ectopic foci**. Ectopic arrythmia occurs only pathological conditions.

Ectopic arrhythmia is divided into two subtypes:

A. **Homotopic** arrhythmia, in which the impulses for heartbeat arise from any part of conductive system.
B. **Heterotopic** arrhythmia, in which the impulses arise from the musculature of heart other than conductive system.

Different ectopic arrhythmia:

1. Heart block.
2. Extrasystole.
3. Paroxysmal tachycardia.
4. Atrial flutter.
5. Atrial fibrillation.
6. Ventricular fibrillation.

1. Heart Block

Heart block is the blockage of impulses generated by SA node in the conductive system. Because of the blockage, the impulses cannot reach the cardiac musculature, resulting in ectopic arrhythmia. Based on the area affected, the heart block is classified into two types, sinoatrial block and atrioventricular block.

Sinoatrial block

Sinoatrial block is the failure of impulse transmission from SA node to AV node. It is also called sinus block.

Atrioventricular block

Atrioventricular block is the heart block in which the impulses are not transmitted from atria (from AV node) to ventricles because of defective conductive system. Atrioventricular block is of two categories, incomplete heart block and complete heart block.

i. *Incomplete heart block*: Incomplete heart block is the condition in which the transmission of impulses from atria to ventricles is slowed down and not blocked completely. Impulses reach ventricles late.
ii. *Complete heart block*: Complete heart block is the condition in which the impulses produced by SA node cannot reach the ventricles. Because of this, the ventricles beat in their own rhythm, independent of atrial beat. It is called **idioventricular rhythm**.

2. Extrasystole

Extrasystole is the premature contraction of the heart before its normal contraction. It is caused by an ectopic focus (discharge of an impulse from any part of the heart other than the SA node). The ectopic focus produces an extra beat of the heart that is always followed by a **compensatory pause**. Compensatory pause is the period during which the heart stops in relaxed state.

3. Paroxysmal Tachycardia

Paroxysmal tachycardia is the sudden attack of increased heart rate due to ectopic foci arising from atria, AV node or ventricle. The attack lasts for a period of few seconds to few hours. It stops suddenly. After the attack, heart functions normally.

4. Atrial Flutter

Atrial flutter is an arrhythmia characterized by rapid ineffective atrial contractions, caused by ectopic foci originating from atrial musculature. It is often associated with atrial paroxysmal tachycardia. Both the atria beat rapidly like the wings of a bird, hence the name atrial flutter. Atrial rate is about 250 to 350 beats per minute.

5. Atrial Fibrillation

Atrial fibrillation is the type of arrhythmia characterized by rapid and irregular atrial contractions at the rate of 300 to 400 beats per minute.

6. Ventricular Fibrillation

Ventricular fibrillation is the dangerous cardiac arrhythmia, characterized by rapid and irregular twitching of ventricles. Ventricles beat very rapidly and irregularly due to the circus movement of impulses within ventricular muscle. The rate reaches 400 to 500 per minute. This is triggered by ventricular extrasystole. This type of arrhythmia is serious as it may lead to death, since the ventricles cannot pump blood.

■ ABNORMAL PACEMAKER

Abnormal pacemaker is the part of the heart other than SA node that becomes the pacemaker and discharges ectopic foci. Various types of arrhythmia develop when an abnormal pacemaker is activated.

Usual abnormal pacemakers are:

1. Atrioventricular node.
2. Atrial musculature.
3. Ventricular musculature.

■ ARTIFICIAL PACEMAKER

Artificial pacemaker is a small **electronic device** that is surgically implanted to regulate abnormal heartbeat. It contains a battery powered **pulse generator,** which produces electrical impulses capable of stimulating the heart. This pacemaker is implanted under the skin over the chest of the patient. Pulses generated by this device are transmitted to the heart through electrodes. Electrodes connected to the device are inserted and passed through a vein and positioned in the heart chambers.

The device has a **lithium battery** that may last for 10 to 15 years. The outer casing of the pacemaker is usually made of titanium, which is rarely rejected by body's immune system.

Pulse generator of the pacemaker has multiple functions. It is programmed to cope up with the needs of the individual patient.

Chapter 61: Cardiac Output

CHAPTER OUTLINE

- **DEFINITIONS AND NORMAL VALUES**
  - STROKE VOLUME
  - MINUTE VOLUME
  - CARDIAC INDEX
- **EJECTION FRACTION**
- **CARDIAC RESERVE**
- **VARIATIONS IN CARDIAC OUTPUT**
  - PHYSIOLOGICAL VARIATIONS
  - PATHOLOGICAL VARIATIONS
- **DISTRIBUTION OF CARDIAC OUTPUT**
- **FACTORS MAINTAINING CARDIAC OUTPUT**
  - VENOUS RETURN
  - FORCE OF CONTRACTION
  - HEART RATE
  - PERIPHERAL RESISTANCE
- **MEASUREMENT OF CARDIAC OUTPUT**

DEFINITIONS AND NORMAL VALUES

Cardiac output is the amount of blood pumped from each ventricle. Usually, it refers to the left ventricular output through aorta.

Cardiac output is expressed in three ways namely, stroke volume, minute volume and cardiac index. However, in routine clinical practice cardiac output refers to **minute volume**.

1. STROKE VOLUME

It is the amount of blood pumped out by each ventricle during each beat.

Stroke volume =
 End-diastolic volume − End-systolic volume

Normal value of stroke volume:
70 mL (60 to 80 mL) when the heart rate is normal (72/min).

2. MINUTE VOLUME

Minute volume is the amount of blood pumped out by each ventricle in one minute. It is the product of stroke volume and heart rate.

Minute volume = Stroke volume × Heart rate

Normal value of minute volume:
5 liters/ventricle/minute.

3. CARDIAC INDEX

Cardiac index is the minute volume expressed in relation to square meter of body surface area. It is defined as the amount of blood pumped out per ventricle/minute/square meter of the body surface area.

Normal value of cardiac index:
Cardiac index = 2.8 ± 0.3 L/sq m of body surface area/minute.

Average **body surface area** in an adult is 1.734 sq m and normal minute volume is 5 L/min.

EJECTION FRACTION

Ejection fraction is the fraction of end-diastolic volume that is ejected out by each ventricle. Normal ejection fraction is 60 to 65%. Refer Chapter 58 for details.

CARDIAC RESERVE

Cardiac reserve is the maximum amount of blood that can be pumped out by heart above the normal value. Cardiac reserve plays an important role in increasing the cardiac output during the conditions such as exercise. It is essential to withstand the stress of exercise. Cardiac reserve in normal healthy adult is 300 to 400%.

VARIATIONS IN CARDIAC OUTPUT

PHYSIOLOGICAL VARIATIONS

1. *Age:* In children, cardiac output is less. Cardiac index is more than in adults because of less body surface area.
2. *Sex:* In females, cardiac output is less. Cardiac index is more.
3. *Body build:* Greater the body build, more is the cardiac output.

4. *Diurnal variation*: Cardiac output is low in early morning and increases in day time.
5. *Environmental temperature:* Increase in temperature above 30°C raises cardiac output.
6. *Emotional conditions:* Cardiac output increases.
7. *After meals:* During the first 1 hour after taking meals, cardiac output increases.
8. *Exercise:* Cardiac output increases.
9. *High altitude:* Cardiac output increases.
10. *Posture:* Cardiac output increases while changing from recumbent to upright position.
11. *Pregnancy:* Cardiac output increases during the later months of pregnancy.
12. *Sleep:* Cardiac output is slightly decreased or unaltered.

PATHOLOGICAL VARIATIONS

Conditions When Cardiac Output Increases

1. Fever.
2. Anemia.
3. Hyperthyroidism.

Conditions When Cardiac Output Decreases

1. Hypothyroidism.
2. Atrial fibrillation.
3. Heart block.
4. Congestive cardiac failure.
5. Shock.
6. Hemorrhage.

DISTRIBUTION OF CARDIAC OUTPUT

Whole amount of blood pumped out by right ventricle goes to lungs. But the blood pumped by left ventricle is distributed to different parts of the body.

Distribution of Blood Pumped Out of Left Ventricle

Distribution of blood pumped out of left ventricle to different organs and the percentage of cardiac output are given in **Table 61.1**.

Liver receives maximum amount of blood. Heart, which pumps the blood to all the other organs, receives the least amount of blood.

FACTORS MAINTAINING CARDIAC OUTPUT

Cardiac output is maintained (determined) by four factors:

1. Venous return.
2. Force of contraction.
3. Heart rate.
4. Peripheral resistance.

1. VENOUS RETURN

Venus return is amount of blood, which is returned to the heart from different parts of the body. Cardiac output is **directly proportional** to venous return provided the other three factors (force of contraction, heart rate and peripheral resistance) remain constant. Venous return in turn depends upon respiratory pump and muscle pump.

TABLE 61.1: Distribution of blood pumped out of left ventricle.

Organ	Amount of blood (mL/min)	Percentage
Liver	1,500	30
Kidney	1,300	26
Skeletal muscles	900	18
Brain	800	16
Skin, bone and GI tract	300	6
Heart	200	4
Total	5,000	100

Respiratory Pump

Respiratory pump increases venous return during inspiration. During inspiration, thoracic cavity expands and makes the intrapleural pressure more negative. This increases the diameter of inferior vena cava resulting in increased venous return. Same time, descent of diaphragm increases the intra-abdominal pressure which compresses abdominal veins and pushes the blood upward towards heart. Thereby the venous return is increased.

Muscle Pump

Muscle pump is the muscular activity that helps return of the blood back to heart. When muscular activity increases the venous return is more.

2. FORCE OF CONTRACTION

Cardiac output is **directly proportional** to the force of contraction provided other three factors remain constant. Force of contraction depends upon diastolic period and ventricular filling. Frank-Starling law of heart is applicable to this. According to **Frank-Starling law**, the force of contraction of heart is directly proportional to initial length of muscle fibers before the onset of contraction.

Force of contraction depends upon preload and afterload.

Preload

Preload is the stretching of the cardiac muscle fibers at the end of diastole just before contraction. During diastolic period, ventricular filling and ventricular pressure increase and stretch the muscle fibers. This results in increase in length of the muscle fibers which in turn increases the force of contraction and cardiac output.

Thus, force of contraction of heart and cardiac output are **directly proportional** to preload.

Afterload

Afterload is the force against which the ventricles must contract and eject the blood. This force is determined by the arterial pressure. At the end of isometric contraction period, semilunar valves are opened and blood is ejected into the aorta and pulmonary artery. So, the pressure increases in these two vessels. Now, the ventricles have to work against this pressure for further ejection. Thus, the afterload for left ventricle is determined by aortic pressure and afterload for right ventricular pressure is determined by pressure in pulmonary artery.

Force of contraction of heart and cardiac output are **inversely proportional** to afterload.

■ 3. HEART RATE

Cardiac output is **directly proportional** to heart rate provided the other three factors remain constant. Moderate change in heart rate does not alter the cardiac output. If there is a marked increase in heart rate, cardiac output is increased.

If there is marked decrease in heart rate, cardiac output is decreased.

■ 4. PERIPHERAL RESISTANCE

Peripheral resistance is the resistance offered to blood flow at the peripheral blood vessels. It is the resistance or load against which the heart has to pump the blood. So, the cardiac output is **inversely proportional** to peripheral resistance.

Resistance is offered at arterioles. So, the arterioles are called **resistant vessels**. In the body, the maximum peripheral resistance is offered at the **splanchnic region**.

■ MEASUREMENT OF CARDIAC OUTPUT

Methods used to measure cardiac output in human beings are:

1. By using Fick's principle.
2. Indicator (dye) dilution technique.
3. Thermodilution technique.
4. Ultrasonic Doppler transducer technique.
5. Doppler echocardiography.
6. Ballistocardiography.

■ 1. BY USING FICK'S PRINCIPLE

According to Fick's principle, amount of a substance taken up by an organ (or by the whole body) or given out in a unit of time is the product of amount of blood flowing through the organ and arteriovenous difference of that substance across the organ.

$$\text{Amount of substance taken or given} = \text{Amount of blood flow/minute} \times \text{Arteriovenous difference}$$

Modification of Fick Principle to Measure Cardiac Output

Fick's principle is modified to measure the cardiac output or a part of cardiac output (amount of blood to an organ). Thus, cardiac output or amount of blood flowing through an organ in a given unit of time is determined by the formula given below.

$$\text{Cardiac output} = \frac{\text{Amount of substance taken or given by the organ/minute}}{\text{Arteriovenous difference of the substance across the organ}}$$

Fick's principle is used to measure cardiac output by determining the amount of oxygen consumed in body in a given period of time and dividing this value by arteriovenous difference across the lungs.

■ 2. INDICATOR (DYE) DILUTION METHOD

Indicator dilution technique is described in detail in Chapter 5. Marker substance used to measure cardiac output is lithium chloride.

■ 3. THERMODILUTION TECHNIQUE

Cardiac output can also be measured by thermodilution technique or **thermal indicator method**. This method is the modified indicator dilution method. It is the popular method to measure cardiac output.

In this method, a known volume of cold sterile solution is injected into the right atrium by using a catheter. Cardiac output is measured by determining the resultant change in the blood temperature in pulmonary artery. For this purpose, **two thermistors** (**temperature transducers**) are used. One of them is placed in the inferior vena cava and the second one is placed in pulmonary artery.

■ 4. ESOPHAGEAL DOPPLER TRANSDUCER TECHNIQUE

This technique involves insertion of a flexible probe into midthoracic part of esophagus. A pulse wave **ultrasonic Doppler transducer** is fixed at the tip of the probe. This transducer calculates the velocity of blood flow in descending aorta. Diameter of aorta is determined by echocardiography. Cardiac output is calculated by using the values of velocity of blood flow and diameter of aorta.

■ 5. DOPPLER ECHOCARDIOGRAPHY

Doppler echocardiography is a method for detecting the direction and velocity of moving blood within the heart. This is also a popular method to measure cardiac output.

Chapter 62: Heart Rate

CHAPTER OUTLINE

- **HEART RATE**
  - NORMAL HEART RATE
  - TACHYCARDIA
  - BRADYCARDIA
- **REGULATION OF HEART RATE**
- **VASOMOTOR CENTER: CARDIAC CENTER**
  - VASOCONSTRICTOR AREA
  - VASODILATOR AREA
  - SENSORY AREA
- **MOTOR (EFFERENT) NERVE FIBERS TO HEART**
  - PARASYMPATHETIC NERVE FIBERS
  - SYMPATHETIC NERVE FIBERS
- **SENSORY (AFFERENT) NERVE FIBERS FROM HEART**
- **FACTORS AFFECTING VASOMOTOR CENTER: REGULATION OF VAGAL TONE**
  - IMPULSES FROM HIGHER CENTERS
  - IMPULSES FROM RESPIRATORY CENTERS
  - IMPULSES FROM BARORECEPTORS
  - IMPULSES FROM CHEMORECEPTORS
  - IMPULSES FROM RIGHT ATRIUM
  - IMPULSES FROM OTHER AFFERENT NERVES
- **BEZOLD-JARISCH REFLEX**

HEART RATE

NORMAL HEART RATE

Normal heart rate is 72/minute. It ranges between 60 and 80/minute.

TACHYCARDIA

Tachycardia is the increase in heart rate above 100/minute.

Physiological Conditions when Tachycardia Occurs

1. Childhood.
2. Exercise.
3. Pregnancy.
4. Emotional conditions such as anxiety.

Pathological Conditions when Tachycardia Occurs

1. Fever.
2. Anemia.
3. Hypoxia.
4. Hyperthyroidism.
5. Hypersecretion of catecholamines.

BRADYCARDIA

Bradycardia is the decrease in heart rate below 60/minute.

Physiological Conditions when Bradycardia Occurs

1. Sleep.
2. Athletes.

Pathological Conditions when Bradycardia Occurs

1. Hypothermia.
2. Hypothyroidism.
3. Heart attack.
4. Congenital heart disease.
5. Obstructive jaundice.

REGULATION OF HEART RATE

Heart rate is maintained within normal range constantly. It is subjected for variation during conditions such as exercise, emotion, etc. However, under physiological conditions, the altered heart rate is quickly brought back to normal. Heart rate is regulated by the nervous mechanism which consists of three components:

  I. Vasomotor center.
 II. Motor (efferent) nerve fibers to the heart.
III. Sensory (afferent) nerve fibers from the heart.

VASOMOTOR CENTER: CARDIAC CENTER

Vasomotor center is the nervous center that regulates the heart rate. It also regulates the blood pressure. Earlier it was called the **cardiac center**. Vasomotor center is bilaterally situated in the **reticular formation** of medulla oblongata and lower part of pons.

Vasomotor center has three areas:

1. Vasoconstrictor area.
2. Vasodilator area.
3. Sensory area.

■ VASOCONSTRICTOR AREA: CARDIOACCELERATOR CENTER

It is situated in the **reticular formation** of medulla and it forms the lateral portion of vasomotor center. Vasoconstrictor area is otherwise known as **pressor area** or cardioaccelerator center.

Functions of Vasoconstrictor Area

This area increases the heart rate by sending accelerator impulses to heart through sympathetic nerves. It also causes constriction of blood vessels.

Control of Vasoconstrictor Area

Vasoconstrictor area is under the control of cerebral cortex and **hypothalamus**.

■ VASODILATOR AREA: CARDIOINHIBITORY CENTER

It is also situated in the reticular formation of medulla. It forms the medial portion of vasomotor center. It is also called **depressor area** or **cardioinhibitory center**.

Functions of Vasodilator Area

Vasodilator area decreases the heart rate by sending inhibitory impulses to the heart through vagus nerve. It also causes dilatation of blood vessels.

Control of Vasodilator Area

Vasodilator area is under the control of **cerebral cortex** and **hypothalamus**. It is also controlled by the impulses from baroreceptors, chemoreceptors and other sensory impulses via afferent nerves.

■ SENSORY AREA

Sensory area is in **nucleus of tractus solitarius** in medulla. It forms posterior part of vasomotor center.

Functions of Sensory Area

Sensory area receives sensory impulse via glossopharyngeal nerve and vagus nerve from periphery, particularly, from the baroreceptors. In turn, this area controls the vasoconstrictor and vasodilator areas.

■ MOTOR (EFFERENT) NERVE FIBERS TO HEART

Heart receives efferent nerves from both the divisions of autonomic nervous system. Parasympathetic fibers arise from the medulla oblongata and pass through vagus nerve. Sympathetic fibers arise from upper thoracic (T1 to T4) segments of spinal cord **(Fig. 62.1)**.

■ PARASYMPATHETIC NERVE FIBERS

Parasympathetic nerve fibers supplying heart arise from **dorsal nucleus of vagus** situated medulla oblongata. Preganglionic parasympathetic nerve fibers from dorsal nucleus of vagus reach the heart and terminate on postganglionic neurons. Postganglionic fibers from these neurons innervate heart muscle.

Most of the fibers from right vagus terminate in SA node. Remaining fibers supply the atrial muscles and AV node. Most of the fibers from left vagus supply AV node and some fibers supply the atrial muscle and SA node.

Ventricles do not receive the vagus nerve supply.

Functions of Parasympathetic Nerve

Vagus nerve is **cardioinhibitory** in function and carries inhibitory impulses from vasodilator area to heart. These impulses decrease the rate and force contraction of heart.

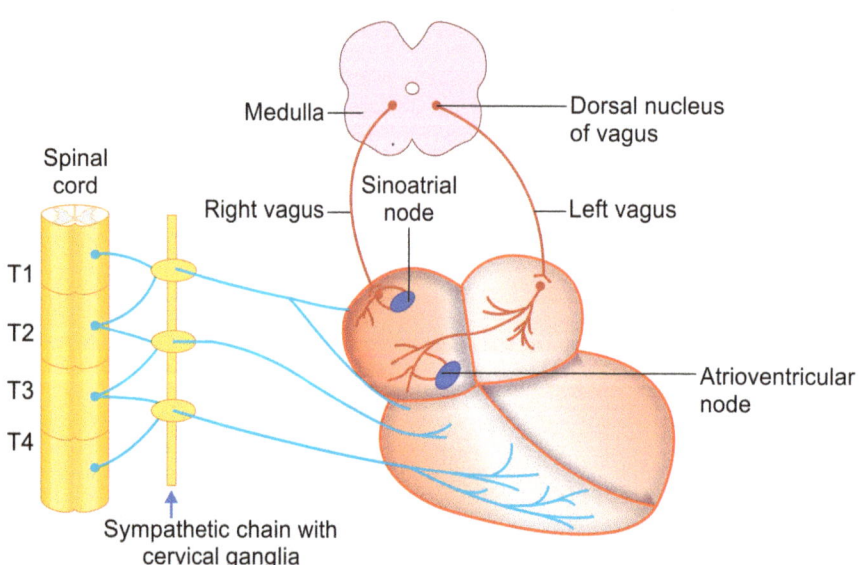

FIGURE 62.1: Nerve supply to heart.

Mode of Action of Vagus Nerve

Vagus nerve inhibits the heart by secreting the neurotransmitter called **acetylcholine**.

Vagal Tone

Vagal tone is the continuous stream of **inhibitory impulses** from vasodilator area to heart via vagus nerve. Heart rate is kept under control because of vagal tone. Vagal tone is also called **cardioinhibitory tone** or **parasympathetic tone**. Heart rate is **inversely proportional** to vagal tone.

SYMPATHETIC NERVE FIBERS

Preganglionic fibers of the sympathetic nerves to heart arise from lateral grey horns of the first 4 thoracic segments (T1 to T4) of the spinal cord. Preganglionic fibers reach the superior, middle and inferior **cervical sympathetic ganglia** situated in the sympathetic chain. From these ganglia, the postganglionic fibers arise. Postganglionic fibers form superior, middle and inferior **cervical sympathetic nerves**.

Nerves Formed by Sympathetic Postganglionic Fibers

1. Superior cervical sympathetic nerve, which innervates larger arteries and base of the heart.
2. Middle cervical sympathetic nerve, which supplies the rest of the heart.
3. Inferior cervical sympathetic nerve, which serves as **sensory (afferent) nerve** from the heart.

Functions of Sympathetic Nerves

Sympathetic nerves are **cardioaccelerator** in function and carry cardioaccelerator impulses from vasoconstrictor area to the heart. These impulses increase the rate and force of contraction of heart.

Mode of Action of Sympathetic Nerves

Sympathetic nerves increase heart rate by secreting the neurotransmitter called **noradrenaline**.

Sympathetic Tone

Sympathetic tone or **cardioaccelerator tone** is the continuous stream of impulses produced by the vasoconstrictor area. These impulses pass through sympathetic nerves and accelerate the heart rate. Heart rate is **directly proportional** to sympathetic tone.

Under normal conditions, vagal tone is dominant over sympathetic tone. Whenever vagal tone is reduced or abolished, the sympathetic tone becomes powerful.

SENSORY (AFFERENT) NERVE FIBERS FROM HEART

Afferent (sensory) nerve fibers from the heart pass through **inferior cervical sympathetic nerve**. These nerve fibers carry sensations of **stretch** and **pain** from the heart to the brain via spinal cord.

FACTORS AFFECTING VASOMOTOR CENTER: REGULATION OF VAGAL TONE

Vasomotor center regulates the cardiac activity by receiving impulses from different sources in the body.

1. IMPULSES FROM HIGHER CENTERS

Vasomotor center is mainly controlled by the impulses from higher centers in the brain.

Cerebral Cortex

Area 13 in cerebral cortex is concerned with emotional reactions of the body. During emotional conditions, this area sends inhibitory impulses to the vasodilator area. This causes reduction in vagal tone leading to cardioacceleration.

Hypothalamus

Hypothalamus influences the heart rate via vasomotor center. Stimulation of posterior and lateral hypothalamic nuclei causes tachycardia. Stimulation of preoptic and anterior nuclei causes bradycardia.

2. IMPULSES FROM RESPIRATORY CENTERS

In forced breathing, heart rate increases during inspiration and decreases during expiration. This variation is called **respiratory sinus arrhythmia**. This is common in some children and in some adults even during quiet breathing.

3. IMPULSES FROM BARORECEPTORS: MAREY'S REFLEX

Baroreceptors or **pressoreceptors** are the receptors, which give response to change in blood pressure. Baroreceptors are of two types, **carotid baroreceptors** and **aortic baroreceptors**. Carotid baroreceptors are situated in the carotid sinus, present in the wall of internal carotid artery. Aortic baroreceptors are situated in the wall of arch of aorta.

Nerve Supply to Baroreceptors

Carotid baroreceptors are supplied by the afferent nerve **Hering's nerve**, a branch of glossopharyngeal nerve. Aortic baroreceptors are supplied by the afferent nerve **aortic nerve**, a branch of vagus nerve (Fig. 62.2). Nerve fibers from the baroreceptors reach the nucleus of tractus solitarius situated adjacent to vasomotor center.

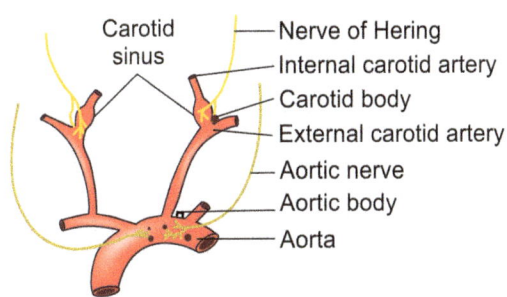

FIGURE 62.2: Nerve supply to baroreceptors and chemoreceptors.

Functions of Baroreceptors: Marey's Reflex

Baroreceptors regulate the heart rate through Marey's reflex. Marey's reflex is a **cardioinhibitory reflex** that decreases heart rate whenever blood pressure increases. Increase in blood pressure stimulate the baroreceptors. Baroreceptors send stimulatory impulses to nucleus of tractus solitarius via afferent. Now, the nucleus of tractus solitarius stimulates the vasodilator area, which in turn increases vagal tone leading to decrease in heart rate.

When pressure is less, the baroreceptors are not stimulated. So, no impulses go to the nucleus of tractus solitaries and heart rate is not decreased. Thus, the heart rate is **inversely proportional** to blood pressure.

Baroreceptors produce the Marey's reflex only during resting conditions. So, in many conditions such as exercise, there is an increase in both blood pressure and heart rate.

Marey's Law

According to Marey's law, the pulse rate (which represents heart rate) is inversely proportional to blood pressure.

■ 4. IMPULSES FROM CHEMORECEPTORS

Chemoreceptors are the receptors giving response to change in chemical constituents of blood, particularly oxygen, carbon dioxide and hydrogen ion concentration. **Peripheral chemoreceptors** are situated in the **carotid body** and **aortic body** adjacent to baroreceptors.

Nerve Supply to Chemoreceptors

Chemoreceptors in carotid body are supplied by **Hering's nerve**, the branch of glossopharyngeal nerve. Chemoreceptors in aortic body are supplied by the **aortic nerve** the branch of vagus nerve (Fig. 62.2).

Functions of Chemoreceptors

Whenever there is hypoxia, hypercapnia, and increased hydrogen ions concentration in the blood, the chemoreceptors are stimulated and inhibitory impulses are sent to vasodilator area. Vagal tone decreases and heart rate increases.

Sinoaortic Mechanism and Buffer Nerves

Sinoaortic mechanism is the mechanism of baroreceptors and chemoreceptors in carotid and aortic regions that regulates heart rate, blood pressure and respiration. The nerves from these receptors are called **buffer nerves**.

■ 5. IMPULSES FROM RIGHT ATRIUM: BAINBRIDGE REFLEX

Bainbridge reflex or **right atrial reflex** is a **cardio-accelerator reflex** that increases the heart rate when venous return is increased.

Wall of right atrium has **stretch receptors**. When venous return increases, the right atrium is distended and stretch receptors are stimulated. Stretch receptors, in turn, send inhibitory impulses through inferior cervical sympathetic nerve to vasodilator area of vasomotor center. Vasodilator area is inhibited resulting in decrease in vagal tone and increase in heart rate.

■ 6. IMPULSES FROM OTHER AFFERENT NERVES

Stimulation of sensory nerves produces varying effects.

Examples

i. Stimulation of **receptors in nasal mucous membrane** causes **bradycardia**. The impulses from nasal mucous membrane pass via the branches of V cranial nerve and decrease the heart rate.
ii. Most of the **painful stimuli** cause tachycardia and some cause **bradycardia**. The impulses are transmitted via pain nerve fibers.

■ BEZOLD-JARISCH REFLEX

Bezold-Jarisch reflex or **coronary chemoreflex** is the reflex characterized by **bradycardia** and **hypotension**, caused by stimulation of **chemoreceptors** present in the wall of left ventricle by substances such as alkaloids. Vagal fibers form the afferent and efferent pathways of this reflex. This reflex occurs in myocardial infarction, hemorrhage, and aortic stenosis (narrowing).

Chapter 63

Blood Pressure

CHAPTER OUTLINE

- **ARTERIAL BLOOD PRESSURE**
  - DEFINITIONS AND NORMAL VALUES
  - VARIATIONS
  - DETERMINANTS OF ARTERIAL BLOOD PRESSURE
  - REGULATION OF ARTERIAL BLOOD PRESSURE
  - NERVOUS MECHANISM
  - RENAL MECHANISM
  - HORMONAL MECHANISM
  - LOCAL MECHANISM
  - MEASUREMENT OF ARTERIAL BLOOD PRESSURE
  - APPLIED PHYSIOLOGY
- **VENOUS BLOOD PRESSURE**
  - DEFINITION
  - NORMAL VALUES
  - EFFECT OF RESPIRATION ON VENOUS BLOOD PRESSURE
- **CAPILLARY BLOOD PRESSURE**
  - DEFINITION, SIGNIFICANCE AND NORMAL VALUES
  - REGIONAL VARIATIONS
  - CAPILLARY ONCOTIC PRESSURE

ARTERIAL BLOOD PRESSURE

DEFINITIONS AND NORMAL VALUES

Arterial blood pressure is defined as the **lateral pressure** exerted by the column of blood on the wall of arteries. This pressure is exerted when blood flows through the arteries. Generally, the term 'blood pressure' refers to arterial blood pressure. Arterial blood pressure is expressed in four different terms:

1. Systolic Blood Pressure

Systolic blood pressure or systolic pressure is defined as the **maximum pressure** exerted in the arteries during systole of heart.

Normal systolic pressure:
  120 mm Hg (110 to 140 mm Hg).

2. Diastolic Blood Pressure

Diastolic blood pressure or diastolic pressure is defined as the **minimum pressure** in the arteries during diastole of heart.

Normal diastolic pressure:
  80 mm Hg (60 to 80 mm Hg).

3. Pulse Pressure

Pulse pressure is the **difference** between systolic pressure and diastolic pressure.

Normal pulse pressure:
  40 mm Hg (120 – 80).

4. Mean Arterial Blood Pressure

It is the average pressure existing in the arteries. It is the diastolic pressure plus one-third of pulse pressure. To determine the mean pressure, diastolic pressure is considered than the systolic pressure. It is because diastolic period of cardiac cycle is longer (0.53 second) than the systolic period (0.27 second).

Normal mean arterial pressure:
  93 mm Hg (80 + 13 = 93).

VARIATIONS OF ARTERIAL BLOOD PRESSURE

Physiological Variations

1. **Age:** Arterial blood pressure increases as age advances **(Table 63.1)**.
2. **Sex:** In females, up to the period of menopause, arterial pressure is about 5 mm Hg less than in males

TABLE 63.1: Arterial blood pressure in different age.

Age	Systolic pressure (mm Hg)	Diastolic pressure (mm Hg)
New born	70	40
After 1 month	85	45
After 6 months	90	50
After 1 year	95	55
After puberty	120	80
After 50 years	140	85
After 70 years	160	90
After 80 years	180	95

of same age. After menopause, the pressure in females becomes equal to that in males of same age.
3. *Body built*: Pressure is more in obese persons than in lean persons.
4. *Diurnal variation*: In early morning, the pressure is slightly low. It gradually increases and reaches the maximum at noon. It becomes low in evening.
5. *After meals*: Arterial blood pressure increases for few hours after meals due to increase in cardiac output.
6. *During sleep*: Usually, the pressure reduces during deep sleep. However, it increases slightly during sleep associated with dreams.
7. *Emotional conditions*: Blood pressure is increases in emotional conditions.
8. *After exercise*: After moderate exercise, systolic pressure increases by 20 to 30 mm Hg above the basal level due to increase in force of contraction and stroke volume. Normally, diastolic pressure is not affected by moderate exercise. It is because the diastolic pressure depends upon peripheral resistance, which is not altered by moderate exercise. More details are given in Chapter 67.

Pathological Variations

Pathological variations of arterial blood pressure are hypertension and hypotension. Refer applied physiology of this chapter for details.

■ DETERMINANTS OF ARTERIAL BLOOD PRESSURE: FACTORS MAINTAINING ARTERIAL BLOOD PRESSURE

Some factors are necessary for the maintenance of normal arterial blood pressure, which are called **local factors**, **mechanical factors** or **determinants** of arterial blood pressure.

Local factors are divided into two types:
I. Central factors which are pertaining to the heart.
II. Peripheral factors which are pertaining to blood and blood vessels.

Central Factors

1. *Cardiac output*

Systolic pressure is **directly proportional** to cardiac output. Whenever the cardiac output increases, the systolic pressure is increased and, when cardiac output is less, the systolic pressure is reduced.

2. *Heart rate*

Moderate changes in heart rate do not affect arterial blood pressure much. However, marked alteration in the heart rate affects the blood pressure by altering cardiac output.

Peripheral Factors

Peripheral resistance is the resistance offered to blood flow at the periphery. Resistance is offered at arterioles, which are called the **resistant vessels**. This is the important factor, which maintains diastolic pressure. Diastolic pressure is **directly proportional** to peripheral resistance.

3. *Blood volume*

Blood pressure is **directly proportional** to blood volume.

4. *Venous return*

Blood pressure is **directly proportional** to venous return.

5. *Elasticity of blood vessels*

Blood pressure is **inversely proportional** to the elasticity of blood vessels. Due to the elastic property, blood vessels are distensible and are able to maintain the pressure. When the elastic property is lost, blood vessels become rigid (**arteriosclerosis**) and pressure increases as in old age.

Deposition of cholesterol, fatty acids and calcium ions cause rigidity of blood vessels (**atherosclerosis**) leading to increased blood pressure.

6. *Velocity of blood flow*

Pressure in a blood vessel is **directly proportional** to the velocity of blood flow. If the velocity of the blood flow increases, the resistance increases. So, the pressure is increased.

7. *Diameter of blood vessels*

Arterial blood pressure is **inversely proportional** to diameter of the blood vessel. If the diameter decreases, the peripheral resistance increases leading to increase in the pressure.

8. *Viscosity of blood*

Arterial blood pressure is **directly proportional** to the viscosity of blood. When viscosity of blood increases, the frictional resistance is increased and this increases the pressure.

■ REGULATION OF ARTERIAL BLOOD PRESSURE

Arterial blood pressure varies even under physiological conditions. However, immediately it is brought back to normal level because of the presence of well-organized regulatory mechanisms in the body. Regulatory mechanisms which maintain the blood pressure within normal limits are:

I. Nervous mechanism or short-term regulatory mechanism.

II. Renal mechanism or long-term regulatory mechanism.
III. Hormonal mechanism.
IV. Local mechanism.

■ NERVOUS MECHANISM FOR REGULATION OF ARTERIAL BLOOD PRESSURE: SHORT-TERM REGULATION

Nervous regulation is rapid among all the mechanisms involved in regulation of arterial blood pressure. When blood pressure is altered, nervous system brings the pressure back to normal within few minutes. Although nervous mechanism is **quick in action**, it operates only for a short period. Nervous mechanism operates through vasomotor system.

Vasomotor system includes three components, vasomotor center, vasoconstrictor center and vasodilator fibers.

1. Vasomotor System

Vasomotor center is bilaterally situated in the **reticular formation** of medulla oblongata and lower part of the pons. Vasomotor center consists of **three areas**:

i. Vasoconstrictor area

Vasoconstrictor area is also called the **pressor area**. It forms the lateral portion of vasomotor center. Vasoconstrictor area sends impulses to blood vessels through sympathetic vasoconstrictor fibers. This area is also concerned with **acceleration of heart rate** (Chapter 62).

ii. Vasodilator area

Vasodilator area is also called **depressor area**. It forms the medial portion of vasomotor center. This area suppresses the vasoconstrictor area and causes vasodilatation. It is also concerned with **inhibition of heart rate** (Chapter 62).

iii. Sensory area

Sensory area is in the nucleus of tractus solitarius situated medulla and pons. This area receives sensory impulses via glossopharyngeal and vagal nerves from the periphery, particularly, from the baroreceptors. Sensory area in turn, controls the vasoconstrictor and vasodilator areas.

2. Vasoconstrictor Fibers

Vasoconstrictor fibers belong to the sympathetic division of autonomic nervous system. These fibers cause vasoconstriction by the release of the neurotransmitter substance, **noradrenaline**.

Vasomotor tone or sympathetic tone

Vasomotor tone or sympathetic tone is the continuous discharge of impulses from vasoconstrictor center through the vasoconstrictor fibers. Vasomotor tone plays an important role in regulating the pressure by producing a constant partial state of constriction of the blood vessels. Thus, the arterial blood pressure is **directly proportional** to vasomotor tone.

3. Vasodilator Fibers

Vasodilator fibers are of **three types**:

i. Parasympathetic vasodilator fibers

Parasympathetic vasodilator fibers cause dilatation of blood vessels by releasing **acetylcholine**.

ii. Sympathetic vasodilator fibers

Some of the sympathetic fibers cause vasodilatation in certain areas by secreting acetylcholine. Such fibers are called sympathetic vasodilator or **sympathetic cholinergic fibers**. Sympathetic cholinergic fibers, which supply the blood vessels of skeletal muscles are important in increasing the blood flow to muscles by vasodilatation during conditions like exercise.

iii. Antidromic vasodilator fibers

Normally, the impulses produced by a cutaneous receptor (like pain receptor) pass through sensory nerve fibers. But, some of these impulses pass through the other branches of the axon in opposite direction and reach the blood vessels supplied by these branches. Now, these impulses dilate the blood vessels. It is called the antidromic or **axon reflex**. And, the nerve fibers are called **antidromic vasodilator fibers**.

Mechanism of Vasomotor System in Regulation of Arterial Blood Pressure

Vasomotor center regulates the arterial blood pressure by causing vasoconstriction or vasodilatation. However, its actions depend upon the impulses it receives from other structures such as baroreceptors, chemoreceptors, higher centers and respiratory centers. Among these structures, baroreceptors and chemoreceptors play a major role in short-term regulation of blood pressure.

1. Baroreceptor mechanism

Baroreceptors are the receptors, which give response to **change in blood pressure**. Baroreceptors are situated in carotid sinus and wall of aorta. Refer Chapter 62 for details of baroreceptors.

Functions of baroreceptors

When arterial blood pressure rises rapidly, the baroreceptors are activated and send stimulatory impulses to nucleus of tractus solitarius through glossopharyngeal and vagus nerves. Now, the nucleus of tractus solitarius acts on both vasoconstrictor area and vasodilator areas of vasomotor center. It inhibits the vasoconstrictor area and excites the vasodilator area.

Inhibition of vasoconstrictor area reduces vasomotor tone. Reduction in vasomotor tone causes vasodilatation resulting in decreased peripheral resistance. Simultaneous excitation of vasodilator center increases vagal tone (Chapter 62). This decreases the rate and force of contraction of heart leading to reduction in cardiac output. These two factors, i.e. decreased peripheral resistance and reduced cardiac output bring the arterial blood pressure back to normal level.

2. Chemoreceptor mechanism

Chemoreceptors are the receptors giving response to change in chemical constituents of blood. Peripheral chemoreceptors are situated in the carotid body and aortic body. Refer Chapter 62 for details of peripheral chemoreceptors.

Function of chemoreceptors

Peripheral chemoreceptors are sensitive to lack of oxygen and excess of carbon dioxide and hydrogen ion concentration in blood. But, lack of oxygen is the most potent stimulus for peripheral chemoreceptors. Whenever blood pressure decreases, the blood flow decreases resulting in decreased oxygen content and excess of carbon dioxide and hydrogen ion. These factors stimulate the chemoreceptors, which send impulses to stimulate the vasoconstrictor center. Blood pressure rises and blood flow increases.

Chemoreceptors play a major role in maintaining respiration (Chapter 73) rather than blood pressure.

Sinoaortic mechanism and Buffer nerves

Mechanism of action of baroreceptors and chemoreceptors in carotid and aortic region constitute sinoaortic mechanism. Nerves from the baroreceptors and chemoreceptors are called buffer nerves because these nerves regulate the heart rate (Chapter 62), blood pressure and respiration (Chapter 73).

3. Higher centers

Vasomotor center is also controlled by the impulses from two higher centers in brain.

i. *Cerebral cortex*

Area 13 in cerebral cortex is concerned with emotional reactions. During emotional conditions, this area sends impulses to vasomotor center. Now, vasomotor center is activated, the vasomotor tone is increased and blood pressure rises.

ii. *Hypothalamus*

Stimulation of posterior and lateral nuclei of hypothalamus causes vasoconstriction and increase in blood pressure. Stimulation of preoptic area causes vasodilatation and decrease in blood pressure. Impulses from hypothalamus are mediated via vasomotor center.

4. Respiratory centers

During the beginning of expiration, arterial blood pressure increases slightly, i.e. by 4 to 6 mm Hg. And it decreases during later part of expiration and during inspiration. It is because of radiation of impulses from respiratory centers towards vasomotor center at different phases of respiratory cycle.

■ RENAL MECHANISM FOR REGULATION OF ARTERIAL BLOOD PRESSURE: LONG-TERM REGULATION

Kidneys play an important role in the long-term regulation of arterial blood pressure. When blood pressure alters slowly in several days/months/years, nervous mechanism adapts to the altered pressure and loses the sensitivity for changes. It cannot regulate the pressure any more. In such conditions, the renal mechanism operates efficiently to regulate the blood pressure. Therefore, it is called long-term regulation.

Kidneys regulate arterial blood pressure by two ways:
1. By regulation of ECF volume.
2. Through renin-angiotensin mechanism.

1. By Regulation of ECF Volume

When the blood pressure increases, kidneys excrete large amounts of water and salt, particularly sodium by means of pressure diuresis and pressure natriuresis.

Pressure diuresis is the excretion of large quantity of water in urine because of increased blood pressure. **Pressure natriuresis** is the excretion of large quantity of sodium in urine.

Because of diuresis and natriuresis, there is decrease in the ECF volume and blood volume, which in turn brings the arterial blood pressure back to normal level.

When blood pressure decreases, the reabsorption of water from renal tubules is increased. This increases ECF volume, blood volume and cardiac output resulting in restoration of blood pressure.

2. Through Renin-Angiotensin Mechanism

Details about source of renin secretion, formation of angiotensin and conditions when renin is secreted are described in Chapter 34.

Actions of angiotensin II

When blood pressure and ECF volume decrease, renin secretion from kidneys is increased. It converts angiotensinogen into angiotensin I. This is converted into angiotensin II by **angiotensin-converting enzyme** (ACE).

Angiotensin II acts in two ways to restore the blood pressure:

i. It causes constriction of arterioles and increases peripheral resistance. So, blood pressure rises. In addition, angiotensin II causes constriction of afferent arterioles in kidneys so that the glomerular filtration reduces. This results in retention of water and salts. This increases ECF volume to normal level. This in turn increases the blood pressure to normal level.
ii. Simultaneously, angiotensin II stimulates the adrenal cortex to secrete aldosterone which increases reabsorption of sodium from renal tubules. Sodium reabsorption is followed by water reabsorption resulting in increased ECF volume and blood volume. It increases the blood pressure to normal level.

Actions of angiotensin III and angiotensin IV

Like angiotensin II, the angiotensins III and IV also increase the blood pressure and stimulate adrenal cortex to secrete aldosterone (Chapter 34).

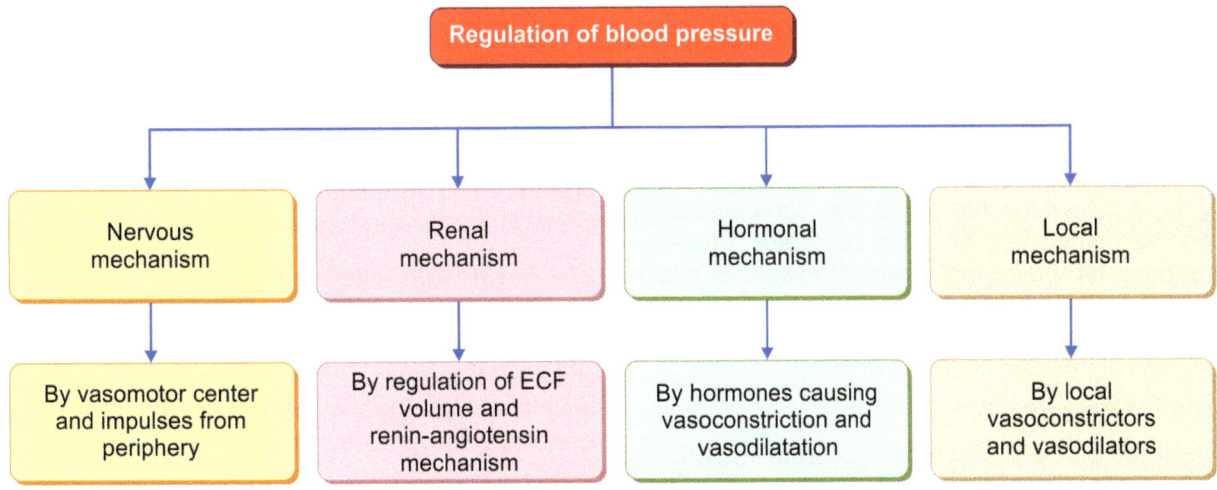

FIGURE 63.1: Regulation of blood pressure.
ECF = Extracellular fluid

■ HORMONAL MECHANISM FOR REGULATION OF ARTERIAL BLOOD PRESSURE

Many hormones are involved in the regulation of blood pressure **(Fig. 63.1)**. Hormones, which increase or decrease the arterial blood pressure are listed in **Table 63.2**.

■ LOCAL MECHANISM FOR REGULATION OF ARTERIAL BLOOD PRESSURE

In addition to nervous, renal and hormonal mechanisms, some local substances also regulate the blood pressure. The local substances regulate the blood pressure by vasoconstriction or vasodilatation.

Local Vasoconstrictors

Local vasoconstrictor substances are of vascular endothelial origin and are known as **endothelins (ET)**. Endothelins are peptides with 21 amino acids. Endothelins are produced by stretching of blood vessels. These peptides act by activating phospholipase, which in turn activates **prostacyclin** and **thromboxane A$_2$**. These two substances cause constriction of blood vessels and increase in blood pressure.

Local Vasodilators

Local vasodilators are of two types:

1. Vasodilators of metabolic origin such as carbon dioxide, lactate, hydrogen ions and **adenosine**.
2. Vasodilators of endothelial origin such as **nitric oxide (NO)**.

■ MEASUREMENT OF ARTERIAL BLOOD PRESSURE

Blood pressure is measured by direct and indirect methods. Direct method which is used in animals only. Indirect method which is used in human beings as well animals. Indirect method is explained below.

TABLE 63.2: Hormones regulating of arterial blood pressure.

Hormones which increase arterial blood pressure	Hormones which decrease arterial blood pressure
1. Adrenaline* 2. Noradrenaline 3. Thyroxine* 4. Aldosterone 5. Vasopressin 6. Angiotensin 7. Serotonin	1. Vasoactive intestinal polypeptide (VIP) 2. Bradykinin 3. Prostaglandin 4. Histamine 5. Acetylcholine 6. Atrial natriuretic peptide 7. Brain natriuretic peptide 8. Ctype natriuretic peptide

*Adrenaline and thyroxine increase systolic pressure but decrease diastolic pressure.

Apparatus

Arterial blood pressure is by apparatus called **sphygmomanometer**. Stethoscope is also necessary to measure blood pressure.

Principle

When an external pressure is applied over the artery, the blood flow through that artery is obstructed. And the pressure required to cause occlusion of blood flow indicates pressure inside the vessel.

Procedure

Brachial artery is usually chosen because of convenience. The arm cuff of sphygmomanometer is tied around upper arm, above the cubital fossa. It is connected to sphygmomanometer. Pressure is measured by two methods, palpatory method and auscultatory method.

1. Palpatory method

First, the **radial pulse** is felt. While feeling the pulse, pressure is increased in the cuff by inflating air into it, with the help of a hand pump. While doing this, mercury column in the sphygmomanometer shows the pressure in the cuff.

When pressure is increased in the arm cuff, brachial artery is compressed and blood flow is obstructed. So, radial pulse disappears. When radial pulse disappears, the pressure is further increased by about 20 mm Hg. Then, the pressure in the cuff is slowly reduced by releasing the valve of the hand pump, i.e. the cuff is deflated slowly. This is done by feeling the pulse and simultaneously watching the mercury column in the apparatus. Pressure is noted when the pulse reappears. Pressure at which pulse reappears indicates the **systolic pressure**.

Disadvantage of palpatory method is that the diastolic pressure cannot be measured.

2. Auscultatory method

Auscultatory method is the most accurate method to determine arterial blood pressure. After determining systolic pressure in palpatory method, the pressure in the cuff is raised by about 20 mm Hg above that level, so that the brachial artery is occluded due to compression. Now, the chest piece of stethoscope is placed over antecubital fossa and the arm cuff is slowly deflated. While doing so, series of sounds are heard through the stethoscope. These sounds are known as Korotkoff sounds. While reducing the pressure, Korotkoff sounds have five phases.

First phase: Tapping sound

While decreasing the pressure from arm cuff, occlusion of the artery is relieved and when blood starts flowing through the artery, first sound appears when the pressure is reduced to 120 mm Hg. It is a clear tapping sound.

Appearance of tapping sound indicates **systolic pressure**. When the pressure is reduced further by 10 mm Hg from the initial level, this sound slowly becomes louder.

Second phase: Murmuring sound

Following the clear taping sound, a soft murmuring sound is heard when the pressure is reduced further by about 15 mm Hg.

Third phase: Gong sound

After the murmuring sound, a very clear and louder sound is heard. It is of gong type. It is heard while reducing the pressure by another 15 mm Hg **(Table 63.3)**.

Fourth phase: Muffled sound

Next to the gong type sound, a mild and muffled sound is heard when the pressure is decreased further by 5 mm Hg.

TABLE 63.3: Phases of Korotkoff sounds.

Phase	Sound
First phase	Tapping sound Indicates systolic pressure
Second phase	Murmuring sound
Third phase	Gong sound
Fourth phase	Muffled sound
Fifth phase	Disappearance of sound Indicates diastolic pressure

Fifth phase: Disappearance of sound

Muffling sound disappears. Disappearance of the sound indicates **diastolic pressure.**

Thus, in auscultatory method, appearance of clear tapping sound during first phase indicates the **systolic pressure** and disappearance of the muffling sound in fifth phase indicates **diastolic pressure**.

Aneroid sphygmomanometer

Aneroid sphygmomanometer consists of an **aneroid device** instead of mercury column. It is commonly used in hospitals and clinics because of the concerns about environmental **toxicity of mercury**. However, it is less accurate compared to mercury sphygmomanometer.

Automatic blood pressure instrument

Nowadays automatic blood pressure instrument is widely used. However, its accuracy of this instrument is controversial.

■ APPLIED PHYSIOLOGY

Pathological variations of arterial blood pressure are hypertension and hypotension.

Hypertension

Definition

Hypertension is defined as the persistent high arterial blood pressure. Clinically, when the systolic pressure remains elevated above 150 mm Hg and diastolic pressure remains elevated above 90 mm Hg, it is considered as hypertension. If there is increase only in systolic pressure, it is called **systolic hypertension**.

Types of Hypertension

Hypertension is divided into two types:
1. Primary hypertension.
2. Secondary hypertension.

1. Primary hypertension or essential hypertension

Primary hypertension is the elevated blood pressure in the absence of any underlying disease. It is also called essential hypertension. Arterial blood pressure is increased because of increased peripheral resistance, which occurs due to some unknown cause.

2. Secondary hypertension

Secondary hypertension is the high blood pressure due to some underlying disorders.

Different forms of secondary hypertension are:

i. **Cardiovascular hypertension** that is produced due to cardiovascular disorders.
ii. **Endocrine hypertension** which is due to hyperactivity of some endocrine glands.
iii. **Renal hypertension** that is caused by renal diseases.
iv. **Neurogenic hypertension** which is developed by nervous disorders.
v. **Hypertension during pregnancy** which is due to toxemia of pregnancy (Chapter 54).

Hypotension

Definition

Hypotension is the low blood pressure. When the systolic pressure is less than 90 mm Hg, it is considered as hypotension.

Types of Hypotension

Hypotension is of two types, primary hypotension and secondary hypotension.

1. *Primary hypotension*

Primary hypotension or **essential hypotension** is the low blood pressure that develops in the absence of any underlying disease and develops due to some unknown cause.

2. *Secondary hypotension*

Secondary hypotension occurs due to some underlying diseases such as myocardial infarction, hypoactivity of pituitary gland or adrenal glands, tuberculosis and nervous disorders.

Orthostatic hypotension

Orthostatic hypotension is the sudden fall in blood pressure while standing for some time. It is due to the effect of gravity. Gravity causes pooling of blood in lower limbs and decrease in blood pressure. It develops in persons affected by **myasthenia gravis** or some nervous disorders like tabes dorsalis, syringomyelia and diabetic neuropathy. Common symptom of this condition is **orthostatic syncope**. Syncope is described in detail in Chapter 66.

■ VENOUS BLOOD PRESSURE

■ DEFINITION

Venous blood pressure is the pressure exerted by the contained blood in veins. Pressure in vena cava and right atrium is called **central venous pressure**. And the pressure in peripheral veins is called **peripheral venous pressure**.

Pressure is not same in all the veins. It varies in different veins in the extremities of the body and also varies from central veins to peripheral veins.

■ NORMAL VALUES

Venous Blood Pressure in the Extremities of the Body

Venous pressure is less in parts of the body above the level of heart and it is more in parts below the level of heart. Refer **Box 63.1** for values.

Venous Pressure in Central and Peripheral Veins

Pressure is greater in peripheral veins than in central veins. Refer **Box 63.1** for values.

BOX 63.1: Normal values of venous blood pressure.

In extremities of the body
Dorsal venous arch of foot : 13.2 mm Hg (17.9 cm H_2O)
Jugular vein : 5.1 mm Hg (6.9 cm H_2O)

In peripheral and central veins
Antecubital vein : 7.1 mm Hg (9.6 cm H_2O).
Superior vena cava : 4.6 mm Hg (6.2 cm H_2O)

1 mm Hg pressure = 1.359 cm H_2O pressure.

■ EFFECT OF RESPIRATION ON VENOUS BLOOD PRESSURE

Effect of respiration on venous blood pressure is demonstrated by two procedures:

1. Valsalva maneuver or Valsalva experiment.
2. Müller maneuver or Müller experiment.

Valsalva Maneuver or Valsalva Experiment

Valsalva maneuver is the **forced expiratory effort** with closed glottis. It is performed by attempting to exhale forcibly while closing the mouth and nose.

Effects of Valsalva maneuver

During this maneuver, the intrathoracic pressure becomes positive and increases to a greatly. It may reach + 50 mm Hg **(Table 63.4)**.

High intrathoracic pressure produces following effects:

1. Compression of central vein in thorax.
2. Decrease in venous return to right atrium.
3. Increase in peripheral venous blood pressure to about 30 cm H_2O, due to accumulation of blood in peripheral veins such as veins of neck, face and limbs.
4. Decrease in central venous pressure.

Uses of Valsalva maneuver

1. Valsalva maneuver is used as a diagnostic tool to evaluate the cardiovascular disorders. Best example is the 30 minutes endurance test.
2. Valsalva maneuver is practiced to relieve chest pain.
3. It is used to correct the abnormal heart rhythms.

30 Seconds Endurance Test

The subject is asked to blow against **sphygmomanometer**, in which the pressure is maintained at 40 mm Hg for 30 seconds. Then the changes in heart rate, blood pressure or murmurs are observed to evaluate the cardiovascular disorders.

Müller Maneuver or Müller Experiment

Müller maneuver or **reverse Valsalva maneuver** is the **forced inspiratory effort** with closed glottis. It is performed by attempting to inhale forcibly, while closing the mouth and nose.

Effects of Müller maneuver

During this maneuver, the intrathoracic pressure decreases greatly and becomes more negative. It is about − 70 mm Hg **(Table 63.4)**.

TABLE 63.4: Valsalva maneuver vs Müller maneuver.

Features	Valsalva maneuver	Müller maneuver
1. Performance	Forced expiratory effort with closed glottis	Forced inspiratory effort with closed glottis
2. Intrathoracic pressure	Increases up to + 50 mm Hg	Decreases up to – 70 mm Hg
3. Central veins in thorax	Compressed	Dilated and blood rushes
4. Venous return to right atrium	Decreases	Increases
5. Peripheral venous blood pressure	Increases to 30 cm H_2O	Decreases to 3 cm H_2O
6. Central venous blood pressure	Decreases	Increases
7. Uses	To evaluate cardiovascular disorders To relieve chest pain To correct abnormal heart rhythms	To evaluate upper respiratory problems To evaluate sleep apnea syndrome

More negative intrathoracic pressure produces following effects:

1. Dilatation of right atrium and central vein because of increase in negative intrathoracic pressure.
2. Rapid emptying of blood from peripheral veins into the central veins and increase in venous return to right atrium.
3. Decrease in peripheral venous blood pressure to less than 3 to 4 cm H_2O.
4. Increase in central venous blood pressure.

Uses of Müller maneuver

Müller maneuver is used to evaluate:

1. Upper respiratory tract problems.
2. **Sleep apnea syndrome** (temporary stoppage of breathing repeatedly during sleep).

CAPILLARY BLOOD PRESSURE

DEFINITION, SIGNIFICANCE AND NORMAL VALUES

Definition

Capillary blood pressure or **capillary hydrostatic pressure** is the pressure exerted by the blood contained in capillary **(Fig. 63.2)**.

Significance

Capillary blood pressure is responsible for the exchange of various substances between blood and interstitial fluid through capillary wall.

Normal Values

Arterial end of capillary : 30 to 32 mm Hg.
Venous end of capillary : 15 mm Hg.

However, capillary pressure varies depending upon the function of the organ or region of the body.

REGIONAL VARIATIONS OF CAPILLARY BLOOD PESSURE

Capillary blood pressure varies in different organs particularly in kidneys and lungs. Regional variation

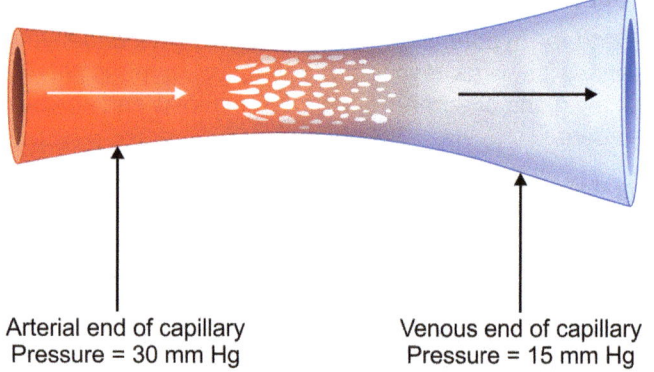

Arterial end of capillary Pressure = 30 mm Hg

Venous end of capillary Pressure = 15 mm Hg

FIGURE 63.2: Capillary blood pressure.

in capillary pressure is in relation to the physiological activities of the particular region. So, it has some functional significance.

Capillary Blood Pressure in Kidney

In kidney, the glomerular capillaries form **high pressure bed** with a pressure of 60 to 70 mm Hg. This high capillary pressure is responsible for glomerular filtration. Peritubular capillaries form **low pressure bed** with a pressure of 8 to 10 mm Hg. This low pressure helps tubular reabsorption.

Capillary Blood Pressure in Lungs

In lungs, the pulmonary capillaries form **low pressure bed**. Capillary pressure of about 7 mm Hg favors exchange of gases between blood and alveoli.

CAPILLARY ONCOTIC PRESSURE

Capillary oncotic pressure or **colloidal pressure** is the pressure exerted by plasma protein which stay within capillaries because of impermeability of capillary membrane to plasma proteins. Normal oncotic pressure is about 25 mm Hg. Among the plasma proteins, albumin exerts 70% of oncotic pressure.

Oncotic pressure plays an important role in regulating filtration across capillary membrane, particularly in renal glomerular capillaries.

CHAPTER 64

Arterial Pulse and Venous Pulse

CHAPTER OUTLINE

- **ARTERIAL PULSE**
  - DEFINITION AND FORMATION
  - TRANSMISSION OF PULSE
  - ARTERIAL PULSE TRACING
  - PULSE POINTS
  - EXAMINATION OF RADIAL PULSE
  - APPLIED PHYSIOLOGY: ABNORMAL ARTERIAL PULSE

- **VENOUS PULSE**
  - DEFINITION AND IMPORTANCE
  - EXAMIANTION OF VENOUS PULSE
  - JUGULAR VENOUS PULSE TRACING
  - APPLIED PHYSIOLOGY: ABNORMAL VENOUS PULSE

ARTERIAL PULSE

DEFINITION AND FORMATION

Arterial pulse is defined as the pressure changes transmitted in the form of waves through arterial wall and blood column from heart to periphery.

During contraction of left ventricle, the blood is ejected forcefully into aorta. It causes distension of aorta and rise in pressure. So, a pressure wave is produced on the elastic wall of aorta. It travels rapidly from the heart towards periphery. And it can be felt after a brief interval, at any superficial peripheral artery such as radial artery at wrist.

Pulse rate is the accurate measure of heart rate except in conditions like **pulses deficit**.

TRANSMISSION OF PULSE

Central arterial pulse is transmitted to the peripheral arteries as **peripheral arterial pulse.** Formation and transmission of pulse wave depends upon the elasticity of blood vessels. Thus, when the walls of arteries are more distensible, the pressure rise is less and so transmission of pulse is less. When the arterial wall loses its elastic property and becomes rigid as in old age, the pressure rise is more and the transmission of pulse is also more.

Pulse is not transmitted to capillaries because capillaries do not have elastic tissues.

Velocity of Transmission of Pulse

Average velocity at which the pulse wave is transmitted varies between 7 and 9 m/sec. Pulse wave travels faster than blood flow. Maximum velocity of blood flow in the body (in larger arteries) is only 50 cm/sec.

ARTERIAL PULSE TRACING

Arterial pulse is recorded by using **polygraph**. Pulse recorded in radial artery or femoral artery is the typical peripheral pulse **(Fig. 64.1)**. Peripheral pulse tracing has three main features.

1. Anacrotic Limb

Anacrotic limb or ascending limb is due to the rise in pressure during systole.

2. Catacrotic Limb

Catacrotic limb or descending limb is due to the fall in pressure during diastole.

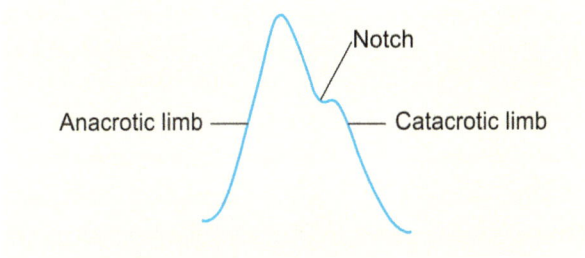

FIGURE 64.1: Radial pulse tracing.

3. Catacrotic Notch

In the upper part of the catacrotic limb of pulse tracing, a small notch appears. It is known as catacrotic notch or **incisura**. This notch is produced by the backflow of blood during the closure of semilunar valves at the beginning of diastolic period, which produces slight increase in the pressure.

4. Pre- and Post-catacrotic Waves

The wave appearing before the notch is called **precatacrotic wave**. The wave appearing after the notch is called **postcatacrotic wave**.

■ PULSE POINTS

Usually, pulse is palpated on the radial artery because it is easily approachable and placed superficially. However, arterial pulse can be felt in different areas on the body. These areas are called pulse points. Pulse points and the area of palpation are given in **Table 64.1**.

■ EXAMINATION OF RADIAL PULSE

Examination of pulse is a valuable clinical procedure. Pulse represents the heartbeat. By examining pulse, important information regarding cardiac function such as rate of contraction, rhythmicity, etc. can be obtained.

Method of Examining Radial Pulse

Subject is made to sit comfortably with forearm placed in mid- or semi-prone position, with wrist slightly flexed. The observer must stand by the right side of subject. Tips of the middle three fingers (index finger, middle finger and ring finger) of the observer are placed over the radial artery of the subject at wrist below the base of thumb. Light pressure is applied by the fingers until the pulse is felt. If necessary, fingers are moved around till the pulse is felt.

Index finger is used to occlude blood flow from radial artery. **Ring finger** is used to occlude retrograde flow of blood from ulnar artery through palmar arch. **Middle finger** is used to assess the pulse.

Observations during Examination of Pulse

1. Rate

Pulse rate is the number of pulses per minute. It has to be counted at least for 30 seconds. Pulse rate in adults is 72/min. Pulse rate at different age is given in **Table 64.2**.

2. Rhythm

Rhythm is the regularity of pulse. Under normal conditions, the pulse appears at regular intervals. Rhythm of the pulse becomes irregular in some pathological conditions. Irregular rhythm of pulse is of two types, regularly irregular and irregularly irregular.

3. Character

Character of pulse is observed while examining the pulse. It denotes the tension on vessel wall produced by the waves of pulse.

4. Volume

Volume is the determination of movement of the vessel wall produced by transmission of pulse wave. It is also a measure of pulse pressure. It depends upon condition of the blood vessel.

5. Condition of wall of the blood vessel

Condition of wall of the blood vessel is assessed by feeling and rolling the radial artery against the underlying bones. Normally, wall of the vessel is not palpable in children and young adults. However, in old age wall of the vessel becomes rigid and palpable. In abnormal conditions such as arteriosclerosis, it is felt as a hard rope.

6. Delayed pulse

Sometimes the arrival of pulse in certain peripheral arteries is delayed. It is an important feature to be noted because it is useful in diagnosis of certain diseases. For example, while palpating radial pulse and femoral pulse simultaneously,

TABLE 64.1: Pulse points.

Pulse point	Area of palpation
1. Temporal pulse	Over the temple, in front of ear on superficial temporal artery
2. Facial pulse	On facial artery at the angle of jaw
3. Carotid pulse	In the neck along anterior border of sternocleidomastoid muscle on common carotid artery
4. Axillary pulse	In axilla on axillary artery
5. Brachial pulse	In cubital fossa along medial border of biceps muscle on brachial artery
6. Radial pulse	Over the thumb side of wrist between tendons of brachioradialis and flexor carpi radialis muscles on radial artery
7. Ulnar pulse	Over the little finger side of wrist on ulnar artery
8. Femoral pulse	In the groin on femoral artery
9. Popliteal pulse	Behind knee, in the popliteal fossa on popliteal artery
10. Dorsalis pedis pulse	Over the dorsum of foot on dorsalis pedis artery
11. Tibialis pulse	Over the back of the ankle behind medial malleolus on posterior tibial artery

TABLE 64.2: Pulse rate at different age.

Age	Pulse rate (per min)
In fetus	150 to 180
At birth	130 to 140
At 10 years of age	90
After puberty	72

there is a short delay in the arrival of femoral pulse wave. It is called femoral delay, radial femoral delay or radiofemoral delay.

■ APPLIED PHYSIOLOGY: ABNORMAL ARTERIAL PULSE

1. Pulsus Deficit

Pulsus deficit is the abnormal condition in which the pulse rate is less than the heart rate. Pulsus deficit is the only condition in which pulse rate is less than the heart rate. It occurs during atrial fibrillation. **Atrial fibrillation** is the type of arrhythmia (irregular heart beat) characterized by rapid and irregular atrial contractions at the rate of 300 to 400 beats per minute.

2. Pulsus Alternans

Pulsus alternans is the abnormal condition characterized by alternation of strong and week pulse. It is common in severe myocardial diseases.

3. Anacrotic Pulse

Anacrotic pulse is the abnormal pulse, characterized by a slow ascending limb which has a notch called anacrotic notch. It is produced in aortic stenosis (narrowing).

4. Thready Pulse

Thready or weak pulse is the abnormally weak and very feeble pulse because of its low volume. And it is hardly felt at the arteries. It usually occurs during severe hemorrhage or severe chills.

5. Pulsus Paradoxus

Pulsus paradoxus is the condition characterized by a weak pulse with marked decrease in volume during inspiration caused by fall in systolic blood pressure by 10 mm Hg. The pulse becomes normal or stronger with increase in volume during expiration. It occurs in many cardiac and respiratory diseases.

6. Water Hammer Pulse

Water hammer pulse or **collapsing pulse is** the abnormal pulse, characterized by a rapid upstroke and an equally rapid downstroke. In other words, it is a bounding and forceful pulse that quickly increases in volume and subsequently and decreases in volume resulting in collapse. It is seen in patent ductus arteriosus, aortic regurgitation (see below) and arteriovenous fistula.

7. Abnormal Pulse in Patent Ductus Arteriosus

Pulse during patent ductus arteriosus is a strong water hammer pulse. Patent ductus arteriosus is the permanent existence of ductus arteriosus.

8. Abnormal Pulse in Aortic Regurgitation

Pulse during aortic regurgitation also is a strong water hammer pulse. **Aortic regurgitation** is the backflow of blood from aorta into left ventricle. It is common during **incompetence** of **semilunar valve** in aorta.

■ VENOUS PULSE

■ DEFINITION AND IMPORTANCE

Venous pulse is defined as the pressure changes transmitted in the form of waves from right atrium to the veins near the heart. Venous pulse is observed only in larger veins near the heart such as jugular vein.

Evaluation of the venous pulse is an integral part of the physical examination because it reflects right atrial pressure and **hemodynamic events** in **right atrium**. Venous pulse recording is used to determine rate of atrial contraction, just as the record of arterial pulse is used to determine rate of ventricular contraction.

In addition, many phases of cardiac cycle can be recognized by means of venous pulse tracing. It is the simple and accurate method to measure duration of different phases in diastole. It also represents the atrial pressure changes taking place during cardiac cycle.

■ EXAMINATION OF VENOUS PULSE

Inspection of jugular vein pulsations is routinely done by bedside examination of neck veins. It provides valuable information about the cardiac function.

To observe the pulsation of internal jugular vein, head of the subject is tilted upwards at 45°. However, in patients with increased venous pressure, the head should be tilted as much as 90°. Pulsations of jugular vein can be noticed when light is passed across the skin overlying internal jugular vein with relaxed neck muscles. Simultaneous palpation of the left carotid artery helps the examiner confirm the venous pulsations.

■ JUGULAR VENOUS PULSE TRACING

Recording of jugular venous pulse is also called **phlebogram**. It is similar to intra-atrial pressure curve **(Fig. 64.2)**.

Phlebogram has three positive waves and three negative waves:
Positive waves: a, c, and v.
Negative waves: x, x_1 and y.

'a' Wave

It is the first wave and is a positive wave. It is due to rise in atrial pressure during atrial systole.

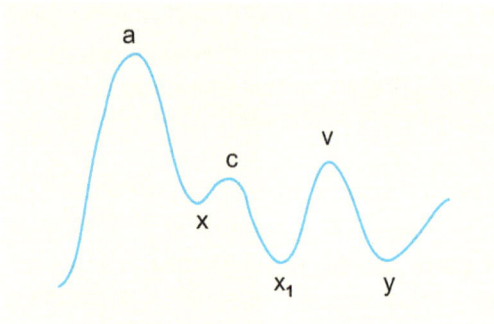

FIGURE 64.2: Phlebogram.

'x' Wave

This negative wave is due to fall of pressure in atrium and coincides with atrial diastole and beginning of ventricular systole.

'c' Wave

This positive wave occurs due to rise in atrial pressure during isometric contraction period. During this period the atrioventricular valves bulge into the atria and increase the pressure in the atria slightly.

'x_1' Wave

It is a negative wave and it is due to fall in pressure during ejection period. During ejection period, the atrioventricular ring is pulled towards ventricles causing fall in atrial pressure.

'v' Wave

This positive wave is due to rise in atrial pressure. The pressure increases because of atrial filling (venous return). It is obtained during isometric relaxation period or during atrial diastole.

'y' Wave

This negative wave denotes fall in pressure in atria. It is due to the opening of atrioventricular valve and emptying of blood into the ventricle. It appears during rapid and slow filling periods. 'y' wave is followed by 'a' wave and the cycle is repeated.

■ APPLIED PHYSIOLOGY: ABNORMAL VENOUS PULSE

1. *Elevated Jugular Venous Pulse*

Elevated jugular venous pulse indicates the rise in right ventricular pressure. It occurs in diseases of heart.

2. *Kussmaul's Sign*

Kussmaul's sign is the increase in venous distention and venous pressure. Normally, it occurs during inspiration. It also occurs in pathological conditions of the heart.

Chapter 65: Regional Circulation and Fetal Circulation

CHAPTER OUTLINE

- REGIONAL CIRCULATION
- CORONARY CIRCULATION
- CEREBRAL CIRCULATION
- SPLANCHNIC CIRCULATION
- CAPILLARY CIRCULATION
- SKELETAL MUSCLE CIRCULATION
- CUTANEOUS CIRCULATION
- FETAL CIRCULATION

REGIONAL CIRCULATION

Circulation of blood through a particular organ or a region of the body is called regional circulation. Blood flow through a region is proportional to the local activity.

Various regional circulations are:

1. Coronary circulation.
2. Cerebral circulation.
3. Splanchnic circulation.
4. Capillary circulation.
5. Skeletal muscle circulation.
6. Cutaneous circulation.
7. Pulmonary circulation.
8. Renal circulation.

Pulmonary circulation is explained in Chapter 68. Renal circulation is explained in Chapter 35. Other regional circulations are given below.

CORONARY CIRCULATION

DISTRIBUTION OF CORONARY BLOOD VESSELS

Coronary Arteries

Heart muscle is supplied by two coronary arteries, the right and left coronary arteries, which are the first branches of aorta. Coronary arteries encircle the heart in the manner of a **crown** hence the name coronary arteries. In Latin corona means crown.

Venous Drainage

Venous drainage from the heart muscle is by three types of vessels namely, coronary sinus, anterior coronary veins and thebesian veins.

Physiological Shunt

Physiological shunt is a **diverted route** (diversion) through which the venous blood is mixed with arterial blood. Deoxygenated blood flowing from thebesian veins into cardiac chambers makes up part of normal physiological shunt. Other component of physiological shunt is the drainage of deoxygenated blood from bronchial circulation into pulmonary vein without being oxygenated (Chapter 68).

NORMAL CORONARY BLOOD FLOW

Normal blood flow through coronary circulation is about 200 mL/min. It forms 4% of cardiac output. It is about 65 mL to 70 mL/min/100 g of cardiac muscle.

PHASIC CHANGES CORONARY BLOOD FLOW

Blood flow through coronary arteries is not constant. It decreases during systole and increases during diastole **(Fig. 65.1)**.

During systole, the coronary blood vessels are compressed and blood flow is reduced. During diastole, the compression is released and the blood vessels are distended. So, the blood flow is increased.

REGULATION OF CORONARY BLOOD FLOW

Like any other organ, heart also has the capacity to regulate its own blood flow by **autoregulation** (Chapter 35). Coronary blood flow is not affected when mean arterial pressure varies between 60 mm Hg and 150 mm Hg. Factors regulating coronary blood flow are:

1. Need for Oxygen

Amount of blood passing through coronary circulation is **directly proportional** to the consumption of oxygen by

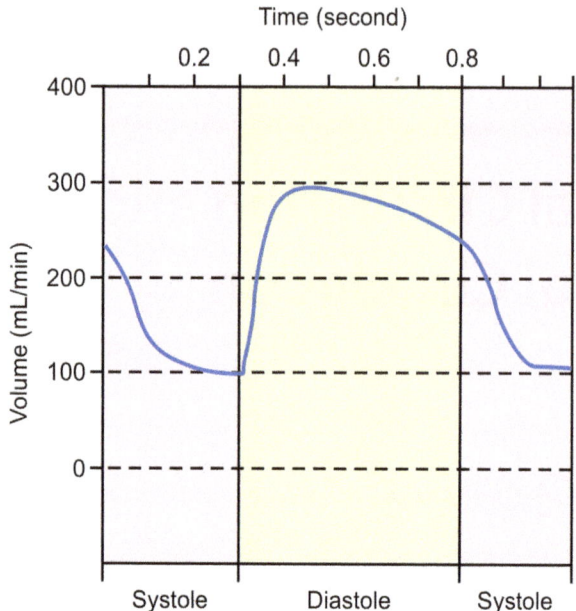

FIGURE 65.1: Phasic changes in coronary blood flow.

cardiac muscle. Even in resting condition, a large amount of oxygen, i.e. 70 to 80% is consumed from the blood by heart muscle than by any other tissues. In conditions associated with increased cardiac activity, the need for oxygen increases enormously. This leads to **coronary vasodilatation** and increase in blood flow to heart.

2. Metabolic Factors

Metabolic products increase coronary blood flow by **coronary vasodilatation** during hypoxic conditions. Such metabolic products are adenosine, potassium, hydrogen, carbon dioxide and adenosine phosphate compounds.

Reactive hyperemia

Reactive hyperemia is the increase in blood flow due to vasodilator effects of metabolites.

3. Coronary Perfusion Pressure

Coronary perfusion pressure is the balance between mean arterial pressure in aorta and the right atrial pressure. Since right atrial pressure is low, the mean arterial pressure becomes the major factor that maintains coronary blood flow.

4. Nervous Factors

Coronary blood vessels are innervated both by parasympathetic and sympathetic divisions of autonomic nervous system. These nerves influence the coronary blood flow only indirectly by acting on the musculature of heart.

During sympathetic stimulation, the rate and force of contraction of heart are increased resulting in liberation of metabolites. The metabolites dilate the blood vessels and increase the coronary blood flow. During parasympathetic stimulation, cardiac functions are inhibited and the liberation of metabolites is less. And coronary blood flow decreases

■ APPLIED PHYSIOLOGY: CORONARY ARTERY DISEASE

Coronary artery disease (CAD) or **coronary heart disease** is a heart disease caused by inadequate blood supply to cardiac muscle due to occlusion of coronary artery.

Coronary Occlusion

Coronary occlusion means the partial or complete obstruction of the coronary artery. Occlusion occurs because of **atherosclerosis**, a condition associated with deposition of cholesterol on the walls of the artery. In due course, this part of the arterial wall becomes **fibrotic** and it is called **atherosclerotic plaque**. The plaque is made up of cholesterol, calcium and other substances from blood.

Because of the atherosclerotic plaque the lumen of the coronary artery becomes narrow. In severe conditions, the artery is completely occluded.

Smaller blood vessels are occluded by the **thrombus** or part of atherosclerotic plaque detached from coronary artery. This thrombus or part of the plaque is called **embolus**.

Myocardial Ischemia

Myocardial ischemia is the reaction of a part of myocardium in response to hypoxia. Hypoxia develops when blood flow to a part of myocardium decreases severely due to occlusion of a coronary artery.

When the ischemia is mild due to obstruction of smaller blood vessel, the blood flow can be restored by rapid development of **coronary collateral arteries**.

Necrosis

Necrosis is the death of cells or tissues by injury or disease in a localized area. When coronary occlusion is severe involving larger blood vessels, severe ischemia develops and it leads to **necrosis of myocardium**. Necrosis is irreversible.

Myocardial Infarction: Heart Attack

Myocardial infarction is the necrosis of myocardium caused by insufficient blood flow due to embolus, thrombus or vascular spasm. It is also called heart attack. In myocardial infarction, death occurs rapidly due to ventricular fibrillation.

Common symptoms of myocardial infarction are:

1. Cardiac pain.
2. Nausea and vomiting.
3. Palpitations.
4. Difficulty in breathing.
5. Extreme weakness.
6. Sweating.

Cardiac Pain: Angina Pectoris

Cardiac pain is the **chest pain** caused by **myocardial ischemia**. It is also called angina pectoris. It is the common manifestation of coronary artery disease. Pain starts beneath the sternum and radiates to the surface of

Chapter 65: Regional Circulation and Fetal Circulation

left arm and left shoulder. Cardiac pain is a **referred pain** (Chapter 83).

CEREBRAL CIRCULATION

Cerebral circulation means flow of blood through the blood vessels of brain.

IMPORTANCE OF CEREBRAL CIRCULATION

Brain tissues need adequate blood supply continuously. Stoppage of blood flow for 5 seconds leads to **unconsciousness** and for 5 minutes leads to **irreparable damage** to the brain cells.

CEREBRAL BLOOD VESSELS

Brain receives blood from the **basilar artery** and **internal carotid artery**. Branches from these arteries form **circle of Willis**. The venous drainage is by sinuses, which open into internal jugular vein.

NORMAL CEREBRAL BLOOD FLOW

Normally, brain receives 750 to 800 mL of blood per minute. It is about 15 to 16% of total cardiac output and about 50 to 55 mL/100 g of brain tissue per minute.

REGULATION OF CEREBRAL BLOOD FLOW

Cerebral circulation is regulated by **three factors**:

1. Autoregulation

Like any other vital organ, brain also regulates its own blood flow by means of autoregulation (Chapter 99). However, the autoregulation in brain has got its own limitations.

2. Chemical Factors

Chemical factors which increase the cerebral blood flow:

i. Decreased oxygen tension.
ii. Increased carbon dioxide tension.
iii. Increased hydrogen ion concentration.

3. Nervous Factors

Cerebral blood vessels are supplied by sympathetic vasoconstrictor fibers. But these fibers do not regulate cerebral blood flow under normal conditions. In pathological conditions like hypertension, the sympathetic nerves cause constriction of cerebral blood vessels, leading to reduction in blood flow. It prevents cerebral vascular hemorrhage and cerebral stroke.

APPLIED PHYSIOLOGY: STROKE

Definition

Stroke is the sudden death of neurons in localized area of brain due to inadequate blood supply. It is characterized by reversible or irreversible paralysis with other symptoms. Stroke is also called **cardiovascular accident** (CVA) or **brain attack**.

Causes of Stroke

1. Heart disease.
2. Hypertension.
3. High cholesterol in blood.
4. High blood sugar (diabetes mellitus).
5. Heavy smoking.
6. Heavy alcohol consumption.

Symptoms of Stroke

Symptoms of stroke depend upon the area of brain that is damaged.

Common symptoms of stroke are:

1. Weakness.
2. Numbness or paralysis particularly on one side of the body.
3. Impairment of speech.
4. Emotional disturbances.
5. Loss of coordination.
6. Loss of memory.
7. Dizziness.
8. Loss of consciousness.
9. Coma or death.

SPLANCHNIC CIRCULATION

INTRODUCTION

Splanchnic or visceral circulation constitutes three portions:

1. Mesenteric circulation supplying blood to GI tract.
2. Splenic circulation supplying blood to spleen.
3. Hepatic circulation supplying blood to liver.

Unique feature of splanchnic circulation is that, the blood from mesenteric bed and spleen forms a major amount of blood flowing to liver. Blood flows to liver from GI tract and spleen through portal system.

MESENTERIC CIRCULATION

Distribution of Blood Flow in Mesenteric Circulation

Stomach : 35 mL/100 g/min
Intestine : 50 mL/100 g/min
Pancreas : 80 mL/100 g/min

SPLENIC CIRCULATION

Importance of Splenic Circulation

Spleen is the main **reservoir for blood**. Due to the dilatation of blood vessels, a large amount of blood is stored in spleen. And the constriction of blood vessels by sympathetic stimulation releases blood into circulation.

Storage of Blood in Spleen

Two structures are involved in spleen in storage of blood namely, splenic venous sinuses and splenic pulp.

Small arteries and arterioles open directly into the venous sinuses. When spleen expands, the sinuses swell and large quantity of blood is stored. The capillaries of splenic pulp are highly permeable. So, most of the blood cells pass through capillary membrane and are stored in the pulp.

HEPATIC CIRCULATION

Hepatic Blood Vessels

Liver receives blood from two sources:

1. Hepatic artery from aorta.
2. Portal vein from mesenteric and splenic vascular bed.

More details are given in Chapter 29.

Normal Blood Flow

Liver receives maximum amount of blood as compared to any other organ in the body since, most of the metabolic activities are carried out in the liver. Blood flow to liver is 1,500 mL/min, which forms 30% of cardiac output. It is about 100 mL/100 g of tissue per minute.

CAPILLARY CIRCULATION

MICROCIRCULATION

Microcirculation is the flow of blood through the minute blood vessels such as arterioles, capillaries and venules. Capillary circulation forms the major part of microcirculation. Capillaries are formed by single layer of endothelial cells which are wrapped around by pericytes.

SALIENT FEATURES OF CAPILLARIES

1. Capillaries arise from arterioles and form the area for exchange of materials between blood and tissues.
2. Capillaries outnumber the other blood vessels. About **10 billion capillaries** are present in the body.
3. Each capillary lies in a very close proximity to the cells of the tissues at a distance of about 20 to 30 mm. This enables easy and rapid exchange of substances between blood and the tissues through interstitial fluid.

PATTERN OF CAPILLARY SYSTEM

Capillaries are disposed between arterioles and venules. From the arterioles, the **meta-arterioles** take origin **(Fig. 65.2)**. From meta-arterioles, two types of capillaries arise.

1. Preferential Channels or Continuous Capillaries

After arising from the meta-arterioles, the preferential channels form a network and finally join the venules.

2. True Capillaries

After arising from meta-arterioles, the true capillaries also form a network and join the venules. Smooth muscle fibers encircle the beginning of true capillaries forming a sphincter called **precapillary sphincter**. This sphincter controls the blood flow through true capillaries.

ANATOMICAL AND PHYSIOLOGICAL SHUNTS

Anatomical Shunt: Arteriovenous Shunt

Anatomical shunt or arteriovenous shunt is the direct link between arterioles and venules. Flow of blood through the capillaries where exchange of nutrients, gases and other substances takes place is called **nutritional flow**. Flow of blood through anatomical shunt is called **non-nutritional flow**. Non-nutritional blood flow occurs in many tissues of the body particularly during resting conditions when metabolic activities are low.

Physiological Shunt

Physiological shunt is the link between arterial and venous side of circulation provided by meta-arteriole. Many tissues of the body such as muscles do not have anatomical shunts. However, the meta-arteriole in these tissues acts as the physiological shunt between arterial and venous sides of the circulation. Non-nutritional blood flow occurs through physiological shunt under resting conditions.

Shunt in Capillaries vs Shunt in Heart

Physiological shunt in capillaries is different from physiological shunt in heart. In capillaries the oxygenated blood flows towards deoxygenated blood. But in heart, the deoxygenated blood flows towards the oxygenated blood (see above).

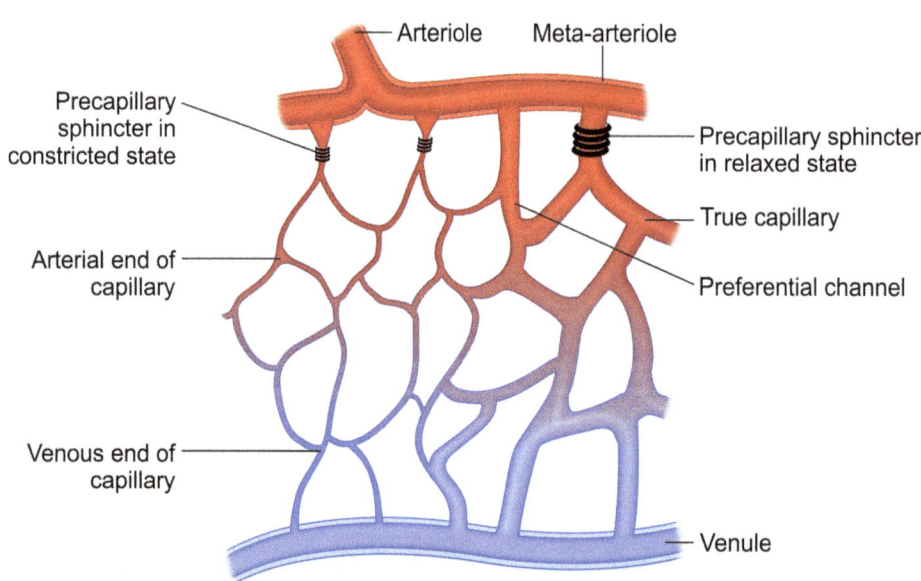

FIGURE 65.2: Capillary bed.

PECULIARITIES OF CAPILLARY BLOOD FLOW

1. Blood does not pass through the capillary system continuously. It is because of the alternate constriction and dilatation of meta-arterioles and alternate opening and closure of precapillary sphincters.
2. In capillaries, blood flows as a single pile or single row of blood cells. In other blood vessels, the blood flows in either axial stream containing mainly blood cells or peripheral stream containing plasma.
3. Under resting conditions, most of the capillaries lie in collapsed state. Only during activity, all the capillaries open up and increase the vascularity.
4. Amount of blood flowing through the capillary system throughout the body is very low. It is only about 150 mL/min.
5. Velocity of blood flow is least in capillaries. It is only about 0.5 to 1 mm/sec. It facilitates exchange of substances between the capillaries and tissues.

FUNCTIONS OF CAPILLARIES

Most important function of capillaries is the exchange of substances between blood and tissues. Oxygen, nutrients and other essential substances enter the tissues from capillary blood; carbon dioxide, metabolites and other unwanted substances are removed from the tissues by capillary blood.

Exchange of materials across the capillary endothelium occurs primarily by **diffusion**. It also occurs by means of filtration and **pinocytosis**.

SKELETAL MUSCLE CIRCULATION
BLOOD FLOW TO SKELETAL MUSCLES

During resting condition, blood flow to skeletal muscle is 4 to 7 mL/100 g/min. During exercise, it increases to about 100 mL/100 g/min.

MUSCULAR CONTRACTION AND BLOOD FLOW

During contraction of muscle, the blood vessels are compressed and the blood flow decreases. And during relaxation of muscle, the compression of blood vessels is relieved and the blood flow increases.

In severe muscular exercise, blood flow increases in between the muscular contractions.

APPLIED PHYSIOLOGY: VARICOSE VEINS

Varicose vein is the vein that becomes irregularly swollen (twisted or tortuous) and enlarged. Superficial veins of the leg are mostly affected.

Causes for Varicose Vein

1. Permanent dilatation of veins due to **incompetence** of the valves of the veins or absence of muscular activity for long periods. So, varicose veins are common in the individuals with occupations, which require standing for long periods.
2. **Thrombophlebitis:** Inflammation of vein associated with formation of thrombus.

CUTANEOUS CIRCULATION
ARCHITECTURE OF CUTANEOUS BLOOD VESSELS

1. **Arterioles** arising from the smaller arteries reach the dermis.
2. After taking origin, the arterioles turn horizontally and give rise to **meta-arterioles**.
3. From meta-arterioles, hairpin-shaped **capillary loops** arise. Arterial limb of the loop ascends vertically and turns to form a venous limb, which descends down.

   After reaching the base of dermis, few venous limbs of neighboring papillae unite to form the **collecting venule**.
4. Collecting venules anastomose with one another to form the **subpapillary venous plexus**.
5. Subpapillary plexus runs horizontally and drain into the **deeper veins**.

FUNCTIONS OF CUTANEOUS CIRCULATION

Cutaneous blood flow performs two functions:

1. Supply of nutrition to skin.
2. Loss of heat from the body and regulation of body temperature.

NORMAL BLOOD FLOW TO SKIN

Under normal conditions, the blood flow to skin is about 250 mL/sq m/min. When the body temperature increases, cutaneous blood flow increases up to 2,800 mL/sq m/min because of cutaneous vasodilatation.

FETAL CIRCULATION
FETAL HEART AND PLACENTA

Development of heart is completed at fourth week of intrauterine life and, it starts beating at the rate of 65 per minute. Along with heart, the blood vessels also develop. Heart rate gradually increases and reaches the maximum rate of about 140 beats per minute just before birth.

Fetal circulation is different from that of adults because of the presence of **placenta**. Since **fetal lungs** are **nonfunctioning**, placenta is responsible for exchange of gases between fetal blood and mother's blood. So, the blood from right ventricle is diverted to placenta.

Fetus is connected with the mother through placenta. Fetal blood passes to placenta through **umbilical vessels** and the maternal blood runs through **uterine vessels**. These two sets of blood vessels lie in close proximity in the placenta through which the exchange of substances takes place between mother's blood and fetal blood. However, there is **no direct admixture** of maternal and fetal blood **(Fig. 65.3)**.

BLOOD VESSELS IN FETUS

Due to nonfunctioning of fetal lungs, fetal heart pumps large quantity of blood into the placenta for exchange

322 Section 8: Cardiovascular System

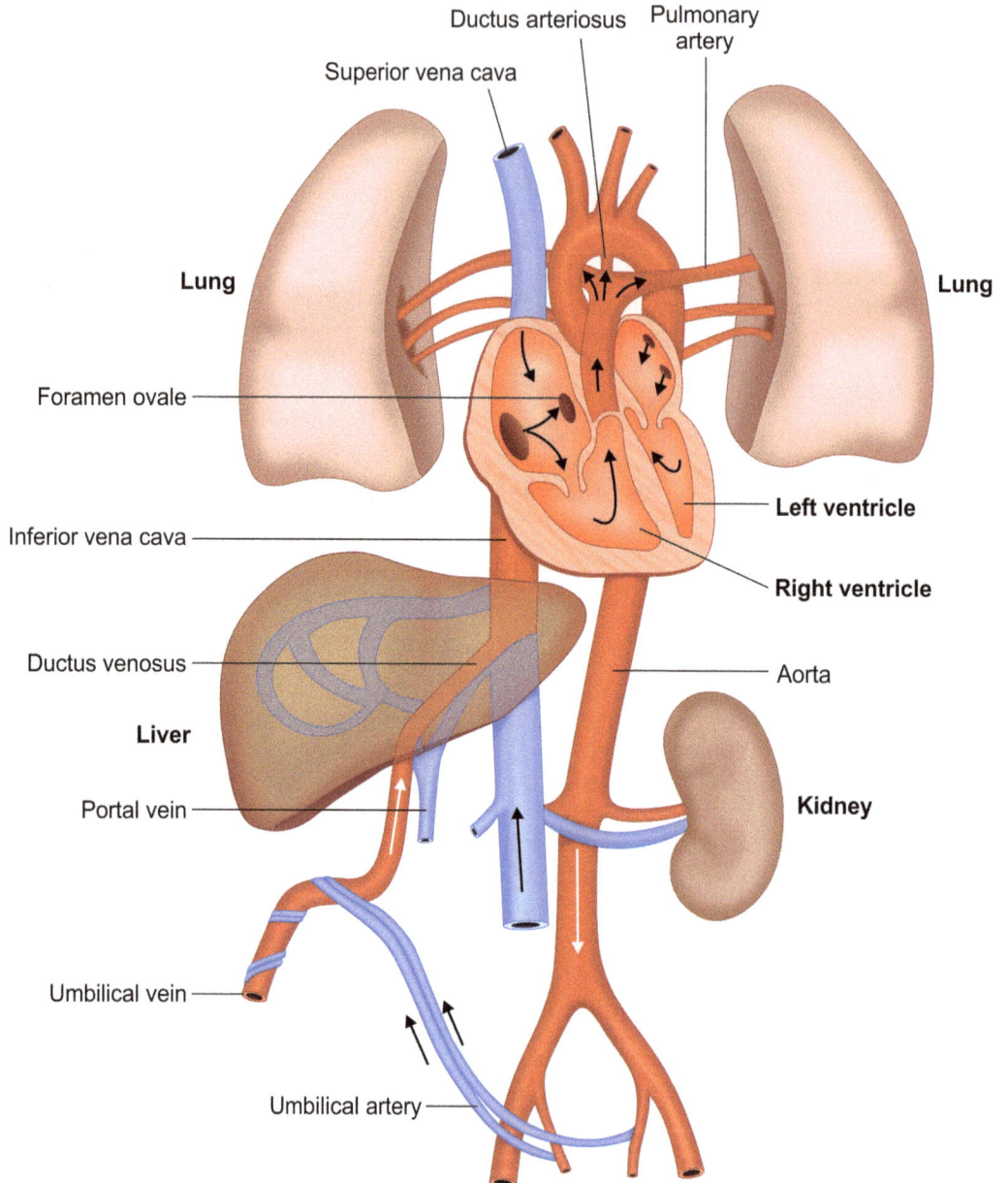

FIGURE 65.3: Fetal circulation.

of substances. From placenta, the umbilical veins collect the blood, which has more oxygen and nutrients. **Umbilical vein** passes through liver. Some amount of blood is supplied to liver from umbilical vein. However, a large quantity of blood is diverted from umbilical vein into the inferior vena cava through **ductus venosus**. Liver receives blood from **portal vein** also.

In liver, the oxygenated blood mixes slightly with deoxygenated blood and enters the right atrium via inferior vena cava. From right atrium, major portion of blood is diverted into left atrium via **foramen ovale**. Foramen ovale is an opening in intra-atrial septum.

Blood from upper part of the body enters the right atrium through superior vena cava. From right atrium, blood enters right ventricle. From here, blood is pumped into pulmonary artery. From pulmonary artery, blood enters the systemic aorta through **ductus arteriosus**. Only a small quantity of blood is supplied to fetal lungs. Blood from left ventricle is pumped into aorta. About 50% of blood from aorta reaches the placenta through umbilical arteries.

■ FETAL LUNGS

Pulmonary vascular resistance is the resistance offered to blood flow through pulmonary vascular bed. This resistance is very high in fetus because of the **nonfunctioning of fetal lungs**. High resistance in fetal lungs increases the pressure in the blood vessels of lungs. Because of the high pressure, the blood is diverted from pulmonary artery into aorta via **ductus arteriosus**.

■ CHANGES IN CIRCULATION AND RESPIRATION AFTER BIRTH: NEONATAL CIRCULATION AND RESPIRATION

1. *First Breath of the Child*

When fetus is delivered and umbilical cord is cut and tied, the lungs start functioning. When placental blood flow is cut off, there is sudden hypoxia and hypercapnia. Now, the respiratory center is strongly stimulated by these two factors and, the respiration starts. Initially, there is gasping, which is followed by normal respiration.

2. Blood Flow to Lungs

Lungs expand during the first breath of the infant. Expansion of lungs causes immediate reduction in the pulmonary vascular resistance and a sudden fall in pressure in the blood vessels of lungs. Therefore, the blood flow from pulmonary artery to lungs increases **(Fig. 65.4)**.

3. Closure of Foramen Ovale

When blood starts flowing through the pulmonary circulation, the oxygenated blood from lungs returns to left atrium. It causes increase in the left atrial pressure. Simultaneously, due to stoppage of blood from placenta, pressure in inferior vena cava is decreased. It leads to fall in right atrial pressure. Thus, the pressure in right atrium is less and the pressure in left atrium is already high. This causes the closure of foramen ovale. Within few days after birth, the foramen ovale closes completely and fuses with the atrial wall.

4. Reversal of Blood Flow in Ductus Arteriosus

In fetus, since pulmonary arterial pressure is very high, the blood passes from pulmonary artery into aorta via ductus arteriosus. However, in neonatal life, since the systemic arterial pressure is more than pulmonary arterial pressure, the blood passes in opposite direction in ductus arteriosus, i.e. from systemic aorta into pulmonary aorta **(Fig. 65.4)**. The reversed flow in ductus arteriosus is heard as **continuous murmur** in infants.

5. Closure of Ductus Venosus

Due to the contraction of smooth muscle near junction between umbilical vein and ductus venosus, the constriction and closure of ductus venosus occurs. Later, the ductus venosus becomes **fibrous band**.

6. Closure of Ductus Arteriosus

Ductus arteriosus starts closing due to narrowing. It closes completely after 2 days and the adult type of circulation starts. In some rare cases, the ductus arteriosus does not close. It remains intact producing a continuous murmur. The condition with intact ductus arteriosus is known as **patent ductus arteriosus**.

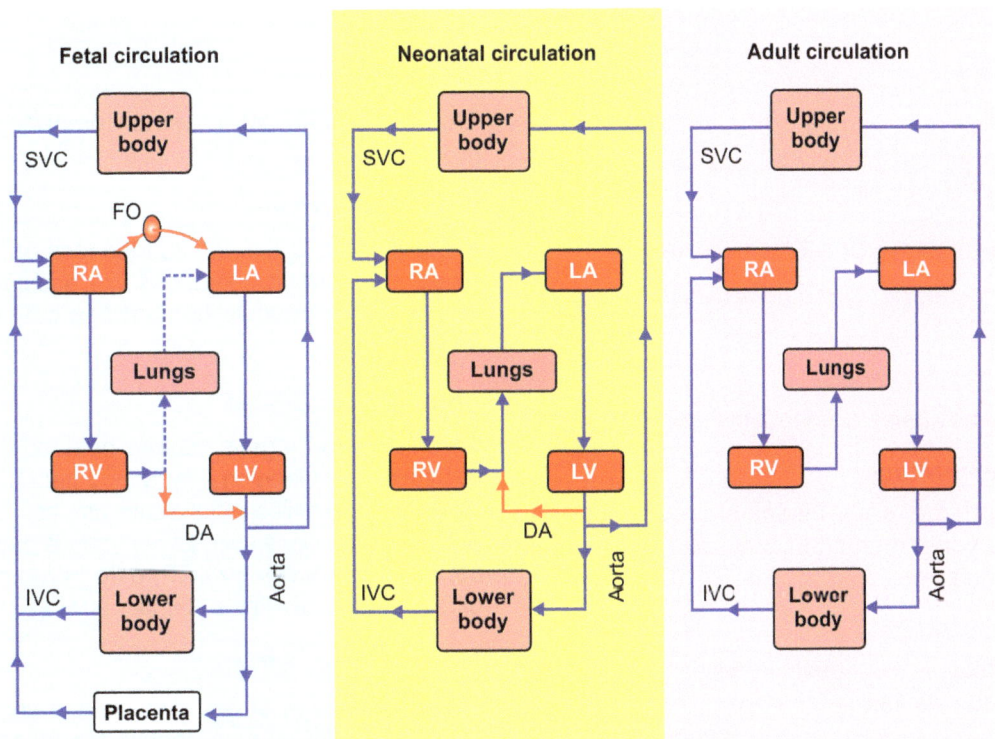

FIGURE 65.4: Fetal, neonatal and adult circulation.
RA = Right atrium, LA = Left atrium, RV = Right ventricle, LV = Left ventricle, FO = Foramen ovale,
DA = Ductus arteriosus, SVC = Superior vena cava, IVC = Inferior vena cava,
Dashed blue line in fetal circulation = Flow of very less quantity of blood.

Chapter 66: Hemorrhage, Circulatory Shock and Heart Failure

CHAPTER OUTLINE

- **HEMORRHAGE**
  - DEFINITION
  - TYPES AND CAUSES
  - EFFECTS OF HEMORRHAGE
- **CIRCULATORY SHOCK**
  - DEFINITION
  - MANIFESTATIONS OF CIRCULATORY SHOCK
- TYPES OF CIRCULATORY SHOCK
- SYNCOPE: FAINTING
- **HEART FAILURE**
  - INTRODUCTION
  - CAUSES
  - SIGNS AND SYMPTOMS

HEMORRHAGE

DEFINITION

Hemorrhage is defined as excess loss of blood due to rupture of the blood vessels.

TYPES AND CAUSES OF HEMORRHAGE

Based on the cause, hemorrhage is classified into **five categories**:

1. Accidental Hemorrhage

It occurs in road accidents and industrial accidents.

2. Capillary Hemorrhage

Capillary hemorrhage is the bleeding due to rupture of capillaries. It is very common in brain and heart during cardiovascular diseases.

3. Internal Hemorrhage

Internal hemorrhage is the bleeding in viscera. It is caused by rupture of blood vessels in the viscera.

4. Postpartum Hemorrhage

Postpartum hemorrhage is the excess bleeding that occurs immediately after labor.

5. Hemorrhage due to Premature Detachment of Placenta

In some cases, the placenta is detached from the uterus of mother before the due date of delivery causing severe hemorrhage.

EFFECTS OF HEMORRHAGE

Effects are different in acute hemorrhage and chronic hemorrhage.

Acute Hemorrhage

Acute hemorrhage is the sudden loss of large quantity of blood. It occurs in conditions like accidents. Decreased blood volume in acute hemorrhage causes hypovolemic shock.

Chronic Hemorrhage

Chronic hemorrhage is the loss of blood either by internal or by external bleeding over a long period of time. Internal bleeding occurs in conditions such as ulcer. External bleeding occurs in conditions such as hemophilia and excess vaginal bleeding (menorrhagia). Chronic hemorrhage produces different types of effects such as anemia.

Compensatory Effects

After hemorrhage, series of compensatory reactions develop in the body to cope up with the blood loss. Some of the compensatory reactions take place immediately after hemorrhage and others at a later period.

CIRCULATORY SHOCK

DEFINITION

Shock is a general term that means depression or suppression of body functions produced by any disorder. Circulatory shock is the shock developed by inadequate blood flow throughout the body. It is a life-threatening condition and if the affected person is not treated immediately, it may result in death.

■ MANIFESTATIONS OF SHOCK

Cardiovascular System

Common feature of circulatory shock is fall in arterial blood pressure which results decreased blood flow to all organs.

Respiratory System

Breathing becomes rapid and shallow resulting in hypoventilation. Some persons may develop **respiratory distress syndrome**.

Kidneys

Initially, urinary output is reduced. Later **tubular necrosis** develops resulting in **acute renal failure**.

Skin

Because of stagnant hypoxia, skin becomes **pale** and cold. **Cyanosis** develops in many parts of the body, particularly in earlobes and fingertips. There is excess sweating.

Vital Organs

Vital organs such as **liver** and endocrine gland fail to function due to necrosis.

Brain

Lack of blood flow to brain tissues produces **ischemia** resulting in **fainting** and irreparable damage of brain tissues.

Finally, the **brain damage** and **cardiac arrest** cause death of the victim.

■ TYPES OF CIRCULATORY SHOCK

Circulatory shock is primarily classified into four types:
  I. Shock due to decreased blood volume.
  II. Shock due to increased vascular capacity.
  III. Shock due to cardiac disease.
  IV. Shock due to obstruction to blood flow.

I. Shock due to Decreased Blood Volume: Hypovolemic Shock

Shock due to decreased blood volume is called hypovolemic shock. It occurs when there is acute loss of at least 10 to 15% of blood. Important manifestations of hypovolemic shock are decrease in cardiac output, low blood pressure, increase in respiratory rate, and restlessness or lethargy.

Some common types of hypovolemic shock are given below.

1. *Hemorrhagic shock*: Occurs due to hemorrhage.
2. *Traumatic shock*: Develops due to trauma (serious injury or wound caused by some external force)
3. *Surgical shock*: Occurs during or after surgical procedures.
4. *Burn shock*: Caused by the effects of burn.
5. *Dehydration shock*: Develops during severe dehydration.

II. Shock due to Increased Vascular Capacity: Vasogenic Shock

Shock occurs because of inadequate blood supply to the tissues due to increased vascular capacity. Capacity of the vascular system increases by the extensive dilatation of blood vessels. It is also known as vasogenic shock (Fig. 66.1). Types of vasogenic shock are:

1. *Neurogenic shock*: Characterized by sudden depression of nervous system due to extensive vasodilatation caused by loss of vasomotor tone. Common feature of neurogenic shock is **syncope** (see below).
2. *Anaphylactic shock*: Anaphylaxis means exaggerated allergic reaction to a foreign protein or antigen or any other substance to which the person has been previously sensitized. Shock due to anaphylaxis is called anaphylactic shock.

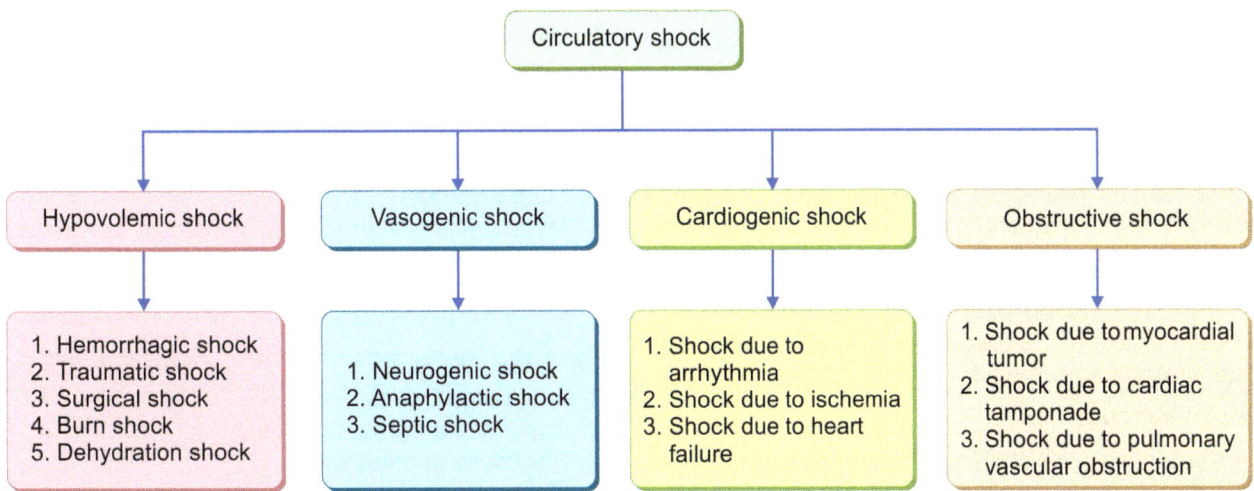

FIGURE 66.1: Different types of circulatory shock.

3. *Septic shock*: Sepsis is the condition characterized by the presence of pathogenic organisms or their toxins in blood or tissues. Shock developed during sepsis is known as septic shock or blood poisoning.

III. Shock due to Cardiac Diseases: Cardiogenic Shock

Shock due to cardiac disease is called cardiogenic shock.

Types of cardiogenic shock

1. Shock due to arrhythmia (abnormal heart beat)
2. Shock due to myocardial ischemia.
3. Shock due to congestive heart failure.

IV. Shock due to Obstruction of Blood Flow: Obstructive Shock

Shock developed due to the obstruction to blood flow through circulatory system is called obstructive shock.

Causes of obstructive shock

1. Tumor in myocardium.
2. **Cardiac tamponade** (compression of heart due to accumulation of fluid in pericardial space).
3. Obstruction of blood vessels in lungs due to embolism.

■ SYNCOPE: FAINTING

Syncope or fainting is the sudden and transient (short-time) loss of consciousness and postural tone with spontaneous recovery. It occurs due to temporary inadequate cerebral blood flow.

Types of Syncope

1. Vasovagal syncope or emotional fainting

Fainting is caused by sudden stimulation of **vagus nerve**. It is also called **neurocardiogenic syncope**. Vasovagal syncope is common in conditions such as severe emotional distress and exertion.

2. Postural syncope

It is caused by loss of consciousness because of **prolonged standing**. It is due to pooling of blood in lower limbs during prolonged standing resulting in decreased blood supply to the brain.

3. Micturition syncope

It is the fainting during micturition. It is common in the patients who suffer from **orthostatic hypotension** (Chapter 63).

4. Effort syncope

Fainting caused **during exercise** or any other **strain** is called effort syncope. It is the common symptom in patients with stenosis of semilunar valves.

5. Cough syncope

This is the fainting while coughing. Severe cough increases intrathoracic pressure, which reduces the venous return and cardiac output leading to fainting.

6. Carotid sinus syncope

Fainting in persons wearing **tight collar dress**. Tight collar of the dress exerts pressure over the region of carotid sinus. This leads to reduction in heart rate, vasodilatation and fainting.

■ HEART FAILURE

■ DEFINITION AND TYPES

Definition of Heart Failure

Heart failure or **cardiac failure** is defined as the condition in which the heart loses the ability to pump sufficient amount of blood to all parts of the body. Heart failure may involve left ventricle or right ventricle or both. It may be acute or chronic.

Acute Heart Failure

Acute heart failure is the sudden and rapid onset of signs and symptoms of abnormal heart functions. Its symptoms are severe initially. However, the symptoms last for a very short time and the condition improves rapidly.

Chronic Heart Failure

Chronic heart failure is the heart failure that is characterized by the symptoms that appear slowly over a period of time and become worst gradually.

Congestive Heart Failure

It is a general term used to describe heart failure resulting in **accumulation of fluid** in lungs and other tissues. When heart is not able to pump blood through aorta, the blood remains in heart. It results in dilatation of the chambers and accumulation of blood in veins (**vascular congestion**). This condition is also manifested by **fluid retention** and **pulmonary edema**.

■ CAUSES OF HEART FAILURE

Common causes of heart failure are:

1. Coronary artery disease.
2. Defective heart valves.
3. Arrhythmia.
4. Cardiac muscle disease such as cardiomyopathy.
5. Hypertension.
6. Congenital heart disease.
7. Diabetes.
8. Hyperthyroidism.
9. Anemia.
10. Lung disorders.
11. Myocarditis (inflammation of cardiac muscle due to viral infection, drugs, alcohol, etc.).

■ SIGNS AND SYMPTOMS OF HEART FAILURE

Signs and Symptoms of Chronic Heart Failure

1. Fatigue and weakness.
2. Rapid and irregular heartbeat.
3. Shortness of breathing.
4. Fluid retention and weight gain.
5. Loss of appetite, nausea and vomiting.

6. Cough.
7. Chest pain, if developed by myocardial infarction.

Signs and Symptoms of Acute Heart Failure

Signs and symptoms of acute heart failure may be same as chronic heart failure. But the signs and symptoms appear suddenly and severely. When heart starts to fail suddenly, the fluid accumulates in lungs causing pulmonary edema. It results in sudden and severe shortness of breath, cough with pink, foamy mucus and heart palpitations. It may lead to sudden death, if not attended immediately.

Chapter 67: Cardiovascular Adjustments during Exercise

CHAPTER OUTLINE

- **EXERCISE**
- **TYPES OF EXERCISE**
  - DYNAMIC EXERCISE
  - STATIC EXERCISE
- **AEROBIC AND ANAEROBIC EXERCISES**
  - AEROBIC EXERCISE
  - ANAEROBIC EXERCISE
  - METABOLISM IN AEROBIC AND ANAEROBIC EXERCISES
- **SEVERITY OF EXERCISE**
  - MILD EXERCISE
  - MODERATE EXERCISE
  - SEVERE EXERCISE
- **EFFECTS OF EXERCISE ON CARDIOVASCULAR SYSTEM**
  - ON BLOOD
  - ON BODY FLUIDS
  - ON HEART RATE
  - ON CARDIAC OUTPUT
  - ON VENOUS RETURN
  - ON BLOOD FLOW TO SKELETAL MUSCLES
  - ON BLOOD PRESSURE

TYPES OF EXERCISE

Exercise is generally classified into two types depending upon the type of muscular contraction, dynamic exercise and static exercise.

DYNAMIC EXERCISE

Dynamic exercise involves **isotonic contraction** of muscles and keeps the joints and muscles moving. Examples are swimming, bicycling, walking, etc. External work is involved in this type of exercise. External work is the shortening of muscle fibers against load.

In this type of exercise, the heart rate, force of contraction, cardiac output and systolic blood pressure increases. However, the diastolic blood pressure is unaltered or decreased. It is because, during dynamic exercise, the peripheral resistance is unaltered or decreased.

STATIC EXERCISE

Static exercise involves **isometric contraction** of muscles without movement of joints. Example is pushing heavy object. This is a type of exercise without the performance of external work. During this exercise, apart from increase in heart rate, force of contraction, cardiac output and systolic blood pressure, the diastolic blood pressure also increases. It is because of increase in peripheral resistance during static exercise.

AEROBIC AND ANAEROBIC EXERCISES

Based on the type of metabolism (energy producing process) involved, the exercise is classified into two types, aerobic exercise and anaerobic exercise.

AEROBIC EXERCISE

Aerobic means 'with air' or 'with oxygen'. The energy is obtained by utilizing nutrients in the presence of oxygen. Aerobic exercise involves activities with **lower intensity**, which is performed for **longer period** (see below).

Examples of Aerobic Exercise

1. Fast walking.
2. Jogging.
3. Running.
4. Bicycling.
5. Skiing.
6. Skating.
7. Hockey.

8. Soccer.
9. Tennis.
10. Badminton.
11. Swimming.
12. Rowing.

ANAEROBIC EXERCISE

Anaerobic means 'without air' or 'without oxygen'. Body obtains energy by burning glycogen stored in the muscles without oxygen. Anaerobic exercise involves **exertion** for **short periods** followed by periods of rest. It uses the muscles at high intensity and a high rate of work for a short period.

Burning glycogen without oxygen liberates lactic acid. Accumulation of lactic acid leads to fatigue. Therefore, this type of exercise cannot be performed for longer period. And a recovery period is essential before going for another burst of anaerobic exercise. Anaerobic exercise helps to increase the muscle strength.

Examples of Anaerobic Exercise

1. Pull ups.
2. Push ups.
3. Weightlifting.
4. Sprinting.
5. Any other rapid burst of strenuous exercise.

METABOLISM IN AEROBIC AND ANAEROBIC EXERCISES

When a person starts doing some exercise like jogging, bicycling or swimming, the muscles start utilizing energy. In order to have quick energy during the first few minutes, the muscles burn glycogen stored in them. During this period, fat is not burnt. Only glycogen is burnt and it is burnt without using oxygen. This is called **anaerobic metabolism.** Lactic acid is produced during this period. Presence of lactic acid causes some sort of **burning sensation** in the muscles particularly the muscles of arms, legs and back.

Muscles burn all the muscle glycogen within 3 to 5 minutes. If the person continues the exercise beyond this, glycogen stored in liver is converted into glucose, which is transported to muscles through blood. Now the body moves into **aerobic metabolism**. Glucose obtained from liver is burnt in the presence of oxygen. No more lactic acid is produced. So, the burning sensation in the muscles disappears. Proper breathing is essential during this period so that adequate oxygen is supplied to the muscles to extract the energy from glucose. Supply of glucose from liver in combination with adequate availability of oxygen allows the person to continue the exercise.

Utilization of all the glycogen stored in liver is completed by about 20 minutes. If the exercise is continued beyond this, the body starts utilizing the fat. The stored fat called body fat is converted into carbohydrate, which is utilized by the muscles. This allows the person to do the exercise for a longer period.

SEVERITY OF EXERCISE

Cardiovascular and other changes in the body depend upon the severity of exercise also. Based on severity, the exercise is classified into three types:

1. MILD EXERCISE

It is the very simple form of exercise like slow walking. Little or no change occurs in cardiovascular system during mild exercise.

2. MODERATE EXERCISE

Moderate exercise does not involve strenuous muscular activity and it can be performed for a longer period. Exhaustion does not occur at the end of moderate exercise. The examples of this type of exercise are fast walking and slow running.

3. SEVERE EXERCISE

Severe exercise involves strenuous muscular activity and it can be performed only for short duration. Fast running for a distance of 100 or 400 meters is the best example of this type of exercise. Complete exhaustion occurs at the end of severe exercise.

EFFECTS OF EXERCISE ON CARDIOVASCULAR SYSTEM

1. ON BLOOD

Red blood cell count increases because of release of **erythropoietin** from kidney due to hypoxia. The pH of blood decreases due to increased carbon dioxide content.

2. ON BODY FLUIDS

More heat is produced during exercise and the **thermoregulatory system** is activated. This in turn, causes secretion of large amount of **sweat** leading to:

i. Fluid loss.
ii. Reduced blood volume.
iii. Hemoconcentration.
iv. Sometimes, severe exercise leads to dehydration.

3. ON HEART RATE

Heart rate increases during exercise. Even the thought of exercise or preparation for exercise increases the heart rate. It is because of impulses from cerebral cortex to medullary centers, which reduces vagal tone.

In moderate exercise, the heart rate increases to 180 beats/minute. In severe muscular exercise it reaches 240 to 260 beats/minute. Increased heart rate during exercise is mainly due to **vagal withdrawal** and **increase in sympathetic tone**.

4. ON CARDIAC OUTPUT

Cardiac output increases up to 20 L/minute in moderate exercise and up to 35 L/minute during severe exercise. Increase in cardiac output is directly proportional to the increase in amount of oxygen consumed during exercise.

5. ON VENOUS RETURN

Venous return increases during exercise because of muscle pump, respiratory pump and splanchnic vasoconstriction.

6. ON BLOOD FLOW TO SKELETAL MUSCLES

There is increase in the amount of blood flowing to skeletal muscles during exercise. In resting condition, the blood supply to the skeletal muscles is 3 to 4 mL/100 gram of the muscle/minute. It increases up to 60 to 80 mL in moderate exercise and up to 90 to 120 mL in severe exercise.

During the muscular activity, stoppage of blood flow occurs when the muscles contract. It is because of compression of blood vessels during contraction. And in between the contractions, the blood flow increases.

7. ON BLOOD PRESSURE

During moderate **isotonic exercise**, the systolic pressure is increased. It is due to increase in heart rate and stroke volume. Diastolic pressure is not altered because peripheral resistance is not affected during moderate isotonic exercise.

In severe exercise involving isotonic muscular contraction, the systolic pressure enormously increases, but the diastolic pressure decreases. Decrease in diastolic pressure is because of the decrease in peripheral resistance. Decrease in peripheral resistance is due to vasodilatation caused by metabolites.

During exercise involving **isometric contraction**, the peripheral resistance increases. So, the diastolic pressure also increases along with systolic pressure.

Blood Pressure After Exercise

After exercise, the blood pressure falls below the resting level. It is because of vasodilatation caused by metabolic end products accumulated in muscles during exercise. However, the pressure returns to resting level quickly as soon as the metabolic end products are removed from muscles.

MODEL QUESTIONS IN CARDIOVASCULAR SYSTEM

■ LONG QUESTIONS

1. Define cardiac cycle. Describe various events of cardiac cycle.
2. Define electrocardiogram. Describe the waves, segments and intervals of normal ECG. Add a note on ECG leads.
3. Give the definitions, normal values and variations of cardiac output. Explain the factors regulating cardiac output.
4. What is cardiac output? Enumerate the various methods to measure cardiac output and, explain the measurement of cardiac output by applying Fick's principle.
5. Describe the innervation of heart and the regulation of heart rate.
6. Define arterial blood pressure. Describe the nervous regulation (short-term) of arterial blood pressure.
7. Describe renal mechanism of (long-term) regulation of arterial blood pressure.
8. Describe the cardiovascular and respiratory changes during exercise.

■ SHORT QUESTIONS

1. Action potential in cardiac muscle.
2. Pacemaker.
3. Conductive system in heart.
4. Isometric contraction period.
5. Heart sounds.
6. Waves of normal ECG.
7. ECG leads.
8. Nerve supply to heart.
9. Vagal tone.
10. Baroreceptors/Chemoreceptors.
11. Determinants of arterial blood pressure.
12. Renal regulation of blood pressure.
13. Hypertension.
14. Venous pressure.
15. Arterial pulse.
16. Phlebogram/Venous pulse.
17. Coronary circulation.
18. Cerebral circulation.
19. Fetal/Neonatal circulation.
20. Stroke.
21. Capillary circulation (microcirculation).
22. Hypovolemic shock.
23. Syncope.
24. Heart failure.
25. Effect of exercise on blood pressure.

■ VERY SHORT ANSWER QUESTIONS

1. Pericardium.
2. Valves of the heart.
3. Actions of heart.
4. Divisions of circulation.
5. Velocity of impulse at different parts of conductive system.
6. Refractory period in cardiac muscle.
7. End systolic volume, end diastolic volume and ejection fraction.
8. Auscultation areas.
9. Cardiac murmurs.
10. P wave/QRS complex/T wave of ECG.
11. Definitions and normal values of cardiac output.
12. Respiratory pump/Muscle pump.
13. Peripheral resistance.
14. Vagal tone/Sympathetic tone.
15. Role of baroreceptors in regulating heart rate.
16. Role of baroreceptors in regulation of arterial blood pressure.
17. Renin-angiotensin mechanism.
18. List the hormones which increase, and hormones which decrease the arterial blood pressure.
19. Korotkoff sounds.
20. Hypotension.
21. Valsalva maneuver.
22. Müller maneuver.
23. Physiological shunt in heart.
24. Myocardial infarction.
25. Angina pectoris/cardiac pain.
26. Importance of cerebral circulation.
27. Hepatic circulation.
28. Physiological shunt.
29. Peculiarities of capillary circulation.
30. Circulation through skeletal muscles.
31. Definition, types and causes of hemorrhage.
32. Heart block.
33. Aerobic and anaerobic exercise.

SECTION 9: RESPIRATORY SYSTEM AND ENVIRONMENTAL PHYSIOLOGY

Chapter 68: Respiratory Tract and Pulmonary Circulation

CHAPTER OUTLINE

- INTRODUCTION
  - TYPES OF RESPIRATION
  - PHASES OF RESPIRATION
- FUNCTIONAL ANATOMY OF RESPIRATORY TRACT
- RESPIRATORY UNIT
  - STRUCTURE OF RESPIRATORY UNIT
  - RESPIRATORY MEMBRANE
- NON-RESPIRATORY FUNCTIONS OF RESPIRATORY TRACT
  - OLFACTION
  - VOCALIZATION
  - PREVENTION OF DUST PARTICLES
  - DEFENSE MECHANISM
  - MAINTENANCE OF WATER BALANCE
  - REGULATION OF BODY TEMPERATURE
  - REGULATION OF ACID-BASE BALANCE
  - ANTICOAGULANT FUNCTION
  - SECRETION OF ANGIOTENSIN-CONVERTING ENZYME
  - SYNTHESIS OF HORMONAL SUBSTANCES
- RESPIRATORY PROTECTIVE REFLEXES
  - COUGH REFLEX
  - SNEEZING REFLEX
  - SWALLOWING REFLEX
- PULMONARY CIRCULATION
  - PULMONARY BLOOD VESSELS
  - PHYSIOLOGICAL SHUNT
  - SALIENT FEATURES OF PULMONARY CIRCULATION
  - PULMONARY BLOOD FLOW
  - PULMONARY BLOOD PRESSURE
  - MEASUREMENT OF PULMONARY BLOOD FLOW
  - REGULATION OF PULMONARY BLOOD FLOW

RESPIRATION

Respiration is the process by which oxygen is taken in and carbon dioxide is given out. The **first breath** takes place only after birth. **Fetal lungs** are **nonfunctional.** So, during intrauterine life the exchange of gases between fetal blood and mother's blood occurs through **placenta**.

After the first breath, the respiratory process continues throughout the life. Permanent stoppage of respiration occurs only at death.

Normal Respiratory Rate at Different Age

Newborn   : 30 to 60/min
Early childhood : 20 to 40/min
Late childhood : 15 to 25/min
Adult   : 12 to 16/min

TYPES OF RESPIRATION

Respiration is often classified into two types:

1. **External respiration** that involves exchange of respiratory gases, i.e. oxygen and carbon dioxide between lungs and blood.
2. **Internal respiration** which involves exchange of gases between blood and tissues.

PHASES OF RESPIRATION

Respiration occurs in two phases:

1. **Inspiration** during which the air enters the lungs from atmosphere.
2. **Expiration** during which the air leaves the lungs.

FUNCTIONAL ANATOMY OF RESPIRATORY TRACT

Respiratory tract is the anatomical structure through which air moves in and out. It consists of nose, pharynx, larynx, trachea, bronchi and lungs **(Fig. 68.1)**.

Covering of Lungs: Pleura

Each lung is covered by a bilayered serous membrane called pleura or **pleural sac**. Pleura is formed two layers, **visceral layer** and **parietal layer**. Visceral (inner) layer lines the surface of the lungs. At hilum, it is continuous

Section 9: Respiratory System and Environmental Physiology

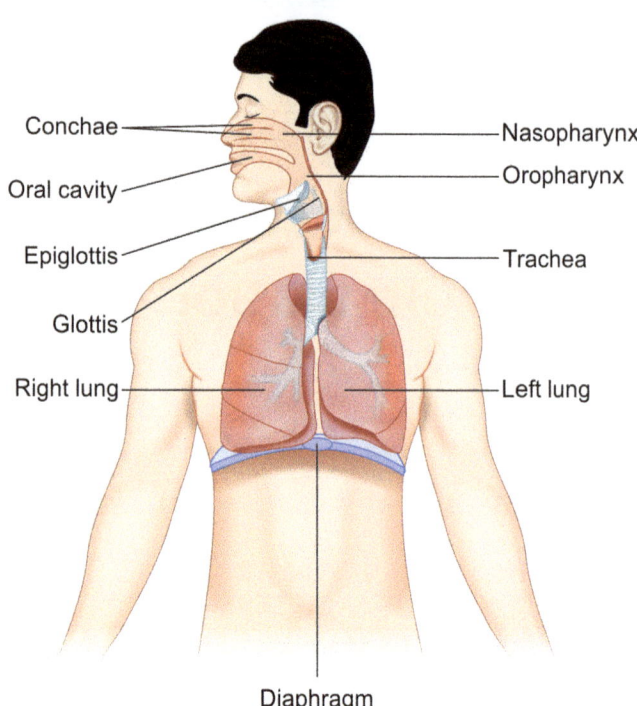

FIGURE 68.1: Respiratory tract.

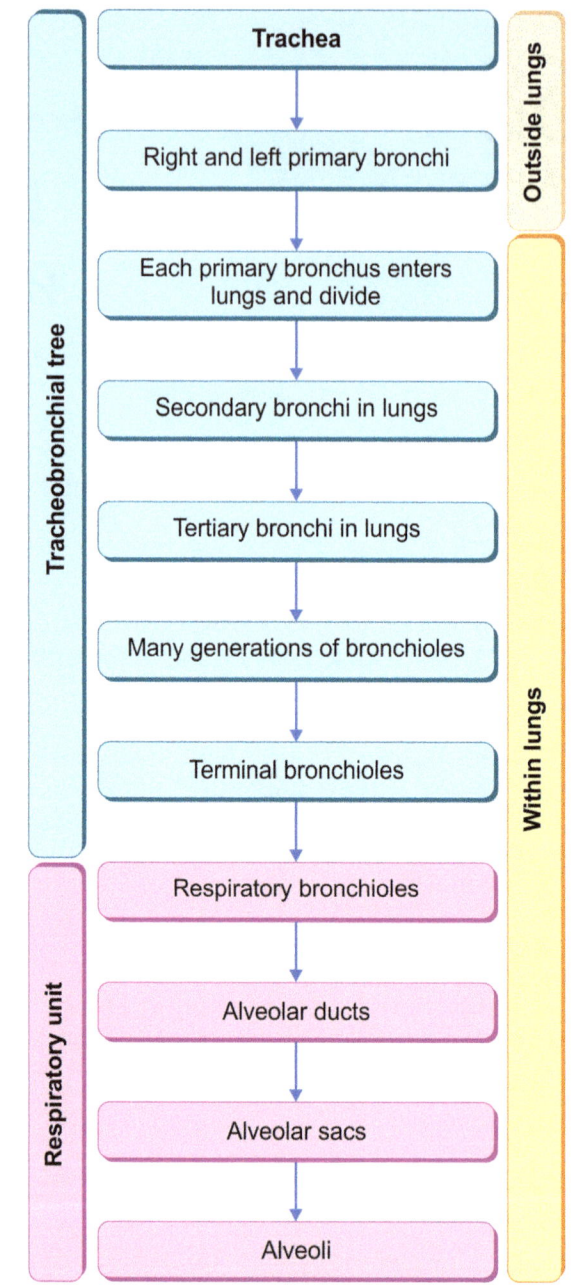

FIGURE 68.2: Schematic representation of tracheobronchial tree and respiratory unit.

with parietal (outer) layer, which is attached to the wall of the thoracic cavity.

Intrapleural Space or Pleural Cavity

The narrow space in between the two layers of pleura is called intrapleural space or pleural cavity.

Intrapleural Fluid

Intrapleural space contains thin film of serous fluid called intrapleural fluid. This fluid is secreted by visceral layer of pleura.

Functions of intrapleural fluid

1. It functions as the lubricant and **prevents friction** between two layers of pleura.
2. It is involved in creating the negative pressure called **intrapleural pressure** within intrapleural space.

Tracheobronchial Tree

Tracheobronchial tree is a part of air passage formed by trachea and bronchi.

Components of tracheobronchial tree

1. Trachea bifurcates into two main or **primary bronchi** called right and primary left bronchi **(Fig. 68.2)**.
2. Each primary bronchus enters the lungs and divides into **secondary bronchi**.
3. Secondary bronchi divide into **tertiary bronchi**. In right lung, there are 10 tertiary bronchi and, in left lung, there are 8 tertiary bronchi.
4. Tertiary bronchi divide several times with reduction in length and diameter into many generations of **bronchioles**.
5. When the diameter of bronchioles becomes 1 mm or less, it is called **terminal bronchiole**.
6. Terminal bronchiole continues or divides into **respiratory bronchiole**, which has a diameter of 0.5 mm.

Upper and Lower Respiratory Tracts

Generally, respiratory tract is divided into two parts:
1. **Upper respiratory tract** which includes all the structures from nose up to vocal cords.
2. **Lower respiratory tract** that includes trachea, bronchi and lungs.

■ RESPIRATORY UNIT

Lung parenchyma is formed by respiratory unit that forms the **terminal portion** of respiratory tract. Respiratory unit is defined as the structural and functional unit of lung. Exchange of gases occurs only in this part of the respiratory tract.

■ STRUCTURE OF RESPIRATORY UNIT

Respiratory unit starts from the respiratory bronchioles **(Fig. 68.3)**. Each **respiratory bronchiole** divides into **alveolar ducts**. Each alveolar duct enters an enlarged structure called the **alveolar sac**. Space inside the alveolar sac is called antrum. Alveolar sac consists of a cluster of **alveoli**. Few alveoli are present in the wall of alveolar duct also.

Thus, respiratory unit includes:

1. Respiratory bronchioles.
2. Alveolar ducts.
3. Alveolar sacs.
4. Alveoli.

Each alveolus is like a pouch with the diameter of about 0.2 to 0.5 mm. It is lined by epithelial cells.

Alveolar Cells or Pneumocytes

Alveolar epithelium consists of alveolar cells or pneumocytes.

Alveolar cells are of two types:
 i. Type I alveolar cells which form the site of gaseous exchange between alveolus and blood.
 ii. Type II alveolar cells which secrete the alveolar fluid and surfactant.

■ RESPIRATORY MEMBRANE

Respiratory membrane is the membranous structure through which exchange of gases occurs in lungs. Respiratory membrane separates air in the alveoli from blood in capillary **(Fig. 72.1)**. Refer Chapter 72 for details of respiratory membrane.

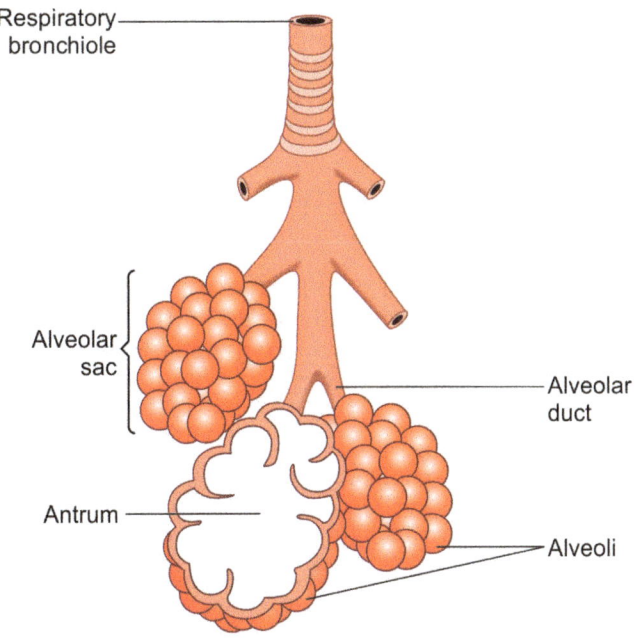

FIGURE 68.3: Structure of respiratory unit.

■ NON-RESPIRATORY FUNCTIONS OF RESPIRATORY TRACT

Besides the primary function of gaseous exchange, the respiratory tract is involved in several non-respiratory functions of the body.

■ 1. OLFACTION

Olfactory receptors present in the mucous membrane of nostril are responsible for **olfactory sensation**.

■ 2. VOCALIZATION

Along with other structures, larynx forms the **speech apparatus**. However, larynx alone is involved in the process of vocalization. Therefore, it is called **sound box**.

■ 3. PREVENTION OF DUST PARTICLES

Dust particles, which enter the nostrils from air, are prevented from reaching the lungs by **filtration action** of hairs in nasal mucous membrane. The small particles, which escape the hairs, are held by the **mucus** secreted by nasal mucous membrane. Those dust particles, which escape the nasal hairs and nasal mucous membrane, are removed by the phagocytic action of **macrophages** in alveoli. Particles which escape the protective mechanisms in nose and alveoli are thrown out by **cough reflex** and **sneezing reflex**.

■ 4. DEFENSE MECHANISM

Defense functions of the lungs are performed by their own defenses and by the presence of various types of cells in mucous membrane lining the alveoli of lungs.

i. Lung's Own Defenses

Epithelial cells lining the air passage secrete some innate immune factors called **defensins** and **cathelicidins**. These two substances are antimicrobial peptides and help lung's natural defenses.

ii. Defense Through Leukocytes

Leukocytes, particularly the neutrophils and lymphocytes present in alveoli of lungs provide defense mechanism against bacteria and virus. **Neutrophils** kill the bacteria by phagocytosis. **Lymphocytes** develop immunity against bacteria.

iii. Defense Through Macrophages

Macrophages engulf dust particles and pathogens, which enter the alveoli and thereby act as **scavengers** in lungs. Macrophages are also involved in the development of immunity by functioning as **antigen presenting cells**.

iv. Defense Through Mast Cells

Mast cells are responsible for allergic reactions.

v. Defense Through Natural Killer Cell

Natural killer (NK) cell destroys the **microorganisms** such as viruses and the viral infected or damaged cells, which may form the tumors. It also destroys the **malignant cells** and prevents development of cancer.

vi. Defense Through Dendritic Cells

Dendritic cells in the lungs function as **antigen presenting cells**.

5. MAINTENANCE OF WATER BALANCE

Respiratory tract plays a role in **water loss mechanism**. During expiration, water evaporates through the expired air and some amount of body water is lost by this process.

6. REGULATION OF BODY TEMPERATURE

During expiration, along with water, heat is also lost from the body. Thus, respiratory tract helps in **heat loss mechanism**.

7. REGULATION OF ACID-BASE BALANCE

Lungs play a role in maintenance of acid-base balance of the body by regulating the carbon dioxide content in blood. Carbon dioxide is produced during various metabolic reactions in the tissues of the body. When it enters the blood, **carbon dioxide** combines with water to form **carbonic acid**. Since carbonic acid is unstable, it splits into hydrogen and bicarbonate ions.

$$CO_2 + H_2O \longrightarrow H_2CO_3 \longrightarrow H^+ + HCO_3^-$$

The entire reaction is reversed in lungs when carbon dioxide is removed from blood into the alveoli of lungs.

$$H^+ + HCO_3^- \longrightarrow H_2CO_3 \longrightarrow CO_2 + H_2O$$

As carbon dioxide is a volatile gas, it is practically blown out by ventilation.

8. ANTICOAGULANT FUNCTION

Mast cells in lungs secrete **heparin**. Heparin is an anticoagulant and it prevents the intravascular clotting.

9. SECRETION OF ANGIOTENSIN CONVERTING ENZYME

Endothelial cells of the pulmonary capillaries secrete the angiotensin-converting enzyme (ACE). It converts the angiotensin I into active angiotensin II which plays an important role in the regulation of ECF volume and blood pressure (Chapter 34).

10. SYNTHESIS OF HORMONAL SUBSTANCES

Lung tissues are also known to synthesize the hormonal substances, prostaglandins, acetylcholine and serotonin which have many physiological actions in the body including regulation of blood pressure (Chapter 50).

RESPIRATORY PROTECTIVE REFLEXES

Respiratory protective reflexes are the reflexes that protect the lungs and air passage from foreign particles. Respiratory protective reflexes are detailed below.

1. COUGH REFLEX

Cough is a modified respiratory process characterized by **forced expiration**. It is the protective reflex that occurs because of irritation of respiratory tract and some other areas such as external auditory meatus.

Causes of Cough Reflex

Cough is produced mainly by irritant agents. It is also produced by cardiac disorders such as congestive **heart failure**, pulmonary disorders such as **chronic obstructive pulmonary disease (COPD)** and tumor in thorax, which may exert pressure on larynx, trachea, bronchi or lungs.

Mechanism of Cough Reflex

Cough begins with **deep inspiration** followed by **forced expiration** with **closed glottis**. This increases the intrapleural pressure above 100 mm Hg. Then, glottis opens suddenly with explosive outflow of air at a high velocity. The velocity of the airflow may reach 960 km/h. It causes expulsion of irritants out of the respiratory tract.

2. SNEEZING REFLEX

Sneezing is also a modified respiratory process characterized by **forced expiration**. It is the protective reflex caused by irritation of nasal mucous membrane.

Causes of Sneezing Reflex

Irritation of the nasal mucous membrane occurs because of dust particles, debris, mechanical obstruction of the airway, and excess fluid accumulation in the nasal passages.

Mechanism Sneezing Reflex

Sneezing starts with **deep inspiration**, followed by **forceful expiration** with **opened glottis** resulting in expulsion of irritant agents out of respiratory tract.

3. SWALLOWING (DEGLUTITION) REFLEX

Swallowing is a respiratory protective reflex that prevents entrance of food particles into the air passage during swallowing.

While swallowing of the food, the respiration is arrested for a while. The temporary arrest of respiration is called **apnea**. The arrest of breathing during swallowing is called swallowing apnea or **deglutition apnea**. It takes place during pharyngeal stage, i.e. II stage of deglutition and prevents entry of food particles into the respiratory tract (Chapter 31).

PULMONARY CIRCULATION

PULMONARY BLOOD VESSELS

Pulmonary blood vessels include **pulmonary artery** which carries **deoxygenated blood** to alveoli of lungs and **bronchial artery** which supply **oxygenated blood** to other structures of lungs (see below).

Pulmonary Artery

Pulmonary artery supplies deoxygenated blood pumped from right ventricle to alveoli of lungs (pulmonary circulation). After leaving the right ventricle, it divides into right and left branches. Each branch enters the corresponding lung along with primary bronchus. After entering the lung, the branch of the pulmonary artery divides into small vessels and finally forms the **capillary**

plexus that is in intimate relationship to alveoli. Capillary plexus is solely concerned with alveolar gas exchange. Oxygenated blood from the alveoli is carried to left atrium by one pulmonary vein from each side.

Bronchial Artery

Bronchial artery arises from descending thoracic aorta. It supplies arterial blood to bronchi, connective tissue and other structures of lung stroma, visceral pleura and pulmonary lymph nodes. Venous blood from these structures is drained by two **bronchial veins** from each side. However, the blood from distal portion of bronchial circulation is drained directly into the tributaries of pulmonary veins.

■ PHYSIOLOGICAL SHUNT

Physiological shunt is defined as a connection between arterial and venous side of circulation (Chapter 65). In lungs, the physiological shunt provides a diversion through which the venous blood is mixed with arterial blood.

Components of Physiological Shunt

Physiological shunt has two components:

1. Flow of deoxygenated blood from **bronchial circulation** into **pulmonary veins** without being oxygenated makes up part of normal physiological shunt.
2. Flow of deoxygenated blood from **thebesian veins** into **cardiac chambers** directly (Chapter 65).

Venous Admixture and Wasted Blood

Venous admixture is the mixing of deoxygenated blood with oxygenated blood. It is caused by physiological shunt.

Fraction of venous blood, which is not fully oxygenated, is generally considered as wasted blood.

■ SALIENT (CHARACTERISTIC) FEATURES OF PULMONARY CIRCULATION

1. Pulmonary artery has a thin wall and it has only about one-third of thickness of the systemic aortic wall. Wall of other pulmonary blood vessels is also thin.
2. Pulmonary blood vessels are highly elastic and more distensible.
3. Smooth muscle coat is not well developed in the pulmonary blood vessels.
4. True arterioles have less smooth muscle fibers.
5. Pulmonary capillaries are larger than systemic capillaries.
6. Vascular resistance in pulmonary circulation is very less; it is only one-tenth of systemic circulation.
7. Pulmonary vascular system is a low-pressure system (see below). Pulmonary capillary pressure is only 7 mm Hg.
8. Pulmonary artery carries deoxygenated blood from heart to lungs and pulmonary veins carry oxygenated blood from lungs to heart.
9. Physiological shunt is present.

■ PULMONARY BLOOD FLOW

Both the lungs receive whole amount of blood that is pumped out from right ventricle. Output of blood per minute is same in both the right and left ventricle. It is about 5 liters.

■ PULMONARY BLOOD PRESSURE

Pulmonary blood pressure is less than systemic blood pressure because the pulmonary blood vessels are more distensible than systemic blood vessels. Thus, the entire pulmonary vascular system is a low-pressure bed.

Pulmonary Arterial Pressure

Systolic pressure : 25 mm Hg
Diastolic pressure : 10 mm Hg
Mean arterial pressure : 15 mm Hg

Mean pulmonary arterial pressure is not calculated by using the same formula for mean systemic arterial pressure.

Mean pulmonary arterial pressure = 2/3 of pulmonary diastolic pressure + 1/3 pulmonary systolic pressure.

Pulmonary Capillary Pressure

Pulmonary capillary pressure is about 7 mm Hg.

■ MEASUREMENT OF PULMONARY CIRCULATION

Pulmonary blood flow is measured by applying **Fick principle**. Details are given in Chapter 61.

■ REGULATION OF PULMONARY CIRCULATION

Under normal conditions, pulmonary blood flow is regulated by the following factors:

1. Cardiac Output

Pulmonary blood flow is **directly proportional** to cardiac output.

Cardiac output is in turn is regulated by four other factors:

1. Venous return.
2. Force of contraction.
3. Heart rate.
4. Peripheral resistance.

Refer Chapter 61 for details of factors affecting cardiac output.

2. Vascular Resistance

Pulmonary blood flow is **inversely proportional** to the pulmonary vascular resistance. Pulmonary vascular resistance is low compared to systemic vascular resistance.

3. Nervous Factors

Stimulation of **sympathetic nerves** under experimental conditions increases the pulmonary vascular resistance by **vasoconstriction**. Stimulation of **parasympathetic nerve** decreases the vascular resistance by **vasodilatation**.

However, under physiological conditions, it is doubtful whether autonomic nerves play any role in regulating the blood flow to lungs.

Chapter 69: Mechanics of Respiration

CHAPTER OUTLINE

- **RESPIRATORY MOVEMENTS**
  - MUSCLES OF RESPIRATION
  - MOVEMENTS OF THORACIC CAGE
  - MOVEMENTS OF LUNGS
- **RESPIRATORY PRESSURES**
  - INTRAPLEURAL PRESSURE
  - INTRA-ALVEOLAR PRESSURE
- **COMPLIANCE**
  - DEFINITION
  - NORMAL VALUES
  - TYPES
  - MEASUREMENT
  - APPLIED PHYSIOLOGY
- **WORK OF BREATHING**

RESPIRATORY MOVEMENTS

During normal quiet breathing, inspiration is the **active process** and expiration is the **passive process**. During inspiration, thoracic cage enlarges and lungs expand so that air enters the lungs easily. During expiration, the thoracic cage and lungs decrease in size and attain the **preinspiratory position** so that air leaves the lungs easily.

MUSCLES OF RESPIRATION

Muscles involved in respiratory movements are inspiratory muscles and expiratory muscles. However, the respiratory muscles are generally classified into two types:

1. Primary or major respiratory muscles which are responsible for change in size of thoracic cage during normal quiet breathing.
2. Accessory respiratory muscles that help primary respiratory muscles during forced respiration.

Inspiratory Muscles

Muscles involved in inspiratory movements are known as inspiratory muscles which are primary or accessory muscles.

1. Primary inspiratory muscles are the diaphragm, which is supplied by phrenic nerve (C3 to C5) and external intercostal muscles, supplied by intercostal nerves (T1 to T11).
2. Accessory inspiratory muscles are sternocleidomastoid, scalene, anterior serrati, elevators of scapulae and pectorals.

Expiratory Muscles

Muscles involved in expiratory movements are known as expiratory muscles which are primary or accessory muscles.

1. Primary expiratory muscles are the internal intercostal muscles, which are innervated by intercostal nerves.
2. Accessory expiratory muscles are the abdominal muscles.

MOVEMENTS OF THORACIC CAGE

During inspiration, thoracic cage enlarges in all axis, viz. anteroposterior, transverse and vertical axis. Increase in anteroposterior and transverse diameters occurs due to the elevation of ribs. Vertical diameter of thoracic cage is increased by the descent of diaphragm.

Change in the size of thoracic cavity occurs because of the movements of four units of structures:

1. Thoracic lid.
2. Upper costal series.
3. Lower costal series.
4. Diaphragm.

1. Thoracic Lid

Thoracic lid is formed by manubrium sterni and the first pair of ribs. Movement of thoracic lid increases the **anteroposterior diameter** of thoracic cage.

2. Upper Costal Series

Upper costal series is constituted by second to sixth pairs of ribs. Upper costal series increases the **anteroposterior**

diameter and **transverse diameter** of the thoracic cage by pump handle movement and bucket handle movements.

Pump handle movement

During inspiration, there is elevation of upper costal series of ribs and upward and forward movement of sternum. This movement is called pump handle movement. It increases **anteroposterior diameter** of the thoracic cage.

Bucket handle movement

Simultaneously, central portions of these ribs (arches of ribs) move upwards and outwards to a more horizontal position. This movement is called bucket handle movement and it increases the **transverse diameter** of thoracic cage.

3. Lower Costal Series

It is formed by the seventh to tenth pairs of ribs. Movement of lower costal series increases the **transverse diameter** of the thoracic cage. These ribs also show bucket handle movement by swinging outward and upward.

Eleventh and twelfth pairs of ribs are the **floating ribs**, which are not involved in changing the size of thoracic cage.

4. Diaphragm

Movement of diaphragm increases the **vertical diameter** of thoracic cage. Normally, before inspiration diaphragm is dome-shaped with convexity facing upwards. During inspiration, due to the contraction of muscle fibers the central tendinous portion is drawn downwards so the diaphragm is flattened and increases the vertical diameter of the thoracic cage.

MOVEMENTS OF LUNGS

During inspiration, due to the enlargement of thoracic cage, negative pressure is increased in the thoracic cavity. It causes **expansion of lungs**. During expiration, the thoracic cavity decreases in size to the preinspiratory position. Pressure in the thoracic cage also comes back to the preinspiratory level. It compresses the lung tissues so that, the air is expelled out of lungs.

Collapsing Tendency of Lungs

Lungs are under constant threat to collapse even under resting conditions because of certain factors.

Factors causing collapsing tendency of lungs

Two factors are responsible for the collapsing tendency of lungs:

1. Elastic property of lung tissues.
2. Surface tension exerted on the surface of alveolar membrane by the fluid secreted from alveolar epithelium.

Fortunately, there are some factors which save the lungs from collapsing.

Factors Preventing Collapsing Tendency of Lungs

In spite of elastic property of the lungs and surface tension in the alveoli of lungs, collapsing tendency of lungs is prevented by two factors:

1. *Intrapleural pressure*

Intrapleural pressure which is always negative (see below) keeps the lungs expanded and prevents the collapsing tendency.

2. *Surfactant*

Surfactant is a surface acting material or agent that is responsible for lowering the surface tension of a fluid and thereby prevents collapsing tendency of lungs. Surfactant that lines the epithelium of alveoli in lungs is known as **pulmonary surfactant** and it decreases the **surface tension** on the alveolar membrane.

Source of secretion of pulmonary surfactant

Pulmonary surfactant is secreted by two types of cells:

  i. **Type II alveolar epithelial cells** in lungs.
  ii. **Clara cells** in bronchioles.

Chemistry of surfactant

Surfactant is a lipoprotein complex formed by lipids especially phospholipids, proteins and ions. The phospholipid called **dipalmitoylphosphatidylcholine** (DPPC) is the major component of surfactant.

Effect of deficiency of surfactant:
Respiratory distress syndrome

Deficiency or absence of surfactant in infants causes collapse of lungs. This condition is called respiratory distress syndrome or hyaline membrane disease. Deficiency of surfactant occurs in adults also and it is called **adult respiratory distress syndrome** (**ARDS**).

RESPIRATORY PRESSURES

Two types of pressures are exerted in thoracic cavity and lungs, intrapleural pressure and intra-alveolar pressure.

INTRAPLEURAL PRESSURE

Definition

Intrapleural pressure or **intrathoracic pressure** is the pressure existing in pleural cavity, that is, in between the visceral and parietal layers of pleura **(Fig. 69.1)**.

Normal Values of Intrapleural Pressure

Respiratory pressures are always expressed in relation to atmospheric pressure, which is 760 mm Hg. Under physiological conditions, the intrapleural pressure is always negative. Normal values of intrapleural pressure are given in **Table 69.1**.

Cause for Negativity of Intrapleural Pressure

Pleural cavity is always lined by a thin layer of fluid that is secreted by the visceral layer of pleura. This fluid is constantly pumped from the pleural cavity into the lymphatic vessels. The pumping of fluid creates the negative pressure in the pleural cavity.

Significance of Intrapleural Pressure

1. It prevents the collapsing tendency of lungs.

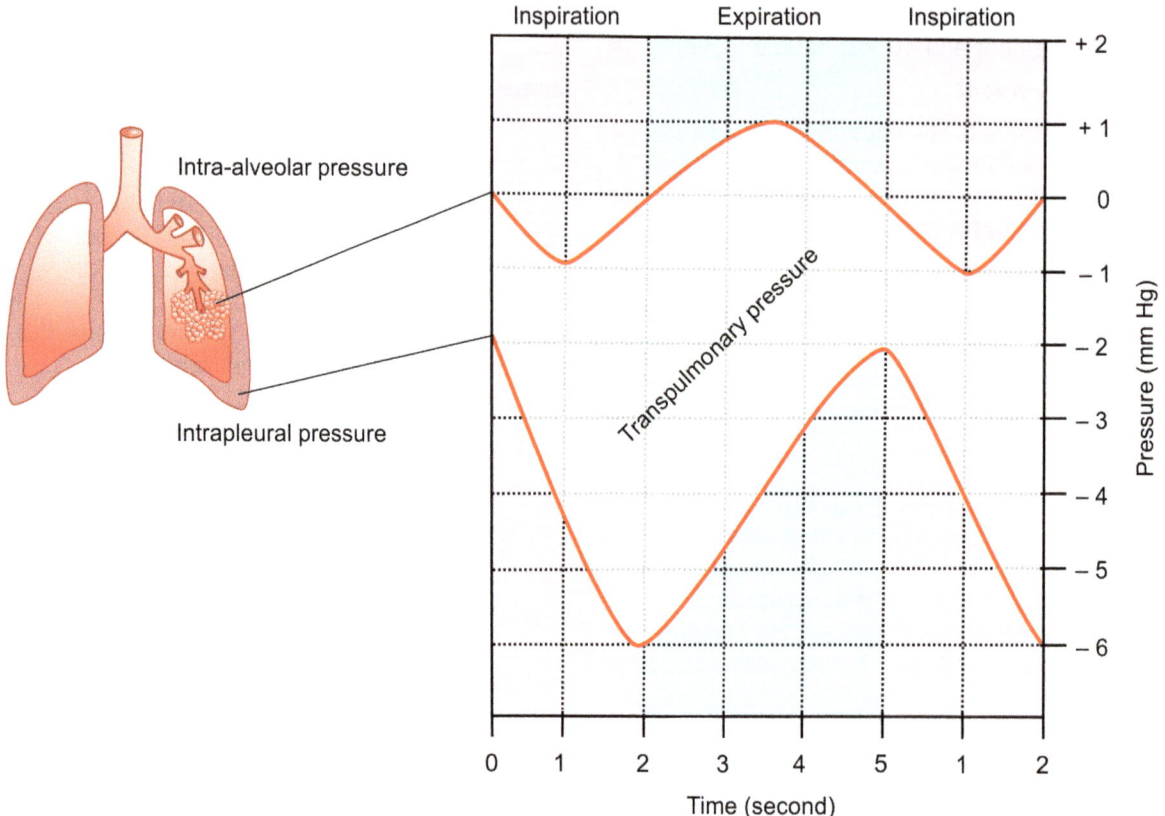

FIGURE 69.1: Changes in respiratory pressures during inspiration and expiration. '0' = Normal atmospheric pressure (760 mm Hg).

TABLE 69.1: Normal values of intrapleural pressure.

Condition	Intrapleural pressure
At the end of normal inspiration	– 6 mm Hg (760 – 6 = 754 mm Hg)
At the end of normal expiration	– 2 mm Hg (760 – 2 = 758 mm Hg)
At the end of forced inspiration	– 30 mm Hg
During forced inspiration with closed glottis: Müller maneuver	– 70 mm Hg
During forced expiration with closed glottis: Valsalva maneuver	+ 50 mm Hg

2. It causes dilatation of vena cava and larger veins in thorax. Also, the negative pressure acts like suction pump and pulls the venous blood from lower part of body towards the heart against gravity. Thus, the intrapleural pressure helps in venous return by acting like **respiratory pump** (Chapter 61).

■ INTRA-ALVEOLAR PRESSURE

Definition

Intra-alveolar pressure or **intrapulmonary pressure** is the pressure existing in the alveoli of the lungs.

Normal Values of Intra-alveolar Pressure

Normally, intra-alveolar pressure is equal to the atmospheric pressure, which is 760 mm Hg. It becomes negative during inspiration and positive during expiration. Normal values are:

Normal values of intra-alveolar pressure are given in **Table 69.2**.

Significance of Intra-alveolar Pressure

1. It causes flow of air in and out of alveoli. During inspiration, the intra-alveolar pressure becomes negative, so the atmospheric air enters the alveoli. And, during expiration, the air is expelled out of alveoli.
2. It also helps in the exchange of gases between the alveolar air and the blood.

■ TRANSPULMONARY PRESSURE

Transpulmonary pressure is the difference between intra-alveolar pressure and intrapleural pressure. It is the measure of elastic forces in lungs, which is responsible for collapsing tendency of lungs.

■ COMPLIANCE
■ DEFINITION AND NORMAL VALUES

Compliance is the ability of lungs and thorax to expand or it is the **expansibility** of lungs and thorax. It is defined

TABLE 69.2: Normal values of intra-alveolar pressure.

Condition	Intra-alveolar pressure
During normal inspiration	– 1 mm Hg (760 – 1 = 759 mm Hg)
During normal expiration	+ 1 mm Hg (760 + 1 = 761 mm Hg)
At the end of inspiration and expiration	Equal to atmospheric pressure: 760 mm Hg
During forced inspiration with closed glottis: Müller maneuver	– 80 mm Hg
During forced expiration with closed glottis: Valsalva maneuver	+ 100 mm Hg

as the change in volume per unit change in the pressure. Determination of compliance is useful as it is the measure of stiffness of lungs. Compliance is expressed in relation to respiratory pressures.

Compliance in Relation to Intra-alveolar Pressure

Compliance is the volume increase in lungs per unit increase in the intra-alveolar pressure:

1. Compliance of lungs and thorax together: 130 mL/ 1 cm H_2O pressure.
2. Compliance of lungs alone: 220 mL/1 cm H_2O pressure.

Compliance in Relation to Intrapleural Pressure

Compliance is the volume increase in lungs per unit decrease in the intrapleural pressure:

1. Compliance of lungs and thorax together = 100 mL/ 1 cm H_2O pressure.
2. Compliance of lungs alone = 200 mL/1 cm H_2O pressure.

Thus, if lungs are removed from thorax, the expansibility (compliance) of lungs alone is doubled. It is because of the restriction exerted by structures of thoracic cage, which interfere with expansion of lungs.

■ APPLIED PHYSIOLOGY: VARIATIONS IN COMPLIANCE

Increase in Compliance

Compliance increases in physiological and pathological conditions:

1. In old age, lung compliance increases due to loss of elastic property of lung tissues.
2. In **emphysema** (obstructive respiratory disease), lung compliance increases because of damage of alveolar membrane **(Fig. 69.2)**.

Decrease in Compliance

Compliance decreases in pathological conditions such as:

1. Deformities of thorax like **kyphosis** and **scoliosis** (Chapter 46).
2. Paralysis of respiratory muscles.
3. **Pleural effusion** (accumulation of fluid in pleural cavity).

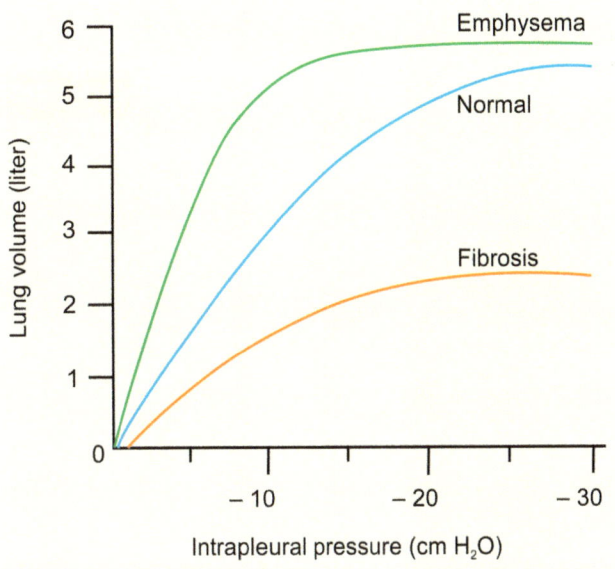

FIGURE 69.2: Variations in lung compliance.

4. **Fibrotic pleurisy** (inflammation of pleura resulting in fibrosis).
5. **Abnormal thorax** due to presence air (**pneumothorax**), fluid (**hydrothorax**), blood (**hemothorax**) and pus (**pyothorax**) in pleural space.

■ WORK OF BREATHING

Work done by respiratory muscles during breathing to overcome the resistance in the thorax and respiratory tract is known as work of breathing.

Work Done by Respiratory Muscles

During the respiratory processes, inspiration is active process and the expiration is a passive process. So, during quiet breathing, the respiratory muscles perform the work only during inspiration and not during expiration.

Energy obtained during the work of breathing is utilized to overcome three types of resistance:

1. Airway resistance: Resistance offered to the passage of air through respiratory tract.
2. Elastic resistance of lungs and thorax.
3. Non-elastic viscous resistance.

Chapter 70

Pulmonary Function Tests

CHAPTER OUTLINE

- TYPES OF LUNG FUNCTION TESTS
- LUNG VOLUMES
- LUNG CAPACITIES
- MEASURMENT OF LUNG VOLUMES AND CAPACITIES
- MEASUREMENT OF FUNCTIONAL RESIDUAL CAPACITY AND RESIDUAL VOLUME
- VITAL CAPACITY
- FORCED EXPIRATORY VOLUME (FEV) OR TIMED VITAL CAPACITY
- RESPIRATORY MINUTE VOLUME (RMV)
- MAXIMUM BREATHING CAPACITY (MBC) OR MAXIMUM VENTILATION VOLUME (MVV)
- PEAK EXPIRATORY FLOW RATE
- RESTRICTIVE AND OBSTRUCTIVE RESPIRATORY DISEASES

TYPES OF LUNG FUNCTION TESTS

Pulmonary function tests or **lung function tests** are useful in assessing the functional status of respiratory system. Pulmonary function tests are carried out mostly by using spirometer. Lung function tests are of two types, static lung function tests and dynamic lung function tests.

Static Lung Function Tests

Static lung function tests are based on **volume of air that flows** into or out of lungs. These tests do not depend upon the rate at which air flows.

Static lung function tests are static **lung volumes** and static **lung capacities**.

Dynamic Lung Function Tests

Dynamic lung function tests are based on time, i.e. the **rate at which air flows** into or out of lungs. These tests are useful in determining the severity of obstructive and restrictive lung diseases.

Dynamic lung function tests are, forced vital capacity, forced expiratory volume, maximum ventilation volume and peak expiratory flow.

LUNG VOLUMES

Lung volumes are the static volumes of air breathed by an individual. Lung volumes are of four types.

1. TIDAL VOLUME (TV)

Tidal volume is the volume of air breathed in and out of lungs in a single normal quiet respiration. Tidal volume signifies the normal depth of breathing.

Normal value = 500 mL (0.5 L)

2. INSPIRATORY RESERVE VOLUME (IRV)

Inspiratory reserve volume is an additional volume of air that can be inspired forcefully after **normal inspiration**.

Normal value = 3,300 mL (3.3 L)

3. EXPIRATORY RESERVE VOLUME (ERV)

Expiratory reserve volume is the additional volume of air that can be expired out forcefully after **normal expiration**.

Normal value = 1,000 mL (1 L)

4. RESIDUAL VOLUME (RV)

Residual volume is the volume of air remaining in the lungs even after **forced expiration**.

Normal value = 1,200 mL (1.2 L)

LUNG CAPACITIES

Lung capacities are the combination of two or more lung volumes. Lung capacities are of four types **(Figs 70.1 to 70.3)**.

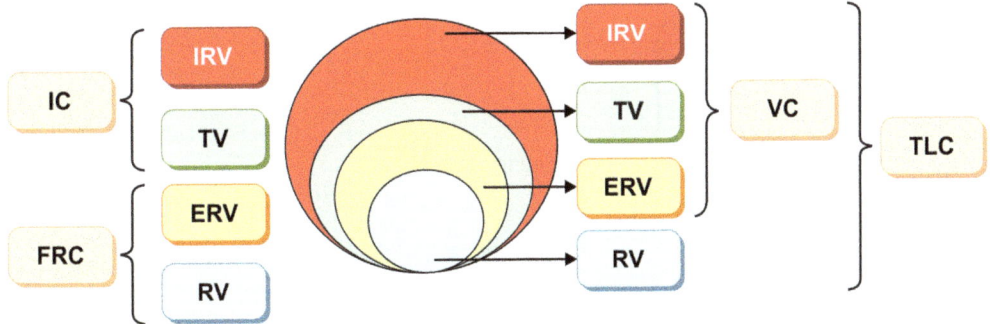

FIGURE 70.1: Lung volumes and capacities.
TV = Tidal volume, IRV = Inspiratory reserve volume, ERV = Expiratory reserve volume, RV = Residual volume, IC = Inspiratory capacity, FRC = Functional residual capacity, VC = Vital capacity, TLC = Total lung capacity

■ 1. INSPIRATORY CAPACITY (IC)

Inspiratory capacity is the maximum volume of air that is inspired after **normal expiration**. It includes tidal volume and inspiratory reserve volume.

$$IC = TV + IRV$$
$$= 500 + 3,300 = 3,800 \text{ mL}$$

■ 2. VITAL CAPACITY (VC)

It is the maximum volume of air that can be expelled out forcefully after a maximal or **deep inspiration**. Vital capacity includes inspiratory reserve volume, tidal volume and expiratory reserve volume.

$$VC = IRV + TV + ERV$$
$$= 3,300 + 500 + 1,000 = 4,800 \text{ mL}$$

■ 3. FUNCTIONAL RESIDUAL CAPACITY (FRC)

It is the volume of air remaining in the lungs after **normal expiration** (after normal tidal expiration). Functional residual capacity includes expiratory reserve volume and residual volume. Functional residual capacity helps to aerate the blood in between breathing and during expiration.

$$FRC = ERV + RV$$
$$= 1,000 + 1,200 = 2,200 \text{ mL}$$

■ 4. TOTAL LUNG CAPACITY (TLC)

Total lung capacity is the volume of air present in the lungs after a maximal or **deep inspiration**. It includes all the volumes.

$$TLC = IRV + TV + ERV + RV$$
$$= 3,300 + 500 + 1,000 + 1,200$$
$$= 6,000 \text{ mL}$$

■ MEASUREMENT OF LUNG VOLUMES AND CAPACITIES

Spirometry is the method to measure lung volumes and capacities. Instrument used for this purpose is called **spirometer**. Modified spirometer is known as **respirometer**. Nowadays **plethysmograph** is also used to measure lung volumes and capacities.

■ SPIROMETER

Spirometer contains two chambers, the outer and inner chambers **(Fig. 70.2)**. Outer chamber is filled with water. A **floating drum** is immersed in the water in an inverted position. Drum is counter balanced by a **weight.** Weight is attached to the top of inverted drum by a chain. A **pen with ink** is attached to the counter weight. Pen is made to write on a **calibrated paper,** which is fixed to a recording device.

Inner chamber is inverted and has a small hole at the top. A **rubber tube** is connected to bottom of inner chamber via a metal tube. A mouthpiece is attached to the other end of this rubber tube. Subject respires through this mouthpiece by closing the nose with a **nose clip**.

When the subject breathes with spirometer, during expiration drum moves up and the counter weight comes down. Reverse of this occurs when the subject breathes the air from the spirometer, i.e. during inspiration. Upward and downward movements of the counter weight are recorded in the form of a graph.

Spirogram

Spirogram is the graphical record of lung volumes and capacities using spirometer. In spirogram upward curve indicates **inspiration** and the downward curve indicates **expiration (Fig. 70.3)**.

Computerized Spirometer

Computerized spirometer is the solid-state electronic equipment. It does not contain a drum or water chamber. Subject has to respire into a sophisticated transducer, which is connected to the instrument by means of a cable.

Disadvantages of Spirometry

Spirometer is used only for a **single breath**. Repeated cycles of respiration cannot be recorded by using this instrument because carbon dioxide accumulates in the spirometer and oxygen or fresh air cannot be provided to the subject.

So, by using simple spirometer, or computerized spirometer, not all the lung volumes and lung capacities can be measured. Volume, which cannot be measured

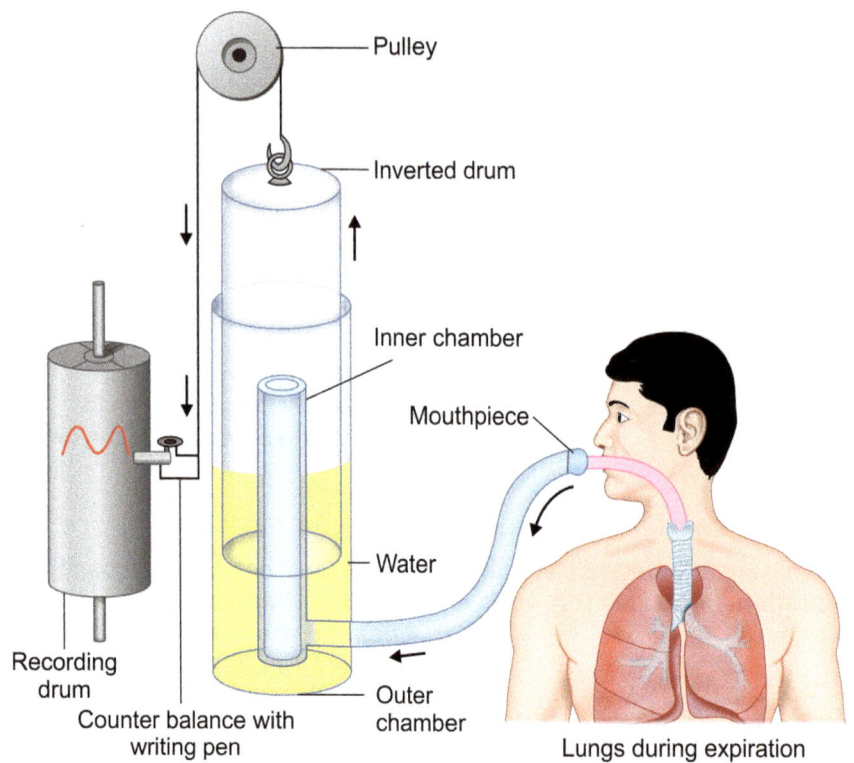

FIGURE 70.2: Spirometer: During expiration, air enters the spirometer from lungs. Inverted drum moves up and the pen draws a downward curve on the recording drum.

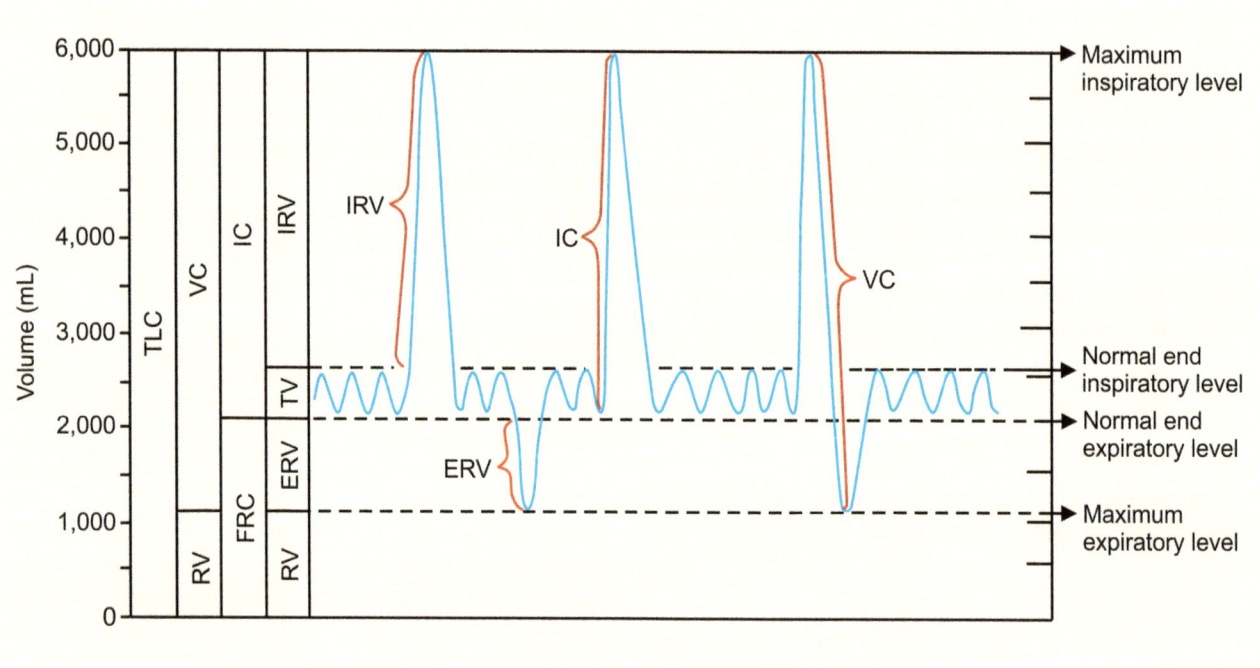

FIGURE 70.3: Spirogram.
TV = Tidal volume, IRV = Inspiratory reserve volume, ERV = Expiratory reserve volume, RV = Residual volume,
IC = Inspiratory capacity, FRC = Functional residual capacity, VC = Vital capacity, TLC = Total lung capacity

by spirometry, is the **residual volume.** Capacities, which include residual volume, also cannot be measured. Capacities that include residual volume are **functional residual capacity** and **total lung capacity.**

Volume and capacities, which cannot be measured by spirometry, are measured by **nitrogen washout** technique or **helium dilution technique** or by body **plethysmograph.**

RESPIROMETER

Respirometer is the modified spirometer. It has provision for removal of carbon dioxide and supply of oxygen.

Carbon dioxide is removed by placing soda lime inside the instrument. Oxygen is supplied to the instrument from the oxygen cylinder, by a suitable valve system.

PLETHYSMOGRAPHY

Plethysmography is another technique used to measure all the lung volumes and capacities (see below).

MEASUREMENT OF FUNCTIONAL RESIDUAL CAPACITY AND RESIDUAL VOLUME

Residual volume and the functional residual capacity cannot be measured by spirometer and can be determined by three methods:

1. HELIUM DILUTION TECHNIQUE

Respirometer is filled with air containing, a known quantity of **helium**. Initially, the subject breathes normally. Then, after the end of expiration, subject breathes from respirometer. Helium from respirometer enters the lungs and mixes with air in lungs. After few minutes of breathing, concentration of helium in the respirometer becomes equal to concentration of helium in the lungs of subject. It is called the equilibration of helium. After **equilibration**, concentration of helium in respirometer is determined. Functional residual capacity is calculated by using the data such as initial volume of air in respirometer, initial concentration of helium in respirometer and final concentration of helium in respirometer.

To determine functional residual capacity, the subject starts breathing with respirometer **after normal expiration**. To measure residual volume, the subject should start breathing from the respirometer **after forced expiration**.

2. NITROGEN WASHOUT METHOD

Normally, concentration of nitrogen in air is 80%. So, if total quantity of nitrogen in the lungs is measured, the volume of air present in lungs can be calculated.

Subject is asked to breathe normally. At the end of normal expiration, the subject inspires **pure oxygen** through a valve and expires into a Douglas bag. This procedure is repeated for 6 to 7 minutes, until the **nitrogen** in lungs is displaced by oxygen. Nitrogen comes to the **Douglas bag**. Afterwards, functional residual capacity is calculated from the data such as volume of air collected in Douglas bag and concentration of nitrogen in Douglas bag.

To measure the functional residual capacity, the subject starts inhaling pure oxygen **after normal expiration** and to determine the residual volume, the subject starts breathing pure oxygen **after forceful expiration**.

3. PLETHYSMOGRAPHY

Plethysmography is a technique to study the variations in the size or volume of a part of the body such as limb. **Plethysmograph** is the instrument used for this purpose. Whole body plethysmograph is the instrument used to measure the lung volumes including residual volume.

VITAL CAPACITY

DEFINITION AND NORMAL VALUE

Definition and normal value of vital capacity are already given.

VARIATIONS OF VITAL CAPACITY

Physiological Variations

1. *Sex:* In females, vital capacity is less than in males.
2. *Body built:* Vital capacity is slightly more in heavily built persons.
3. *Posture:* Vital capacity is more in standing position and less in lying position.
4. *Athletes:* Vital capacity is more.
5. *Occupation:* Vital capacity is decreased in people with sedentary jobs. It is increased in persons who play musical wind instruments such as bugle and flute.

Pathological Variations

Vital capacity is reduced in the following respiratory diseases:

1. Asthma.
2. Emphysema.
3. Weakness or paralysis of respiratory muscle.
4. Pulmonary congestion.
5. Pneumonia.
6. Pneumothorax.
7. Hemothorax.
8. Pyothorax.
9. Hydrothorax.
10. Pulmonary edema.
11. Pulmonary tuberculosis.

FORCED EXPIRATORY VOLUME (FEV) OR TIMED VITAL CAPACITY

DEFINITION

Forced expiratory volume (FEV) is the volume of air, which can be **expired forcefully** in a given unit of time after a **deep inspiration**. It is also called timed vital capacity.

FEV_1 = Volume of air expired forcefully in 1 second
FEV_2 = Volume of air expired forcefully in 2 seconds
FEV_3 = Volume of air expired forcefully in 3 seconds

NORMAL VALUES

Forced expiratory volume in persons with normal respiratory functions is as follows:

FEV_1 = 83% of total vital capacity
FEV_2 = 94% of total vital capacity
FEV_3 = 97% of total vital capacity
After 3rd second = 100% of total vital capacity

SIGNIFICANCE OF DETERMINING FEV

Vital capacity may be almost normal in some of the respiratory diseases. However, the FEV has great diagnostic value, as it is decreased significantly in some respiratory diseases. For example, it is very much decreased in the obstructive diseases like asthma and

TABLE 70.1: Restrictive and obstructive respiratory diseases.

Type	Disease	Structures involved
Restrictive respiratory diseases	Poliomyelitis	CNS
	Myasthenia gravis	CNS and thoracic cavity
	Flail chest (broken ribs)	Thoracic cavity
	Paralysis of diaphragm	CNS
	Spinal cord diseases	CNS
	Pleural effusion	Thoracic cavity
Obstructive respiratory diseases	Asthma Chronic bronchitis Emphysema Cystic fibrosis	Lower respiratory tract
	Laryngotracheobronchitis Epiglottis Tumors Severe cough and cold with phlegm	Upper respiratory tract

emphysema. It is slightly reduced in some of the restrictive respiratory diseases like fibrosis.

RESPIRATORY MINUTE VOLUME (RMV)

Respiratory minute volume is the volume of air breathed in and out of lungs every minute. It is the product of tidal volume (TV) and respiratory rate (RR).

$$RMV = TV \times RR$$
$$= 500 \times 12 = 6,000 \text{ mL}$$

Normal respiratory minute volume is 6 L. It increases in physiological conditions such as voluntary hyperventilation, exercise and emotional conditions. It is reduced in respiratory diseases.

MAXIMUM BREATHING CAPACITY (MBC) OR MAXIMUM VENTILATION VOLUME (MVV)

Maximum breathing capacity (MBC) is the maximum volume of air which can be breathed in and out of lungs by rapid and forceful respiration per minute. It is also called maximum ventilation volume (MVV).

Subject is asked to breathe forcefully and rapidly with a **respirometer** for 15 seconds. Volume of air inspired and expired is measured from the spirogram. From this value, the MBC is calculated for 1 minute.

Normal value:

In adult male : 150 to 170 L/min.
In adult female : 80 to 100 L/min.

Maximum breathing capacity is reduced in respiratory diseases.

PEAK EXPIRATORY FLOW RATE (PEFR)

Peak expiratory flow rate (PEFR) is the maximum rate at which the air can be expired after deep inspiration. It is measured by **Wright's peak flowmeter** or a **mini peak flowmeter**.

Normal value: 400 L/min.

SIGNIFICANCE OF DETERMINING PEFR

Determination of peak expiratory flow rate is useful to diagnose respiratory diseases especially the obstructive respiratory diseases. Generally, PEFR is reduced in all type of respiratory disease. However, reduction is more significant in the obstructive diseases than in restrictive diseases.

Thus, in restrictive diseases, the PEFR is 200 L/min and in obstructive diseases, it is only 100 L/min.

RESTRICTIVE AND OBSTRUCTIVE RESPIRATORY DISEASES

Diseases of respiratory tract are classified into two types:
1. Restrictive respiratory disease.
2. Obstructive respiratory disease.

These two types of respiratory diseases are determined by lung functions tests, particularly FEV.

RESTRICTIVE RESPIRATORY DISEASE

Restrictive respiratory disease is the abnormal respiratory condition characterized by **difficulty in inspiration**. Expiration is not affected. Restrictive respiratory disease may be because of abnormality of lungs, thoracic cavity or/and nervous system.

OBSTRUCTIVE RESPIRATORY DISEASE

Obstructive respiratory disease is the abnormal respiratory condition characterized by **difficulty in expiration**.

The obstructive and respiratory diseases are listed in **Table 70.1**.

Chapter 71: Ventilation and Dead Space

CHAPTER OUTLINE

- **PULMONARY VENTILATION**
  - DEFINITION
  - NORMAL VALUE AND CALCULATION
- **ALVEOLAR VENTILATION**
  - DEFINITION
  - NORMAL VALUE AND CALCULATION
- **DEAD SPACE**
  - DEFINITION AND TYPES
  - NORMAL VALUE
  - MEASUREMENT
- **VENTILATION-PERFUSION RATIO**
  - DEFINITION
  - NORMAL VALUE AND CALCULATION
  - SIGNIFICANCE
- **INSPIRED AIR**
- **ALVEOLAR AIR**
- **EXPIRED AIR**

PULMONARY VENTILATION

DEFINITION

Pulmonary ventilation is the volume of air moving in and out of lungs per minute in quiet breathing. It is also called **respiratory minute volume** (RMV).

NORMAL VALUE AND CALCULATION

Normal value of pulmonary ventilation is 6 L/minute. It is the product of tidal volume (TV) and the rate of respiration (RR). Pulmonary ventilation is calculated by the following formula:

Pulmonary ventilation
= Tidal volume × Respiratory rate
= 500 mL × 12/minute
= 6,000 mL = 6 L/minute

ALVEOLAR VENTILATION

DEFINITION

Alveolar ventilation is the amount of air utilized for gaseous exchange every minute. Alveolar ventilation is different from pulmonary ventilation. In pulmonary ventilation, 6 L of air moves in and out of lungs in every minute. But the whole volume of air is not utilized for exchange of gases. Volume of air subjected for exchange of gases is the alveolar ventilation. Air that is trapped in the respiratory passage (dead space) does not take part in gaseous exchange.

NORMAL VALUE AND CALCULATION

Normal value of alveolar ventilation is 4,200 mL (4.2 L)/minute. Alveolar ventilation is calculated by the following formula:

Alveolar ventilation
= (Tidal volume – Dead space) × Respiratory rate
= (500 – 150) mL × 12/min
= 4,200 mL (4.2 L)/min

DEAD SPACE

DEFINITION AND TYPES OF DEAD SPACE

Dead space is defined as the part of respiratory tract, where gaseous exchange does not take place. Air present in the dead space is called **dead space air**. Dead space is of two types, anatomical dead space and physiological dead space.

Anatomical Dead Space

Anatomical dead space includes nose, pharynx, trachea, bronchi and branches of bronchi up to terminal bronchioles.

Physiological Dead Space

Physiological dead space includes the anatomical dead space plus two additional volumes:

1. *Air in the alveoli, which are nonfunctioning:* In some respiratory diseases, alveoli do not function because of destruction of alveolar membrane.

2. *Air in the alveoli, which do not receive adequate blood flow:* Gaseous exchange does not take place during inadequate blood supply.

Wasted ventilation and wasted air

Wasted ventilation is the volume of air that occupies physiological dead space. Wasted air is the air that is not utilized for gaseous exchange. Dead space air is considered as wasted air.

■ NORMAL VALUE OF DEAD SPACE

Under normal conditions, physiological dead space is equal to anatomical dead space. It is because, all the alveoli are functioning and all alveoli receive adequate blood flow in normal conditions. Volume of normal dead space is 150 mL.

In respiratory disorders, which affect the pulmonary blood flow or the alveoli, the dead space increases. It is associated with reduction in alveolar ventilation.

■ MEASUREMENT OF DEAD SPACE

Dead space is measured by single breath **nitrogen wash-out method**. Subject respires normally for few minutes. Then, he takes a sudden inhalation of pure oxygen. Oxygen replaces the air in dead space (air passage), i.e. the dead space air contains only oxygen and it pushes the other gases into alveoli.

Now, the subject exhales through a **nitrogen meter**. Nitrogen meter determines the concentration of nitrogen in expired air continuously.

First portion of expired air comes from upper part of respiratory tract or air passage, which contains only **oxygen**. Next portion of expired air comes from the alveoli, which contains **nitrogen**. Now, the nitrogen meter shows the nitrogen concentration, which rises sharply and reaches the plateau soon. By using data obtained from nitrogen meter, a graph is plotted. From this graph, the dead space is calculated **(Fig. 71.1)**.

The graph has two areas, area without nitrogen and area with nitrogen. Area of the graph is measured by planimeter or by computer. Area without nitrogen indicates dead space air.

It is calculated by the formula:

$$\text{Dead space} = \frac{\text{Area without } N_2}{\text{Area with } N_2 + \text{Area without } N_2} \times \text{Volume of expired air}$$

For example, in a subject:

Area with nitrogen = 70 sq cm
Area without nitrogen = 30 sq cm
Volume of air expired = 500 mL

$$\text{Dead space} = \frac{30}{70+30} \times 500$$

$$= \frac{30}{100} \times 500$$

$$= 150 \text{ mL}$$

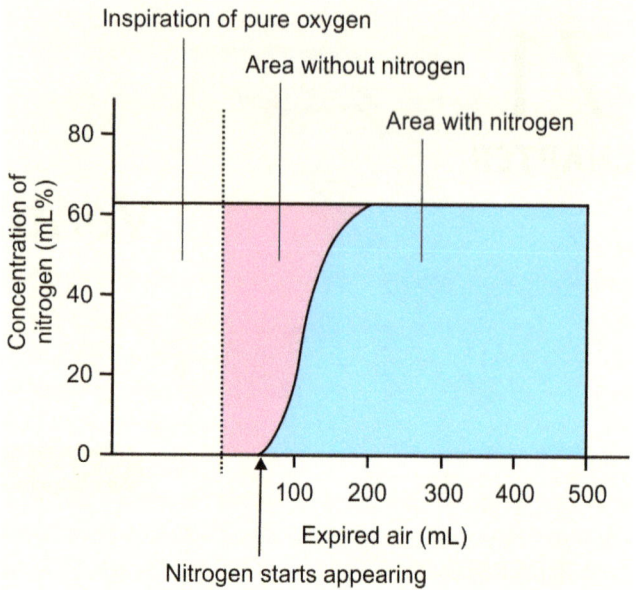

FIGURE 71.1: Measurement of dead space.

■ VENTILATION-PERFUSION RATIO

■ DEFINITION

Ventilation-perfusion ratio is the ratio of alveolar ventilation and amount of blood that perfuse the alveoli.

It is expressed as V_A/Q. V_A is alveolar ventilation and Q is the blood flow (perfusion).

■ NORMAL VALUE OF VENTILATION-PERFUSION RATIO

Normal value of ventilation-perfusion ratio is about 0.84.
Ventilation-perfusion ratio is calculated by the formula:

$$\text{Ventilation-perfusion ration} = \frac{\text{Alveolar ventilation}}{\text{Pulmonary blood flow}}$$

Alveolar ventilation
 = (Tidal volume – Dead space) × Respiratory rate
 = (500 – 150 mL) × 12/min
 = 4,200 mL/min

Blood flow through alveoli
 (pulmonary blood flow) = 5,000 mL/min

Therefore,

$$\text{Ventilation-perfusion ratio} = \frac{4,200}{5,000}$$

$$= 0.84$$

■ SIGNIFICANCE OF VENTILATION-PERFUSION RATIO

Ventilation-perfusion ratio signifies the **gaseous exchange**. It is affected if there is any change in alveolar ventilation or in blood flow. In respiratory disorders such as **chronic obstructive pulmonary diseases (COPD)**, ventilation is affected because of destruction of alveolar membrane. So, the ventilation-perfusion ratio reduces greatly.

TABLE 71.1: Composition of alveolar air, inspired air and expired air.

Components	Inspired (atmospheric) air		Alveolar air		Expired air	
	Volume (mL%)	Partial pressure (mm Hg)	Volume (mL%)	Partial pressure (mm Hg)	Volume (mL%)	Partial pressure (mm Hg)
Oxygen	20.84	159.00	13.60	104.00	15.70	120.00
Carbon dioxide	0.04	0.30	5.30	40.00	3.60	27.00
Nitrogen	78.62	596.90	74.90	569.00	74.50	566.00
Water vapor, etc.	0.50	3.80	6.20	47.00	6.20	47.00
Total	100.00	760.00	100.00	760.00	100.00	760.00

■ INSPIRED AIR

Inspired air is the atmospheric air, which is inhaled during inspiration. Composition of inspired air is given in **Table 71.1**.

■ ALVEOLAR AIR

Alveolar air is the air present in the alveoli of lungs. It is collected by **Haldane-Priestly tube**.

Importance of Alveolar Air

1. Alveolar air is different from the inspired air or atmospheric air. Alveolar air is partially replaced by atmospheric air during each breath.
2. Oxygen diffuses from alveolar air into pulmonary capillaries constantly.
3. Carbon dioxide diffuses from pulmonary blood into alveolar air constantly.
4. Dry atmospheric air is humidified, while passing through respiratory passage just before entering the alveoli **(Table 71.1)**.

■ EXPIRED AIR

Expired air is the amount of air that is exhaled during expiration. It is a combination of dead space air and alveolar air. Expired air is collected by using **Douglas bag**.

Concentration of gases in expired air is somewhere between inspired air and alveolar air. Composition of expired air is given in **Table 71.1**.

Chapter 72: Exchange and Transport of Respiratory Gases

CHAPTER OUTLINE

- EXCHANGE OF GASES
- EXCHANGE OF RESPIRATORY GASES IN LUNGS
  - RESPIRATORY MEMBRANE
  - DIFFUSING CAPACITY
  - DIFFUSION OF OXYGEN
  - DIFFUSION OF CARBON DIOXIDE
- EXCHANGE OF RESPIRATORY GASES AT TISSUE LEVEL
  - DIFFUSION OF OXYGEN FROM BLOOD INTO THE TISSUES
  - DIFFUSION OF CARBON DIOXIDE FROM TISSUES INTO BLOOD
  - RESPIRATORY EXCHANGE RATIO
  - RESPIRATORY QUOTIENT
- TRANSPORT OF GASES
- TRANSPORT OF OXYGEN
  - AS SIMPLE SOLUTION
  - IN COMBINATION WITH HEMOGLOBIN
  - OXYGEN-HEMOGLOBIN DISSOCIATION CURVE
- TRANSPORT OF CARBON DIOXIDE
  - AS DISSOLVED FORM
  - AS CARBONIC ACID
  - AS BICARBONATE
  - AS CARBAMINO COMPOUNDS
  - CARBON DIOXIDE DISSOCIATION CURVE

■ EXCHANGE OF GASES

Oxygen is essential for the cells. Carbon dioxide, which is produced as waste product in the cells must be expelled from the cells and body. Lungs serve to exchange these two gases with blood.

■ EXCHANGE OF RESPIRATORY GASES IN LUNGS

In the lungs, exchange of respiratory gases takes place between the alveoli and the blood. Exchange of gases occurs through **bulk flow** diffusion (Chapter 3).

Respiratory unit is the structure through which the exchange of gases between blood and alveoli takes place. Refer Chapter 68 for details.

■ RESPIRATORY MEMBRANE

Exchange of respiratory gases takes place through respiratory membrane. It is formed by **epithelium** of the respiratory unit and **endothelium** of pulmonary capillary (Fig. 72.1).

Respiratory membrane is formed by different layers of structures belonging to the alveoli and capillaries.

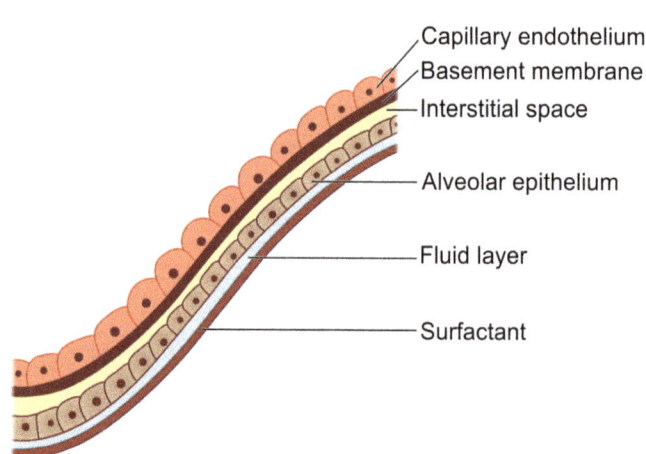

FIGURE 72.1: Structure of respiratory membrane.

Layers of Respiratory Membrane

Different layers of respiratory membrane from within outside are given in **Table 72.1**.

TABLE 72.1: Layers of respiratory membrane.

Parts of respiratory membrane	Different layers
Alveolar part	1. Layer of surfactant 2. Thin layer of alveolar fluid 3. Layer of alveolar epithelium 4. Basement membrane of alveolar epithelial
Between alveolar and capillary parts	5. Interstitial space
Capillary part	6. Basement membrane of capillary endothelium 7. Capillary endothelium

■ DIFFUSING CAPACITY

Diffusing capacity is defined as the volume of gas that diffuses through the respiratory membrane each minute for a pressure gradient of 1 mm Hg.

Diffusing Capacity for Oxygen and Carbon Dioxide

Diffusing capacity for oxygen is 21 mL/min/1 mm Hg. Diffusing capacity for carbon dioxide is 400 mL/min/1 mm Hg. Thus, the diffusing capacity for carbon dioxide is about 20 times more than that of oxygen.

Factors Affecting Diffusing Capacity

1. *Pressure gradient*: Diffusing capacity is **directly proportional** to the pressure gradient. Pressure gradient is the difference between partial pressure of a gas in the alveoli and pulmonary capillary blood (see below).
2. *Solubility of gas in fluid medium*: Diffusing capacity is **directly proportional** to solubility of the gas.
3. *Total surface area of respiratory membrane*: Diffusing capacity is **directly proportional** to surface area of respiratory membrane. Surface area of respiratory membrane in each lung is about 70 sq. m.
4. *Molecular weight of the gas*: Diffusing capacity is inversely **proportional** to molecular weight of the gas.
5. *Thickness of respiratory membrane*: Diffusing capacity is **inversely proportional** to the thickness of respiratory membrane.

■ DIFFUSION OF OXYGEN

Entrance of Oxygen from Atmospheric Air into the Alveoli

Partial pressure of oxygen in the atmospheric air is 159 mm Hg and, in the alveoli, it is 104 mm Hg. Because of the pressure gradient of 55 mm Hg, oxygen easily enters from atmospheric air into the alveoli **(Table 72.2)**.

Diffusion of Oxygen from Alveoli into the Blood

Partial pressure of oxygen in the pulmonary capillary is 40 mm Hg and, in the alveoli, it is 104 mm Hg. The pressure gradient is 64 mm Hg. It facilitates the diffusion of oxygen from alveoli into the blood **(Fig. 72.2)**.

■ DIFFUSION OF CARBON DIOXIDE

Diffusion of Carbon Dioxide from Blood into Alveoli

Partial pressure of carbon dioxide in alveoli is 40 mm Hg, whereas in the blood it is 46 mm Hg. Pressure gradient of 6 mm Hg is responsible for the diffusion of carbon dioxide from blood into the alveoli **(Fig. 72.3)**.

Diffusion of Carbon Dioxide from the Alveoli into the Atmospheric Air

In the atmospheric air, partial pressure of carbon dioxide is very insignificant and is only about 0.3 mm Hg, whereas in the alveoli, it is 40 mm Hg. So, carbon dioxide passes to atmosphere from alveoli easily.

■ EXCHANGE OF RESPIRATORY GASES AT TISSUE LEVEL

■ DIFFUSION OF OXYGEN FROM BLOOD INTO TISSUES

Partial pressure of oxygen in arterial end of systemic capillary is 95 mm Hg. Average oxygen tension in the tissues is 40 mm Hg. It is because of continuous metabolic activity and constant utilization of oxygen. Pressure gradient of about 55 mm Hg between capillary blood and the tissues is responsible for diffusion of oxygen into the tissues **(Fig. 72.4)**.

Oxygen content in arterial blood is 19 mL%, and in the venous blood, it is 14 mL%. Thus, the diffusion of oxygen from blood to the tissues is 5 mL/100 mL of blood.

■ DIFFUSION OF CARBON DIOXIDE FROM TISSUES INTO THE BLOOD

Partial pressure of carbon dioxide is high in the cells and is about 46 mm Hg. The partial pressure of carbon dioxide in arterial blood is 40 mm Hg. Pressure gradient of 6 mm Hg is responsible for the diffusion of carbon dioxide from tissues to the blood **(Fig. 72.5)**.

Carbon dioxide content in arterial blood is 48 mL%. And, in the venous blood, it is 52 mL%. So, the diffusion

TABLE 72.2: Partial pressure, and content of oxygen and carbon dioxide in alveoli, capillaries and tissue.

Gas	Arterial end of pulmonary capillary	Alveoli	Venous end of pulmonary capillary	Arterial end of systemic capillary	Tissue	Venous end of systemic capillary
pO_2 (mm Hg)	40	104	104	95	40	40
Oxygen content (mL%)	14	–	19	19	–	14
pCO_2 (mm Hg)	46	40	40	40	46	46
Carbon dioxide content (mL%)	52	–	48	48	–	52

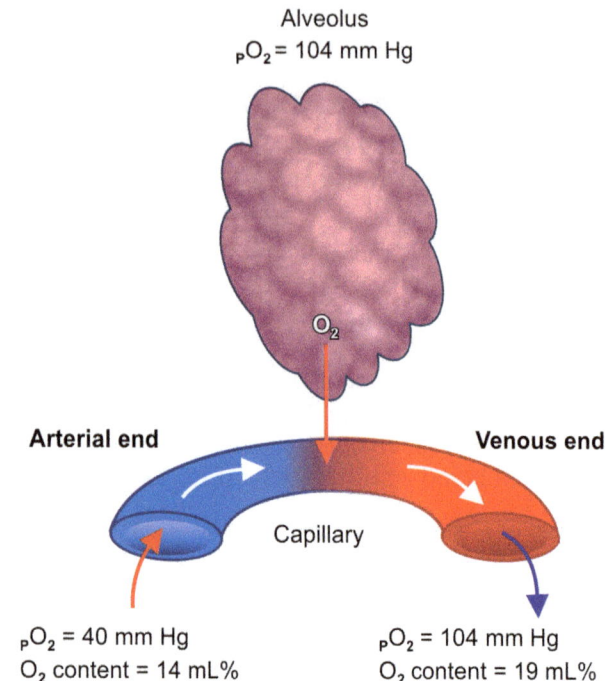

FIGURE 72.2: Diffusion of oxygen from alveolus to pulmonary capillary.

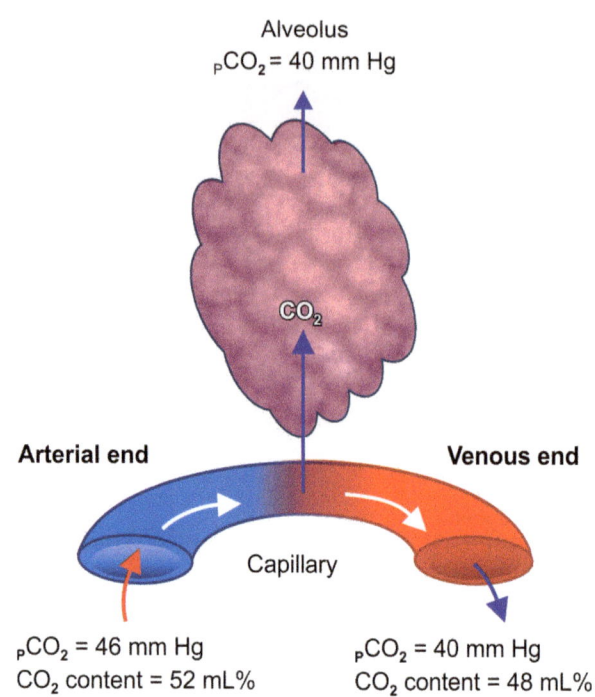

FIGURE 72.3: Diffusion of carbon dioxide from pulmonary capillary to alveolus.

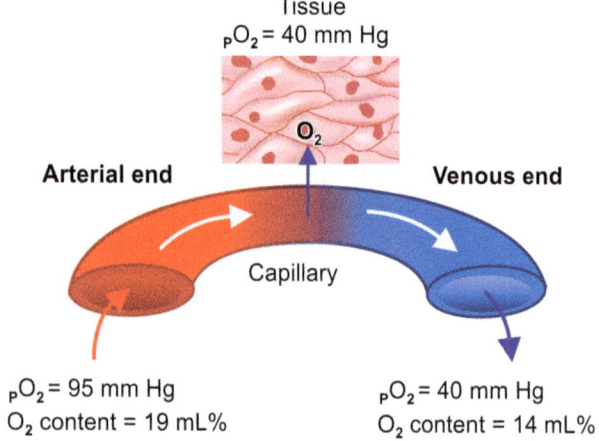

FIGURE 72.4: Diffusion of oxygen from capillary to tissue.

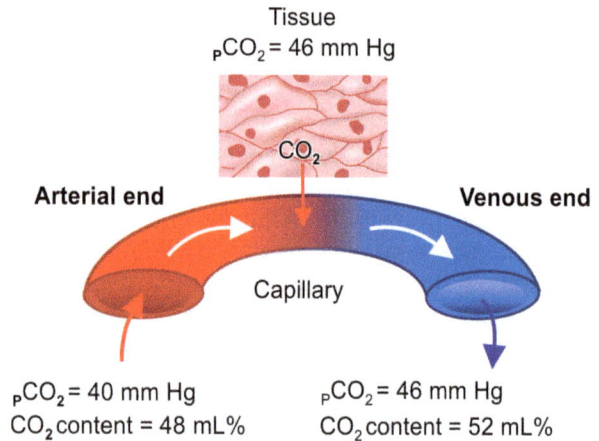

FIGURE 72.5: Diffusion of carbon dioxide from tissue to capillary.

of carbon dioxide from tissues to the blood is 4 mL/ 100 mL of blood.

■ RESPIRATORY EXCHANGE RATIO

Respiratory exchange ratio (R) is the ratio between net output of carbon dioxide from tissues to simultaneous net uptake of oxygen by the tissues.

$$R = \frac{CO_2 \text{ output}}{O_2 \text{ uptake}}$$

Respiratory exchange ratio depends upon the type of food substance that is metabolized. However, when a balanced diet containing average quantity of proteins, carbohydrates and lipids is utilized, the R is about 0.825.

■ RESPIRATORY QUOTIENT

Respiratory quotient is the molar ratio of carbon dioxide production to oxygen consumption. It is used to determine the utilization of different foodstuffs. For about 1 hour after meals, the respiratory quotient is 1.0.

■ TRANSPORT OF GASES

Blood transports the respiratory gases. Oxygen is transported from alveoli of lungs to cells. Carbon dioxide, is transported from cells to alveoli of lungs.

■ TRANSPORT OF OXYGEN

Oxygen is transported from alveoli to the tissue by the blood in two forms:

1. As simple physical solution.
2. In combination with hemoglobin.

TRANSPORT OF OXYGEN AS SIMPLE SOLUTION

Oxygen dissolves in water of plasma and is transported in this **physical form**. Amount of oxygen transported in this way is very negligible. It is only 0.3 mL/100 mL of plasma. It is about 3% of total oxygen in blood.

IN COMBINATION WITH HEMOGLOBIN

Oxygen combines with hemoglobin in blood and is transported as **oxyhemoglobin**. Transport of oxygen in this form is important, because maximum amount (97%) of oxygen is transported by this method.

Oxygen combines with the iron in heme part of hemoglobin. Oxygen combines with hemoglobin only as a physical combination. It is only **oxygenation** and not oxidation. Because of this type of combination oxygen can be readily released from hemoglobin when it is needed.

Oxygen Carrying Capacity of Blood

Oxygen carrying capacity of blood is the amount of oxygen transported by blood. One gram of hemoglobin carries 1.34 mL of oxygen. It is called oxygen carrying capacity of hemoglobin. Normal hemoglobin content in blood is 15 g%. So, the blood with 15 g% of hemoglobin should carry 20.1 mL% of oxygen, i.e. 20.1 mL of oxygen in 100 mL of blood. But, the blood with 15 g% of hemoglobin carries only 19 mL% of oxygen, i.e. 19 mL of oxygen is carried by 100 mL of blood **(Table 72.3)**. Oxygen carrying capacity of blood is only 19 mL% because the hemoglobin is not fully saturated with oxygen. It is saturated only for about 95%.

OXYGEN-HEMOGLOBIN DISSOCIATION CURVE

Oxygenhemoglobin dissociation curve is the curve that demonstrates the relationship between partial pressure of oxygen and percentage saturation of hemoglobin with oxygen. It explains the affinity of hemoglobin for oxygen.

Normally in the blood, hemoglobin is saturated with oxygen only up to 95%. Saturation of hemoglobin with oxygen depends upon the partial pressure of oxygen. When the partial pressure of oxygen is more, hemoglobin accepts oxygen and when the partial pressure of oxygen is less, hemoglobin releases oxygen.

Normal Oxygen-Hemoglobin Dissociation Curve

Under normal conditions, the oxygen-hemoglobin dissociation curve is 'S' shaped or sigmoid shaped

TABLE 72.3: Gases in arterial and venous blood.

Gas		Arterial blood	Venous blood
Oxygen	Partial pressure (mm Hg)	95	40
	Content (mL%)	19	14
Carbon dioxide	Partial pressure (mm Hg)	40	46
	Content (mL%)	48	52

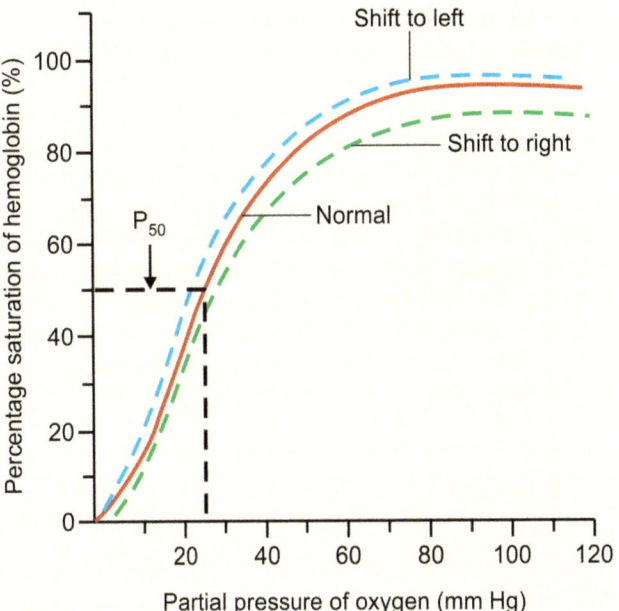

FIGURE 72.6: Oxygen-hemoglobin dissociation curve.

(Fig. 72.6). Lower part of the curve indicates dissociation of oxygen from hemoglobin. Upper part of the curve indicates the acceptance of oxygen by hemoglobin depending upon the partial pressure of oxygen.

P_{50}

P_{50} is the partial pressure of oxygen at which hemoglobin saturation with oxygen is 50%. When the partial pressure of oxygen is 25 to 27 mm Hg, the hemoglobin is saturated to about 50%. That is, the blood contains 50% of oxygen. At 40 mm Hg of partial pressure of oxygen, the saturation is 75%. It becomes 95% when the partial pressure of oxygen is 100 mm Hg.

Factors Affecting Oxygen-Hemoglobin Dissociation Curve

Oxygen-hemoglobin dissociation curve is shifted to left or right by various factors:
I. Shift to left indicates acceptance (association) of oxygen by hemoglobin.
II. Shift to right indicates dissociation of oxygen from hemoglobin.

I. Conditions when shift to left occurs

1. In fetal blood, because fetal hemoglobin has got more affinity for oxygen than the adult hemoglobin.
2. Decrease in hydrogen ion concentration and increase in pH (alkalinity).

II. Conditions when shift to right occurs

1. Decrease in partial pressure of oxygen.
2. Increase in partial pressure of carbon dioxide (Bohr effect).
3. Increase in hydrogen ion concentration and decrease in pH (acidity).

4. Increased body temperature.
5. Excess of 2,3-diphosphoglycerate (DPG) which is a byproduct of carbohydrate metabolism present in red blood corpuscles.

Bohr Effect

Bohr effect is the effect by which presence of carbon dioxide decreases the affinity of hemoglobin for oxygen. In the tissues, due to continuous metabolic activities, the partial pressure of carbon dioxide is high. Because of this, carbon dioxide enters the blood. Presence of carbon dioxide in blood decreases the affinity of hemoglobin for oxygen. So, oxygen is released from the blood to the tissues. And, oxygen dissociation curve is shifted to right.

■ TRANSPORT OF CARBON DIOXIDE

Carbon dioxide is transported by the blood from tissues to the alveoli. Partial pressure and content of carbon dioxide in arterial blood and venous blood are given in **Table 72.3**.

Carbon dioxide is transported in the blood in four ways:

1. As dissolved form : 7%
2. As carbonic acid : Negligible
3. As bicarbonates : 63%
4. As carbamino compounds : 30%.

■ TRANSPORT OF CARBON DIOXIDE AS DISSOLVED FORM

Carbon dioxide diffuses into blood and dissolves in the fluid of plasma forming a **simple solution**. Only about 3 mL/100 mL of plasma of carbon dioxide is transported as dissolved state. It is about 7% of total carbon dioxide in the blood.

■ TRANSPORT OF CARBON DIOXIDE AS CARBONIC ACID

Part of dissolved carbon dioxide in plasma combines with the water to form carbonic acid. This reaction is very slow and the transport of carbon dioxide in this form is negligible.

■ TRANSPORT OF CARBON DIOXIDE AS BICARBONATE

About 63% of carbon dioxide is transported as bicarbonate. From plasma, the carbon dioxide enters the RBCs. In the RBCs, carbon dioxide combines with water to form carbonic acid in the presence of an enzyme called **carbonic anhydrase**. Carbonic anhydrase is present only inside the RBCs and not in the plasma. That is why the carbonic acid formation is at least 200 to 300 times more in the RBCs than in plasma.

Carbonic acid is very unstable. Almost all carbonic acid (99.9%) formed in RBCs, dissociates into bicarbonate and hydrogen ions. Concentration of bicarbonate ions in RBC increases more and more. Due to concentration gradient, bicarbonate ions diffuse through the cell membrane into the plasma.

Chloride Shift or Hamburger Phenomenon

Chloride shift or Hamburger phenomenon is the exchange of a chloride ion for a bicarbonate ion across the erythrocyte membrane.

Chloride shift occurs when carbon dioxide enters the blood from tissues. In plasma, plenty of sodium chloride is present. It dissociates into sodium and chloride ions **(Fig. 72.7)**. When the negatively charged bicarbonate, ions move out of RBC into the plasma, the negatively charged

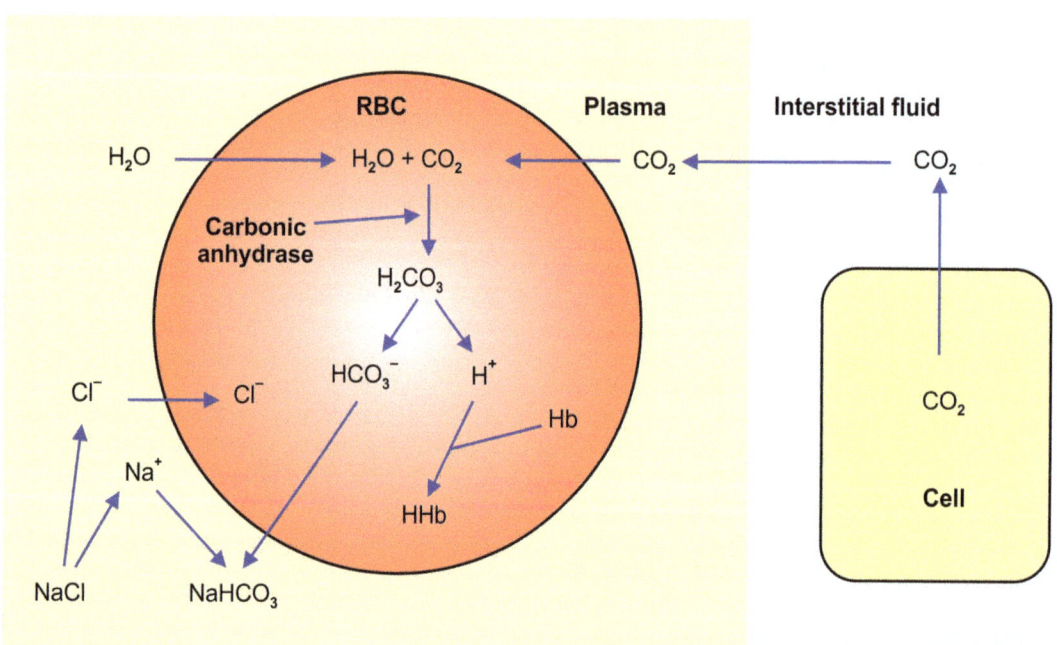

FIGURE 72.7: Transport of carbon dioxide in blood in the form of bicarbonate and chloride shift.

chloride ions move into the RBC in order to maintain the **electrolyte equilibrium** (ionic balance).

Reverse Chloride Shift

Reverse chloride shift is the process by which the chloride ions are moved back into plasma from RBC. This occurs in lungs.

When the blood reaches the alveoli, sodium bicarbonate in the plasma dissociates into the sodium and bicarbonate ions. Bicarbonate ion moves into the RBC. It makes chloride ion to move out of the RBC into the plasma, where it combines with sodium and forms sodium chloride.

Bicarbonate ion inside the RBC combines with hydrogen ion, forms carbonic acid, which dissociates into water and carbon dioxide. Carbon dioxide is then expelled out.

Thus, **chloride shift** occurs in tissues and **reverse chloride shift** occurs in lungs.

TRANSPORT OF CARBON DIOXIDE AS CARBAMINO COMPOUNDS

About 30% of carbon dioxide is transported as carbamino compounds. Carbon dioxide is transported in blood in combination with hemoglobin and plasma proteins. Carbon dioxide combines with hemoglobin to form carbamino hemoglobin or **carbhemoglobin**. And, it combines with plasma proteins to form carbamino proteins. Carbamino hemoglobin and **carbamino proteins** are together called carbamino compounds.

CARBON DIOXIDE DISSOCIATION CURVE

Carbon dioxide is transported in blood as physical solution and in combination with water, plasma proteins and hemoglobin. Amount of carbon dioxide combining with blood depends upon the partial pressure of carbon dioxide.

Carbon dioxide dissociation curve is the curve that demonstrates the relationship between partial pressure of carbon dioxide and quantity of carbon dioxide that combines with blood.

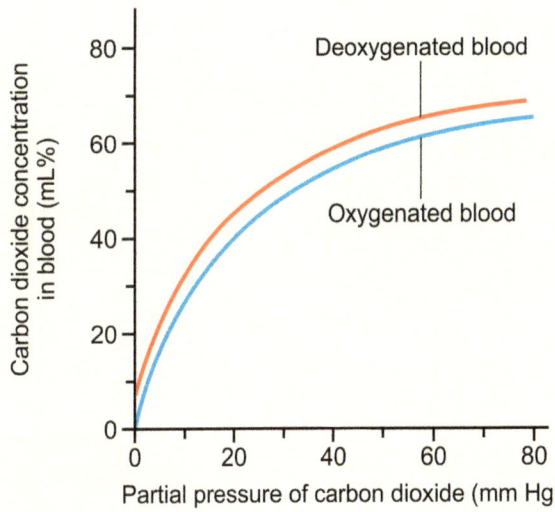

FIGURE 72.8: Carbon dioxide dissociation curve.

Normal Carbon Dioxide Dissociation Curve

Normal carbon dioxide dissociation curve shows that the carbon dioxide content in the blood is 48 mL% when the partial pressure of carbon dioxide is 40 mm Hg. It becomes 52 mL% when the partial pressure of carbon dioxide is 48 mm Hg. Carbon dioxide content becomes 70 mL% when the partial pressure is about 100 mm Hg **(Fig. 72.8)**.

Haldane Effect

Haldane effect is the effect by which combination of oxygen with hemoglobin displaces carbon dioxide from hemoglobin. Excess of oxygen content in blood causes shift of the carbon dioxide dissociation curve to the right.

Significance of Haldane effect

Haldane's effect is essential for release of carbon dioxide from blood into the alveoli of lungs and uptake of oxygen by the blood.

Chapter 73

Regulation of Respiration

CHAPTER OUTLINE

- **REGULATORY MECHANISMS**
- **NERVOUS MECHANISM**
  - RESPIRATORY CENTERS
  - MEDULLARY CENTERS
  - PONTINE CENTERS
  - CONNECTIONS OF RESPIRATORY CENTERS
- **INTEGRATION OF RESPIRATORY CENTERS**
- **FACTORS AFFECTING RESPIRATORY CENTERS**
- **CHEMICAL MECHANISM**
  - CENTRAL CHEMORECEPTORS
  - PERIPHERAL CHEMORECEPTORS

■ REGULATORY MECHANISMS

Respiration is a reflex process. But it can be controlled voluntarily (**voluntary breath holding**) for a short period. **Breath holding time** in a normal healthy adult is 45 to 55 seconds. However, by practice, breathing can be withheld for a long period.

Respiration is subjected to variation, even under normal physiological conditions. But the altered pattern of respiration is brought back to normal, within a short time by some regulatory mechanisms in the body. Regulatory mechanisms responsible for quiet regular breathing are nervous or neural mechanism and chemical mechanism.

■ NERVOUS MECHANISM

Nervous mechanism that regulates respiration includes respiratory centers, afferent nerves and efferent nerves.

■ RESPIRATORY CENTERS

Respiratory centers are group of neurons, which control the rate, rhythm and force of respiration. These centers are bilaterally situated in reticular formation of brainstem **(Fig. 73.1)**. Depending upon the situation in brainstem, respiratory centers are classified into two groups:

I. Medullary centers:
 1. Dorsal respiratory group of neurons.
 2. Ventral respiratory group of neurons.

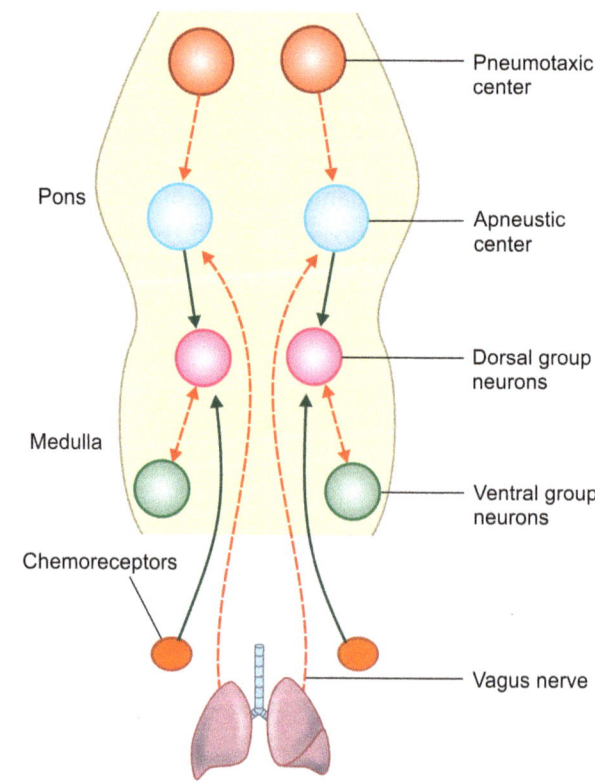

FIGURE 73.1: Nervous regulation of respiration.
Solid green line = Stimulation, Dotted red line = Inhibition.

II. Pontine centers:
   1. Pneumotaxic center.
   2. Apneustic center.

■ MEDULLARY CENTERS

1. Dorsal Respiratory Group of Neurons

Dorsal respiratory group of neurons are situated in nucleus of tractus solitarius of upper medulla oblongata (Fig. 73.1). Usually, these neurons are collectively called **inspiratory center**. All the neurons of dorsal respiratory group are **inspiratory neurons** and generate inspiratory ramp by the virtue of their **autorhythmic property** (Table 73.1).

Function

Dorsal group of neurons are responsible for basic rhythm of respiration (see below for details).

2. Ventral Respiratory Group of Neurons Situation

Ventral respiratory group of neurons are present in nucleus ambiguus and nucleus retroambiguus which are situated in the medulla oblongata. Usually, ventral group neurons were collectively called **expiratory center**. Ventral respiratory group has both **inspiratory** and **expiratory neurons**.

Function

Normally, ventral group neurons are inactive during quiet breathing and become active during forced breathing. During forced breathing, these neurons stimulate both inspiratory muscles and expiratory muscles.

■ PONTINE CENTERS

1. Apneustic Center

Apneustic center is situated in nuclei of reticular formation of lower pons.

Function

Apneustic center increases depth of inspiration by acting directly on dorsal respiratory group of neurons.

2. Pneumotaxic Center

Pneumotaxic center is situated in nuclei of reticular formation in upper pons. It is formed by neurons of medial parabrachial and subparabrachial nuclei.

Function

Primary function of pneumotaxic center is to control the medullary respiratory centers, particularly the dorsal group neurons. It acts through apneustic center. Pneumotaxic center inhibits the apneustic center so that the dorsal group neurons are inhibited. Because of this, inspiration stops and expiration starts. Thus, pneumotaxic center influences the switching between inspiration and expiration. Pneumotaxic center increases respiratory rate by reducing the duration of inspiration.

■ CONNECTIONS OF RESPIRATORY CENTERS

Efferent Pathway

Nerve fibers from respiratory centers leave brainstem and descend in spinal cord and terminate on the motor neurons in the anterior horn cells of cervical and thoracic segments of spinal cord.

From the motor neurons of spinal cord two sets of nerve fibers arise:

1. Phrenic nerve fibers (C3 to C5) which supply the diaphragm.
2. Intercostal nerve fibers (T1 to T11) which supply the external intercostal muscles.

Afferent Pathway

Impulses from peripheral chemoreceptors and baroreceptors are carried to respiratory centers by the branches of glossopharyngeal and vagus nerves. Vagal nerve fibers also carry impulses from stretch receptors of lungs to the respiratory centers.

Thus, the respiratory centers receive afferent impulses from different parts of the body and modulate the movements of thoracic cage and lungs accordingly through efferent nerve fibers.

TABLE 73.1: Respiratory centers.

Features	Medullary centers		Pontine centers	
	Dorsal respiratory group of neurons	Ventral respiratory group of neurons	Apneustic center	Pneumotaxic center
Situation	Nucleus of tractus solitarius	Nucleus ambiguous and Nucleus retroambiguus	Nuclei of reticular formation of lower pons	Nuclei of reticular formation of upper pons
Type of neurons	Inspiratory neurons	Inspiratory neurons and expiratory neurons	Inspiratory neurons	Neurons of parabrachial and subparabrachial nuclei
Function	Generate inspiratory ramp Has autorhythmicity Always active	Inactive during quiet breathing Active during forced breathing	Prolonged inspiration and short expiration	Switching between inspiration and expiration by inhibiting inspiration through apneustic center

INTEGRATION OF RESPIRATORY CENTERS

Role of Medullary Centers

Rhythmic discharge of inspiratory impulses

Dorsal respiratory group neurons maintain the normal rhythm of respiration by discharge of impulses (action potentials) rhythmically. These impulses are transmitted to the respiratory muscles by phrenic and intercostal nerves.

Inspiratory ramp

Inspiratory ramp is the pattern of discharge from dorsal respiratory group neurons characterized by steady increase in amplitude of the action potential. To start with, the amplitude of action potential is low due to the activation of only few neurons. Later, more and more neurons are activated leading to gradual increase in the amplitude of the action potential in a **ramp fashion**. Impulses of this type of firing from dorsal group neurons are called **inspiratory ramp signals**.

Impulses from dorsal group of neurons are produced only for a period of **2 seconds** during which inspiration occurs. After 2 seconds, the ramp signals stop abruptly and do not appear for another **3 seconds**. Switching off ramp signals causes expiration. At the end of 3 seconds, the inspiratory ramp signals reappear in same pattern, and the cycle is repeated.

Normally, during inspiration, dorsal respiratory group neurons inhibit expiratory neurons of ventral group. During expiration, the expiratory neurons inhibit the dorsal group neurons. Thus, the medullary respiratory centers control each other.

Significance of inspiratory ramp signals

Significance of inspiratory ramp signals is that there is a slow and steady inspiration so that, the filling of lungs with air is also steady.

Role of Pontine Centers

Pontine respiratory centers regulate the medullary centers. Apneustic center accelerates the activity of dorsal group of neurons and the stimulation of this center, causes prolonged inspiration.

Pneumotaxic center inhibits the apneustic center and restricts the duration of inspiration.

Pre-Bötzinger Complex

Pre-Bötzinger complex (pre-BötC) is an additional respiratory center found in animals. It is formed by a group of neurons called pacemaker neurons, which generate the rhythmic respiratory impulses. Exact functioning mechanism of this complex is not known.

FACTORS AFFECTING RESPIRATORY CENTERS

Respiratory centers regulate the respiratory movements, by receiving impulses from various sources in the body.

1. *Impulses from Higher Centers*

Higher centers alter the respiration by sending impulses directly to dorsal group neurons. Impulses from various parts of **cerebral cortex** such as anterior cingulate gyrus, olfactory tubercle and posterior orbital gyrus inhibit the respiration. Impulses from motor area and Sylvian area of cerebral cortex produce forced breathing.

2. *Impulses from Stretch Receptors of Lungs: Hering-Breuer Reflex*

Hering-Breuer reflex is a **protective reflex** that restricts the inspiration and prevents **overstretching** of lung tissues. It is initiated by the stimulation of stretch receptors of air passage.

Stretch receptors give response to stretch of the tissues. During inspiration, there is stretching of lungs due to entrance of air resulting in stimulation of stretch receptors on bronchi and bronchioles. Impulses from stretch receptors pass through vagal afferent fibers to respiratory centers and inhibit the dorsal group neurons. So, inspiration stops and expiration starts. Thus, overstretching of lung tissues is prevented.

However, Hering-Breuer reflex does not operate during quiet breathing. It operates, only when the tidal volume increases beyond 1,000 mL.

This reflex is also called Hering-Breuer inflation reflex since occurs due to inflation of lungs during inspiration. The reverse of this reflex is called Hering-Breuer deflation reflex and it takes place during expiration. During expiration as the stretching of lungs is abolished, the deflation of lungs occurs.

3. *Impulses from 'J' Receptors of Lungs*

'J' receptors are **juxtacapillary receptors** which are present on the wall of alveoli and having close contact with pulmonary capillaries.

Stimulation of the 'J' receptors produces a reflex response, which is characterized by apnea followed by hyperventilation, bradycardia, hypotension and weakness of skeletal muscles.

Role of 'J' receptors in physiological conditions is not clear. However, these receptors are responsible for hyperventilation in the patients affected by pulmonary congestion and left heart failure.

4. *Impulses from Irritant Receptors of Lungs*

Besides stretch receptors, there is another type of receptors in the bronchi and bronchioles, called irritant receptors. The irritant receptors are stimulated by irritant chemical agents such as ammonia and sulfur dioxide.

Stimulation of irritant receptors produces reflex hyperventilation along with bronchospasm. Hyperventilation along with bronchospasm prevents further entry of harmful agents into the alveoli.

5. Impulses from Baroreceptors

Baroreceptors are the receptors which give response to change in blood pressure. Refer Chapter 62 for details of baroreceptors.

Whenever arterial blood pressure increases, baroreceptors are activated and send inhibitory impulses to vasomotor center in medulla oblongata. This causes decrease in blood pressure and inhibition of respiration. However, in physiological conditions, the role of baroreceptors in regulation of respiration is insignificant.

6. Impulses from Chemoreceptors

Chemoreceptors play an important role in the chemical regulation of respiration. Details of the chemoreceptors and chemical regulation of respiration are explained later in this chapter.

7. Impulses from Proprioceptors

Proprioceptors are the receptors, which give response to the change in the position of body. These receptors are situated in joints, tendons and muscles.

Proprioceptors are stimulated during the muscular exercise and, send impulses to brain particularly, the cerebral cortex through somatic afferent nerves. Cerebral cortex in turn causes hyperventilation by sending impulses to the medullary respiratory centers.

8. Impulses from Thermoreceptors

Thermoreceptors are the cutaneous receptors, which give response to change in the environmental temperature. There are two types of temperature receptors, namely, the receptors for cold and the receptors for warmth.

When the body is **exposed to cold** or when cold water is applied over the body, cold receptors are stimulated and, send impulses to cerebral cortex via somatic afferent nerves. Cerebral cortex in turn stimulates the respiratory centers and causes hyperventilation.

9. Impulses from Pain Receptors

Pain receptors are the receptors which give response to pain stimulus. Whenever pain receptors are stimulated, the impulses are sent to cerebral cortex via somatic afferent nerves. Cerebral cortex in turn stimulates the respiratory centers and causes hyperventilation

■ CHEMICAL MECHANISM

Chemical mechanism of regulation of respiration is operated through the chemoreceptors which give response to changes in chemical constituents of blood such as hypoxia, hypercapnia and increased hydrogen ion concentration.

Types of Chemoreceptors

Chemoreceptors are classified into two groups namely central chemoreceptors and peripheral chemoreceptors.

■ CENTRAL CHEMORECEPTORS

Chemoreceptors present in the brain are called the central chemoreceptors. These chemoreceptors are situated in medulla oblongata, close to dorsal respiratory group of neurons. This area with chemoreceptors is known as **chemosensitive area**. Chemoreceptors are in close contact with blood and cerebrospinal fluid.

Mechanism of Action

Main stimulant for the central chemoreceptors is the increased hydrogen ion concentration.

Hydrogen ion concentration increases in the blood, it cannot stimulate the central chemoreceptors because, the hydrogen ions from blood cannot cross the blood-brain barrier and blood cerebrospinal fluid barrier.

On the other hand, carbon dioxide can easily cross the blood-brain barrier and blood cerebrospinal fluid barrier and enter the interstitial fluid of brain or the cerebrospinal fluid. There, the carbon dioxide combines with water to form carbonic acid. Since carbonic acid is unstable, it immediately dissociates into hydrogen ion and bicarbonate ion.

$$CO_2 + H_2O \longrightarrow H_2CO_3 \longrightarrow H^+ + HCO_3^-$$

Hydrogen ions stimulate the central chemoreceptors. Chemoreceptors in turn send stimulatory impulses to dorsal respiratory group of neurons causing increased ventilation (increased rate and force of breathing).

■ PERIPHERAL CHEMORECEPTORS

Chemoreceptors present in the carotid and aortic region are called peripheral chemoreceptors. Refer Chapter 62 for details.

Mechanism of Action

Reduction in partial pressure of oxygen is the most potent stimulant for peripheral chemoreceptors. Whenever, partial pressure of oxygen decreases, the chemoreceptors are stimulated and send impulses through aortic and Hering's nerves. These impulses reach the respiratory centers, particularly the dorsal group of neurons and stimulate them. Dorsal group of neurons send stimulatory impulses to respiratory muscles resulting in increased ventilation.

This provides enough oxygen and rectifies the lack of oxygen.

Peripheral chemoreceptors are mildly sensitive to the increased partial pressure of carbon dioxide and increased hydrogen ion concentration.

Chapter 74: Diseases and Disorders of Respiration

CHAPTER OUTLINE

- RESPIRATORY PATTERNS
- APNEA
- HYPERVENTILATION
- HYPOVENTILATION
- HYPOXIA
- OXYGEN TOXICITY (POISONING)
- HYPERCAPNIA
- HYPOCAPNIA
- ASPHYXIA
- DYSPNEA
- PERIODIC BREATHING
- CYANOSIS
- CARBON MONOXIDE POISONING
- BRONCHIAL ASTHMA
- OTHER RESPIRATORY DISORDERS

■ RESPIRATORY PATTERNS

Normal respiratory pattern is called **eupnea**. Respiratory pattern is altered by many ways.

■ ALTERED PATTERNS OF RESPIRATION

1. *Tachypnea*: Increase in rate of respiration.
2. *Bradypnea*: Decrease in rate of respiration.
3. *Polypnea*: Rapid, shallow breathing resembling panting in dogs. In this type of breathing, only the rate of respiration increases but the force does not increase significantly.
4. *Apnea*: Temporary arrest of breathing.
5. *Hyperpnea*: Increase in pulmonary ventilation due to increase in force of breathing with or without increase in rate of respiration.
6. *Hyperventilation*: Abnormal increase in rate and force of respiration. It is also called over breathing and it results in excess removal of carbon dioxide (see below for details).
7. *Hypoventilation*: Decrease in rate and force of respiration.
8. *Dyspnea*: Difficulty in breathing.
9. *Periodic breathing*: Abnormal respiratory rhythm.

■ APNEA

Apnea is defined as temporary arrest of breathing. Apnea can also be produced voluntarily which is called **breath holding** or **voluntary apnea**. The breath holding time is known as **apnea time**. It is about 45 to 55 seconds in a normal adult, after a deep inspiration.

Apnea occurs in the following conditions:

1. Voluntary effort (voluntary breath holding).
2. After hyperventilation.
3. During deglutition (deglutition apnea: Chapter 31).
4. Sleep apnea (apnea during sleep).

■ HYPERVENTILATION

Hyperventilation or **over breathing** or **over ventilation** is increased pulmonary ventilation due to rapid and forced breathing. Both rate and force of breathing are increased.

■ CAUSES OF HYPERVENTILATION

Hyperventilation mostly occurs in conditions like exercise when partial pressure of carbon dioxide is increased. Excess of carbon dioxide stimulates the respiratory centers. Voluntarily also, hyperventilation can be produced. It is called **voluntary hyperventilation**.

■ EFFECTS OF HYPERVENTILATION

Common features of hyperventilation are dizziness, feeling of fainting and chest pain. During hyperventilation, excess carbon dioxide is washed out. In blood, the partial pressure of carbon dioxide is reduced. It causes suppression of respiratory centers, resulting in **apnea**. Apnea is followed

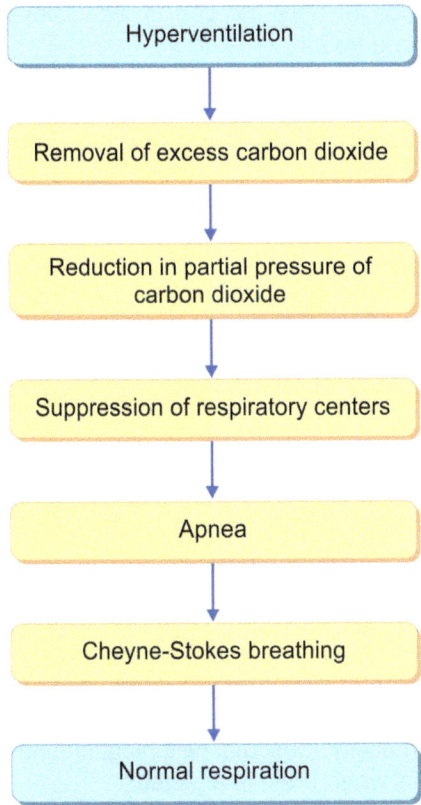

FIGURE 74.1: Effects of hyperventilation.

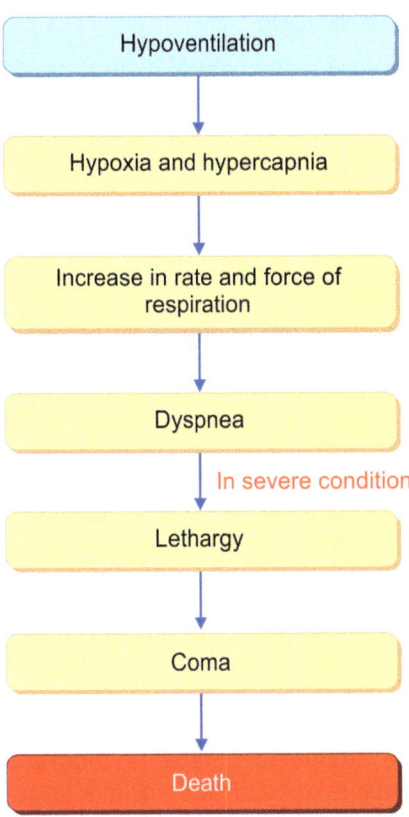

FIGURE 74.2: Effects of hypoventilation.

by Cheyne-Stokes type of periodic breathing. After a period of **Cheyne-Stokes breathing,** normal respiration is restored **(Fig. 74.1)**.

■ HYPOVENTILATION

Hypoventilation is the decrease in pulmonary ventilation caused by decrease in rate or force of breathing. Thus, the amount of air moving in and out of lungs is reduced.

■ CAUSES OF HYPOVENTILATION

Hypoventilation occurs when respiratory centers are suppressed or by administration of some drugs. It also occurs during partial **paralysis** of respiratory muscles.

■ EFFECTS OF HYPOVENTILATION

Hypoventilation results in development of **hypoxia** along with **hypercapnia**. It increases the rate and force of respiration, leading to **dyspnea**. Severe conditions result in lethargy, coma and death **(Fig. 74.2)**.

■ HYPOXIA

Hypoxia is defined as the reduced availability of oxygen to the tissues.

■ CAUSES OF HYPOXIA

Four important causes of hypoxia are:
1. Decreased oxygen tension in arterial blood.
2. Decreased oxygen carrying capacity of blood.
3. Decreased velocity of blood flow.
4. Decreased utilization of oxygen by the cells.

■ CLASSIFICATION OF HYPOXIA

On the basis of these factors, hypoxia is classified into four types:

I. Hypoxic hypoxia.
II. Anemic hypoxia.
III. Stagnant hypoxia.
IV. Histotoxic hypoxia.

I. *Hypoxic Hypoxia*

Hypoxic hypoxia or arterial hypoxia means the decreased **oxygen content** in the blood. Hypoxic hypoxia is caused by low oxygen tension in inspired (atmospheric), respiratory disorders and cardiac disorders.

II. *Anemic Hypoxia*

Anemic hypoxia is the condition characterized by decreased **oxygen carrying capacity** of blood. The oxygen availability is normal. But the blood is not able to take up sufficient amount of oxygen due to anemic condition.

Any condition that causes anemia can cause anemic hypoxia. Common causes for anemic hypoxia are decreased RBC count, decreased hemoglobin content in the blood.

III. *Stagnant Hypoxia*

Stagnant hypoxia or hypokinetic hypoxia is the hypoxia caused by decreased **velocity of blood flow**. Stagnant hypoxia is due to reduction in velocity of blood flow which occurs in conditions such as congestive cardiac failure and hemorrhage.

IV. Histotoxic Hypoxia

Histotoxic hypoxia is the type of hypoxia produced by the inability of tissues for **utilization of oxygen**. Histotoxic hypoxia occurs due to cyanide or sulfide poisoning. These substances destroy the cellular oxidative enzymes. So, even if oxygen is supplied, the tissues are not able to utilize it.

■ EFFECTS OF HYPOXIA

1. *Effects on blood*

Hypoxia stimulates the secretion of erythropoietin from kidney. Erythropoietin increases production of RBCs. Thus, the oxygen carrying capacity of blood is improved by increase in RBC count and hemoglobin content.

2. *Effects on cardiovascular system*

Initially, due to the reflex stimulation of cardiac and vasomotor centers, there is increase in rate and force of contraction of heart, cardiac output and blood pressure. Later, there is reduction in the rate and force of contraction of heart. Cardiac output and blood pressure are also decreased.

3. *Effects on respiration*

Initially, the respiratory rate is increased due to chemoreceptor reflex. Because of this large amount of carbon dioxide is washed out leading to alkalemia. Later, the respiration tends to be shallow and periodic. Finally, the rate and force of breathing are reduced to a great extent due to the failure of respiratory centers.

4. *Effects on digestive system*

Hypoxia is associated with loss of appetite, nausea and vomiting. Mouth becomes dry and there is a feeling of thirst.

5. *Effects on kidney*

Juxtaglomerular apparatus of kidney secretes erythropoietin. Alkaline urine is excreted.

6. *Effects on central nervous system*

In mild hypoxia, the symptoms are similar to those of **alcoholic intoxication**. The individual is depressed, with loss of self-control. Person becomes talkative, quarrelsome, ill-tempered and rude. Memory is impaired. Muscles become fatigued.

If hypoxia is acute and severe, there is sudden loss of consciousness. If not treated immediately, coma occurs which leads to death.

■ TREATMENT FOR HYPOXIA: OXYGEN THERAPY

Best treatment for hypoxia is oxygen therapy, i.e. treating the affected person with oxygen. Pure oxygen or oxygen combined with another gas is administered. Depending upon the situation, oxygen therapy can be given either under normal atmospheric pressure or under high pressure (**hyperbaric oxygen**).

In Normal Atmospheric Pressure

Pure oxygen is administered with normal atmospheric pressure, i.e. at one atmosphere (760 mm Hg). Administration of pure oxygen is well tolerated by the patient for long hours.

In High Atmospheric Pressure: Hyperbaric Oxygen

Hyperbaric oxygen is the pure oxygen with high atmospheric pressure of 2 or more than 2 atmospheres. Hyperbaric oxygen therapy with 2 to 3 atmospheres is tolerated by the patient for about 5 hours. Refer oxygen toxicity below.

■ OXYGEN TOXICITY

Oxygen toxicity or **oxygen poisoning** is the increased oxygen content in tissues beyond certain critical level.

■ CAUSE OF OXYGEN TOXICITY

Oxygen toxicity is caused by breathing **hyperbaric oxygen** (pure oxygen with a high pressure of 2 to 3 atmosphere).

■ EFFECTS OF OXYGEN TOXICITY

1. Irritation of lung tissues and pulmonary edema.
2. Destruction of cytochrome system leading to damage of tissues due to increase metabolic rate.
3. Hyperirritability, muscular twitching, ringing in ears and dizziness when brain is affected.
4. Finally, convulsions, coma and death.

■ HYPERCAPNIA

Hypercapnia is the increased carbon dioxide content of blood.

■ CAUSES OF HYPERCAPNIA

It occurs in conditions such as asphyxia and breathing air containing excess carbon dioxide.

■ EFFECTS OF HYPERCAPNIA

1. Dyspnea.
2. Reduction in pH of blood.
3. Increase in heart rate and blood pressure.
4. Headache, depression and laziness.
5. Muscular rigidity, tremors and convulsions.
6. Giddiness and loss of consciousness.

■ HYPOCAPNIA

Hypocapnia is the decreased carbon dioxide content in blood.

■ CONDITIONS WHEN HYPOCAPNIA OCCURS

It occurs in conditions associated with hypoventilation. It also occurs after prolonged hyperventilation.

■ EFFECTS OF HYPOCAPNIA

1. Rate and force of respiration decrease.
2. Increase in pH of blood leading to respiratory alkalosis.
3. Calcium concentration decreases resulting in tetany.
4. Dizziness, mental confusion, muscular twitching and loss of consciousness.

ASPHYXIA

Asphyxia is the condition characterized by combination of hypoxia and hypercapnia due to obstruction of air passage.

CONDITIONS WHEN ASPHYXIA OCCURS

Asphyxia develops in conditions characterized by acute obstruction of air passage such as, hanging, strangulation and drowning.

EFFECTS OF ASPHYXIA

Effects of asphyxia develop in three stages:

1. Stage of Hyperpnea

Hyperpnea is the first stage of asphyxia. It extends for about 1 minute. In this stage, breathing becomes deep and rapid. It is due to the powerful stimulation of respiratory centers by carbon dioxide accumulated. Hyperpnea is followed by **dyspnea** and **cyanosis**. The eyes become more prominent.

2. Stage of Convulsions

This stage is characterized by **convulsions** (uncontrolled involuntary muscular contractions). Duration of this stage is less than one minute. Following effects develop in this stage due to the effect of hypercapnia on brain and spinal cord:

i. Expiratory efforts become more violent.
ii. Generalized convulsions appear.
iii. Heart rate increases.
iv. Arterial blood pressure increases.
v. Consciousness is lost.

3. Stage of Collapse

This stage lasts for about three minutes. Effects developed in this stage are:

i. Depression of brain centers due to lack of oxygen. So, convulsions disappear.
ii. Respiratory gasping occurs with stretching of the body and opening of mouth as if gasping for breath.
iii. Dilatation of pupils.
iv. Reduction in heart rate.
v. Loss of all reflexes.
vi. Gradual increase in the duration between the gasps.
vii. Finally, the death.

All together asphyxia extends only for 5 minutes. The person can be saved by timely help such as relieving the respiratory obstruction, good aeration, etc. Otherwise, death occurs.

DYSPNEA

Dyspnea or air hunger means **difficulty in breathing**. Normally, breathing goes on without our consciousness. When breathing enters the consciousness and produces discomfort, it is called dyspnea. Dyspnea is also defined as consciousness of necessity for increased respiratory effort.

DYSPNEA POINT

Dyspnea point is the level at which there is increased ventilation with severe breathing discomfort.

CONDITIONS WHEN DYSPNEA OCCURS

Physiologically, dyspnea occurs during severe muscular exercise.

Pathological conditions when dyspnea occurs are the following:

1. Obstructive respiratory disorders.
2. Cardiac disorders such as left ventricular failure.
3. Metabolic disorders such as diabetic acidosis.

PERIODIC BREATHING

Periodic breathing is the abnormal or uneven respiratory rhythm. It is of two types, Cheyne-Stokes breathing and Biot breathing.

CHEYNE-STOKES BREATHING

Cheyne-Stokes breathing is the periodic breathing characterized by rhythmic hyperpnea and apnea. It is the most common type of periodic breathing.

Features of Cheyne-Stokes Breathing

Cheyne-Stokes breathing is marked by two alternate patterns of respiration, hyperpneic period and apneic period.

1. Hyperpneic Period: Waxing and Waning of Breathing

To begin with, the breathing is shallow. Force of respiration increases gradually and reaches the maximum (hyperpnea). From there, breathing decreases gradually and reaches minimum. Then it is followed by apnea. The gradual increase followed by gradual decrease in force of respiration is called waxing and waning of breathing (Fig. 74.3).

2. Apneic Period

When, the force of breathing is reduced to minimum, cessation of breathing occurs for a short period. It is again followed by hyperpneic period and the cycle is repeated.

Causes for waxing and waning

Initially, during forced breathing, large quantity of carbon dioxide is washed out from blood leading to inactivation of respiratory centers. It causes apnea. During apnea, there is accumulation of carbon dioxide with reduction in oxygen tension resulting in activation of respiratory centers. This causes gradual increase in the force of breathing to the maximum. And the cycle is repeated.

Conditions when Cheyne-Stokes Breathing Occurs

Cheyne-Stokes breathing occurs in both physiological and pathological conditions.

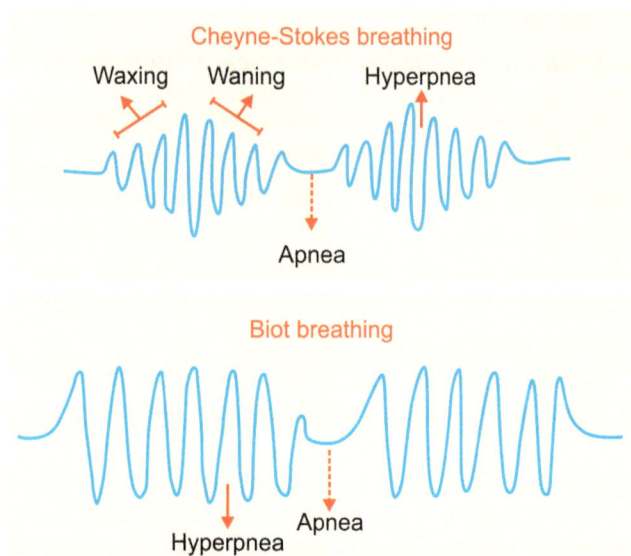

FIGURE 74.3: Periodic breathing.

Physiological conditions when Cheyne-Stokes breathing occurs

1. During deep sleep.
2. In high altitude.
3. After prolonged voluntary hyperventilation.
4. In newborn babies.
5. After severe muscular exercise.

Pathological conditions when Cheyne-Stokes breathing occurs

1. During increased intracranial pressure.
2. During cardiac failure.
3. During renal diseases.
4. Poisoning by narcotics.
5. In premature infants.

BIOT BREATHING

Biot breathing is another form of periodic breathing characterized by period of apnea and hyperpnea.

Features of Biot Breathing

There is no waxing and waning of breathing **(Fig. 74.3)**. After apneic period, hyperpnea occurs abruptly.

Causes of Abrupt Apnea and Hyperpnea

Due to apnea, carbon dioxide accumulates and it stimulates the respiratory centers leading to hyperpnea. During hyperpnea, lot of carbon dioxide is washed out. So, the respiratory centers are not stimulated and apnea occurs.

Conditions when Biot's Breathing Occurs

Biot's breathing occurs only in pathological conditions such as nervous disorders involving lesions in respiratory centers.

CYANOSIS

Cyanosis is defined as diffused **bluish coloration** of skin and mucus membrane.

CAUSE FOR CYANOSIS

Cyanosis is caused by the presence of large amount of reduced hemoglobin in the blood. Quantity of reduced hemoglobin should be at least 5 to 7 g/dL in the blood to cause cyanosis.

CONDITIONS WHEN CYANOSIS OCCURS

1. Any condition which leads to arterial hypoxia and stagnant hypoxia.
2. Conditions when altered hemoglobin such as methemoglobin or sulfhemoglobin is formed.
3. Conditions like polycythemia when blood flow is slow.

CARBON MONOXIDE POISONING

Carbon monoxide is a dangerous gas because it displaces oxygen from hemoglobin. Common sources for carbon monoxide are exhaust of gasoline engines, coal mines, gases from guns, deep wells and underground drainage system.

EFFECTS OF CARBON MONOXIDE

Carbon monoxide binds with same site in hemoglobin for oxygen. More over hemoglobin has 200 times more affinity for carbon monoxide than oxygen. So, oxygen transport and oxygen carrying capacity of the blood are decreased.

SYMPTOMS OF CARBON MONOXIDE POISONING

Symptoms of carbon monoxide poisoning depend upon its concentration in air:

1. While breathing air with 1% of carbon monoxide, mild symptoms like headache and nausea appear.
2. While breathing air containing carbon monoxide above 1% causes convulsions, cardiorespiratory arrest, loss of consciousness and coma occur.
3. High carbon monoxide content in air causes death.

BRONCHIAL ASTHMA

Bronchial asthma is the inflammatory disease of respiratory tract characterized by recurrent attacks of difficult breathing with **wheezing**. Asthma is a **paroxysmal order** because the attack commences suddenly.

Wheezing

Wheezing is a high-pitched **whistling** sound produced while breathing. It is associated with difficult breathing.

Wheezing occurs due to obstruction of air passage because of bronchiolar constriction.

CAUSES OF BRONCHIAL ASTHMA

1. Leukotrienes released from eosinophils and mast cells during inflammation cause bronchoconstriction (bronchospasm).
2. Asthma is caused by exposure allergic substances which produce hypersensitivity of nerve fibers to larynx and nose.
3. Pulmonary edema and congestion of lungs caused by left ventricular failure also leads to asthma. Asthma developed in this condition is called cardiac asthma.

FEATURES OF BRONCHIAL ASTHMA

1. During the asthma attack, the difficulty is felt both during inspiration and expiration. More difficulty is experienced during expiration.
2. Because of difficulty during expiration, the lungs are not deflated completely, so that the residual volume and functional residual capacity are increased.
3. Tidal volume, vital capacity, FEV_1 and alveolar ventilation are decreased.
4. Carbon dioxide accumulates, resulting in acidosis, dyspnea and cyanosis.

OTHER RESPIRATORY DISORDERS

ATELECTASIS

Atelectasis is the partial or complete **collapse of lungs**. When a large portion of lung is collapsed, the partial pressure of oxygen is reduced in blood, leading to dyspnea and death.

Atelectasis is caused by deficiency of surfactant, obstruction of bronchus or bronchiole. It is also caused by presence of air **(pneumothorax)**, fluid **(hydrothorax)**, blood **(hemothorax)** or pus **(pyothorax)** in the pleural space.

PNEUMONIA

Pneumonia is the **inflammation** of lung tissues, followed by the accumulation of blood cells, fibrin and exudates in the alveoli. Affected part of the lungs becomes **consolidated**. Inflammation of lung is caused by bacterial or viral infection and inhaling noxious chemical substance.

PULMONARY EDEMA

Pulmonary edema is the accumulation of serous fluid in the alveoli and the interstitial tissue of lungs. It is caused by increased pulmonary capillary pressure (due to left ventricular failure or mitral valve disease), pneumonia and breathing harmful chemicals.

PLEURAL EFFUSION

Pleural effusion is the accumulation of large amount of fluid in pleural cavity. Pleural effusion occurs because of blockage of lymphatic drainage, flow of fluid from pulmonary capillaries and inflammation of pleural membrane.

PULMONARY TUBERCULOSIS

Tuberculosis is the disease caused by **tubercle bacilli**. This disease can affect any organ in the body. However, the lungs are affected more commonly. Infected tissue is invaded by macrophages and later it becomes fibrous. Affected tissue is called **tubercle**. In severe conditions, the destruction of the lung tissue is followed by formation of large **abscess cavities**.

EMPHYSEMA

Emphysema is an **obstructive respiratory disease** characterized by extensive **damage of lung tissues**. It is caused by cigarette smoking, oxidant gases and untreated bronchitis.

Chapter 75: High Altitude, Deep Sea Physiology and Exposure to Cold and Heat

CHAPTER OUTLINE

- **HIGH ALTITUDE PHYSIOLOGY**
  - BAROMETRIC PRESSURE AND PARTIAL PRESSURE OF OXYGEN AT DIFFERENT ALTITUDES
  - CHANGES IN THE BODY AT HIGH ALTITUDE
  - MOUNTAIN SICKNESS
  - ACCLIMATIZATION
  - AVIATION PHYSIOLOGY
  - SPACE PHYSIOLOGY
- **DEEP SEA PHYSIOLOGY**
  - BAROMETRIC PRESSURE AT DIFFERENT DEPTHS
  - EFFECT OF HIGH BAROMETRIC PRESSURE: NITROGEN NARCOSIS
  - DECOMPRESSION SICKNESS
- **EFFECTS OF EXPOSURE TO COLD**
  - HEAT PRODUCTION
  - PREVENTION OF HEAT LOSS
- **EFFECTS OF EXPOSURE TO SEVERE COLD**
  - LOSS OF TEMPERATURE REGULATING CAPACITY
  - FROSTBITE
- **EFFECTS OF EXPOSURE TO HEAT**
  - HEAT EXHAUSTION
  - DEHYDRATION EXHAUSTION
  - HEAT CRAMPS
  - HEATSTROKE: SUNSTROKE

HIGH ALTITUDE PHYSIOLOGY

Any altitude above 8,000 ft from mean sea level is called high altitude. People can ascend up to this level without any adverse effect.

At high altitudes, amount of oxygen available in the atmosphere is same as in sea level. But the barometric pressure is low. So, the partial pressure of gases, particularly oxygen decreases leading to hypoxia. Carbon dioxide in high altitude is very much negligible and it does not create any problem.

BAROMETRIC PRESSURE AND PARTIAL PRESSURE OF OXYGEN AT DIFFERENT ALTITUDES

Barometric pressure and partial pressure of oxygen at different altitudes and their common effects on the body are given in **Table 75.1**.

CHANGES IN THE BODY AT HIGH ALTITUDE

During exposure to high altitude, most of changes occur in the body because of rapid ascent. Besides hypoxia, some other factors are also responsible for changes in the functions of the body at high altitude.

Factors Affecting Physiological Functions at High Altitude

1. Hypoxia.
2. Expansion of gases.
3. Fall in atmospheric temperature.
4. Light rays.

1. Effect of Hypoxia

Refer Chapter 74 for effects of hypoxia on physiological functions.

2. Effects of Expansion of Gases

Volume of gases increases when the barometric pressure is reduced. So, at high altitude, volume of all gases increases in atmospheric air, as well as in the body. Expansion of gases in GI tract causes painful distention of stomach and intestine. It is minimized by supporting the abdomen with a belt or by evacuation of the gases. Expansion of gases also destroys the alveoli.

During very rapid ascent from sea level to over 30,000 feet height, the gases evolve as bubbles, particularly nitrogen, resulting in decompression sickness (see below).

TABLE 75.1: Barometric pressure, partial pressure of oxygen and common effects at different altitudes.

Altitude (feet)	Barometric pressure (mm Hg)	Partial pressure of oxygen (mm Hg)	Common effects
Sea level	760	159	–
5,000	600	132	No hypoxia
10,000	523	110	Mild symptoms of hypoxia start appearing
15,000	400	90	Moderate hypoxia develops with following symptoms: 1. Reduction in visual acuity 2. Effects on mental functions 3. Improper judgment 4. Feeling of overconfidence
20,000	349	73	Severe hypoxia appears with cardiorespiratory symptoms such as: 1. Increase in heart rate and cardiac output 2. Increase in respiratory rate and respiratory minute volume This is the highest level for permanent inhabitants
25,000	250	62	This is the critical altitude for survival: 1. Hypoxia becomes severe 2. Breathing oxygen becomes essential
29,628	235	49	This is the height of Mount Everest
30,000	226	47	Symptoms become severe even with oxygen
50,000	87	18	Hypoxia becomes more severe even with pure oxygen

3. Effects of Reduced Atmospheric Temperature

Environmental temperature falls gradually at high altitudes. Temperature decreases to about 0°C at the height of 10,000 feet. It becomes – 22°C at the height of 20,000 feet. At the altitude of 40,000 feet, the temperature falls to – 44°C. Injury or **frostbite** occurs if the body is not adequately protected by warm clothing.

4. Effects of Light Rays

Skin becomes susceptible for injury due to many harmful rays such as **ultraviolet rays** of sunlight. Moreover, the sunrays reflected by the snow might injure the retina of the eye, if it is not protected with suitable tinted glasses.

■ MOUNTAIN SICKNESS

Mountain sickness is the condition characterized by adverse effects of hypoxia at high altitude. It develops in persons going to high altitude for the first time. It occurs within a day in these persons before they get acclimatized to high altitude.

Symptoms of Mountain Sickness

1. *Digestive system*: Loss of appetite, nausea and vomiting occur because of expansion of gases in the gastrointestinal tract.
2. *Cardiovascular system:* Heart rate increases.
3. *Respiratory system*: Pulmonary blood pressure increases due to hypoxia-nduced vasodilatation and increased blood flow. Increased pulmonary blood pressure results in pulmonary edema and breathlessness.
4. *Nervous system*: Symptoms of nervous system are weakness, fatigue, headache, depression, disorientation, irritability, lack of sleep.

Treatment for Mountain Sickness

Treatment depends upon severity of sickness. Symptoms can be reverted by returning to lower altitude or by breathing oxygen. Medical attention is required if symptoms are very severe.

■ ACCLIMATIZATION

Acclimatization is defined as adaptations or the adjustments by the body in high altitude. While staying at high altitudes for several days to several weeks, a person slowly gets adapted or adjusted to low oxygen tension.

Changes During Acclimatization

During acclimatization, various changes occur in the body to cope with the adverse effects of hypoxia at high altitude.

1. Changes in blood

RBC count and packed cell volume increase. Hemoglobin content in the blood rises to 20 g%. So, the oxygen carrying capacity of the blood is increased. Thus, more oxygen can be carried to tissues in spite of hypoxia. All these changes in blood are due to release of erythropoietin from kidney which is induced by hypoxia.

2. Changes in cardiovascular system

Overall activity of cardiovascular system is increased in high altitude. There is increase in rate and force of contraction of heart, cardiac output and blood pressure. Hypoxia-induced vasodilatation increases the vascularity in the body. So, blood flow to the vital organs such as heart, brain, muscles, etc. increases.

3. Respiratory system

i. Pulmonary ventilation increases up to 65% due to the stimulation of chemoreceptors.

ii. **Pulmonary hypertension** develops due to increased cardiac output and pulmonary blood flow.
iii. Diffusing capacity of gases increases in the alveoli due to the increase in pulmonary blood flow and pulmonary ventilation. It enables more diffusion of oxygen into the blood.

4. *Changes in tissues*

Both in human beings and animals residing at high altitudes permanently, the cellular oxidative enzymes involved in metabolic reactions are more than in the inhabitants at sea level.

Even, when a sea level inhabitant stays at high altitude for certain period, quantity of the oxidative enzymes is not increased.

■ AVIATION PHYSIOLOGY

Aviation physiology is the study of physiological responses of the body in **aviation environment.**

Flying affects the body through **accelerative forces** and **gravitational forces,** which are developed during the **flight maneuvering.** Pilots and other crew members of aircraft are trained to overcome the effects of these forces.

Accelerative Force

Acceleration means **change in velocity**. Flying straight in horizontal plane with constant velocity has minimum effects on the body. However, changes in velocity produce severe physiological effects. Accelerative forces are developed in the flight during linear, radial or centripetal and angular acceleration.

Gravitational Force: G Unit

Gravitational force (G force) is the major factor that develops accelerative force. Force or pull of gravity upon the body is expressed in **G unit.** On the earth, this pull is responsible for body weight. Force of gravity while sitting, standing or lying position is considered to be equal to body weight and it is referred as 1 G. G unit increases in acceleration.

While traveling in an airplane, elevator or a car, if there is a sudden change in speed or direction, the passengers are thrown or centrifuged in opposite direction. It is because of change in the G unit.

While flying, G unit cause physiological changes in the body. Body can be protected from the effects of G forces, particularly positive G by using abdominal belt and anti-G suit.

■ SPACE PHYSIOLOGY

Space physiology is the study of physiological responses of the body in space and space crafts.

Major differences between the environments of earth and space are atmospheric factors, radiation and gravity. These three factors challenge the human survival in space. Atmospheric factors include atmospheric pressure, temperature, humidity and gas composition.

Spacecraft or **spacelab** is provided with stable and sophisticated environmental control system, which maintains all the atmospheric factors close to earth's environment. **Astronauts** also wear **launch and entry suit (LES)** which is a pressurized suit that protects the body from space environment.

Another factor which affects the body in the space is **weightlessness**, which is due to absence of gravity (microgravity).

■ DEEP SEA PHYSIOLOGY

In high altitude, the problem is with low atmospheric (barometric) pressure. In deep sea or mines, the problem is with high barometric pressure. Increased barometric pressure in deep sea produce two major problems:

1. Compression effect on the body and internal organs.
2. Decrease in volume of gases.

■ BAROMETRIC PRESSURE AT DIFFERENT DEPTHS

At sea level, the barometric pressure is 760 mm Hg, which is referred as 1 atmosphere. At the depth of every 33 feet (about 10 m), the pressure increases by 1 atmosphere.

Thus, at the depth of 33 feet, the pressure is 2 atmospheres. It is due to the air above water and the weight of water itself. Pressure at different depths is given in **Table 75.2**.

TABLE 75.2: Barometric pressure and the effects at different depth.

Depth (feet)	Atmospheric pressure (atmosphere)	Effects on the subject
Sea level	1	–
33	2	–
66	3	–
100	4	Symptoms of nitrogen narcosis appear
133	5	Lack of concentration Becomes jovial and careless
166	6	Starts feeling drowsy
200	7	Feels fatigued and weak Becomes very careless
233	8	Loses power of judgment Unable to do skilled work
266	9	Becomes unconscious

Chapter 75: High Altitude, Deep Sea Physiology and Exposure to Cold and Heat

■ EFFECT OF HIGH BAROMETRIC PRESSURE: NITROGEN NARCOSIS

Narcosis means unconsciousness or **stupor** (lethargy with suppression of sensations and feelings) produced by drugs. **Nitrogen narcosis** means narcotic effect produced by nitrogen at high pressure. Nitrogen narcosis is common in deep sea divers.

Mechanism of Nitrogen Narcosis

Nitrogen is soluble in fat. During compression by high barometric pressure in deep sea, nitrogen escapes from blood vessels and gets dissolved in the fat present in various parts of the body, especially the neuronal membranes. The dissolved nitrogen acts like an anesthetic agent suppressing the neuronal excitability. Nitrogen remains in dissolved form in the fat till the person remains in the deep sea. When the ascends up, decompression sickness develops.

Symptoms of Nitrogen Narcosis

1. First symptom starts appearing at a depth of 120 feet. The person becomes very jovial, careless and does not understand the seriousness of the conditions.
2. At the depth of 150 to 200 feet, the person becomes drowsy.
3. At 200 to 250 feet depth, the person becomes extremely fatigued and weak. There is loss of concentration and judgment. Ability to perform skilled work or movements is also lost.
4. Beyond the depth of 250 feet, the person becomes unconscious.

■ DECOMPRESSION SICKNESS

Decompression sickness is the disorder that occurs when a person returns rapidly to normal surroundings (atmospheric pressure) from the area of high atmospheric pressure such as deep sea. It is also known as dysbarism, compressed air sickness, caisson disease, bends or diver's palsy.

Causes of Decompression Sickness

High barometric pressure at deep sea leads to compression of gases in the body. Compression reduces the volume of gases.

Among the respiratory gases, oxygen is utilized by tissues. Carbon dioxide can be exhaled out. But, nitrogen, which is present in high concentration, i.e. 80% is an inert gas. So, it is neither utilized nor exhaled. When nitrogen is compressed by high atmospheric pressure in deep sea, it escapes from blood vessels and enters the organs. As it is fat soluble, it gets dissolved in the fat of the tissues and tissue fluids. It is very common in the brain tissues.

As long as the person remains in deep sea, nitrogen remains in solution and does not cause any problem. But, if the person ascends rapidly and returns to atmospheric pressure, decompression sickness occurs.

Due to sudden return to atmospheric pressure, the nitrogen is decompressed and escapes from the tissues at a faster rate. Being a gas, it forms **bubbles** while escaping rapidly. The bubbles travel through blood vessels and ducts. In many places, the bubbles obstruct the blood flow and produce air **embolism,** leading to decompression sickness.

Symptoms of Decompression Sickness

Symptoms of decompression sickness are:
1. Severe pain in tissues, particularly the joints, produced by nitrogen bubbles in the myelin sheath of sensory nerve fibers.
2. Sensation of numbness, tingling or pricking (paresthesia) and itching.
3. Temporary paralysis due to nitrogen bubbles in the myelin sheath of motor nerve fibers.
4. Muscle cramps associated with severe pain.
5. Occlusion of coronary arteries followed by coronary ischemia, caused by bubbles in the blood.
6. Occlusion of blood vessels in brain and spinal cord also.
7. Damage of tissues of brain and spinal cord because of obstruction of blood vessels by the bubbles.
8. Dizziness, paralysis of muscle, shortness of breath and choking.
9. Finally, fatigue, unconsciousness and death.

Prevention of Decompression Sickness

Decompression sickness is prevented by taking proper precautionary measures. While returning to mean sea level, the ascent should be very slow with short stay at regular intervals. Stepwise ascent allows nitrogen to come back to the blood without forming bubbles. It prevents the decompression sickness.

Treatment

If a person is affected by decompression sickness, first **recompression** should be done. It is done by keeping the person in a **recompression chamber**. Then, he is brought back to atmospheric pressure by reducing the pressure slowly. Oxygen therapy may be useful.

■ EFFECTS OF EXPOSURE TO COLD

During exposure to cold, the body temperature is maintained by two mechanisms:
A. Heat production.
B. Prevention of heat loss.

■ HEAT PRODUCTION

When the body is exposed to cold, the heat is produced by the following activities.

1. By Accelerating Metabolic Activities

During exposure to cold, **heat gain center** in hypothalamus is stimulated. It causes secretion of adrenaline and noradrenaline by sympathetic centers. These hormones, especially adrenaline increase heat production by accelerating cellular metabolic activities.

2. By Shivering

Shivering is the increased **involuntary muscular activity** with slight vibration of the body in response to fear, onset of fever or exposure to cold. Shivering occurs when the body temperature falls to about 25°C (77°F).

During exposure to cold, the heat gain center activates the motor center for shivering situated in posterior hypothalamus leading to shivering. Enormous heat is produced during shivering due to severe muscular activities.

■ PREVENTION OF HEAT LOSS

When the body is exposed to cold, the heat gain center in hypothalamus is stimulated. It activates the sympathetic centers in posterior hypothalamus resulting in **cutaneous vasoconstriction** and decrease in blood flow. Due to decrease in cutaneous blood flow, sweat secretion is decreased and heat loss is prevented.

■ EFFECTS OF EXPOSURE TO SEVERE COLD

Exposure of body to severe cold leads to death if quick remedy is not provided. Survival time depends upon the temperature of the environment.

If a person is exposed to ice cold water, i.e. 0°C for 20 to 30 minutes, the body temperature falls below 25°C (77°F) and the person can survive if he is placed immediately in hot water tub with a temperature of 43°C (110°F). The survival time at 9°C (28°F) is about 1 hour and the survival time at 15.5°C (60°F) is about 5 hours.

Effects of exposure of body to extreme cold are:
1. Loss of temperature regulating capacity.
2. Frostbite.

■ LOSS OF TEMPERATURE REGULATING CAPACITY

Temperature regulating capacity of hypothalamus is affected when the body temperature reduces to about 34.4°C (94°F). Hypothalamus totally loses the power of temperature regulation when body temperature falls below 25°C (77°F). Shivering does not occur.

In addition to loss of hypothalamic function, the metabolic activities are also suppressed. Sleep or coma develops due to depression of the central nervous system.

■ FROSTBITE

Frostbite is the **freezing** of the surface of the body when it is exposed to cold. It occurs due to sluggishness of blood flow. Most commonly the exposed areas such as ear lobes and digits of hands and feet are affected. Frostbite is common in mountaineers. Prolonged exposure will lead to permanent damage of the cells followed by thawing and **gangrene** (death and decay of tissues) formation.

■ EFFECTS OF EXPOSURE TO HEAT

Effects of exposure to heat are:
1. Heat exhaustion.
2. Dehydration exhaustion.
3. Heat cramps.
4. Heatstroke: Sunstroke.

■ HEAT EXHAUSTION

Heat exhaustion is the body's response to excess loss of water and salt through sweat caused by exposure to hot environmental conditions. In fact, it is the warning that body is getting too hot. Heat exhaustion results in loss of consciousness and collapse.

■ DEHYDRATION EXHAUSTION

Prolonged exposure to heat results in dehydration. It is due to excess sweating. Dehydration leads to fall in cardiac output, and blood pressure. Collapse occurs if treatment is not given immediately.

■ HEAT CRAMPS

Severe **muscle cramps** (sudden painful involuntary spasmodic contractions of muscles involving chest, abdomen and legs) occur. Cramps are due to reduction in the quantity of salts and water as a result of increased sweating during the continuous exposure to heat.

■ HEATSTROKE: SUNSTROKE

Heatstroke is an abnormal increase in body temperature that occurs during exposure to extreme heat. It is characterized by increase in body temperature above 41°C (106°F) accompanied by some physical and neurological symptoms. Heatstroke is very severe and often becomes fatal if not treated immediately. Hypothalamus loses the power of regulating body temperature.

Sunstroke is the heatstroke that is caused by prolonged exposure to sun during summer in desert or tropical areas.

Features

Common features of heatstroke or sunstroke are:
1. Nausea and vomiting.
2. Dizziness.
3. Headache.
4. Abdominal pain.
5. Difficulty in breathing.
6. Vertigo.
7. Confusion.
8. Muscle cramps and convulsions.
9. Paralysis.
10. Unconsciousness.

If immediate and vigorous treatment is not given, the damage of brain tissues occurs, resulting in coma and death.

Treatment

Person affected by heatstroke or sunstroke must be treated before the damage of organs. The subject should be immediately moved from hot environment and **hospitalized** as soon as possible. Immediate cooling of the body is the usual treatment. The person must be immersed in **cold water** or cold water may be sprayed on the skin. If water supply is not sufficient, cooling the head and neck of the subject should be done first. Ice cubes can be rubbed on head and neck. Ice packs must be kept under armpits and groin. Cooling efforts should be continued till the body temperature falls to about 35°C.

Chapter 76: Artificial Respiration

CHAPTER OUTLINE

- CONDITIONS WHEN ARTIFICIAL RESPIRATION IS REQUIRED
- METHODS OF ARTIFICIAL RESPIRATION
  - MANUAL METHODS
  - MECHANICAL METHODS

CONDITIONS WHEN ARTIFICIAL RESPIRATION IS REQUIRED

Artificial respiration is required whenever there is arrest of breathing without cardiac failure.

Arrest of breathing occurs in the following conditions:

1. Accidents.
2. Drowning.
3. Gas poisoning.
4. Electric shock.
5. Anesthesia.

Stoppage of oxygen supply for 5 minutes causes **irreversible changes** in tissues of brain, particularly tissues of cerebral cortex. So, the artificial respiration (resuscitation) must be started quickly without any delay, before the development of cardiac failure.

Purpose of artificial respiration is to ventilate the alveoli and to stimulate the respiratory centers.

METHODS OF ARTIFICIAL RESPIRATION

Methods of artificial respiration are of two types:

I. Manual methods.
II. Mechanical methods.

MANUAL METHODS

Manual methods of **resuscitation** (process carried out to revive someone from unconsciousness or apparent death) can be applied quickly without waiting for the availability of any mechanical aids.

Affected person must be provided with clear air. The clothes around neck and chest regions must be loosened. Mouth, face and throat should be cleared off mucus, saliva, foreign particles, etc. Tongue must be drawn forward and, it must be prevented from falling posteriorly which may cause airway obstruction.

Manual methods are of two types:

1. Mouth-to-mouth method.
2. Holger-Nielsen method.

1. Mouth-to-Mouth Method

1. Subject is kept in supine position and the **resuscitator** (person who give resuscitation) kneels at the side of the subject.
2. By keeping the thumb on subject's mouth, the lower jaw is pulled downwards. Nostrils of the subject are closed with thumb and index finger of the other hand.
3. Resuscitator then takes a deep inspiration and exhales into the subject's mouth forcefully. Volume of exhaled air must be twice the normal tidal volume. This expands the subject's lungs **(Fig. 76.1)**.
4. Then, the resuscitator removes his mouth from that of the subject. Now, a passive expiration occurs in the subject due to elastic recoil of the lungs.

This procedure is repeated at a rate of 12 to 14 times a minute, till normal respiration is restored.

Mouth-to-mouth method is the most effective manual method because carbon dioxide in expired air of the resuscitator directly stimulates the respiratory centers and facilitates onset of respiration.

Only disadvantage is that the close contact between the mouths of resuscitator and subject may not be acceptable for various reasons.

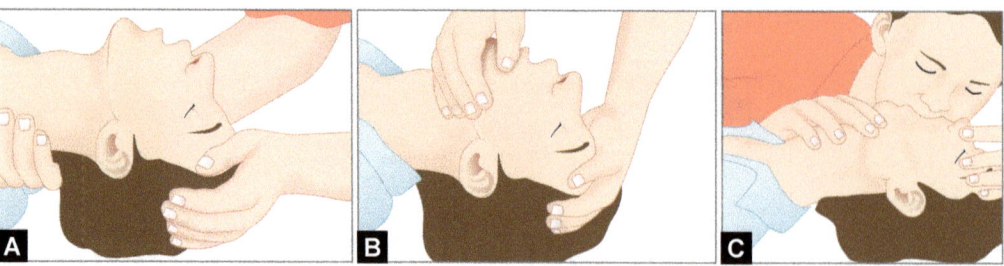

FIGURE 76.1: Mouth-to-mouth method of artificial respiration.
A. Resuscitator kneels by the side of subject.
B. Subject's lower jaw is pulled down and nostrils are closed.
C. Resuscitator takes a deep inspiration and exhales into subject's mouth.
(*Courtesy:* Dr CL Ghai)

Holger-Nielsen Method or Back Pressure Arm Lift Method

1. Subject is placed in prone position with head turned to one side. Hands are placed under the cheeks with flexion at elbow joint and abduction of arms at the shoulders. Resuscitator kneels beside the head of the subject and places the palm of hands over back of the subject.
2. Now, the resuscitator bends forward with straight arms (without flexion at elbow) and applies pressure on the back of the subject. Weight of the resuscitator and pressure on back of the subject compresses his chest and expels air from the lungs.
3. Later, the resuscitator leans back. At the same time, he draws the subject's arm forward by holding it just above elbow **(Fig. 76.2)**.

This procedure causes expansion of thoracic cage and flow of air into the lungs. The movements are repeated at the rate of 12 per minute, till the normal respiration is restored.

■ MECHANICAL METHODS

Mechanical methods of artificial respiration become necessary when the subject needs artificial respiration for long periods. It is essential during the respiratory failure due to paralysis of respiratory muscles or any other cause.

Mechanical methods are of two types:

1. Drinker method.
2. Ventilation method.

1. *Drinker Method*

The machine used in this method is called **iron lung chamber** or **tank respirator**. This equipment has an airtight chamber made of iron or steel. The subject is placed inside this chamber with head outside the chamber.

By means of some pumps, the pressure inside the chamber is made positive and negative alternately. During the negative pressure in chamber, the subject's thoracic cage expands and inspiration occurs. And, during positive pressure the expiration occurs.

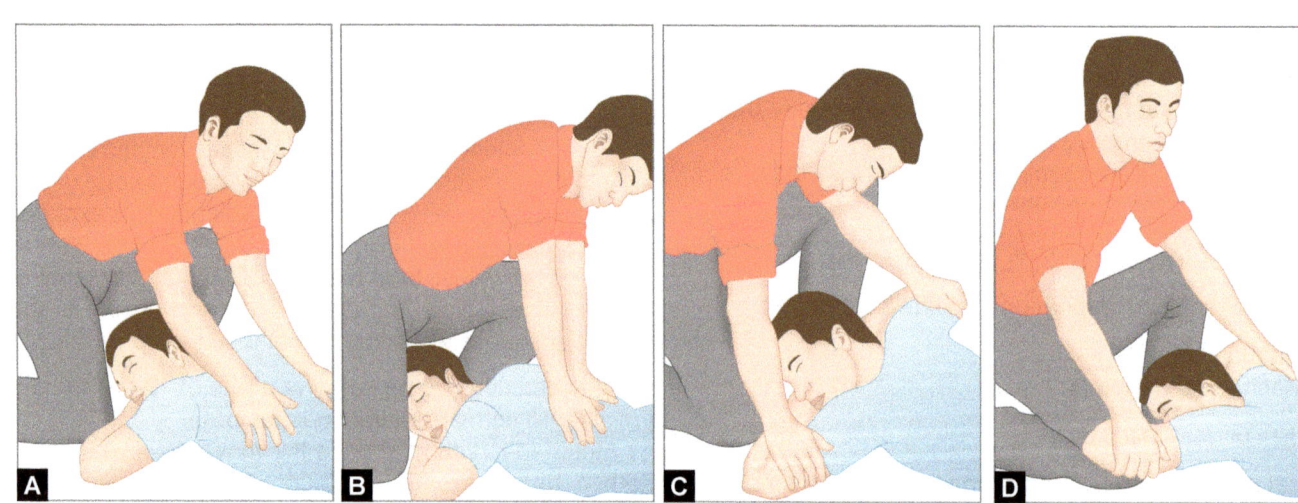

FIGURE 76.2: Holger-Nielsen method of artificial respiration.
A. Resuscitator places his palm over back of subject.
B. Applying pressure on back of subject for expiration.
C. Resuscitator leans back and holds subject's arm.
D. He draws subject's arm forward for inspiration.
(*Courtesy:* Dr CL Ghai)

By using the tank respirator, the patient can survive for a longer time, even up to the period of 1 year till the natural respiratory functions are restored.

2. Ventilation Method

A rubber tube is introduced into the trachea of the patient through the mouth. By using a pump, air or oxygen is pumped into the lungs with pressure intermittently. When air is pumped, inflation of lungs occurs. When it is stopped, expiration occurs and the cycle is repeated.

The apparatus used for ventilation is called ventilator.

Ventilator is of two types:
  i. Volume ventilator.
  ii. Pressure ventilator.

i. *Volume ventilator*

By volume ventilator, a constant volume of air is pumped into the lungs of patients intermittently with minimum pressure.

ii. *Pressure ventilator*

By pressure ventilator, air is pumped into the lungs of subject with constant high pressure.

Chapter 77

Effects of Exercise on Respiration

CHAPTER OUTLINE

- **EFFECTS OF EXERCISE ON RESPIRATION**
  - **PULMONARY VENTILATION**
  - **DIFFUSING CAPACITY FOR OXYGEN**
  - **CONSUMPTION OF OXYGEN**
- **OXYGEN DEBT**
- **VO$_2$ MAX**
- **RESPIRATORY QUOTIENT**

■ EFFECTS OF EXERCISE ON RESPIRATION

Muscular exercise brings about many changes on various systems of the body. The degree of changes depends upon the severity of exercise. Refer Chapter 67 for types and severity of exercise.

■ EFFECT ON PULMONARY VENTILATION

During exercise, **hyperventilation** occurs. In moderate exercise, respiratory rate increases to about 30 per minute and tidal volume increases to about 2,000 mL. Thus, the pulmonary ventilation increases to about 60 L/min during moderate exercise. In severe muscular exercise, it rises still further up to 100 L/min.

■ EFFECT ON DIFFUSING CAPACITY FOR OXYGEN

Diffusing capacity for oxygen is about 21 mL/min/1 mm Hg at resting condition. It rises to 45 to 50 mL/min/1 mm Hg during moderate exercise due to increase in blood flow through the pulmonary capillaries.

■ EFFECT ON CONSUMPTION OF OXYGEN

Oxygen consumed by the tissues, particularly the skeletal muscles is greatly enhanced during exercise. Because of vasodilatation in muscles during exercise, more amount of blood flows through the muscles and more amount of oxygen diffuses into the muscles from blood. The amount of oxygen utilized by the muscles is directly proportional to the amount of oxygen available.

■ OXYGEN DEBT

Oxygen debt is the **extra amount of oxygen** required by the muscles during recovery from severe muscular exercise. After a period of severe muscular exercise, amount of oxygen consumed is greatly increased. Oxygen required is more than the quantity available to the muscle. This much of oxygen is required not only for the activity of the muscle but also for reversal of some metabolic processes such as:

1. Reformation of glucose from lactic acid, accumulated during exercise.
2. Resynthesis of ATP and creatine phosphate.
3. Restoration of amount of oxygen dissociated from hemoglobin and myoglobin.

Thus, for the above reversal phenomena, an extra amount of oxygen must be made available in the body after severe muscular exercise. Oxygen debt is about six times more than the amount of oxygen consumed under resting conditions.

■ VO$_2$ MAX

VO$_2$ max is the amount of oxygen consumed under maximal aerobic metabolism. It is the product of maximal cardiac output and maximal amount of oxygen consumed by the muscle.

In a normal active and healthy male, the VO$_2$ max is 35 to 40 mL/kg body weight/minute. In females, it is 30 to 35 mL/kg/min.

There is an increase of VO$_2$ max by 50% during exercise.

■ RESPIRATORY QUOTIENT

Respiratory quotient is the molar ratio of carbon dioxide production to oxygen consumption. Respiratory quotient in resting condition is 1.0 and during exercise it increases to 1.5 to 2. However, at the end of exercise, respiratory quotient reduces to 0.5.

MODEL QUESTIONS IN RESPIRATORY SYSTEM AND ENVIRONMENTAL PHYSIOLOGY

LONG QUESTIONS

1. Explain the transport of oxygen in blood.
2. Explain the transport of carbon dioxide in blood.
3. Describe the nervous regulation of respiration.
4. Describe the chemical regulation of respiration.
5. What is hypoxia? Describe the types, causes and effects of hypoxia. Add a note on oxygen therapy.
6. Describe changes in the body at high altitude and explain the acclimatization.
7. Describe in detail the respiratory and cardiovascular changes during exercise.

SHORT QUESTIONS

1. Respiratory unit.
2. Nonrespiratory functions of respiratory tract.
3. Salient features of pulmonary circulation.
4. Respiratory pressures.
5. Compliance.
6. Lung volumes.
7. Lung capacities.
8. Dead space.
9. Oxygen hemoglobin dissociation curve.
10. Carbon dioxide dissociation curve.
11. Exchange of gases between alveoli and blood.
12. Exchange of gases between blood and tissues.
13. Respiratory centers.
14. Chemoreceptors.
15. Hypoxia.
16. Asphyxia.
17. Periodic breathing.
18. Mountain sickness.
19. Acclimatization.
20. Decompression sickness.
21. Effects of sudden exposure to cold.
22. Effects of sudden exposure to heat.
23. Heatstroke or sunstroke.
24. Artificial respiration.
25. Respiratory changes during exercise.

VERY SHORT ANSWER QUESTIONS

1. Upper and lower respiratory tract.
2. Intrapleural cavity and intrapleural fluid.
3. Tracheobronchial tree.
4. Role of lungs in defense mechanism.
5. Cough reflex.
6. Sneezing reflex
7. Physiological shunt and physiological dead space.
8. Pulmonary blood pressure.
9. Respiratory muscles.
10. Pump handle and bucket handle movements.
11. Surfactant.
12. Respiratory distress syndrome.
13. Intrapleural and intra-alveolar pressure.
14. Any one lung volume/lung capacity.
15. Vital capacity.
16. Forced expiratory volume or timed vital capacity.
17. Respiratory minute volume.
18. Maximum breathing capacity or maximum ventilation volume.
19. Peak expiratory flow meter.
20. Define ventilation and describe pulmonary ventilation and alveolar ventilation.
21. Ventilation-perfusion ratio.
22. Differences between inspired air and alveolar air.
23. Respiratory membrane.
24. Diffusion capacity and factors affecting it.
25. P_{50}.
26. Oxygen carrying capacity of hemoglobin and blood.
27. What is indicated by shift to the right of oxygen hemoglobin dissociation curve? Name some of the factors causing it.
28. What is indicated by shift to the left of oxygen hemoglobin dissociation curve? Name some of the factors causing it.
29. Chloride shift or Hamburger phenomenon.
30. Bohr effect.
31. Haldane effect.
32. Any one respiratory center.
33. Inspiratory ramp.
34. Hering-Breuer reflex.
35. Different types of receptors in lungs which alter the respiration.
36. Apnea.
37. Oxygen toxicity.
38. Dyspnea.
39. Cheyne-Stokes breathing
40. Biot breathing.
41. Pneumothorax/Hydrothorax/Hemothorax/Pyothorax.
43. Pneumonia.
43. Pulmonary edema.
44. Pleural effusion.
45. Nitrogen narcosis.
46. Frostbite.
47. Ventilator.
48. Oxygen debt.
49. VO_2 max.
50. Mouth-to-mouth method of resuscitation.

SECTION 10 NERVOUS SYSTEM

Chapter 78: Overview of Nervous System, Neuron and Neuroglia

CHAPTER OUTLINE

- DIVISIONS OF NERVOUS SYSTEM
- NEURON AND ITS CLASSIFICATION
- CLASSIFICATION OF NERVE FIBERS
- PROPERTIES OF NERVE FIBERS
- DEGENERATION OF NERVE FIBERS
- REGENERATION OF NERVE FIBER
- NEUROGLIA

■ DIVISIONS OF NERVOUS SYSTEM

Nervous system controls all the activities of the body. It is quicker than the other control system in the body namely, endocrine system.

Nervous system is divided into two parts:

I. Central nervous system.
II. Peripheral nervous system.

● CENTRAL NERVOUS SYSTEM

Central nervous system (CNS) includes **brain** and **spinal cord**. It is formed by **neurons** and the supporting cells called **neuroglia**. Structures of brain and spinal cord are arranged in two layers namely, the gray matter and white matter. **Gray matter** is formed by nerve cell bodies and proximal parts of nerve fibers arising from the nerve cell body. **White matter** is formed by nerve fibers.

In brain, white matter is in inner part and gray matter is placed in the outer part. In spinal cord, white matter is placed in the outer part and gray matter is in inner part.

Brain is situated in the skull. It is continued as spinal cord in the vertebral canal through the **foramen magnum** of the skull bone. Brain and spinal cord are surrounded by three layers of meninges called the outer **dura mater**, middle **arachnoid mater** and inner **pia mater**. The space between the arachnoid mater and pia mater is known as **subarachnoid space**. This space is filled with a fluid called **cerebrospinal fluid (CSF)**. Both, the brain and spinal cord are actually suspended in CSF. Important parts of brain and segments of the spinal cord are shown in **Figure 78.1**.

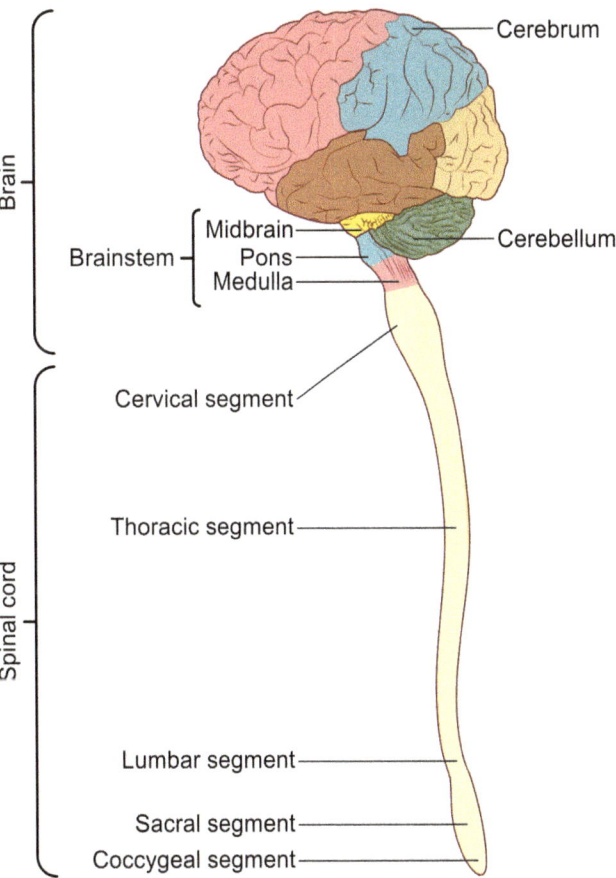

FIGURE 78.1: Parts of central nervous system.

Parts of Brain

Brain consists of three major divisions:

1. Prosencephalon.

2. Mesencephalon.
3. Rhombencephalon.

1. Prosencephalon

Prosencephalon or **forebrain** is subdivided into two parts:
  i. **Telencephalon** which includes cerebral hemispheres, basal ganglia, hippocampus and amygdaloid nucleus.
  ii. **Diencephalon** which consists of thalamus, hypothalamus, metathalamus and subthalamus.

2. Mesencephalon

Mesencephalon is also known as **midbrain**.

3. Rhombencephalon

Rhombencephalon or **hindbrain** is subdivided into two portions:
  i. **Metencephalon** formed by pons and cerebellum.
  ii. **Myelencephalon** or medulla oblongata **(Fig. 78.2)**.

Midbrain, pons and medulla oblongata are together called the **brainstem**.

PERIPHERAL NERVOUS SYSTEM

Peripheral nervous system (PNS) is formed by the neurons and their processes present in all regions of the body. It consists of cranial nerves arising from brain and spinal nerves arising from the spinal cord. It is again divided into two subdivisions:

1. Somatic nervous system.
2. Autonomic nervous system.

1. Somatic Nervous System

Somatic nervous system is concerned with **somatic functions**. It includes the nerves supplying the skeletal muscles. Somatic nervous system controls the movements of the body by acting on skeletal muscles **(Fig. 78.3)**.

2. Autonomic Nervous System

Autonomic nervous system is concerned with regulation of visceral or vegetative functions. So, it is otherwise called vegetative or involuntary nervous system.

Autonomic nervous system consists of two divisions:
  I. Sympathetic division.
  ii. Parasympathetic division.

NEURON AND ITS CLASSIFICATION

Neuron or nerve cell is defined as the structural and functional unit of the nervous system. Like any other cell in the body, neuron has nucleus and all the organelles in the cytoplasm. However, it is different from other cells by two ways:

1. Neuron has branches or processes called **axon** and **dendrites**.
2. Neuron has **no centrosome**. So, it cannot undergo division.

CLASSIFICATION OF NEURON

Neurons are classified by three different methods:
  I. Depending upon number of poles.
  II. Depending upon function.
  III. Depending upon length of the axon.

I. Depending upon Number of Poles

Based on the number of poles from which the nerve fibers arise, neurons are divided into three types:

1. **Unipolar neurons** that have only **one pole** from which, both the axon and dendrite arise **(Fig. 78.4)**.

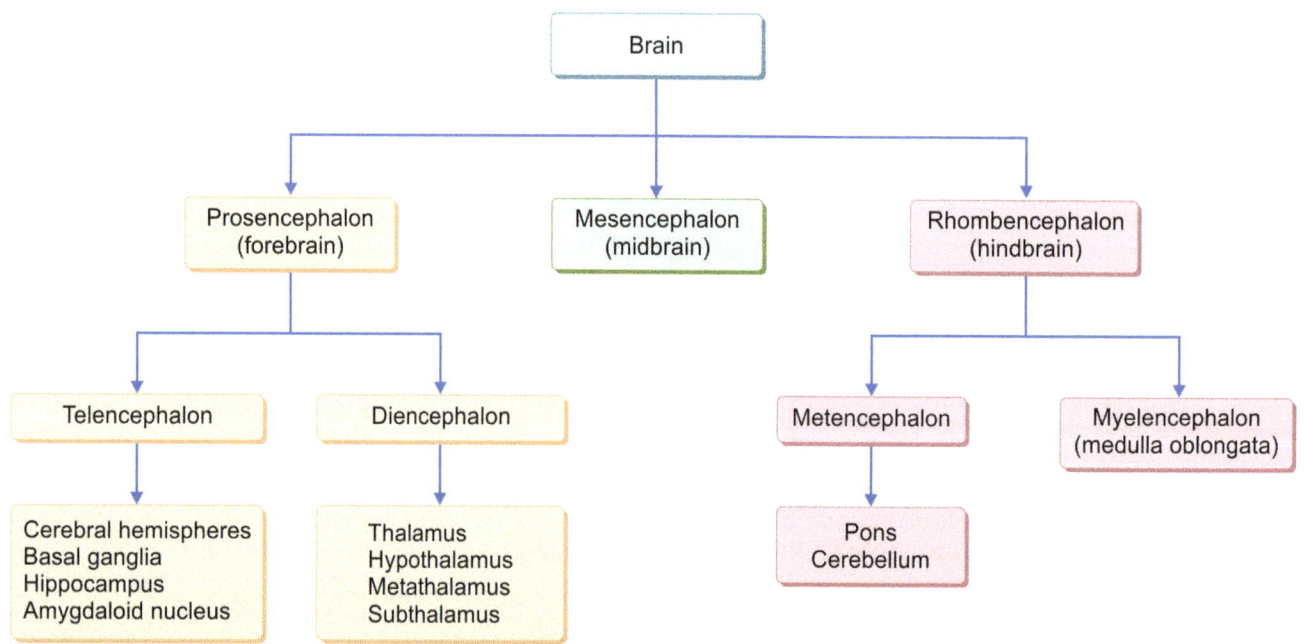

FIGURE 78.2: Parts of brain.

Chapter 78: Overview of Nervous System, Neuron and Neuroglia

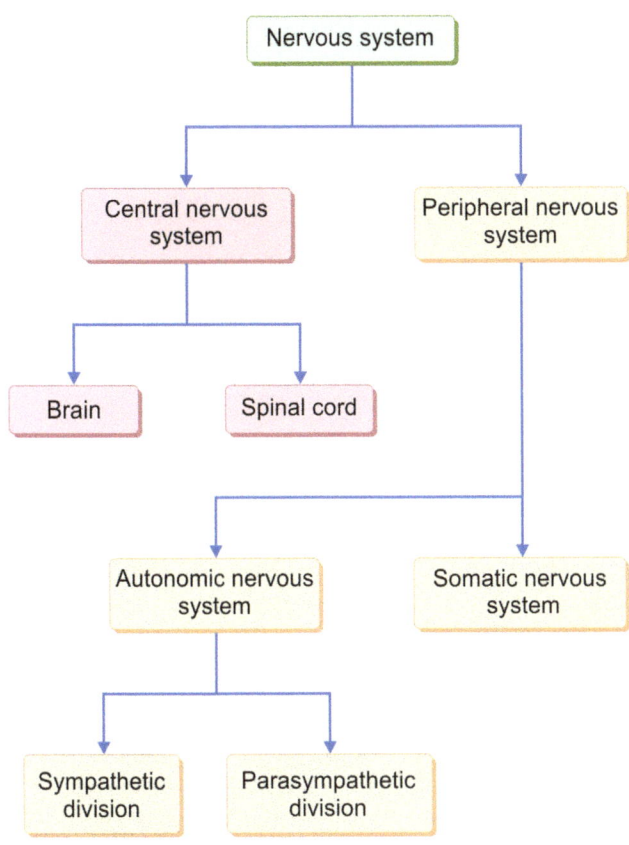

FIGURE 78.3: Organization of nervous system.

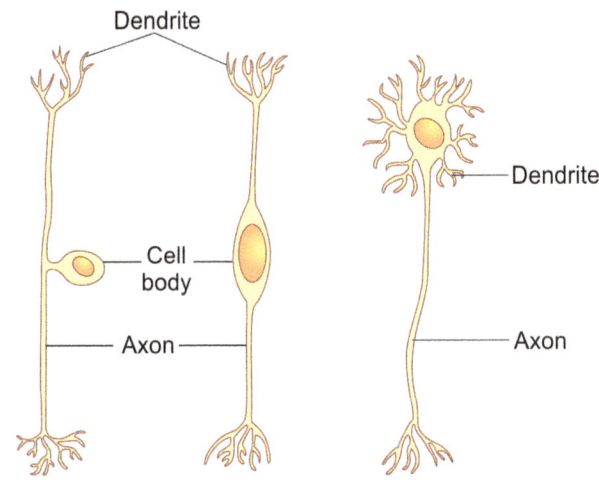

FIGURE 78.4: Types of neuron.

2. **Bipolar neurons** which have **two poles**. Axon arises from one pole and dendrites arise from the other pole.
3. **Multipolar neurons** which have **many poles**. One of the poles gives rise to axon and, all other poles give rise to dendrites.

II. *Depending upon Function*

On the basis of function, the nerve cells are classified into two types:

1. **Motor** or **efferent neurons** which carry the **motor impulses** from central nervous system to the peripheral effector organs such as muscles, glands, blood vessels, etc.
2. **Sensory** or **afferent neurons** which carry the **sensory impulses** from periphery to the central nervous system.

III. *Depending upon Length of Axon*

Depending upon the length of axon, neurons are divided into two types:

1. **Golgi type I neurons** that have **long axons**. Cell body of these neurons is in central nervous system and their axons leave the central nervous system and reach the remote peripheral organs.
2. **Golgi type II neurons** that have **short axons**. These neurons are present in large numbers in cerebral cortex and cerebellar cortex.

■ STRUCTURE OF NEURON

Neuron is made up of three parts:

1. Nerve cell body.
2. Dendrite.
3. Axon.

Dendrite and axon together form the **processes of neuron (Fig. 78.5)**. In general, the dendrites are short processes and the axons are long processes. The dendrites and axons are usually called **nerve fibers**.

1. Nerve Cell Body

Nerve cell body is also known as **soma** or **perikaryon**. It is irregular in shape and, it is constituted by a mass of cytoplasm called **neuroplasm** which is covered by a cell membrane. Neuroplasm contains a large nucleus, Nissl bodies, neurofibrils, mitochondria and Golgi apparatus. Nissl bodies and neurofibrils are found only in nerve cell and not in other cells.

Centrioles are absent in nerve cell. So, the nerve cells can not multiply.

Nucleus

Each neuron has one nucleus which is centrally placed in the nerve cell body. Nucleus has one or two prominent nucleoli.

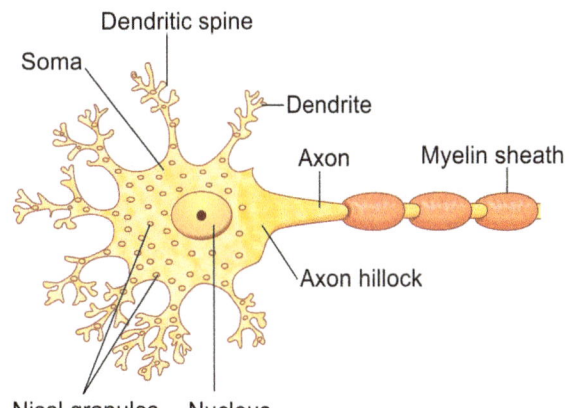

FIGURE 78.5: Structure of a neuron.

Nissl bodies or Nissl granules

Nissl bodies are small basophilic granules found in neuroplasm of neurons and are named after the discoverer. These bodies are present in the soma **except axon hillock**. Nissl granules are present in dendrites also but not in axon. Nissl bodies have ribosomes which are concerned with synthesis of proteins. The proteins formed in soma are transported to the axon by **axonal flow**.

Neurofibrils

Neurofibrils are thread-like structures present in the form of network in the soma and the nerve processes.

Mitochondria

Mitochondria are present in the soma and in axon. As in other cells, mitochondria form the **powerhouse** of nerve cell, where ATP is produced (Chapter 1).

Golgi apparatus

Golgi apparatus of the nerve cell body is similar to that of other cells. It is concerned with processing and packaging of proteins into granules (Chapter 1).

2. Dendrite of Neuron

Dendrite of neuron are is branched repeatedly. Dendrite may be present or absent. If present, it may be one or many in number. Dendrite has Nissl granules and neurofibrils.

3. Axon of Neuron

Axon is longer than dendrite. Each neuron has only one axon. Axon arises from **axon hillock** of the nerve cell body. Axon extends for a long distance away from the nerve cell body. Length of the longest axon is about 1 meter.

Organization of nerve

Many axons together form a bundle called **fasciculus**. Many fasciculi together form a **nerve**.

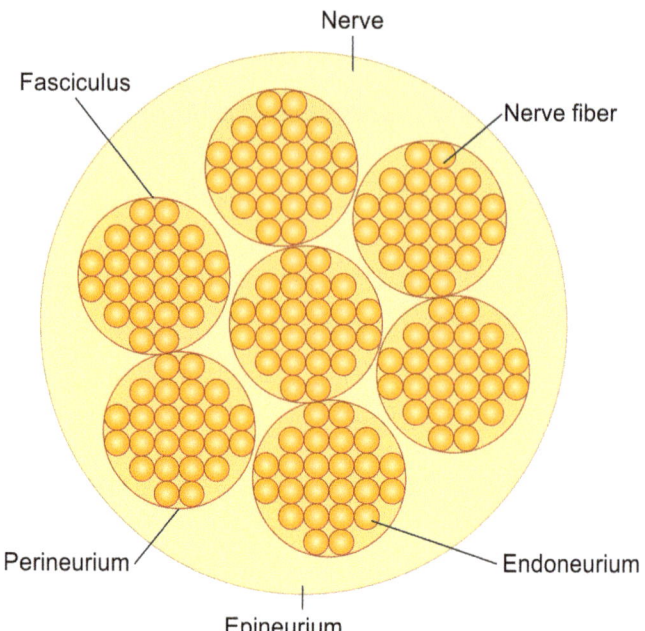

FIGURE 78.6: Cross-section of a nerve.

Coverings of nerve

Whole nerve is covered by tubular sheath, called **epineurium**. Each fasciculus is covered by **perineurium** and each nerve fiber (axon) is covered by **endoneurium** (Fig. 78.6).

Internal structure of axon: Axis cylinder

Axon has a long central core of cytoplasm called **axoplasm**. Axoplasm is covered by the tubular sheath like membrane called **axolemma** which is the continuation of the cell membrane of nerve cell body. The axoplasm along with axolemma is called the **axis cylinder** of the nerve fiber (Fig. 78.7). Axoplasm contains mitochondria, neurofibrils and axoplasmic vesicles. But Nissl bodies are absent in the axon. Axis cylinder of the nerve fiber is covered by **neurilemma** (cell membrane; see below).

Non-myelinated nerve fiber

Nerve fiber described above is the non-myelinated nerve fiber which is not covered by myelin sheath.

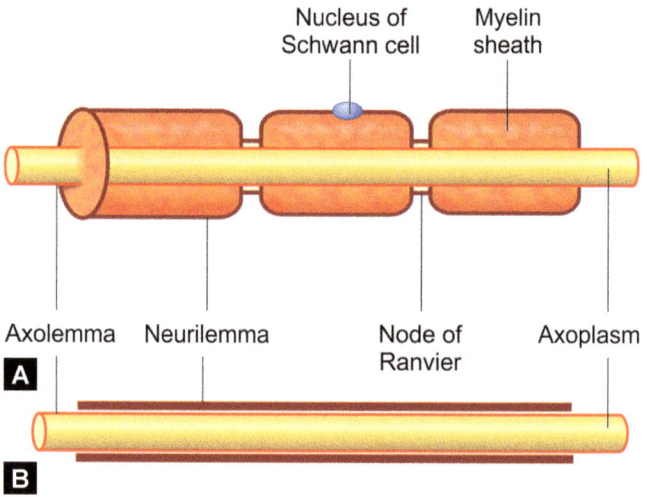

FIGURE 78.7: A. Myelinated nerve fiber. B. Non-myelinated nerve fiber.

Myelinated nerve fiber

Nerve fibers which are insulated by myelin sheath are called myelinated nerve fibers.

Myelin Sheath

Myelin sheath is a thick lipoprotein sheath that insulates the myelinated nerve fiber. Myelin sheath is not a continuous sheath and it is absent at regular intervals. The area where the myelin sheath is absent is called **node of Ranvier**. The segment of the nerve fiber between two nodes is called **internode**.

Formation of myelin sheath: Myelinogenesis

Formation of myelin sheath around the axon is called the myelinogenesis. It is formed by **Schwann cells** in neurilemma.

Chapter 78: Overview of Nervous System, Neuron and Neuroglia

Functions of myelin sheath

1. *Faster conduction:* Myelin sheath is responsible for faster conduction of impulse through the nerve fibers. In the myelinated nerve fibers, the impulses jump from one node to another node by **saltatory conduction** (see below).
2. *Insulating capacity:* Myelin sheath has a high insulating capacity. Because of this quality, the myelin sheath restricts the nerve impulse within the single nerve fiber, and prevents the stimulation of neighboring nerve fibers.

Neurilemma or Sheath of Schwann

Neurilemma is a thin membrane which surrounds the axis cylinder. It contains **Schwann cells** whose nucleus is situated between myelin sheath and neurilemma.

In non-myelinated nerve fiber, the neurilemma continuously surrounds axolemma. In myelinated nerve fiber, it covers the myelin sheath. At the node of Ranvier (where myelin sheath is absent), the neurilemma invaginates and runs up to axolemma in the form of a finger like process.

Functions of neurilemma

i. In non-myelinated nerve fiber, the neurilemma serves as a covering membrane.
ii. In myelinated nerve fiber, it is necessary for **myelinogenesis**.

■ NEUROTROPHINS: NEUROTROPHIC FACTORS

Neurotrophins or neurotrophic factors are the protein substances, which play important role in growth and functioning of nervous tissue. Neurotrophins are secreted by many tissues in the body, particularly muscles, neurons and astrocytes (neuroglial cells).

Functions of Neurotrophins

Neurotrophins:

1. Facilitate initial growth and development of nerve cells in central and peripheral nervous system.
2. Promote survival and repair of the nerve cells.
3. Play an important role in the maintenance of nervous tissue and neural transmission.

Commercial preparations of neurotrophins are used for the treatment of neural diseases

Types of Neurotrophins

Many types of neurotophic factors are identified.

Nerve growth factor

Nerve growth factor (NGF) is was the first neurotrophin protein substance identified as neurotrophin. It is found in many tissues. It promotes early growth and development of neurons.

Commercial preparation of NGF extracted from animals is used to treat many nervous disorders such as Alzheimer's disease, neuron degeneration in aging and neuron regeneration in spinal cord injury.

Other neurotrophins

1. Brain-derived neurotrophic growth factor (BDGF) found in brain and human sperm.
2. Ciliary neurotrophic factor (CNTF).
3. Glial cell line-derived neurotrophic factor (GDNF).
4. Fibroblast growth factor (FGF).
5. Neurotrophin-3, 4 and 5 (NT-3, NT-4 and NT-5).

■ CLASSIFICATION OF NERVE FIBERS

Nerve fibers are classified by six methods.

■ 1. DEPENDING UPON STRUCTURE

Based on the structure, the nerve fibers are classified into two types:

i. **Myelinated nerve fibers** that are covered by myelin sheath.
ii. **Nonmyelinated nerve fibers** which are not covered by myelin sheath.

■ 2. DEPENDING UPON DISTRIBUTION

Nerve fibers are classified into two types on the basis of the distribution:

i. **Somatic nerve fibers** which supply the skeletal muscles of the body.
ii. **Visceral** or **autonomic nerve fibers** which supply internal organs of the body.

■ 3. DEPENDING UPON ORIGIN

On the basis of origin, the nerve fibers are divided into two types:

i. **Cranial nerves** arising from **brain**.
ii. **Spinal nerves** arising from **spinal cord**.

■ 4. DEPENDING UPON FUNCTION

On the basis of functions, the nerve fibers are of two types:

i. **Sensory** or **afferent nerve fibers** which carry **sensory impulses** from different parts of the body to the central nervous system.
ii. **Motor** or **efferent nerve fibers** which carry **motor impulses** from central nervous system to different parts of the body **(Box 78.1)**.

■ 5. DEPENDING UPON SECRETION OF NEUROTRANSMITTER

Depending upon the neurotransmitter substance secreted, the nerve fibers are divided into two types:

BOX 78.1: Afferent and efferent nerve fibers.

Efferent nerve fiber
Carry motor information from central nervous system to different parts of the body
Afferent nerve fiber
Carry sensory information from different parts of the body to central nervous system

i. **Adrenergic nerve fibers** that secrete **noradrenaline**.
ii. **Cholinergic nerve fibers** that secrete **acetylcholine**.

6. DEPENDING UPON DIAMETER AND CONDUCTION OF IMPULSE: ERLANGERGASSER CLASSIFICATION

Erlanger and Gasser classified the nerve fibers into three major types on the basis of diameter of the fibers and the rate of conduction of impulses:

i. Type A nerve fibers.
ii. Type B nerve fibers.
iii. Type C nerve fibers.

Among these fibers, type A nerve fibers are the **thickest fibers** and type C nerve fibers are the **thinnest fibers**. Type A nerve fibers are divided into four subtypes. Except 'C' type of fibers, all the nerve fibers are myelinated.

Velocity of impulse through a nerve fiber is directly proportional to the **thickness** of the fibers.

Different types of nerve fibers along with diameter and velocity of conduction are given in the **Table 78.1**.

PROPERTIES OF NERVE FIBERS

EXCITABILITY

Details of excitability and stimulus are given in Chapter 21.

Response to Stimulus

When a nerve fiber is stimulated, based on the strength of stimulus, two types of response develop.

1. Action potential or nerve impulse.
2. Electrotonic potential or local potential.

Action Potential or Nerve Impulse

Action potential or nerve impulse develops in a nerve fiber when it is stimulated by a stimulus with adequate strength. Stimulus with adequate strength necessary for producing the action potential in a nerve fiber is known as **threshold** or **minimal stimulus**. Action potential is **propagated**.

Action potential in a nerve fiber is similar to that in a muscle, except for some minor differences **(Table 78.2)**. The action potential in a skeletal muscle fiber is described in Chapter 22.

Resting membrane potential in the nerve fiber is –70 mV. The firing level is at – 55 mV. Depolarization ends

TABLE 78.1: Types of nerve fibers.

Type	Diameter (μ)	Velocity of conduction (m/sec)
A alpha	12 to 24	70 to 120
A beta	6 to 12	30 to 70
A gamma	5 to 6	15 to 30
A delta	2 to 5	12 to 15
B	1 to 2	3 to 10
C	<1.5	0.5 to 2

TABLE 78.2: Differences in electrical potentials between nerve fiber and skeletal muscle fiber.

Event	Nerve fiber	Skeletal muscle fiber
Resting membrane potential	– 70 mV	– 90 mV
Firing level	– 55 mV	– 75 mV
End of depolarization	+ 35 mV	+ 55 mV

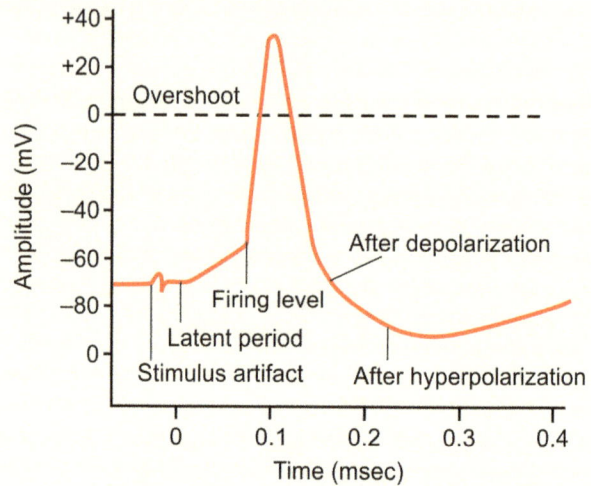

FIGURE 78.8: Action potential in nerve fiber.

at + 35 mV **(Fig. 78.8)**. Usually, the action potential starts in the initial segment of nerve fiber.

Electrotonic Potential or Local Potential

When the stimulus with **subliminal strength** is applied, only electrotonic potential develops and the action potential does not develop. Electrotonic potential is **non-propagated**.

Cathelectrotonic and anelectrotonic potentials

While recording electrical potential in a nerve fiber, two electrodes, namely **cathode** and **anode** are used. Potential change that is produced at cathode is called cathelectrotonic potential. Potential that is developed at anode is known as anelectrotonic potential.

Only the cathelectrotonic potential can be transformed into action potential or electrotonic potential.

CONDUCTIVITY

Conductivity is the ability of nerve fibers to transmit the impulse from area of stimulation to the other areas. Action potential is transmitted through the nerve fiber as **nerve impulse**. Normally, action potential is transmitted through the nerve fiber in only **one direction**.

Mechanism of Conduction of Action Potential

Depolarization occurs first at the site of stimulation in the nerve fiber. It causes depolarization of the neighboring areas. Like this, depolarization travels throughout the nerve fiber. Depolarization is followed by **repolarization**.

Chapter 78: Overview of Nervous System, Neuron and Neuroglia

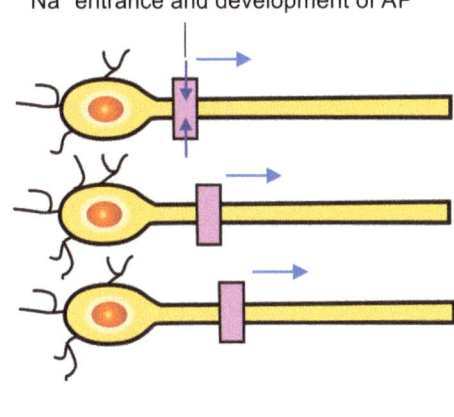

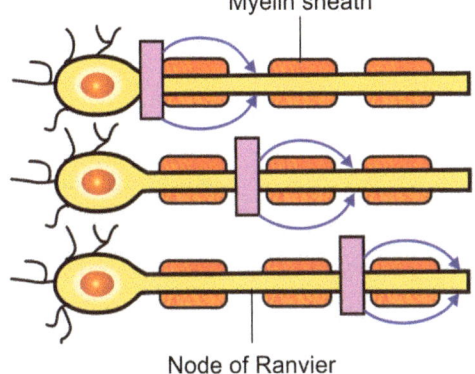

FIGURE 78.9: Mode of conduction through nerve fibers. **A.** Non-myelinated nerve fiber: Continuous conduction. **B.** Myelinated nerve fiber: Saltatory conduction (impulse jumps from node to node).

AP = Action potential

Conduction Through Myelinated Nerve Fiber: Saltatory Conduction

Saltatory conduction is a form of conduction of nerve impulse in which, the impulse jumps from one node to another. Conduction of impulse through a myelinated nerve fiber is about 50 times faster than through a nonmyelinated fiber. It is because the action potential jumps from one node to another **node of Ranvier** instead of traveling through the entire nerve fiber (Fig. 78.9).

Mechanism of saltatory conduction

Myelin sheath is not permeable to ions. So, the entry of sodium from extracellular fluid into nerve fiber occurs only in the node of Ranvier, where the myelin sheath is absent. It causes depolarization in the node, and not in the internode. Thus, the depolarization occurs at **successive nodes**. So, the action potential jumps from one node to another. Hence, it is called saltatory conduction (saltare = jumping).

■ REFRACTORY PERIOD

Refractory period is the period at which the nerve does not give any response to a stimulus. Refractory period is of two types.

1. Absolute Refractory Period

Absolute refractory period is the period during which the nerve does not show any response at all, whatever may be the strength of stimulus.

2. Relative Refractory Period

It is the period, during which the nerve fiber shows response, if the strength of stimulus is increased to maximum.

■ SUMMATION

One **subliminal stimulus** does not produce any response in the nerve fiber because, the subliminal stimulus is very weak. However, if two or more subliminal stimuli are applied within a short interval of about 0.5 m/sec, the response is produced. It is because the subliminal stimuli are summed up together to become strong enough to produce the response. This phenomenon is known as summation.

■ ADAPTATION

While stimulating a nerve fiber continuously, excitability of the nerve fiber is greater in the beginning. Later the response decreases slowly and finally the nerve fiber does not show any response at all. This phenomenon is known as adaptation or **accommodation**.

Causes for adaptation are:

1. When a nerve fiber is stimulated continuously, depolarization occurs continuously.
2. Continuous depolarization inactivates the sodium pump and increases the efflux of potassium ions.

■ INFATIGABILITY

A nerve fiber cannot be fatigued, even if it is stimulated continuously for a long time. Reason for this is the nerve fiber can conduct only **one action potential** at a time. At that time, it is completely **refractory** and does not conduct another action potential.

■ ALL-OR-NONE LAW

All-or-none law states that when a nerve is stimulated by a stimulus it gives maximum response or does not give response at all. Refer Chapter 57 for details of all-or-none law.

■ DEGENERATION OF NERVE FIBERS

When a nerve fiber is injured, various changes occur in the nerve fiber and nerve cell body. All these changes are together called the **degenerative changes**. Injury to a nerve fiber occurs due to obstruction of blood flow, crushing of nerve fiber or transection of nerve fiber.

■ DEGREES OF INJURY

According to **Sunderland**, injury to nerve fibers is classified into five types depending upon the order of **severity**.

First Degree Injury

First degree injury is caused by **pressure applied** over a nerve for a short period leading to occlusion of blood flow and hypoxia. Axon loses the function temporarily for a short time, which is called **conduction block**. The function returns within few hours to few weeks. First degree of injury is called **Seddon neuropraxia**.

Second Degree Injury

Second degree is due to the **prolonged severe pressure,** which causes **Wallerian degeneration** (see below). However, the endoneurium is intact. Repair and restoration of function take about 18 months. Second degree of injury is called **axonotmesis**.

Third Degree Injury

In this case, the **endoneurium** is interrupted. Epineurium and perineurium are intact. After degeneration, the recovery is slow and poor or incomplete. Third, fourth and fifth degrees of injury are called **neurotmesis**.

Fourth Degree Injury

This type of injury is more severe. Epineurium and perineurium are also interrupted. Fasciculi of nerve fibers are disturbed and disorganized. Regeneration is poor or incomplete.

Fifth Degree Injury

Fifth degree of injury involves **complete transaction** of the nerve trunk with loss of continuity. Useful regeneration is not possible unless the cut ends are rearranged and approximated quickly by surgery.

■ DEGENERATIVE CHANGES IN NEURON

Degeneration means deterioration or impairment or pathological changes of an injured tissue. When a peripheral nerve fiber is injured, the degenerative changes occur in the nerve cell body and the nerve fiber of same neuron and the adjoining neuron.

Accordingly, the degenerative changes are classified into three types:

1. Wallerian degeneration.
2. Retrograde degeneration.
3. Transneural degeneration.

■ 1. WALLERIAN OR ORTHOGRADE DEGENERATION

Wallerian or **orthograde degeneration** is the pathological change that occurs in the distal cut end of nerve fiber (axon). It is named after the discoverer **Waller**. Wallerian degeneration starts within 24 hours of injury. The change occurs throughout the length of distal part of nerve fiber simultaneously.

Changes in nerve

i. Axis cylinder swells and breaks up into small pieces. After few days, the broken pieces appear as debris in the space occupied by axis cylinder **(Fig. 78.10)**.
ii. Myelin sheath is slowly disintegrated into fat droplets. The changes in myelin sheath occur from 8th to 35th day.

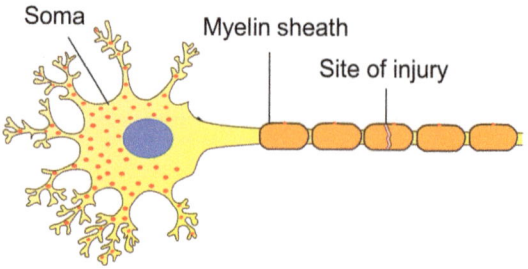
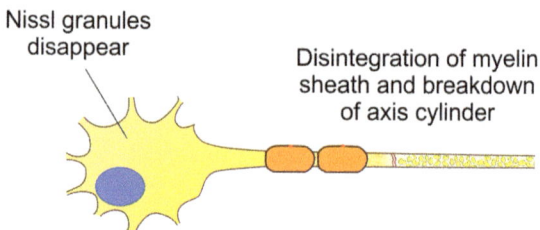
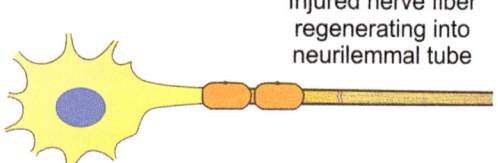
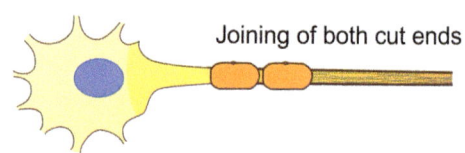
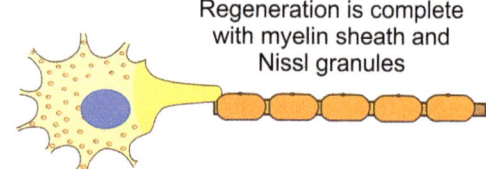

FIGURE 78.10: Degeneration and regeneration of nerve fiber.

iii. Neurilemmal sheath is unaffected, but the Schwann cells multiply rapidly. The macrophages invade from outside. Macrophages remove the debris of axis cylinder and the fat droplets of disintegrated myelin sheath.
iv. So, the neurilemmal tube becomes empty. Later it is filled by the cytoplasm of Schwann cell. All these changes take place for about 2 months from the day of injury.

■ 2. RETROGRADE DEGENERATION

Retrograde degeneration is the pathological changes which occur in the nerve cell body and axon proximal to the cut end.

Changes in nerve cell body

Changes in the nerve cell body commence within 48 hours after the section of nerve.

Changes in nerve cell body are:
 i. First, Nissl granules disintegrate into fragments by **chromatolysis**.
 ii. Golgi apparatus is disintegrated.
 iii. Nerve cell body swells due to accumulation of fluid and becomes round.
 iv. Neurofibrils disappear followed by displacement of the nucleus towards the periphery.
 v. Sometimes, the nucleus is **extruded** out of the cell. In this case, death of the neuron occurs and regeneration of the injured nerve is not possible.

Changes in axon proximal to cut end

In the axon, changes occur only up to first node of Ranvier from the site of injury. Degenerative changes that occur in proximal cut end of axon are similar to those changes occurring in distal cut end of the nerve fiber.

3. TRANSNEURONAL DEGENERATION

If an afferent nerve fiber is cut, the degenerative changes occur in another neuron with which the afferent nerve fiber synapses. It is called transneuronal degeneration.

REGENERATION OF NERVE FIBER

Regeneration is the **regrowth** of lost or destroyed part of a tissue. The injured and degenerated nerve fiber can regenerate. It starts as early as 4th day after injury, but, becomes more effective only after 30 days and is completed in about 80 days.

CRITERIA FOR REGENERATION

Regeneration is possible only if certain criteria are fulfilled by the degenerated nerve fiber:

1. Gap between the cut ends of the nerve should not exceed 3 mm.
2. Neurilemma should be present.
3. Nucleus must be intact.
4. Two cut ends should remain in the same line.

STAGES OF REGENERATION

1. First, some pseudopodia-like extensions called **fibrils** or **regenerative sprouts** grow from the proximal cut end of the nerve.
2. Fibrils move towards the distal cut end of the nerve fiber.
3. Some of the fibrils enter the neurilemmal tube of distal end and form axis cylinder.
4. Schwann cells line up in the neurilemmal tube and actually guide the fibrils into the tube. Schwann cells also synthesize nerve growth factors, which attract the fibrils from proximal segment.
5. Axis cylinder is fully established inside the neurilemmal tube. These processes are completed in about 3 months after injury.
6. Myelin sheath is formed by Schwann cells slowly. Myelination is completed in 1 year.
7. Diameter of the nerve fiber gradually increases. However, the degenerated nerve fiber has only 80% of original diameter.
8. In the nerve cell body, first the Nissl granules appear followed by Golgi apparatus.
9. Cell loses the excess fluid and nucleus occupies the central portion.

Though anatomical regeneration occurs in the nerve, functional recovery occurs after a long period.

NEUROGLIA

DEFINITION

Neuroglia or **glial cell** or glia (glia = glue) is the **supporting cell** of the nervous system. Neuroglial cells are **non-excitable** and do not transmit nerve impulse (action potential). So, these cells are also called **nonneural cells.**

CLASSIFICATION OF NEUROGLIAL CELLS

Neuroglial cells are distributed in central nervous system (CNS) as well as peripheral nervous system (PNS). Refer **Table 78.3** for functions of different types of neuroglia.

Central Neuroglial Cells

1. *Astrocytes*: Two types, fibrous and protoplasmic astrocytes **(Fig. 78.11)**.
2. *Microglia*.
3. *Oligodendrocytes*.

Peripheral Neuroglial Cells

1. Schwann cells.
2. Satellite cells.

FUNCTIONS OF NEUROGLIAL CELLS

Refer **Table 78.3** for functions of different types of neuroglia.

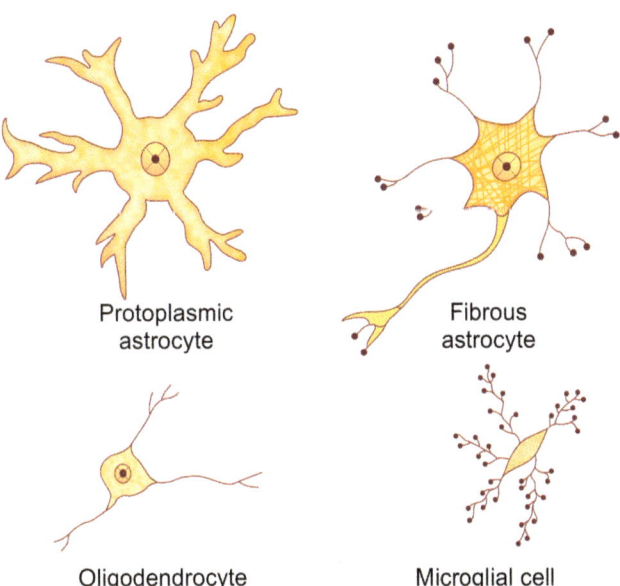

FIGURE 78.11: Neuroglial cells in CNS.

TABLE 78.3: Situation, types and functions of neuroglia.

Classification	Situation	Types	Functions
Central neuroglia	Central nervous system	Astrocytes	1. Form blood-brain barrier 2. Provide supporting network 3. Maintain the ECF status around neurons 4. Regulate calcium and potassium level in ECF 5. Regulate the level and recycling of neurotransmitters at synaptic level 6. Secrete neurotrophins
		Microglia	1. Function as macrophages 2. Protect brain from microorganisms by phagocytic action 3. Provide immune and inflammatory response in brain damage
		Oligodendrocytes	1. Provide myelination 2. Form supporting network
Peripheral neuroglia	Peripheral nervous system	Schwann cells	1. Provide myelination 2. Help in regeneration of injured nerve fibers 3. Scavenge cellular debris by phagocytosis
		Satellite cells	1. Provide supporting network 2. Maintain the ECF status around neurons

Chapter 79: Receptors, Synapse and Neurotransmitters

CHAPTER OUTLINE

- RECEPTORS
- CLASSIFICATION OF RECEPTORS
- PROPERTIES OF RECEPTORS
- SYNAPSE
- CLASSIFICATION OF SYNAPSE
- FUNCTIONAL ANATOMY OF SYNAPSE
- FUNCTIONS OF SYNAPSE
- PROPERTIES OF SYNAPSE
- CONVERGENCE AND DIVERGENCE
- NEUROTRANSMITTERS
- NEUROMODULATORS

RECEPTORS

Receptors are specialized sensory nerve endings which give response to sensory stimuli. These sensory nerve endings terminate in periphery as **unmyelinated endings** or in the form of specialized **capsulated structures**.

When stimulated, receptors produce a series of impulses, which are transmitted through the sensory nerves.

Biological Transducers

Actually receptors function like a transducer. **Transducer** is a device, which converts one form of energy into another.

So, receptors are often defined as the **biological transducers** which convert various forms of energy (stimuli) in the environment into action potentials in nerve fiber.

CLASSIFICATION OF RECEPTORS

Receptors are classified into two types:

I. Exteroceptors.
II. Interoceptors.

EXTEROCEPTORS

Exteroceptors are the receptors which give response to stimuli arising **from outside** the body. Exteroceptors are divided into three groups.

1. Cutaneous Receptors

Receptors situated in the **skin** are called the cutaneous receptors. Cutaneous receptors are also called **mechanoreceptors** because of their response to **mechanical stimuli** such as touch, pressure and pain (**Figs. 79.1** and **79.2**). Touch and pressure receptors give response to vibration also. Different types of cutaneous receptors are given in **Table 79.1**.

2. Chemoreceptors

Receptors, which give response to **chemical stimuli**, are called the chemoreceptors (**Fig. 79.2**).

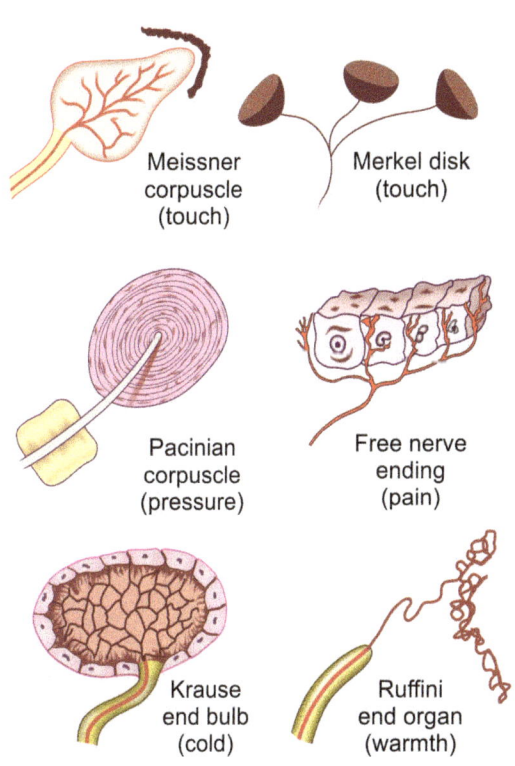

FIGURE 79.1: Cutaneous receptors.

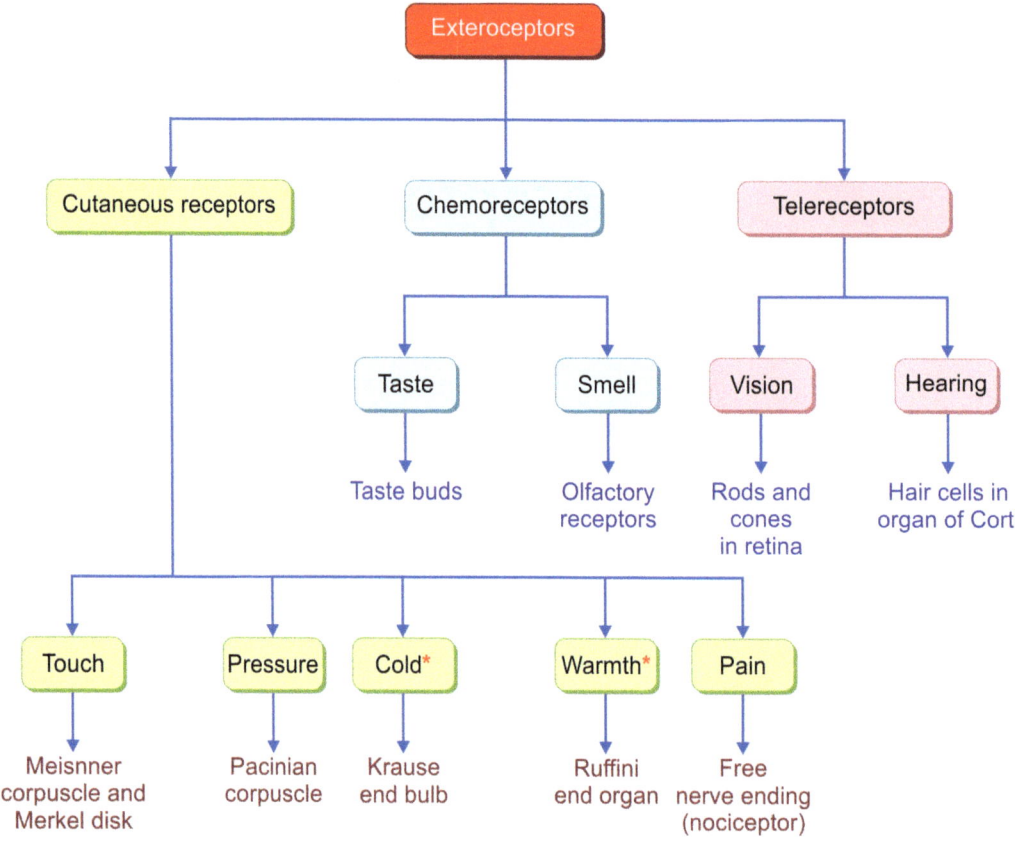

FIGURE 79.2: Exteroceptors.

*Receptors of cold and warmth are together called temperature receptors (thermoreceptors)

TABLE 79.1: Cutaneous receptors.

Receptor	Situation	Structure	Type of nerve Fiber	Sensation
Meisnner corpuscle	Upper dermis between papillae	Encapsulated with collagen fiber network	Aβ	Touch
Merkel disk	Base of epidermis	Branched dendrite. Each branch is expanded like a disk and not encapsulated	Aβ	Touch
Pacinian corpuscle	Deeper layer of dermis Fascia over muscles Tendons Tissues around joint capsule	Onion like concentric laminae encapsulated with connective tissue	C	Pressure Vibration
Krause end bulb	Dermis	Encapsulated with collagen fiber network	Aδ	Cold temperature
Ruffini end organ	Deeper layer of dermis	Covered by elongated cylindrical capsule	C	Warm temperature
Free nerve ending	Skin Muscle Fascia Joints	Uncapsulated ramified nerve fibers	Aδ C	Pain

3. Telereceptors

Telereceptors or **distance receptors** are the receptors which give response to stimuli arising **away from body**. Examples are given in **Figure 79.2**.

■ INTEROCEPTORS

Interoceptors are the receptors which give response to stimuli arising **from within** the body. Interoceptors are of two types.

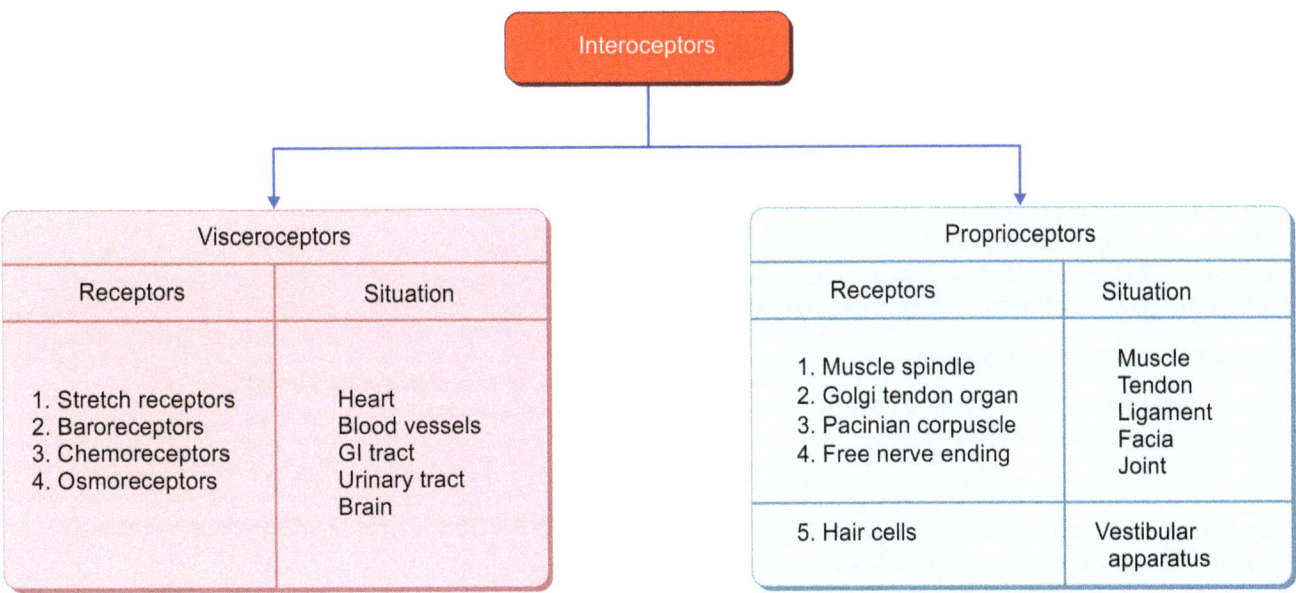

FIGURE 79.3: Interoceptors.

1. *Visceroceptors*

Receptors situated in the viscera are called visceroceptors. Visceroceptors are listed in **Figure 79.3**.

2. *Proprioceptors*

Proprioceptors are the receptors which give response to **change in the position** of different parts of the body (Chapter 88). Proprioceptors are listed in **Figure 79.3**.

■ PROPERTIES OF RECEPTORS

■ 1. SPECIFICITY OF RESPONSE: MÜLLER LAW

According to Müller law, each type of receptor gives response only to one **specific sensation**. This phenomenon called specificity of response. For example, pain receptors give response only to pain sensation.

■ 2. ADAPTATION: SENSORY ADAPTATION

Adaptation is the decrease in discharge of sensory impulses from a receptor when it is stimulated continuously with constant strength. Depending upon adaptation time, the receptors are divided into two types:

i. Phasic receptors, which get adapted rapidly. Examples are touch and pressure receptors.
ii. Tonic receptors, which get adapted slowly. Examples are muscle spindle, pain receptors and cold receptor.

■ 3. RESPONSE TO INCREASE IN STRENGTH OF STIMULUS

During the stimulation of a receptor, if the response given by the receptor is to be doubled, strength of stimulus must be increased 100 times. This phenomenon is called **Weber-Fechner law**, which states that the change in response of a receptor is directly proportional to the logarithmic increase in the intensity of stimulus.

■ 4. SENSORY TRANSDUCTION

Sensory transduction in a receptor is a process by which the energy (stimulus) in the environment is converted into electrical impulses (action potentials) in nerve fiber. **Transduction** means conversion of one form of energy into another.

Sensory transduction varies depending upon the type of receptor. For example, the **chemoreceptor** converts **chemical energy** into action potential in the sensory nerve fiber. The **touch receptor** converts **mechanical energy** into action potential in the sensory nerve fiber.

■ 5. RECEPTOR POTENTIAL

Receptor potential is a nonpropagated transmembrane potential difference that develops when a receptor is stimulated. It is also called **generator potential**. Receptor potential is not action potential. It is a **graded potential** (Chapter 22).

Properties of Receptor Potential

Receptor potential has two important properties:

i. Receptor potential is non-propagated. It is confined within the receptor itself.
ii. It does not obey all-or-none law.

Significance of Receptor Potential

When the receptor potential is sufficiently strong (when the magnitude is about 10 mV), it causes development of action potential in the sensory nerve.

Mechanism of Development of Receptor Potential

Pacinian corpuscles are generally used to study the receptor potential because of their large size and anatomical configuration.

Pacinian corpuscles give response to **pressure** stimulus. When pressure stimulus is applied, Pacinian corpuscle is compressed. This results in the opening of mechanically gated sodium channels. So, the positively charged sodium ions enter the interior of fiber and produces a **mild depolarization**, i.e. receptor potential.

SYNAPSE

Synapse is the **junction** between the two neurons through which the nerve impulse passes from one neuron to another neuron. It is not the anatomical continuation. It is only a **physiological continuity** between two nerve cells.

CLASSIFICATION OF SYNAPSE

Synapse is classified by two methods, anatomical classification and functional classification.

ANATOMICAL CLASSIFICATION

Synapse is formed by axon of one neuron ending on the cell body, dendrite or axon of the next neuron. First neuron from which the axon arises is called the **presynaptic neuron**. Second neuron on which the axon of first neuron ends is called **postsynaptic neuron**.

Depending upon ending of axon, synapse is classified into three types:

1. *Axoaxonic synapse*: Axon of presynaptic neuron terminates on **axon** of postsynaptic neuron.
2. *Axodendritic synapse*: Axon of presynaptic neuron terminates on **dendrite** of postsynaptic neuron.
3. *Axosomatic synapse*: Axon of presynaptic neuron ends on **soma** (cell body) of postsynaptic neuron (Fig. 79.4).

FUNCTIONAL CLASSIFICATION

On the basis of function, synapse is classified into two types.

1. Electrical Synapse

Electrical synapse is a type of synapse in which the physiological continuity between presynaptic and

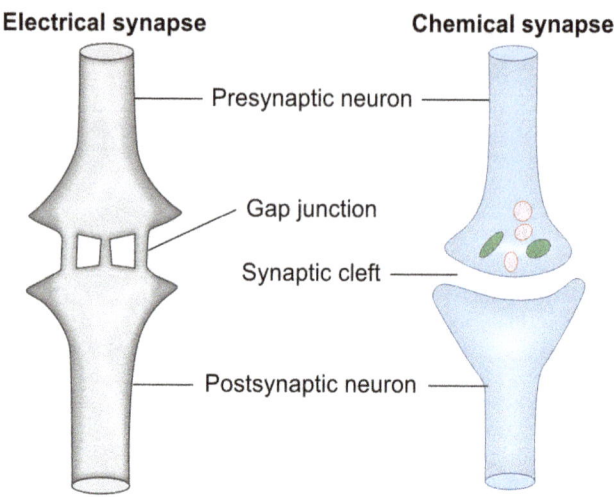

FIGURE 79.5: Electrical and chemical synapse.

postsynaptic neurons is provided by **gap junction (Fig. 79.5)**. There is direct exchange of ions between the two neurons though the gap junction. So, the action potential reaching the terminal portion of presynaptic neuron directly enters the postsynaptic neuron.

2. Chemical Synapse

Chemical synapse is the junction between a nerve fiber and a muscle fiber or between two nerve fibers, through which the signals are transmitted by the release of chemical transmitter. In the chemical synapse, there is no continuity between the presynaptic and postsynaptic neurons.

FUNCTIONAL ANATOMY OF CHEMICAL SYNAPSE

Axon of the presynaptic neuron divides into many small branches before forming the synapse. These branches are known as presynaptic **axon terminals**. Membrane of presynaptic axon terminal is called **presynaptic membrane (Fig. 79.6)**.

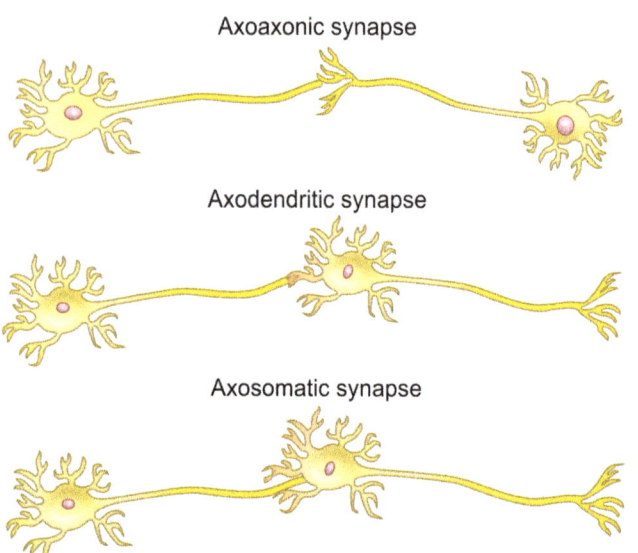

FIGURE 79.4: Anatomical synapses.

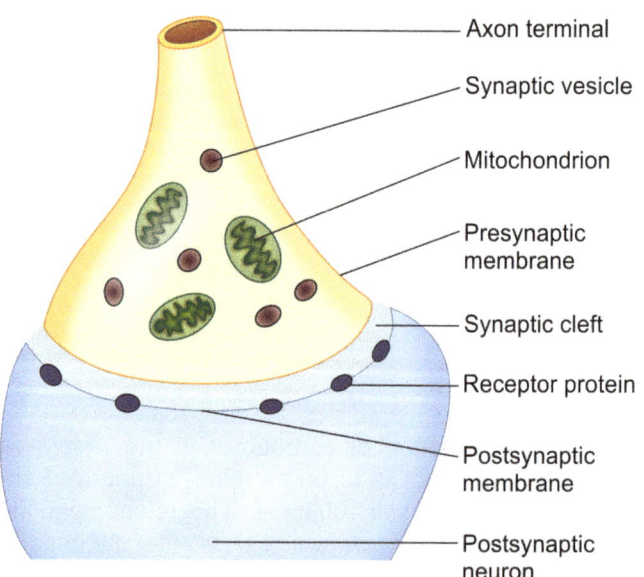

FIGURE 79.6: Structure of chemical synapse.

Presynaptic terminal has two important structures:

1. **Mitochondria**, which help in the synthesis of neurotransmitter substances.
2. **Synaptic vesicles**, which store neurotransmitter substance.

Membrane of the postsynaptic neuron is called **postsynaptic membrane**. It contains some **receptor proteins**. The space in between the presynaptic membrane and the postsynaptic membrane is called **synaptic cleft**. **Basal lamina** of this cleft contains cholinesterase, which destroys acetylcholine.

■ FUNCTIONS OF SYNAPSE

Function of the synapse is to transmit the impulses from one neuron to another. However, some synapses inhibit the impulses. Accordingly, synapse is divided into two types:

1. Excitatory synapses, which transmit the impulses (excitatory function).
2. Inhibitory synapses, which inhibit the transmission of impulses (inhibitory function).

■ EXCITATORY SYNAPSE

Excitatory synapse transmits the impulses from presynaptic neuron to postsynaptic neuron by the development of excitatory postsynaptic potential.

Excitatory Postsynaptic Potential: EPSP

Excitatory postsynaptic potential (EPSP) is a **nonpropagated** electrical potential that develops during the process of synaptic transmission.

When action potential reaches the presynaptic axon terminal, the voltage-gated **calcium channels** at the presynaptic membrane are opened and **calcium ions** enter the axon terminal from ECF. Calcium ions cause bursting of synaptic vesicles and release of **neurotransmitter**. Now, the neurotransmitter diffuses through presynaptic membrane and enters the synaptic cleft **(Fig. 79.7)**. Common neurotransmitter in synapse is **acetylcholine**.

The neurotransmitter binds with receptor protein present in the postsynaptic membrane to form the **neurotransmitter-receptor complex**.

Neurotransmitter-receptor complex causes opening of ligand-gated **sodium channels**. Now, **sodium ions** from ECF enter the cell body of postsynaptic neuron. As the sodium ions are positively charged, resting membrane potential inside the cell body becomes slightly positive and a **mild depolarization** develops. This type of mild depolarization is called **excitatory postsynaptic potential (EPSP)**. EPSP is confined only to the synapse. It is a **graded potential** (Chapter 22).

Properties of EPSP

1. EPSP is nonpropagated.
2. It does not obey all-or-none law.

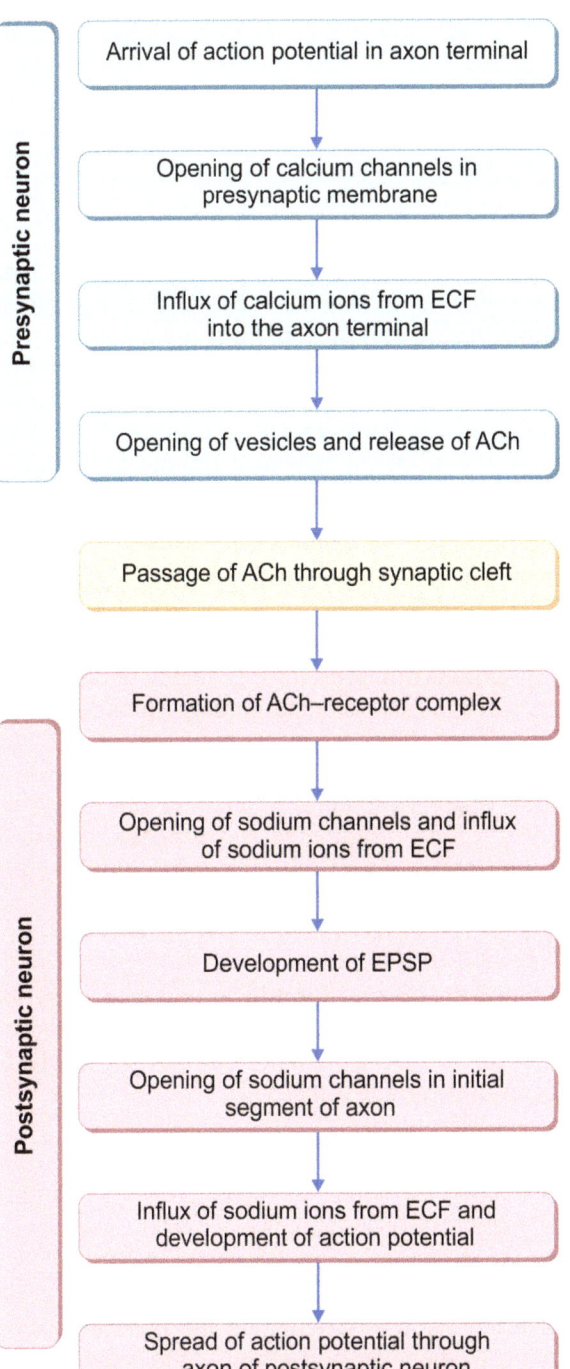

FIGURE 79.7: Sequence of events during synaptic transmission.
ACh = Acetylcholine, ECF = Extracellular fluid, EPSP = Excitatory postsynaptic potential

Significance of EPSP

EPSP is not transmitted into the axon of postsynaptic neuron. However, it causes development of action potential in the axon.

■ INHIBITORY SYNAPSE

Inhibitory synapse does not transmit the impulses from presynaptic neuron to postsynaptic neuron.

Inhibition of synaptic transmission is classified into three types:

1. Postsynaptic inhibition.
2. Presynaptic inhibition.
3. Renshaw cell inhibition.

1. Postsynaptic Inhibition

Postsynaptic inhibition or **direct inhibition** is the type of synaptic inhibition that occurs due to the release of an **inhibitory neurotransmitter** from presynaptic terminal instead of an excitatory neurotransmitter substance. The inhibitory neurotransmitter develops **inhibitory postsynaptic potential (IPSP)** instead of EPSP. Inhibitory neurotransmitters are **gamma-aminobutyric acid** (GABA), dopamine and glycine.

Development of IPSP: Action of GABA

GABA binds with receptor to form neurotransmitter-receptor complex which opens the ligand-gated **potassium channels** instead of sodium channels. Now, the **potassium ions** from cell body of postsynaptic neuron move to ECF. Simultaneously, chloride channels also open and chloride ions (which are more in ECF) move inside the cell body of postsynaptic neuron. Exit of potassium ions and influx of chloride ions cause more negativity inside, leading to **hyperpolarization**. The hyperpolarized state of the synapse inhibits synaptic transmission.

2. Presynaptic Inhibition

Presynaptic or **indirect inhibition** is a type of synaptic inhibition that occurs due to failure of presynaptic axon terminal to release sufficient quantity of **excitatory neurotransmitter** substance.

3. Renshaw Cell Inhibition

This is a type of synaptic inhibition caused by **Renshaw cells** in spinal cord (Chapter 81).

Significance of Synaptic Inhibition

Synaptic inhibition in CNS limits the number of impulses going to muscles and enables the muscles to act **properly and appropriately**.

PROPERTIES OF SYNAPSE

1. ONE WAY CONDUCTION: BELL-MAGENDIE LAW

According to Bell-Magendie law, the impulses are transmitted only in one direction in synapse, i.e. from presynaptic neuron to postsynaptic neuron.

2. SYNAPTIC DELAY

Synaptic delay is a short delay that occurs during the transmission of impulses through the synapse. It is due to the time taken for:

  i. Release and passage of neurotransmitter from axon terminal to postsynaptic membrane.

  ii. Action of the neurotransmitter to open the ionic channels in postsynaptic membrane.

  Normal duration of synaptic delay is 0.3 to 0.5 m/sec.

3. FATIGUE

During continuous muscular activity, synapse forms the seat of fatigue along with Betz cells present in the motor area of frontal lobe of cerebral cortex. Refer Chapter 21 for details of fatigue. Fatigue at the synapse is due to the **depletion of acetylcholine**.

4. SUMMATION

Summation is the **fusion of effects**. Summation is of two types:

  i. **Spatial summation** which occurs when many presynaptic terminals are stimulated simultaneously.
  ii. **Temporal summation** which occurs when one presynaptic terminal is stimulated repeatedly.

5. ELECTRICAL PROPERTY

Electrical properties of the synapse are the EPSP and IPSP, which are already described in this chapter.

CONVERGENCE AND DIVERGENCE

Convergence is the process by which many presynaptic neurons terminate on a single postsynaptic neuron **(Fig. 79.8)**. Divergence is the process by which one presynaptic neuron terminates on many postsynaptic neurons.

NEUROTRANSMITTERS

DEFINITION

Neurotransmitter is a chemical substance that acts as the mediator for the transmission of nerve impulse from one neuron to another neuron through a synapse.

CLASSIFICATION OF NEUROTRANSMITTERS

Depending upon Chemical Nature

Depending upon chemical nature, neurotransmitters are classified into three groups **(Table 79.2)**:

1. Amino acids.
2. Amines.
3. Others.

Depending upon Function

Depending upon function, neurotransmitters are classified into two types:

1. **Excitatory neurotransmitters** which are responsible for the conduction of impulse.
2. **Inhibitory neurotransmitters** which inhibit the conduction of impulse **(Table 79.3)**.

TRANSPORT AND RELEASE OF NEUROTRANSMITTER

Neurotransmitter is produced in the cell body of the neuron and is transported through axon. At the axon terminal, the neurotransmitter is stored in small packets

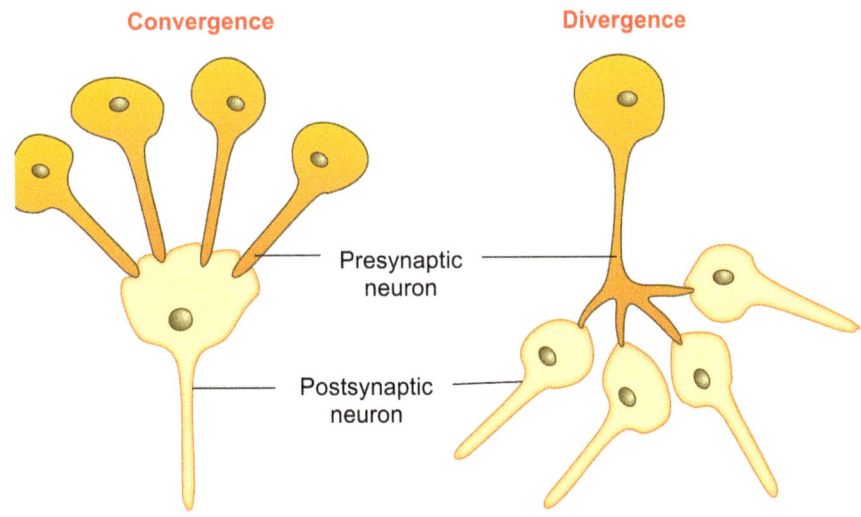

FIGURE 79.8: Convergence and divergence.

TABLE 79.2: Neurotransmitters.

Group	Name	Site of secretion	Action
Amino acids	GABA	Cerebral cortex, cerebellum, basal ganglia, retina and spinal cord	Inhibitory
	Glycine	Forebrain, brainstem, spinal cord and retina	Inhibitory
	Glutamate	Cerebral cortex, brainstem and cerebellum	Excitatory
	Aspartate	Cerebellum, spinal cord and retina	Excitatory
Amines	Noradrenaline	Postganglionic adrenergic sympathetic nerve endings, cerebral cortex, hypothalamus, basal ganglia, brainstem, locus ceruleus and spinal cord	Excitatory and Inhibitory
	Adrenaline	Hypothalamus, thalamus and spinal cord	Excitatory and Inhibitory
	Dopamine	Basal ganglia, hypothalamus, limbic system, neocortex, retina and sympathetic ganglia	Inhibitory
	Serotonin	Hypothalamus, limbic system, cerebellum, spinal cord, retina, gastrointestinal (GI) tract, lungs and platelets	Inhibitory
	Histamine	Hypothalamus, cerebral cortex, GI tract and mast cells	Excitatory
Others	Nitric oxide	Many parts of CNS, neuromuscular junction and GI tract	Excitatory
	Acetylcholine	Neuromuscular junction Synapse Preganglionic parasympathetic nerve and postganglionic parasympathetic nerve Preganglionic sympathetic nerve, postganglionic sympathetic cholinergic nerve Amacrine cells of retina and Many regions of brain	Excitatory

GABA = Gamma-aminobutyric acid, CNS = Central nervous system

TABLE 79.3: Excitatory and inhibitory neurotransmitters.

Excitatory neurotransmitters	Inhibitory neurotransmitters	Neurotransmitters with excitatory and inhibitory actions
1. Acetylcholine 2. Nitric oxide 3. Histamine 4. Glutamate 5. Aspartate	1. Gamma-aminobutyric acid (GABA) 2. Glycine 3. Dopamine 4. Serotonin	1. Noradrenaline 2. Adrenaline

called **vesicles**. Under the influence of a stimulus, these vesicles get ruptured and release the neurotransmitter into synaptic cleft. It binds to receptors on the surface of the postsynaptic cell.

NEUROMODULATORS

Neuromodulator is a chemical messenger, which **modifies and regulates** the activities which take place during synaptic transmission. Neuromodulator does not propagate nerve impulses like neurotransmitter.

CHEMISTRY AND TYPES OF NEUROMODULATORS

Generally, the neuromodulators are **peptides**. So, neuromodulators are often called **neuropeptides**. Almost all the peptides found in nervous tissues are neuromodulators.

Neuromodulators are classified into two types:

1. **Non-opioid neuromodulators** which act by binding with G-protein-coupled receptors.
2. **Opioid neuromodulators** which act by binding with opioid receptors located in nerve endings in brain and GI tract.

ACTIONS OF NEUROMODULATORS

Neurotransmitters cause excitability of neurons or other tissues by producing either **depolarization** or **hyperpolarization**.

But neuromodulators have diverse actions such as:

1. Regulation of synthesis, breakdown or reuptake of neurotransmitter.
2. Excitation or inhibition of membrane receptors by acting independently or together with neurotransmitter.
3. Control of gene expression.
4. Regulation of local blood flow.
5. Promotion of formation of new synapses.
6. Control of glial cell morphology.

Chapter 80: Reflex Activity

CHAPTER OUTLINE

- DEFINITION AND SIGNIFICANCE OF REFLEXES
- REFLEX ARC
- CLASSIFICATION OF REFLEXES
- SUPERFICIAL REFLEXES
- DEEP REFLEXES OR TENDON REFLEXES
- VISCERAL REFLEXES
- PATHOLOGICAL REFLEXES
- PROPERTIES OF REFLEXES
- RECIPROCAL INHIBITION AND RECIPROCAL INNERVATION
- REFLEXES IN MOTOR NEURON LESION

DEFINITION AND SIGNIFICANCE OF REFLEXES

Reflex activity is the **involuntary** response to a stimulus. It is a type of **protective mechanism** and it protects the body from irreparable damages.

For example, when hand is placed on a hot object, it is withdrawn immediately. When a bright light is thrown into the eyes, eyelids are closed and **pupil** is constricted to prevent the damage of retina by entrance of excess light into the eyes.

REFLEX ARC

Reflex arc is the anatomical **nervous pathway** for a reflex action.

Simple reflex arc includes five components:

1. Receptor

Receptor is the **end organ**, which receives the stimulus. When the receptor is stimulated, impulses are generated in afferent nerve.

2. Afferent Nerve

Afferent or **sensory nerve** transmits sensory impulses from the receptor to the center.

3. Center

Center receives the sensory impulses via afferent nerve fibers and in turn, it generates appropriate motor impulses. Center is located in the brain or spinal cord.

In simple reflex arc, the **synapse** between afferent nerve and efferent nerve forms the center.

4. Efferent Nerve

Efferent or **motor nerve** transmits motor impulses from the center to the effector organ **(Fig. 80.1)**.

5. Effector Organ

Effector organ is the structure such as the muscle or gland where the activity occurs in response to the stimulus.

Afferent and efferent nerve fibers may be connected directly to the center. In some places, one or more neurons are interposed between these nerve fibers and the center. Such neurons are called **connector neurons** or **internuncial neurons** or **interneurons**.

CLASSIFICATION OF REFLEXES

Reflexes are classified by six different methods depending upon various factors as given below:

I. Depending upon whether inborn or acquired reflexes.
II. Depending upon situation: **Anatomical classification**.

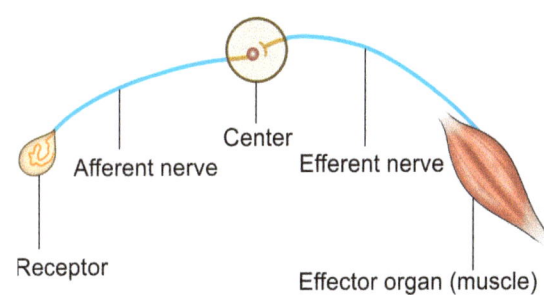

FIGURE 80.1: Simple reflex arc.

III. Depending upon purpose: **Physiological classification**.
IV. Depending upon number of synapses.
V. Depending upon whether visceral or somatic.
VI. Depending upon clinical basis.

■ I. CLASSIFICATION DEPENDING UPON WHETHER INBORN OR ACQUIRED

1. *Inborn Reflexes or Unconditioned Reflexes*

Inborn reflexes or unconditioned reflexes are the natural reflexes which are present since the time of birth. Such reflexes do not require previous learning, training or conditioning.

Example is the secretion of saliva when a drop of honey is kept in the mouth of a newborn baby for the first time. The baby does not know the taste of the honey but still saliva is secreted.

2. *Acquired Reflexes or Conditioned Reflexes*

Acquired reflexes or conditioned reflexes are the reflexes that are developed after conditioning or training. These reflexes are not inborn but acquired after birth. Such reflexes require previous learning, training or conditioning.

Example is the secretion of saliva by the sight, smell, thought or hearing of a known edible substance.

■ II. CLASSIFICATION DEPENDING UPON SITUATION OF CENTER: ANATOMICAL CLASSIFICATION

1. Cerebellar reflexes.
2. Cortical reflexes.
3. Midbrain reflexes.
4. Bulbar or medullary reflexes.
5. Spinal reflexes.

■ III. CLASSIFICATION DEPENDING UPON PURPOSE: PHYSIOLOGICAL CLASSIFICATION

1. *Protective Reflexes or Flexor Reflexes*

Protective reflexes are the reflexes which protect the body from **nociceptive** (harmful) **stimuli**. These reflexes are also called **withdrawal reflexes** or flexor reflexes. Protective reflexes involve flexion at different joints hence the name flexor reflexes.

2. *Antigravity Reflexes or Extensor Reflexes*

Antigravity reflexes are the reflexes which protect the body against **gravitational force**. These reflexes are also called extensor reflexes because, the extensor muscles contract during these reflexes resulting in extension at joints.

■ IV. CLASSIFICATION DEPENDING UPON NUMBER OF SYNAPSE

1. *Monosynaptic Reflexes*

Reflexes having only **one synapse** in the reflex arc are called monosynaptic reflexes. **Stretch reflex** is the best example for monosynaptic reflex and it is elicited by stimulation of muscle spindle.

2. *Polysynaptic Reflexes*

Reflexes having **more than** one synapse in the reflex arc are called polysynaptic reflexes. Examples are **flexor reflexes** (withdrawal reflexes) are the polysynaptic reflexes.

■ V. CLASSIFICATION DEPENDING UPON WHETHER SOMATIC OR VISCERAL REFLEXES

1. *Somatic Reflexes*

Somatic reflexes are the reflexes, for which the reflex arc is formed by **somatic nerve fibers.** These reflexes involve the participation of skeletal muscles. And there may be flexion or extension at different joints during these reflexes.

2. *Visceral or Autonomic Reflexes*

Visceral or autonomic reflexes are the reflexes, for which at least a part of reflex arc is formed by **autonomic nerve fibers.** These reflexes involve participation of smooth muscle or cardiac muscle. Visceral reflexes include pupillary reflexes, gastrointestinal reflexes, cardiovascular reflexes, respiratory reflexes, etc.

Some reflexes such as swallowing, coughing or vomiting are considered as visceral reflexes. However, these reflexes involve some participation of skeletal muscles also.

■ VI. CLASSIFICATION DEPENDING UPON CLINICAL BASIS

Depending upon clinical basis reflexes are classified into four types:

A. Superficial reflexes.
B. Deep reflexes.
C. Visceral reflexes.
D. Pathological reflexes.

■ SUPERFICIAL REFLEXES

Superficial reflexes are the reflexes, which are elicited from the **surface of the body**.

Superficial reflexes are elicited from:

1. Cornea (corneal reflex) and conjunctiva (conjunctival reflex) of eyeball.
2. Mucus membrane (mucus membrane reflexes).
3. Skin (cutaneous reflexes).

Details of superficial reflexes are given in **Tables 80.1** and **80.2**.

■ DEEP REFLEXES OR TENDON REFLEXES

Deep reflexes or tendon reflexes are elicited from deeper structures beneath the skin such as tendon.

Details of deep reflexes are given in **Table 80.3**.

■ VISCERAL REFLEXES

Visceral reflexes are the reflexes arising from the **pupil** and the **visceral organs**.

TABLE 80.1: Superficial reflexes elicited from the eye and the mucous membrane.

Reflex	Method of eliciting reflex	Response	Afferent nerve	Center	Efferent nerve
1. Corneal reflex	Touching cornea with a wisp of cotton	Closing of eyelids (blinking)	Ophthalmic branch of V cranial nerve	Pons: Trigeminal nucleus	VII cranial nerve
2. Conjunctival reflex	Touching conjunctiva with wisp of cotton				
3. Nasal reflex (sneezing reflex)	Stimulating the nasal mucosa with a wisp of cotton	Sneezing	V cranial nerve	Medulla: Nucleus tractus solitarius	V, VII, IX and X cranial nerves
4. Pharyngeal reflex (gag reflex)	Touching roof of mouth, back of tongue, uvula, tonsils or back of throat or pharynx with a wisp of cotton or any other object.	Elevation of soft palate and retching (strong involuntary effort to vomit) or gagging (opening of mouth)	IX cranial nerve	Medulla: Nucleus tractus solitarius	X cranial nerve

TABLE 80.2: Superficial reflexes elicited from the skin (cutaneous reflexes).

Reflex	Method of eliciting reflex	Response	Afferent nerve	Center (spinal segments)	Efferent nerve
1. Scapular reflex	Stroking the skin at interscapular space	Contraction of scapular muscles and Drawing in of scapula	Suprascapular nerve	C5 and C6	Suprascapular nerve
2. Upper abdominal reflex	Stroking the abdominal wall below the costal margin (supraumbilical level)	Ipsilateral contraction of abdominal muscle and Movement of umbilicus towards site of stroke	T7 and T8 spinal nerves	T7 and T8	T7 and T8 spinal nerves
3. Middle abdominal reflex	Scratching the abdominal wall near umbilicus (umbilical level)		T9 and T10 spinal nerves	T9 and T10	T9 and T10 spinal nerves
4. Lower abdominal reflex	Stroking the abdominal wall at umbilical and iliac level (infraumbilical level)		T11 and T12 spinal nerves	T11 and T12	T11 and T12 spinal nerves
5. Cremasteric reflex	Scratching the skin at upper and inner aspect of thigh	Elevation of testicles	L1 and L2 spinal nerves	L1 and L2	L1 and L2 spinal nerves
6. Gluteal reflex	Stroking the skin over buttock	Contraction of gluteus muscles	Posterior femoral cutaneous nerve	S1 to S3	Inferior gluteal nerve
7. Plantar reflex	Stroking the sole	Plantar flexion and adduction of toes	Sciatic nerve	L5 to S1	Sciatic nerve
8. Bulbocavernosus reflex	Stroking the dorsum of glans penis	Contraction of bulbocavernosus	Perineal nerve	S3 and S4	Perineal nerve
9. Anal reflex	Stroking the perianal region	Contraction of anal sphincter	Inferior rectal nerve	S3 and S4	Inferior rectal nerve

C = Cervical, T = Thoracic, L = Lumbar, S = Sacral

Visceral reflexes are:

1. Pupillary reflexes in which, the size of pupil is altered. Details are given in Chapter 96.
2. Oculocardiac reflex in which heart rate decreases due to the pressure applied over eyeball.

TABLE 80.3: Deep (tendon) reflexes.

Reflex	Method of eliciting reflex	Response	Afferent nerve	Center	Efferent nerve
1. Jaw jerk	Tapping the middle of the chin with slightly opened mouth	Closure of mouth	V cranial nerve	Pons: V cranial nerve nuclei	V cranial nerve
2. Biceps jerk	Tapping the biceps tendon	Flexion of forearm	Musculo-cutaneous nerve	5th and 6th cervical spinal segments	Musculo-cutaneous nerve
3. Triceps jerk	Tapping the triceps tendon	Extension of forearm	Radial nerve	6th and 7th cervical spinal segments	Radial nerve
4. Supinator jerk or brachioradialis jerk or radial periosteal reflex	Tapping the tendon over distal end (styloid process) of radius	Supination and flexion of forearm	Radial nerve	5th and 6th cervical spinal segments	Radial nerve
5. Knee jerk or patellar tendon reflex	Tapping the patellar tendon	Extension of knee due to contraction of quadriceps muscle	Femoral nerve	2nd, 3rd and 4th lumbar spinal segments	Femoral nerve
6. Ankle jerk or Achilles tendon reflex	Tapping the Achilles tendon	Plantar flexion of foot	Tibial nerve	1st and 2nd sacral spinal segments	Tibial nerve

3. Carotid sinus reflex in which the pressure over carotid sinus in neck by **tight collar dress** decreases heart rate and blood pressure.

■ PATHOLOGICAL REFLEXES

Pathological reflexes are the reflexes that are elicited only in pathological conditions. Three pathological reflexes are well known.

■ 1. BABINSKI REFLEX

Babinski reflex is the **abnormal plantar reflex**. It is also called **Babinski sign** or **phenomenon**. In normal plantar reflex, a gentle scratch over the outer edge of the sole of the foot causes plantar flexion and adduction of all toes.

But in Babinski reflex, there is dorsiflexion of great toe and fanning of other toes. Babinski reflex is present in **upper motor neuron lesion** particularly in lesion of corticospinal (pyramidal) tracts. It is noticed in some physiological conditions also. It is present in infants up to 2 years because of incomplete myelination of pyramidal tracts. In adults this reflex may be elicited in deep sleep and in old age.

■ 2. CLONUS

Clonus is a series of rapid and repeated involuntary jerky movements, which occur while eliciting a deep reflex. It occurs in **upper motor neuron lesion** (Chapter 82).

When a deep reflex is elicited in a normal person, the contractions of a muscle or group of muscles are smooth and continuous. But in upper motor neuron lesion clonus occurs. It is because of hypertonicity of muscles and exaggeration of deep reflexes.

Clonus is well seen in calf muscles producing **ankle clonus** and quadriceps producing **patella clonus**. Clonus is also seen in wrists, fingers, jaw and elbow.

■ 3. PENDULAR MOVEMENTS

Pendular movements are the slow **oscillatory movements** (instead of brisk movements) that are developed while eliciting a tendon jerk. The pendular movements are very common while eliciting the knee jerk in patients affected by **cerebellar lesion**. Such movements are similar to movements of **clock's pendulum** hence the name pendular movements.

■ PROPERTIES OF REFLEXES
■ ONE WAY CONDUCTION: BELL-MAGENDIE LAW

During any reflex activity, the impulses are transmitted in only one direction through the reflex arc as per Bell-Magendie law. Impulses pass from receptors to the center and then from center to effector organ.

■ REACTION TIME

Reaction time is the **time interval** between application of stimulus and the onset of reflex. It depends upon the length of afferent and efferent nerve fibers, velocity of impulse through these fibers and **synaptic delay** (Chapter 79).

■ SUMMATION

Refer Chapter 79 for details of summation. Summation (fusion of effects) in reflex action is of two types:

1. *Spatial Summation*

When two afferent nerve fibers supplying a muscle are stimulated separately with subliminal stimulus, there is no response. But the muscle contracts when both the nerve fibers are stimulated together with same strength of stimulus. It is called spatial summation.

2. Temporal Summation

When one nerve fiber is stimulated repeatedly with subliminal stimuli, these stimuli are summed up to give response in the muscle. It is called temporal summation.

■ RECRUITMENT

Recruitment is defined as the successive activation of additional motor units with progressive increase in force of muscular contraction.

When an excitatory nerve is stimulated for a long time, there is a gradual increase in the response of reflex activities. It is due to the activation of more and more motor units. Recruitment is similar to the effect of temporal summation.

■ AFTER DISCHARGE

After discharge is the continuation of response for some time even after cessation of stimulus. When a reflex action is elicited continuously for some time and then the stimulation is stopped, the reflex activity (contraction) will be continued for some time even after the stoppage of the stimulus. It is because of the discharge of impulses from the center even after stoppage of stimulus. The internuncial neurons are responsible for after discharge.

■ REBOUND PHENOMENON

Reflex activities can be inhibited forcefully for some time. But, when the inhibition is suddenly removed, the reflex activity becomes more forceful than before inhibition. It is called rebound phenomenon. The reason for this state of over excitation is not known.

■ FATIGUE

When a reflex activity is continuously elicited for a long time, the response is reduced slowly and at one stage, the response does not occur. This type of failure to give response to the stimulus is called fatigue. The center or the synapse of the reflex arc is the **first seat of fatigue**.

■ RECIPROCAL INHIBITION AND RECIPROCAL INNERVATION

■ RECIPROCAL INHIBITION

Reciprocal inhibition is the process during reflex activity, by which there is relaxation of a group of muscles during contraction of their antagonistic muscles.

When a **flexor reflex** is elicited, the **flexor muscles** are excited (contracted) and the **extensor muscles** are inhibited (relaxed) in that side. This phenomenon is called the reciprocal inhibition.

Reciprocal inhibition occurs because of reciprocal innervation.

■ RECIPROCAL INNERVATION

Reciprocal innervation is a type of innervation of muscles, because of which contraction of a group of muscles is accompanied by relaxation of their **antagonistic muscles**.

Afferent nerve fibers, which produce flexor reflex in a limb, have connections with motor neurons supplying flexor muscles and the motor neurons supplying the extensor muscles of same side.

Afferent nerve **excites** the motor neurons, which supply the **flexor muscles**. Simultaneously, it **inhibits** the motor neurons supplying **extensor muscles** through an interneuron. Accordingly, the flexor muscles contract and extensor muscles relax resulting in flexion of the limb.

■ CROSSED EXTENSOR REFLEX

Crossed extensor reflex is the **withdrawal reflex** in which the flexors of the withdrawing limb are excited (contracting) and extensors are inhibited (relaxed), while the opposite occurs in the other limb. For example, while eliciting a flexor reflex activity in a limb, that limb is flexed. Simultaneously the opposite limb is extended **(Fig. 80.2)**.

Flexors are excited and extensors are inhibited in this limb, but in the opposite limb, the flexors are inhibited and extensors are excited. Crossed extensor reflex is because of reciprocal inhibition.

■ SIGNIFICANCE OF RECIPROCAL INHIBITION

Reciprocal inhibition and reciprocal innervation are very important in spinal reflexes, which are involved in **locomotion**. It helps in the forward movement of one limb while causing the backward movement of the opposite limb.

■ REFLEXES IN MOTOR NEURON LESION

■ UPPER MOTOR NEURON LESION

During upper motor neuron lesion, all the superficial reflexes are lost. The deep reflexes are exaggerated and Babinski's sign is present (Chapter 82).

■ LOWER MOTOR NEURON LESION

During lower motor lesion, all the superficial and deep reflexes are lost. Refer Chapter 82 for details.

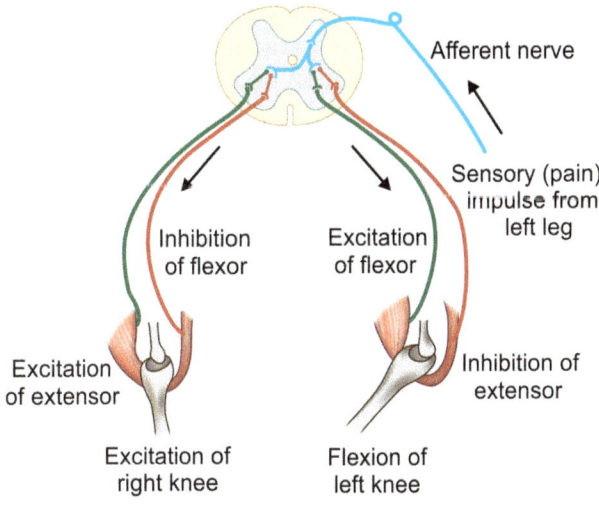

FIGURE 80.2: Crossed extensor reflex.
Green lines = Excitation, Red lines = Inhibition

Chapter 81: Spinal Cord

CHAPTER OUTLINE

- FEATURES OF SPINAL CORD
- INTERNAL STRUCTURE OF SPINAL CORD
- GRAY MATTER
- WHITE MATTER
- TRACTS IN SPINAL CORD
- ASCENDING TRACTS
- DESCENDING TRACTS
- APPLIED PHYSIOLOGY

FEATURES OF SPINAL CORD

Spinal cord is a part of central nervous system, the other part being the brain. Spinal cord is cylindrical in shape. It has a length of about 45 cm in males and about 43 cm in females.

Situation and Extent of Spinal Cord

Spinal cord is situated in the **vertebral canal.** It extends between **foramen magnum** where it is continuous with medulla oblongata of brain, and lower border of first lumbar vertebra.

Coverings of Spinal Cord

Spinal cord is covered by membranous sheaths called **meninges** which continue as coverings of brain. Meninges are **dura mater, pia mater** and **arachnoid mater.** Meninges are responsible for **protection and nourishment** of the nervous tissues.

Enlargements of Spinal Cord

Spinal cord has two spindle-shaped swellings, called **cervical enlargement** and **lumbar enlargement**. Below the lumbar enlargement spinal cord forms a cone-shaped **conus medullaris**. A non-nervous filament called **filum terminale** extends from conus medullaris downward.

Fissure and Sulci in Spinal Cord

A furrow called **anterior median fissure** is present on the anterior surface of spinal cord. Lateral to the anterior median fissure on either side, is a depression called the **anterolateral sulcus**. It denotes the exit of anterior nerve root. **Posterior median sulcus** is on posterior surface of spinal cord. This is continuous with **posterior median septum**.

On either side, lateral to posterior median sulcus, there is **posterior intermediate sulcus**. It is continuous with **posterior intermediate septum**. Lateral to the posterior intermediate sulcus, is the **posterolateral sulcus**. This denotes the entry of posterior nerve root.

SEGMENTS OF SPINAL CORD

Spinal cord is made up of 31 segments, which are listed in **Table 81.1**. Spinal cord is a continuous structure. The appearance of segments is because of spinal nerves arising from spinal cord.

SPINAL NERVES

Spinal nerve is a **mixed nerve** consisting of both motor and sensory fibers. Spinal nerves form a part of **peripheral nervous system**.

In humans, there are 31 pairs of spinal nerves corresponding to the segments of spinal cord in a symmetrical manner. Spinal nerves are listed in **Table 81.1**.

Each spinal nerve is formed by two roots:

1. *Anterior or ventral root*: Formed by efferent (motor) nerve fibers.

TABLE 81.1: Segments of spinal cord and spinal nerve.

Spinal segments/Spinal nerves	Number
Cervical segments/Cervical spinal nerves	8
Thoracic segments/Thoracic spinal nerves	12
Lumbar segments/Lumbar spinal nerves	5
Sacral segments/Sacral spinal nerves	5
Coccygeal segment/Coccygeal spinal nerves	1
Total segments/Spinal nerves	**31**

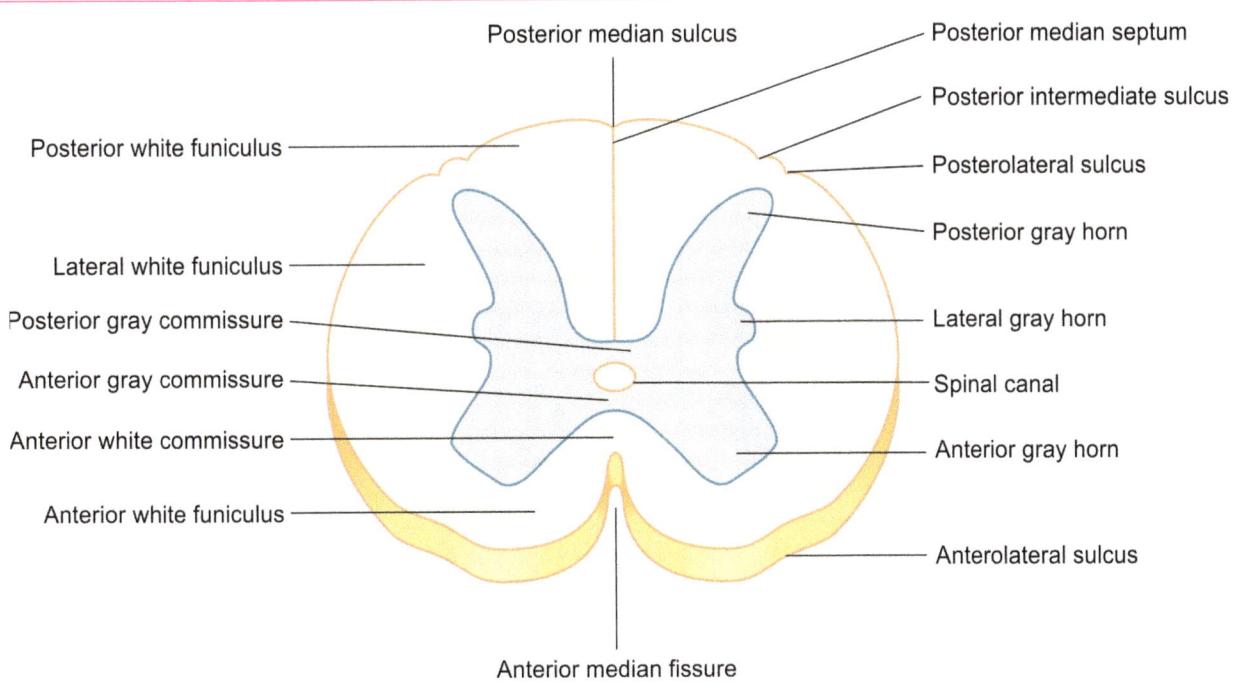

FIGURE 81.1: Section of spinal cord: Thoracic segment.

2. *Posterior or dorsal root:* Formed by afferent (sensory) nerve fibers. This root has posterior root ganglion which contains soma of neurons.

   Both the nerve roots on either side leave the spinal cord and pass through the corresponding intervertebral foramina.

INTERNAL STRUCTURE OF SPINAL CORD

Neural substance of the spinal cord is divided into inner gray matter and outer white matter **(Fig. 81.1)**.

GRAY MATTER OF SPINAL CORD

Gray matter of the spinal cord has nerve cell bodies, dendrites and parts of axons. It is placed centrally in the form of wings of butterfly and it resembles the letter 'H'. In the center of gray matter, is the **spinal canal**.

Each lateral half of gray matter has an **anterior gray horn** and one **posterior gray horn**. In addition, the gray matter forms **lateral gray horn** in all thoracic and first two lumbar segments. Part of the gray matter anterior to central canal is called the **anterior gray commissure** and part of gray matter posterior to the central canal is called the **posterior gray commissure**.

Neurons in Gray Matter of Spinal Cord

Gray matter contains two types of neurons.
1. Golgi type I neurons which have long axons.
2. Golgi type II neurons which have short axons.

Organization of these neurons in the gray matter of spinal cord is described in two methods:
  I. Nuclei or columns.
  II. Laminae or layers.

I. Nuclei in Spinal Cord

Clusters of neurons are present in the form of nuclei or cell column in gray matter **(Fig. 81.2)**.

1. Nuclei in anterior gray horn

Anterior gray horn contains the nuclei of **lower motor neurons** which are of three types:
  i. Alpha motor neurons.
  ii. Gamma motor neurons.
  iii. Renshaw cells.

2. Nuclei in lateral gray horn

Lateral gray horn has **intermediolateral nucleus**. Sympathetic preganglionic fibers which arise from this leave the spinal cord through the anterior nerve root. This nucleus extends between T1 and L2 segments of spinal cord **(Table 81.2)**.

3. Nuclei in posterior gray horn

Posterior gray horn contains the nuclei of **sensory neurons**, which are of four types:
  i. Marginal nucleus.
  ii. Substantia gelatinosa of Rolando.
  iii. Chief sensory nucleus or nucleus proprius.
  iv. Clarke's nucleus.

II. Laminae of Spinal Cord: Rexed Laminae

Neurons of gray matter are distributed in laminae or layers. **Bror Rexed** classified the neurons in 10 laminae hence the name **Rexed laminae**.

Laminae in different gray horns are:

1. *Posterior gray horn*: Laminae I to VI having nuclei of sensory neurons.

Section 10: Nervous System

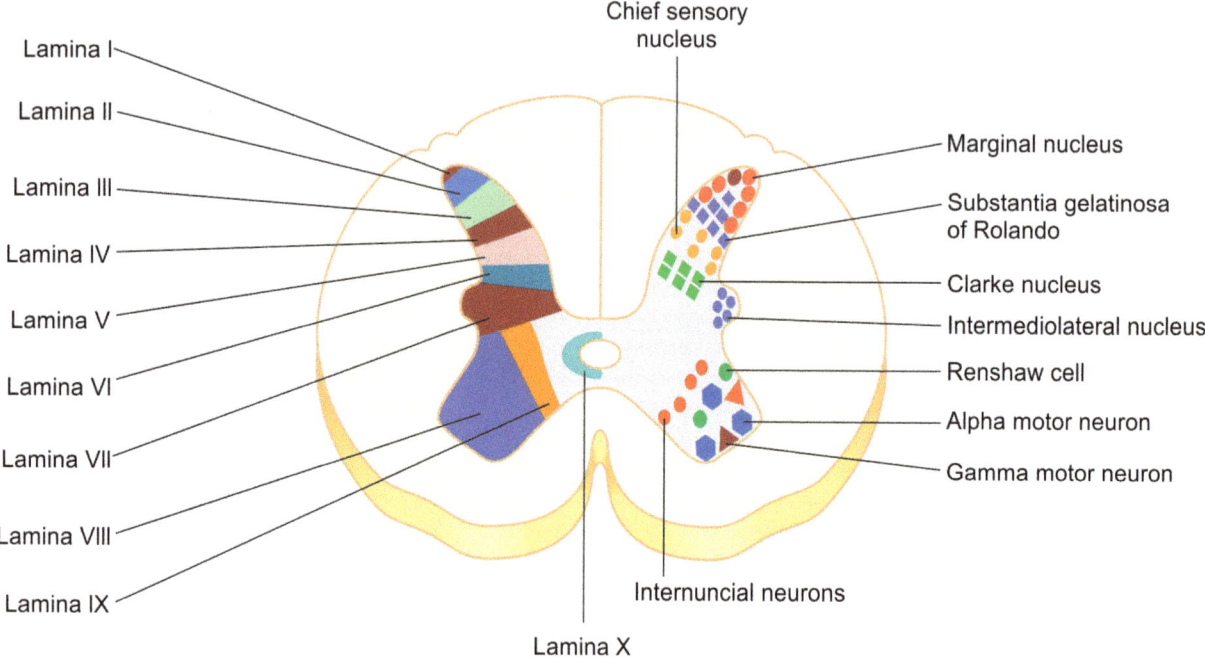

FIGURE 81.2: Nuclei and laminae in gray horn of spinal cord: Thoracic segment.

TABLE 81.2: Neurons in gray horns of spinal cord.

Gray horn	Neurons
Anterior gray horn	1. Alpha motor neurons 2. Gamma motor neurons 3. Renshaw cells
Lateral gray horn	1. Neurons of intermediolateral nucleus
Posterior gray horn	1. Marginal cells 2. Substantia gelatinosa of Rolando 3. Chief sensory nucleus 4. Clarke nucleus

2. *Lateral gray* horn: Lamina VII which contains intermediolateral nucleus.
3. *Anterior gray* horn: Laminae VIII and IX having nuclei of motor neurons.
4. *Around spinal canal*: Lamina X which has neuroglia.

WHITE MATTER OF SPINAL CORD

White matter of spinal cord surrounds the gray matter. It is formed by the bundles of nerve fibers. **Anterior median fissure** and the **posterior median septum** divide the entire mass of white matter into two lateral halves. The band of white matter lying in front of anterior gray commissure is called the **anterior white commissure**.

DIVISIONS OF WHITE MATTER

Anterior and posterior nerve roots divide each lateral half of the white matter into three **white columns** or **funiculi**:

1. Anterior or ventral white column
2. Lateral white column
3. Posterior or dorsal white column

TRACTS IN SPINAL CORD

A **nerve tract** is a collection of nerve fibers. **Spinal tracts** are divided into two main groups namely short tracts and long tracts.

Short Tracts of Spinal Cord

Short tracts which connect different parts of spinal cord itself are of two types:

1. Association or intrinsic tracts, which connect adjacent segments of spinal cord on the same half.
2. Commissural tracts, which connect opposite halves of same segment of spinal cord.

Long Tracts of Spinal Cord

Long tracts or **projection tracts** which connect the spinal cord with other parts of CNS are of two types:

1. Ascending tracts, which carry sensory impulses from the spinal cord to brain.
2. Descending tracts, which carry motor impulses from brain to the spinal cord.

ASCENDING TRACTS OF SPINAL CORD

Ascending tracts of spinal cord carry the impulses of various sensations to the brain. Pathway for each sensation is formed by two or three groups of neurons:

1. First order neurons.
2. Second order neurons.
3. Third order neurons.

First Order Neurons

First order neurons receive sensory impulses from the **receptors** and send them to sensory neurons present in the posterior gray horn of spinal cord through their fibers. Nerve cell bodies of these neurons are located in the **posterior nerve root ganglion** that lies outside the spinal cord.

Second Order Neurons

Second order neurons are the sensory neurons present in **posterior gray horn**. Fibers from these neurons form the **ascending tracts** of spinal cord. These fibers carry sensory impulses from spinal cord to different **subcortical areas** (brain areas below cerebral cortex) such as thalamus, cerebellum, etc.

All the ascending tracts are formed by fibers of second order neurons of the sensory pathways except the ascending tracts in the posterior white column which are formed by the fibers of first order neurons.

Third Order Neurons

Third order neurons are in the **subcortical areas**. The fibers of these neurons carry the sensory impulses from subcortical areas to **cerebral cortex.**

Features of the ascending tracts are given in **Table 81.3**.

■ 1. ANTERIOR SPINOTHALAMIC TRACT

Anterior spinothalamic tract is formed by the fibers of second order neurons of the pathway for **crude touch sensation**. This tract is situated in anterior white column **(Figs. 81.3 and 81.4)**.

Origin

Fibers of this tract arise from **chief sensory nucleus** which form the **second order neurons**.

First order neurons which receive impulses from pressure receptors are situated in the posterior nerve root ganglia. Axons of the first order neurons reach the chief sensory nucleus through the posterior nerve root.

Course

After origin, the fibers **cross** the middle line, enter the anterior white column of opposite side and ascend upwards to reach thalamus.

TABLE 81.3: Ascending tracts of spinal cord.

Situation	Tract	Origin	Course	Termination	Function
Anterior white column	1. Anterior spinothalamic tract	Chief sensory nucleus	Crossing in spinal cord Forms spinal lemniscus	Ventral posterolateral nucleus of thalamus	Crude touch sensation
Lateral white column	2. Lateral spinothalamic tract	Substantia gelatinosa	Crossing in spinal cord Forms spinal lemniscus	Ventral posterolateral nucleus of thalamus	Pain sensation Temperature sensations
	3. Ventral spinocerebellar tract	Marginal nucleus	Crossing in spinal cord	Anterior lobe of cerebellum	Subconscious kinesthetic sensations
	4. Dorsal spinocerebellar tract	Clarke nucleus	Uncrossed fibers	Anterior lobe of cerebellum	Subconscious kinesthetic sensations
	5. Spinotectal tract	Chief sensory nucleus	Crossing in spinal cord	Superior colliculus	Spinovisual reflex
	6. Fasciculus dorsolateralis	Posterior nerve root ganglion	Component of lateral spinothalamic tract	Substantia gelatinosa	Pain sensation Temperature sensations
	7. Spinoreticular tract	Intermediolateral cells	Crossed and uncrossed fibers	Reticular formation of brainstem	Consciousness Awareness
	8. Spino-olivary tract	Non-specific	Uncrossed fibers	Olivary nucleus	Proprioception
	9. Spinovestibular tract	Non-specific	Crossed and uncrossed fibers	Lateral vestibular nucleus	Proprioception
Posterior white column	10. Fasciculus gracilis	Posterior nerve root ganglia	Uncrossed fibers No synapse in spinal cord	Nucleus gracilis in medulla	Tactile sensation Tactile localization Tactile discrimination Vibratory sensation
	11. Fasciculus cuneatus	Posterior nerve root ganglia	Uncrossed fibers No synapse in spinal cord	Nucleus cuneatus in medulla	Conscious kinesthetic sensation Stereognosis

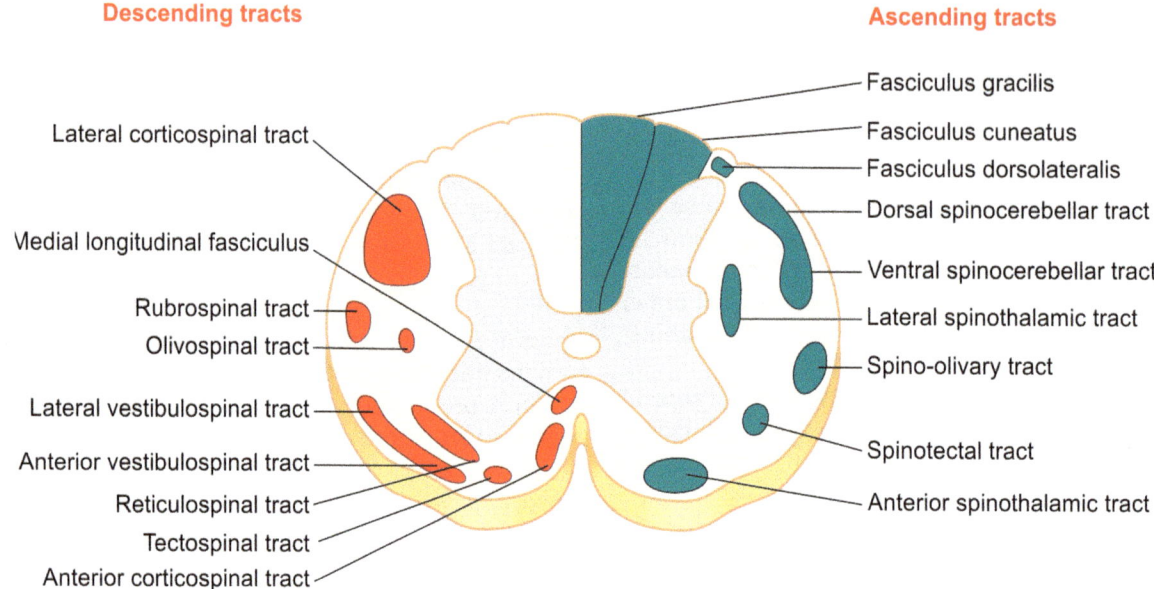

FIGURE 81.3: Tracts of spinal cord.

Termination

Anterior spinothalamic tract terminates in **ventral posterolateral nucleus** of thalamus. From here, fibers of third order neuron carry the impulses to somesthetic area (sensory cortex) of cerebral cortex.

Function

Anterior spinothalamic tract carries impulses of **crude touch** (protopathic) sensation.

Effect of Lesion

Bilateral lesion of this tract leads to loss of crude touch sensation below the level of lesion on both sides. Unilateral lesion of this tract causes loss of crude touch sensation in opposite side.

■ 2. LATERAL SPINOTHALAMIC TRACT

Lateral spinothalamic tract is formed by the fibers from the second order neurons of the pathway for **pain and temperature sensations**. This tract is situated in the lateral white column **(Figs. 81.3 and 81.4)**.

Origin

Fibers of this tract take origin from **substantia gelatinosa of Rolando**. Some fibers arise from marginal nucleus.

Course

After origin, the fibers cross the midline, reach the lateral column of opposite side and ascend upwards to reach thalamus.

Termination

Lateral spinothalamic tract terminates in **ventral posterolateral nucleus** of thalamus. From here, third order neuron fibers relay to the somesthetic area (sensory cortex) of cerebral cortex.

Function

Fibers of this tract carry impulses of **pain and thermal sensations**.

Effect of Lesion

Bilateral lesion of this tract leads to total loss of pain and temperature sensations on both sides below the level of lesion. Unilateral lesion causes loss of pain and temperature sensations in the opposite side.

■ 3. VENTRAL SPINOCEREBELLAR TRACT

Ventral spinocerebellar or **Gower's tract** is formed by the fibers of second order neurons of the pathway for **subconscious kinesthetic sensation**. This tract is situated in lateral white column **(Figs. 81.3 and 81.5)**.

Origin

Fibers of this tract arise from the **marginal nucleus** in posterior gray horn.

Course

Majority of the fibers **cross** the midline and ascend in lateral white column of opposite side. Very few fibers ascend in the lateral white column of the same side. All the fibers ascend and reach the cerebellum via superior cerebellar peduncle.

Termination

These fibers terminate in the **anterior lobe** of cerebellum.

Function

This tract carries the impulses of subconscious kinesthetic sensation (proprioceptive impulses) from muscles, tendons and joints. The impulses of **subconscious kinesthetic sensation** are also called **nonsensory impulses**.

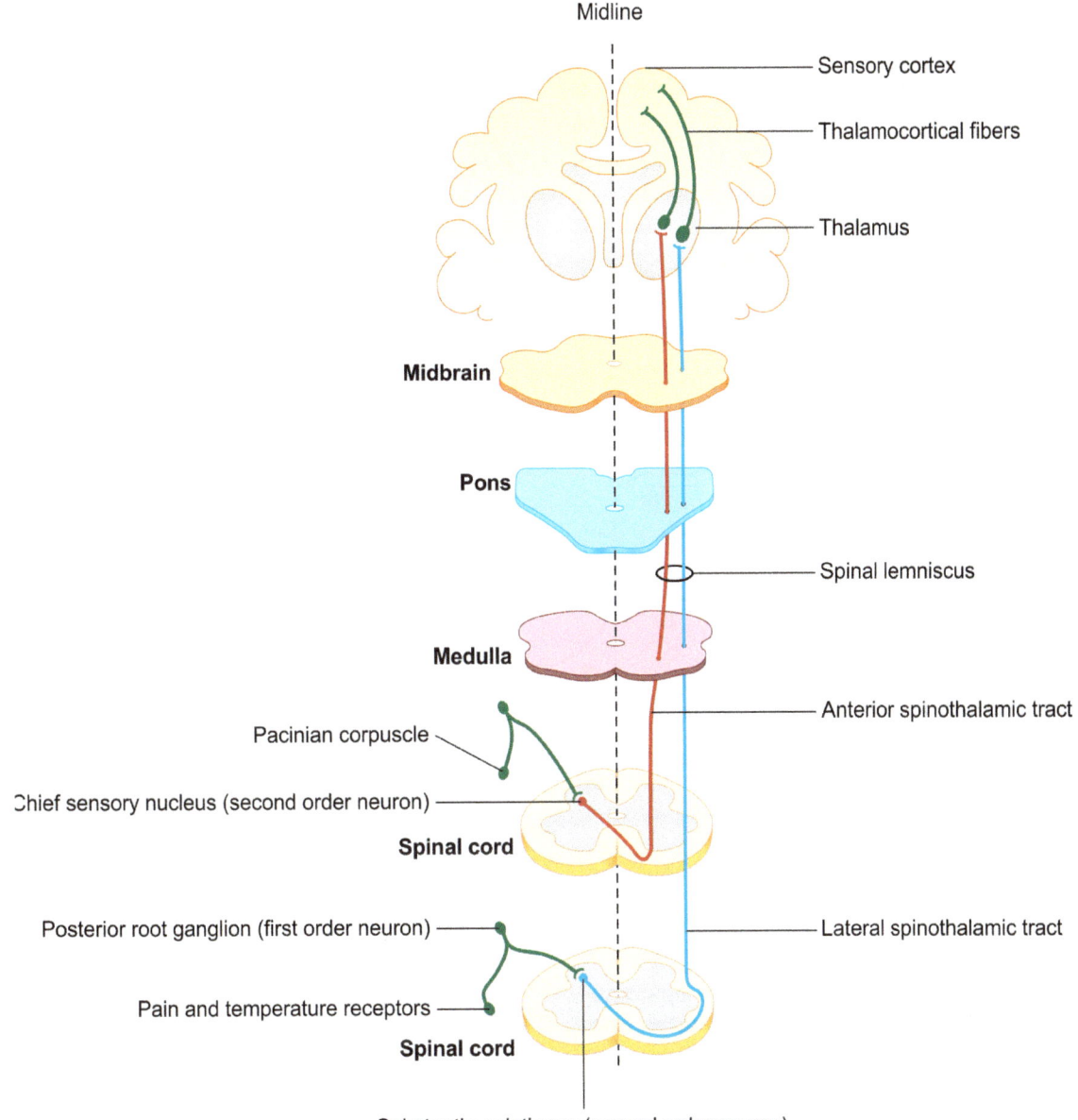

FIGURE 81.4: Spinothalamic tracts and pathways for crude touch, pain and temperature sensations. Anterior spinothalamic tract (red) carries crude touch sensation. Lateral spinothalamic tract (blue) carries pain and temperature sensations.

Effect of Lesion

Lesion of this tract leads to loss of subconscious kinesthetic sensation in the opposite side.

■ 4. DORSAL SPINOCEREBELLAR TRACT

Otherwise called **Flechsig's tract** this tract is formed by the fibers of second order neurons of the pathway for **subconscious kinesthetic sensation (Figs. 81.3 and 81.5)**. It is situated in the lateral white column.

Origin

Fibers of this tract arise from **Clarke's nucleus** in posterior gray matter.

Course

This tract is formed by **uncrossed fibers**. The axons from Clarke's nucleus run to lateral column of same side ascend and reach the cerebellum through inferior cerebellar peduncle.

Termination

Fibers of this tract end in the cortex of anterior lobe of cerebellum along with ventral spinocerebellar tract fibers.

Function

Along with ventral spinocerebellar tract, the dorsal spinocerebellar tract carries the impulses of subconscious kinesthetic sensation (nonsensory impulses).

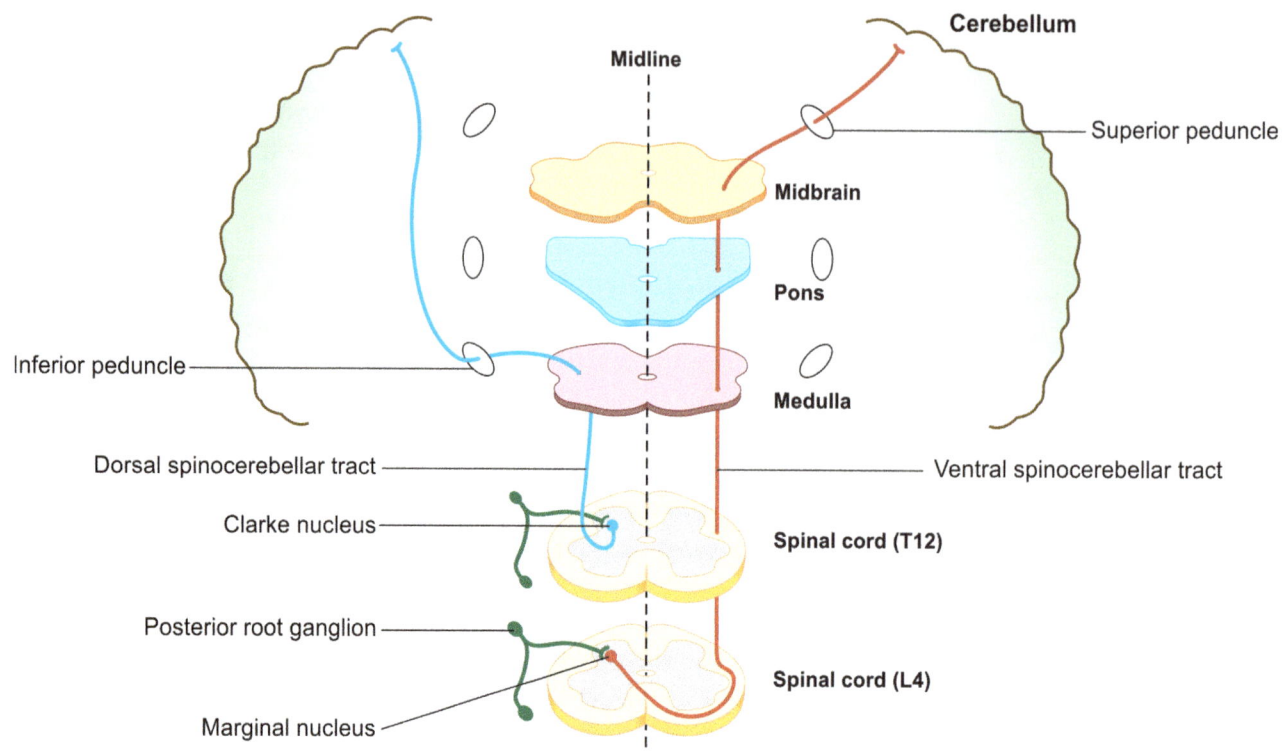

FIGURE 81.5: Spinocerebellar tracts and pathway for subconscious kinesthetic sensation.

Effect of Lesion

Unilateral loss of the subconscious kinesthetic sensation occurs in lesion of this tract on the same side.

5. SPINOTECTAL TRACT

Spinotectal tract is a component of anterior spinothalamic tract **(Fig. 81.3)**. Fibers this tract originates from chief sensory nucleus. After taking origin, the fibers **cross** towards opposite lateral column and ascend to reach midbrain along with anterior spinothalamic tract. Fibers of spinotectal tract terminate in superior colliculus in midbrain. This tract is concerned with **spinovisual reflex**.

6. FASCICULUS DORSOLATERALIS

This tract is also called tract of Lissauer. It is a component of lateral spinothalamic tract. It is situated in the lateral white column **(Fig. 81.3)**. Fibers of this tract arise from posterior root ganglia and enter the spinal cord through lateral division of posterior nerve root. After entering the spinal cord, the fibers pass upwards or downwards for few segments on the same side and synapse with cells of substantia gelatinosa of Rolando. Axons from these cells (second order neurons) join the lateral spinothalamic tract. This tract carries impulses of **pain** and **temperature sensations**.

7. SPINORETICULAR TRACT

Spinoreticular tract is situated in anterolateral white column. Fibers of this tract arise from intermediolateral nucleus. This tract consists of crossed and uncrossed fibers. After taking origin, some of the fibers cross the midline and then ascend upwards. Remaining fibers ascend up in the same side. All the fibers terminate in the reticular formation of brainstem.

Fibers of the spinoreticular tract are the components of **ascending reticular activating system** and are concerned with **consciousness and awareness**.

8. SPINO-OLIVARY TRACT

This tract is situated in anterolateral part of white column. Origin of the fibers of this tract is not specific. However, the fibers terminate in the olivary nucleus of medulla oblongata of the same side. From here, the neurons project into cerebellum. This tract is concerned with **proprioception**.

9. SPINOVESTIBULAR TRACT

Spinovestibular tract is situated in the lateral white column of the spinal cord. The fibers of this tract arise from all the segments of spinal cord and terminate on the lateral vestibular nucleus. This tract is also concerned with **proprioception**.

10. FASCICULUS GRACILIS (TRACT OF GOLL) AND
11. FASCICULUS CUNEATUS (TRACT OF BURDACH)

Both the tracts are together called ascending posterior column tracts because of their situation in posterior column. These two tracts are formed by fibers of **first order neurons** which arise from posterior root ganglia **(Fig. 81.6)**.

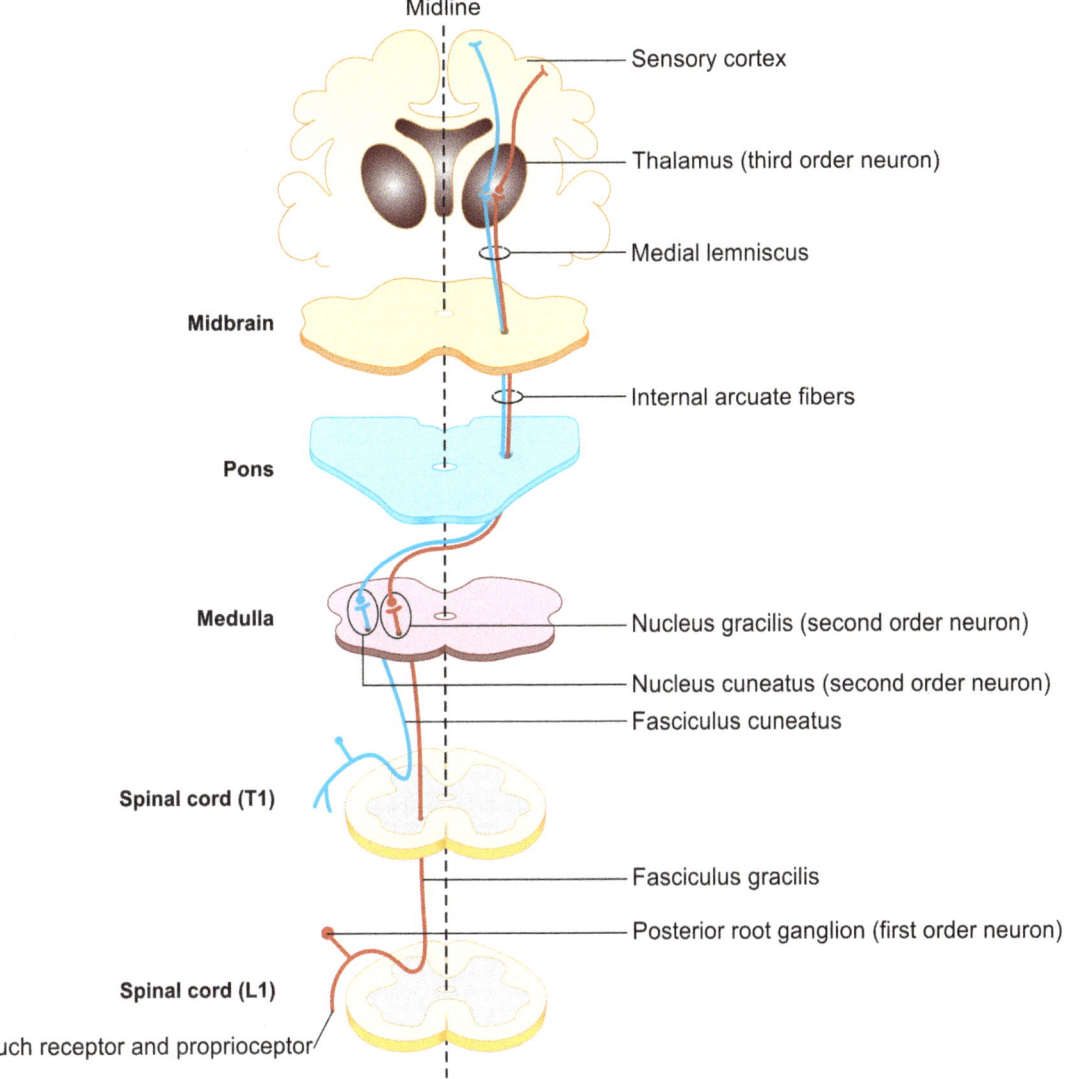

FIGURE 81.6: Ascending tracts in posterior white column of spinal cord and pathway for 1. Fine touch sensation, 2. Tactile localization, 3. Tactile discrimination, 4. Vibratory sensation, 5. Conscious kinesthetic sensation, 6. Stereognosis.

In the cervical and upper thoracic segments of spinal cord, the posterior white column is divided into medial **fasciculus gracilis** and lateral **fasciculus cuneatus**.

Origin

Fibers of these two tracts are the axons of **first order neurons** in the posterior root ganglia.

Course

After entering the spinal cord, the fibers ascend through the posterior white column. Fasciculus gracilis contains the fibers from lower parts of the body, and fasciculus cuneatus contains fibers from upper part of the body.

Termination

These two tracts terminate in the **medulla oblongata** of same side. The fibers of fasciculus gracilis terminate in the **nucleus gracilis** and the fibers of fasciculus cuneatus terminate in the **nucleus cuneatus**. The cells of these medullary nuclei form the **second order neurons**.

Axons of the second order neurons form **internal arcuate fibers**. The internal arcuate fibers from both the sides cross the midline forming **sensory decussation** and then ascend as **medial lemniscus** and terminate in **ventral posterolateral nucleus** of thalamus. From here, fibers of the third order neurons relay to **sensory area** of cerebral cortex.

Functions

Tracts of the posterior white column convey impulses of following sensations:

i. **Fine tactile sensation**.
ii. **Tactile localization:** Ability to locate the area of skin where tactile stimulus is applied with closed eyes.
iii. **Tactile discrimination** (two-point discrimination): Ability to recognize the two stimuli applied over the skin simultaneously with closed eyes.
iv. **Sensation of vibration:** Ability to perceive the vibrations (from a vibrating tuning fork placed over bony prominence) conducted to deep tissues through skin.

v. **Conscious kinesthetic sensation:** Sensation or awareness of muscular activities in the body.
vi. **Stereognosis:** Ability to recognize the known objects by touch with closed eyes.

Effect of Lesion

Lesion in the fibers of these tracts or lesion in the posterior white column leads to the following symptoms on the same side below the lesion:

i. Loss of fine tactile sensation. However, crude touch sensation is normal.
ii. Loss of tactile localization.
iii. Loss of two-point discrimination.
iv. Loss of sensation of vibration.
v. **Astereognosis:** It is the inability to recognize known objects by touch while closing the eyes.
vi. Lack of ability to differentiate the weight of different objects.
vii. Loss of proprioception: It is inability to appreciate the position and movement of different parts of the body.
viii. **Sensory ataxia** or **posterior column ataxia:** It is the condition characterized by uncoordinated, slow and clumsy voluntary movements because of the loss of proprioception.

■ DESCENDING TRACTS OF SPINAL CORD

Descending tracts of the spinal cord are formed by motor nerve fibers arising from brain and descend into the spinal cord. Features of the descending are given in **Table 81.4**. Descending tracts of the spinal cord are of two types:

I. Pyramidal tracts which are concerned with voluntary movements.
II. Extrapyramidal tracts which are concerned with regulation of muscle tone, posture and equilibrium.

■ PYRAMIDAL TRACTS

Pyramidal tracts or **corticospinal tracts**. There are two corticospinal tracts, the anterior corticospinal tract and lateral corticospinal tract.

Origin

Fibers of pyramidal tracts mainly arise from **Giant cells** or **Betz cells** or **pyramidal cells** situated in area 4 (primary motor area) of frontal lobe. Some fibers arise from other

TABLE 81.4: Descending tracts of spinal cord.

	Tract	Situation	Origin	Course	Function
Pyramidal tracts	1. Anterior corticospinal tract	Anterior white column	Primary motor area Premotor area Supplementary motor areas Somatosensory areas	Uncrossed fibers	Control of voluntary movements
	2. Lateral corticospinal tract	Lateral white column		Crossed fibers	Form upper motor neurons
Extrapyramidal tracts	1. Medial longitudinal fasciculus	Anterior white column	Vestibular nucleus Reticular formation Superior colliculus Cells of Cajal	Uncrossed fibers Extend up to upper cervical segments	Coordination of reflex ocular movements Integration of movements of eyes and neck
	2. Anterior vestibulospinal tract	Anterior white column	Medial vestibular nucleus	Uncrossed fibers Extend up to upper thoracic segments	Maintenance of muscle tone and posture
	3. Lateral vestibulospinal tract	Lateral white column	Lateral vestibular nucleus	Mostly uncrossed Extend to all segments	Maintenance of position of head and body during acceleration
	4. Reticulospinal tract	Lateral white fasciculus	Reticular formation of pons and medulla	Mostly uncrossed Extend up to thoracic segments	Coordination of voluntary and reflex movements Control of muscle tone Control of respiration Control of diameter of blood vessels
	5. Tectospinal tract	Anterior white column	Superior colliculus	Crossed fibers Extend up to lower cervical segments	Control of movement of head in response to visual and auditory impulses
	6. Rubrospinal tract	Lateral white column	Red nucleus	Crossed fibers Extend up to thoracic segments	Facilitatory influence on flexor muscle tone
	7. Olivospinal tract	Lateral white column	Inferior olivary nucleus	Mostly crossed Extent: Not clear	Control of movements due to proprioception

Termination: Fibers of all the tracts terminate on motor neurons situated in the anterior gray horn of spinal cord.

areas of frontal lobe and somatosensory area of parietal lobe.

Course

After taking origin, the nerve fibers run downwards through cerebral hemisphere and converge in the form of a fan-like structure called **corona radiata**. Then the fibers descend down and in upper part of medulla these fibers give the appearance of a **pyramid** hence the name pyramidal tracts.

In the lower part of medulla, 80% of fibers from each side cross to the opposite side. While crossing the midline, the fibers of both sides form the **pyramidal decussation**. After crossing and forming pyramidal decussation, these fibers descend through the posterior part of lateral white column of the spinal cord as crossed pyramidal tract or **lateral corticospinal tract** or indirect corticospinal tract.

Remaining 20% of fibers do not cross to the opposite side but descend down through the anterior white column of the spinal cord as uncrossed pyramidal tract or **anterior corticospinal tract** or direct corticospinal tract **(Fig. 81.7)**.

Termination

All the fibers of pyramidal tracts terminate in the **motor neurons** of anterior gray horn. Axons of the motor neurons leave the spinal cord as spinal nerves through anterior nerve roots and supply the skeletal muscles.

Neurons giving origin to the fibers of pyramidal tract are called the **upper motor neurons**. The motor neurons in the spinal cord are called the **lower motor neurons**.

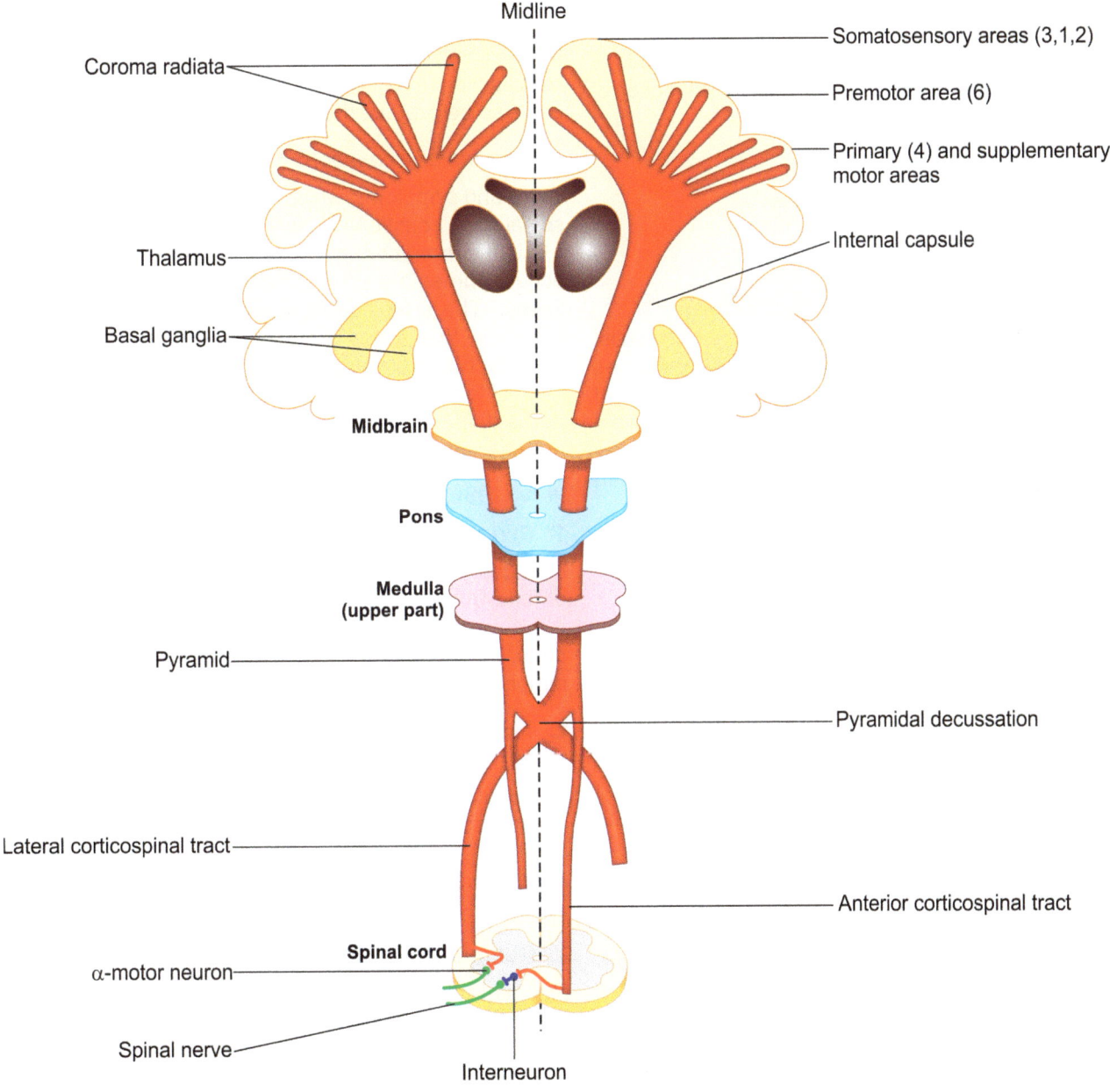

FIGURE 81.7: Pyramidal tracts.

Function

Pyramidal tracts are concerned with **voluntary movements** of the body. Fibers of the pyramidal tracts transmit motor impulses from motor area of cerebral cortex to the anterior motor neurons of the spinal cord. These two tracts are responsible for fine, skilled movements.

Effect of Lesion

Lesion in the neurons of motor cortex and the fibers of pyramidal tracts is called the **upper motor neuron lesion**. Effects of upper motor lesion are given in the next chapter.

■ EXTRAPYRAMIDAL TRACTS

Descending tracts of spinal cord other than pyramidal tracts are called extrapyramidal tracts. Extrapyramidal tracts are listed in **Table 81.4**.

■ APPLIED PHYSIOLOGY

Injury to spinal cord or any disease of spinal cord leads to either temporary or permanent dysfunction. Dysfunction of spinal cord occurs because of:

I. Complete transection.
II. Incomplete transection.
III. Hemisection.
IV. Diseases of spinal cord.

■ I. COMPLETE TRANSECTION OF SPINAL CORD

Complete transection of spinal cord occurs due to bullet injury and accidents. Complete transection causes immediate **loss of sensation** and **voluntary movement** below the level of lesion. In quick transection of spinal cord, the patient feels himself cut into two. Then the effects (symptoms) of complete transection of spinal cord start appearing.

Effects occur in three stages:

1. Stage of spinal shock.
2. Stage of reflex activity.
3. Stage of reflex failure.

1. Stage of Spinal Shock

Common symptoms during this stage are **paralysis of limbs**, **loss of reflexes**, and **loss of sensations**. There is decreased venous return resulting in accumulation of blood in lower limbs. When lesion is at or above T1 segment, the blood pressure falls drastically.

2. Stage of Reflex Activity

Stage of reflex activity is also called **stage of recovery**. After 3 weeks period, depending largely upon the general health of the patient, muscle tone and reflex activity begin to return to the isolated segments of spinal cord below the level of lesion. Tone returns first to flexor muscles.

3. Stage of Reflex Failure

Though the reflex movements return, muscles below the level of injury have less power and less resistance. Usually, general condition of the patient starts **deteriorating**. General infection or **toxemia** becomes common. Due to this, the failure of reflex function develops. The reflexes become more difficult to elicit. Muscles become extremely **flaccid** and undergo **wasting**.

■ II. INCOMPLETE TRANSECTION OF SPINAL CORD

If spinal cord is gravely injured, but does not suffer complete division, the condition is called as incomplete transection.

After incomplete transection of the spinal cord also, all the three stages of complete transection occur:

Features are similar to those of complete transection. In second stage, tone returns first to extensor muscles.

■ III. HEMISECTION OF SPINAL CORD: BROWN-SÉQUARD SYNDROME

Lesion involving one lateral half of the spinal cord is called hemisection. It can occur due to injury during accidents. It can also be produced experimentally in animals.

Symptoms of Hemisection of Spinal Cord

Signs and symptoms, which occur after hemisection of the spinal cord, constitute Brown-Séquard syndrome.

If the hemisection is due to injury, spinal shock occurs immediately. Muscles lose the tone and become flaccid. The reflexes are abolished. In case the patient survives, this stage gradually passes off and certain signs and symptoms develop. Effects occur below the level of lesion and at the level of lesion. Effects in these areas differ on the same side and opposite side. There are changes in sensory and motor functions.

■ IV. DISEASES OF SPINAL CORD

1. Syringomyelia

Syringomyelia is a disorder characterized by the presence of **fluid-filled cavities** in the spinal cord.

It occurs due to the over growth of **neuroglial cells**. Features of this disease are the loss of pain and temperature sensations and muscular weakness.

2. Tabes Dorsalis

Tabes dorsalis is a slowly progressive nervous disorder affecting all functions of spinal cord.

It occurs due to the degeneration of posterior (sensory) nerve roots. It usually occurs in **syphilis**. In tabes dorsalis, both sensory and motor functions are affected.

3. Multiple Sclerosis

Multiple sclerosis (MS) is a chronic and **progressive inflammatory disease** characterized by **demyelination** (destruction of myelin sheath) in brain and spinal cord. The term **sclerosis** refers to **scars** in the myelin sheath.

Initial symptoms include loss of sensations, weakness and disturbances in maintenance of posture. Symptoms when the disease progresses include tremor, fatigue and muscle spasms, speech difficulty, difficulty in performing day-to-day activities, complete blindness and suicidal tendency.

4. Disk Prolapse

Disk prolapse is the rupture of intervertebral disk or **spinal disk** which is the cartilaginous structure of vertebral column that separates each vertebra. During disk prolapse, the soft inner material bulges out and irritates or compresses or damages the nerve root that passes through the gap between the vertebrae. Severity of the condition depends upon the degree of bulging.

Symptoms of disk prolapse include pain and weakness in the area of prolapse. Most common areas of disk prolapse are neck and lower part of vertebral column.

Chapter 82: Somatosensory System and Somatomotor System

CHAPTER OUTLINE

- **SENSATIONS**
- **SOMATOSENSORY SYSTEM**
  - TYPES OF SOMATIC SENSATIONS
  - SENSORY PATHWAYS
  - SENSORY FIBERS PASSING THROUGH SPINAL CORD
  - SENSORY FIBERS PASSING THROUGH TRIGEMINAL NERVE
  - APPLIED PHYSIOLOGY
- **MOTOR ACTIVITIES OF THE BODY**
- **SOMATOMOTOR SYSTEM**
  - ACTIVITIES OF SKELETAL MUSCLES
  - STRUCTURE OF MOTOR SYSTEM
  - MOTOR NEURONS IN SPINAL CORD AND CRANIAL NERVE NUCLEI
  - CLASSIFICATION OF MOTOR PATHWAYS
  - UPPER MOTOR NEURON AND LOWER MOTOR NEURON
  - APPLIED PHYSIOLOGY

■ SENSATIONS

Sensation is a process of detecting and sensing external or internal stimuli received by sensory receptors. It is different from **perception** which means identification and interpretation of sensations.

Sensations are of two types:

1. Somatic Sensations

Somatic sensations are the sensations arising from skin, muscles, tendons, joints and visceral organs. These sensations have **specific receptors**, which respond to a particular type of stimulus.

2. Special Sensations

Special sensations are the **complex sensations** for which the body has some **specialized sense organs**. Such sensations are usually called **special senses**. Special senses are vision, hearing, taste and smell.

Special senses are described in Section 11. This chapter deals only with somatic sensations.

■ SOMATOSENSORY SYSTEM

Somatosensory system is the sensory system associated with different parts of the body. It includes specific receptors, sensory or afferent neurons and the centers.

■ TYPES OF SOMATIC SENSATIONS

Somatic sensations are classified into three types:

1. Epicritic sensations.
2. Protopathic sensations.
3. Deep sensations.

1. Epicritic Sensations

Epicritic sensations are the mild or **light sensations** which are perceived and localized more accurately.

Epicritic sensations are:

i. Fine touch or tactile sensation.
ii. Tactile localization.
iii. Tactile discrimination.
iv. Temperature sensation with finer range between 25 and 40°C.

2. Protopathic Sensations

Protopathic sensations are the **crude sensations** which are primitive type of sensations.

Protopathic sensations are:

i. Pressure sensation.
ii. Pain sensation.
iii. Temperature sensation with a wider range, i.e. below 25°C and above 40°C (Fig. 82.1).

Chapter 82: Somatosensory System and Somatomotor System

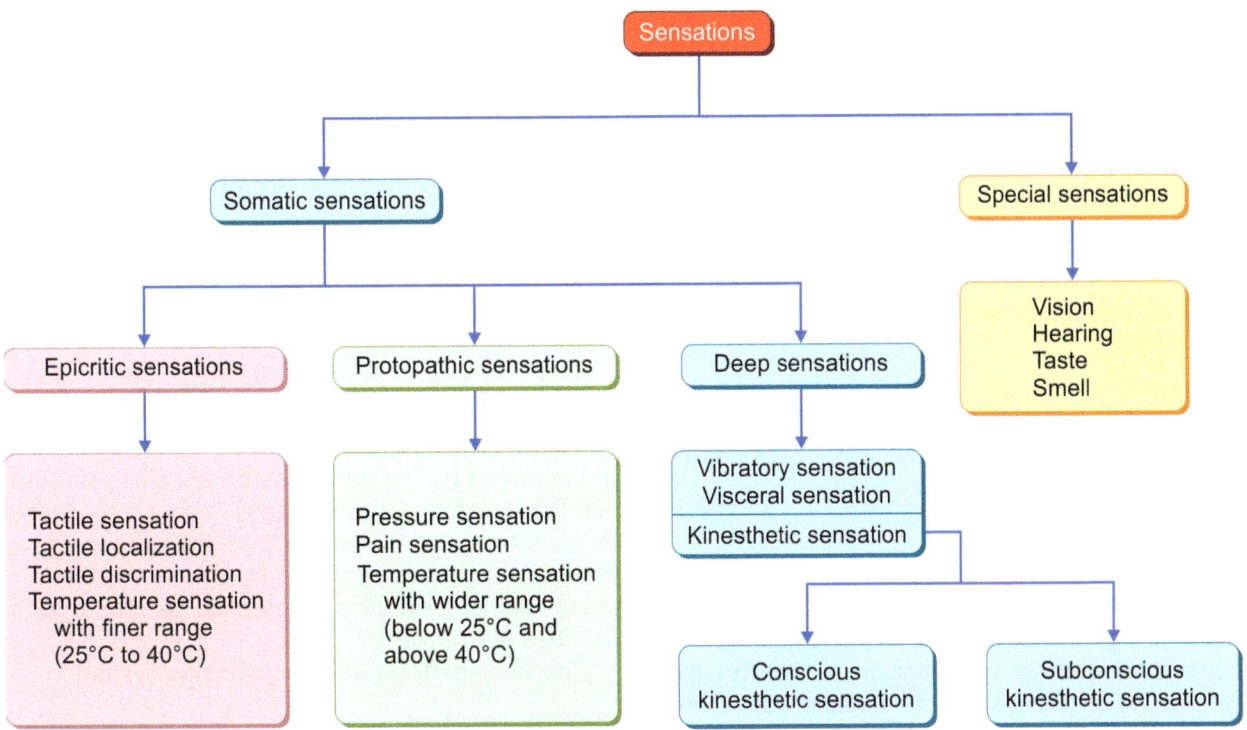

FIGURE 82.1: Classification of sensations.

3. Deep Sensations

Deep sensations are sensations arising from **deeper structures** beneath the skin and visceral organs.

Deep sensations are:

i. Sensation of vibration or pallesthesia: Combination of touch and pressure sensation.
ii. Kinesthetic sensation or kinesthesia: Sensation of position and movements of different parts of the body. Kinesthetic sensation is of two types:
   a. Conscious kinesthetic sensation.
   b. Subconscious kinesthetic sensation. Impulses of this sensation are called nonsensory impulses.
iii. Visceral sensations arising from viscera.

Combined or Synthetic Sensations

Combined or synthetic sensations are the sensations synthesized at cortical level, by combination two or more basic sensations. Examples of synthetic senses are **vibratory sensation** and **stereognosis (Box 82.1)**.

BOX 82.1: Combined sensations.

Vibratory sensation
Ability to perceive vibrations from a vibrating tuning fork placed over bony prominence conducted to deep tissues through skin
Produced by combination of touch and pressure sensations
Stereognosis
Ability to recognize the known objects by touch with closed eyes
Produced by combination of touch and pressure sensations

Paresthesia or Abnormal Sensations

Paresthesia or abnormal sensations are the unusual feelings on skin without any specific stimulus. Examples of abnormal sensations are numbness, pricking, tingling and burning **(Box 82.2)**.

■ SENSORY PATHWAYS

Sensory pathways carry the impulses from receptors in different parts of the body to centers in brain.

Sensory pathways are of two types:

1. Pathways of somatosensory system.
2. Pathways of viscerosensory system.

   Pathways of somatosensory system convey the information from sensory receptors in skin, skeletal muscles and joints. Pathways of this system are constituted by somatic nerve fibers called somatic afferent nerve fibers.

BOX 82.2: Abnormal sensations.

Numbness
Lack of sensation in a part of the body
Pricking
Sensation of being pierced or pricked
Tingling
Sensation of slight prickling or sensation of tapping by several needle-like objects
Burning
Sensation of a type of pain that is different from aching or stabbing pain

Pathways of viscerosensory system convey the information from receptors of the viscera. Pathways of this system are constituted by visceral or autonomic fibers. This chapter deals mainly with the somatosensory system.

Somatosensory fibers from different parts of the body run through:

i. Spinal tracts
ii. Trigeminal nerve.

SENSORY FIBERS PASSING THROUGH SPINAL CORD

Sensory fibers from different parts of the body except face and scalp form the sensory pathways which pass through spinal cord. These sensory pathways are constituted by two or three groups of neurons:

i. First order or primary neurons.
ii. Second order or secondary neurons.
iii. Third order or tertiary neurons.

These three groups of neurons are described along with ascending tracts of spinal cord in Chapter 81. Pathways of some sensations such as kinesthetic sensation have only first and second order neurons.

Details of pathways are given in **Table 82.1**, Diagrams of pathways are given in Chapter 81, along with ascending tracts of spinal cord.

SENSORY FIBERS PASSING THROUGH TRIGEMINAL NERVE

Trigeminal nerve carries somatosensory information from face, teeth, periodontal tissues (tissues around teeth), oral cavity, nasal cavity, cranial dura mater and major part of scalp to sensory cortex. It also conveys proprioceptive impulses from the extrinsic muscles of the eyeball.

Origin

Sensory fibers of trigeminal nerve arise from the **trigeminal ganglion** situated near temporal bone. Peripheral processes of neurons in this ganglion form three divisions of trigeminal nerve, namely **ophthalmic**, **mandibular** and **maxillary** divisions **(Table 82.2)**. Cutaneous distribution of the three divisions of trigeminal nerve is shown in **Figure 82.2**.

Central processes from neurons of trigeminal ganglion enter pons in the form of sensory root.

Termination

After reaching the pons, fibers of sensory root divide into two groups. One group of fibers terminate in ventral posteromedial nucleus of thalamus in the same side or opposite side. From thalamus, the fibers reach the somatosensory areas of cerebral cortex. These fibers carry the sensations of touch, pressure, pain and temperature from the regions mentioned above.

Another group of fibers terminate in spinocerebellum of same side. These fibers carry proprioceptive impulses from facial muscles, muscles of mastication and ocular muscles.

APPLIED PHYSIOLOGY

Lesions or other nervous disorders in sensory pathway affect the sensory functions of the body. Effects are given in **Table 82.3**.

MOTOR ACTIVITIES OF THE BODY

Motor activities of the body are divided into two types:

1. Activities of skeletal muscles which are involved in the posture and movement.
2. Activities of smooth muscles, cardiac muscles and other tissues, which are involved in the functions of various visceral organs.

Activities of the skeletal muscles (voluntary functions) are controlled by the somatomotor system. Activities of other tissues or the visceral organs (involuntary functions) are controlled by the visceral or autonomic nervous system, which is constituted by the sympathetic and parasympathetic systems. Autonomic nervous system is described in Chapter 92.

This chapter deals with somatomotor system.

SOMATOMOTOR SYSTEM

Somatomotor system is the part of nervous system that controls the activities of the skeletal muscles (voluntary functions). It is constituted by somatic motor nerve fibers.

ACTIVITIES OF SKELETAL MUSCLES

Movements of the body depend upon the different groups of skeletal muscles. Various types of movements or the motor activities brought about by these muscles are:

1. Execution of smooth, precise and accurate voluntary movements.
2. Coordination of movements responsible for skilled activities.
3. Coordination of movements responsible for maintenance of posture and equilibrium.

All these motor activities are controlled by different parts of the nervous system, which are together called the motor system.

STRUCTURE OF MOTOR SYSTEM

Motor system includes spinal cord and its nerves, cranial nerves, brainstem, cerebral cortex, cerebellum and basal ganglia. The neuronal circuits between these parts of the nervous system which are responsible for the motor activities are called the **motor pathways**.

MOTOR NEURONS IN SPINAL CORD AND CRANIAL NERVE NUCLEI

Activities of skeletal muscles are executed by the impulses discharged from alpha motor neurons situated in ventral (anterior) gray horn of spinal cord and nuclei of many of the cranial nerves present in brainstem.

Alpha motor neurons in the spinal cord which innervate the **extrafusal fibers** of skeletal muscles are responsible for the **contraction of muscles** in upper

TABLE 82.1: Sensory pathways.

Sensation	Receptor	First order neuron in	Second order neuron in	Third order neuron in	Center
Fine touch Tactile localization Tactile discrimination Vibratory sensation Stereognosis	Meissner corpuscles and Merkel disk	Posterior nerve root ganglion fibers form Fasciculus gracilis and Fasciculus cuneatus	Nucleus gracilis and Nucleus cuneatus: Fibers form internal arcuate fibers	Ventral posterolateral nucleus of thalamus	Sensory cortex
Pressure Crude touch	Pacinian corpuscle	Posterior nerve root ganglion	Chief sensory nucleus Fibers form anterior spinothalamic tract	Ventral posterolateral nucleus of thalamus	Sensory cortex
Temperature	Warmth: Ruffini end bulb Cold: Krause end bulb	Posterior nerve root ganglion	Substantia gelatinosa Fibers form lateral spinothalamic tract	Ventral posterolateral nucleus of thalamus	Sensory cortex
Conscious kinesthetic sensation	Proprioceptors: Muscle spindle Golgi tendon apparatus	Posterior nerve root ganglion Fibers form Fasciculus gracilis and Fasciculus cuneatus	Nucleus gracilis and Nucleus cuneatus: Fibers form internal arcuate fibers	Ventral posterolateral nucleus of thalamus	Sensory cortex
Subconscious kinesthetic sensation	Proprioceptors: Muscle spindle Golgi tendon apparatus	Posterior nerve root ganglion	Nucleus of Clarke and Marginal nucleus Fibers form dorsal and ventral spinocerebellar tracts	—	Anterior lobe of cerebellum
Pain	Free nerve endings	Posterior nerve root ganglion Fast pain: Aδ-fibers Slow pain: C fibers	Fast pain: Marginal nucleus in spinal cord Slow pain: Substantia gelatinosa of Rolando Fibers form lateral spinothalamic tract	Ventral posterolateral nucleus of thalamus, reticular formation and midbrain	Sensory cortex

TABLE 82.2: Functions of three divisions of trigeminal nerve.

Division	Areas supplied	Function
Ophthalmic	Forehead Eye Front portion of nose	Sensory
Maxillary	Upper teeth, gums and lip Lower eyelid Sides of nose	Sensory
Mandibular	Lower teeth, gums and lip	Sensory
	Jaw	Motor

limbs, trunk and lower part of the body. The **gamma motor neurons** which innervate the **intrafusal fibers** of muscle are responsible for the maintenance of **muscle tone**. Motor neurons of the cranial nerve nuclei situated in brainstem send their signals to the muscles of neck and upper part of trunk via cranial nerves.

Final Common Pathway

Alpha motor neurons in spinal cord or cranial nerve nuclei are called **'final common pathway'** of motor

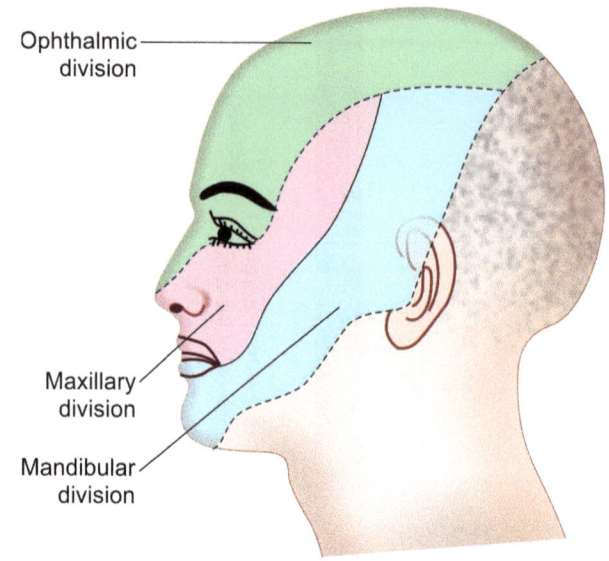

FIGURE 82.2: Cutaneous distribution (sensory) of the three divisions of trigeminal nerve.

TABLE 82.3: Effects of disorders of sensory pathways.

Condition	Definition
1. Anesthesia	Loss of all sensations
2. Hyperesthesia	Increased sensitivity to sensory stimuli
3. Hypoesthesia	Reduction in sensitivity to stimuli
4. Hemianesthesia	Loss of all sensations in one side of body
5. Paresthesia	Abnormal sensations such as tingling, burning, prickling and numbness
6. Hemiparesthesia	Abnormal sensations in one side of body
7. Dissociated anesthesia	Loss of some sensations while other sensations are intact
8. General anesthesia	Loss of all sensations with loss of consciousness produced by general anesthetic agents
9. Local anesthesia	Loss of sensations in a restricted area of the body
10. Spinal anesthesia	Loss of sensations without loss of consciousness due to spinal cord lesion or spinal anesthetic agents injected beneath of coverings spinal cord
11. Tactile anesthesia	Loss of tactile sensations
12. Tactile hyperesthesia	Increased sensitivity to tactile
13. Analgesia	Loss of pain sensation
14. Hyperalgesia	Increased sensitivity to pain
15. Paralgesia	Abnormal pain sensation
16. Thermoanesthesia or thermanesthesia or thermanalgesia	Loss of thermal sensation
17. Pallanesthesia	Loss of sensation of vibration
18. Astereognosis	Loss of ability to recognize known object with closed eyes due to loss of cutaneous sensations
19. Illusion	Mental depression due to misinterpretation of a sensory stimulus
20. Hallucination	Feeling of a sensation without any stimulus

Chapter 82: Somatosensory System and Somatomotor System

TABLE 82.4: Effects of upper motor neuron lesion and lower motor neuron lesion.

	Effects	Upper motor neuron lesion	Lower motor neuron lesion
Clinical observation	1. Muscle tone	Hypertonia	Hypotonia
	2. Paralysis	Spastic type of paralysis	Flaccid type of paralysis
	3. Wastage of muscle	Wastage of muscle occurs	Wastage of muscle occurs
	4. Superficial reflexes	Lost	Lost
	5. Plantar reflex	Abnormal plantar reflex – Babinski sign	Absent
	6. Deep reflexes	Exaggerated	Lost
	7. Clonus	Present	Absent
Clinical confirmation	8. Electrical activity	Normal	Absent
	9. Muscles affected	Groups of muscles are affected	Individual muscles are affected
	10. Fascicular twitch in EMG	Absent	Present

system because the motor impulses from different parts of nervous system reach the muscles only through them.

■ CLASSIFICATION OF MOTOR PATHWAYS

Motor pathways are divided into two types of tracts:

1. Pyramidal tracts which are concerned with voluntary movements.
2. Extrapyramidal tracts which are concerned with coordination muscle tone, posture, equilibrium and integration and the regulation of motor activities.

Details of these tracts are given in Chapter 81.

■ UPPER MOTOR NEURON AND LOWER MOTOR NEURON

Neurons of the motor system are divided into upper motor neurons and lower motor neurons depending upon their location and termination.

Upper Motor Neuron

Upper motor neurons are the neurons in the higher centers of brain, which control the lower motor neurons.

Upper motor neurons are of three types:

1. Motor neurons in the **cerebral cortex**. Fibers of these neurons form corticospinal (pyramidal) and corticobulbar tracts.
2. Neurons in the **basal ganglia** and **brainstem nuclei**.
3. Neurons in the **cerebellum**.

Motor neurons in the cerebral cortex, which give origin to pyramidal tracts, belong to the pyramidal system and the remaining motor neurons belong to extrapyramidal system.

Lower Motor Neuron

Lower motor neurons are the anterior gray horn cells in the **spinal cord** and the motor neurons of the **cranial nerve nuclei** situated in brainstem, which innervate the muscles directly.

Lower motor neurons constitute the '**final common pathway**' of motor system. The lower motor neurons are under the influence of the upper motor neurons.

■ APPLIED PHYSIOLOGY

Effects of Lesion of Motor Neurons

Effects of lesions of upper motor neurons and lower motor neurons are given in **Table 82.4**. The effects of lower motor neuron lesion are the loss of muscle tone and flaccid paralysis.

Effects of upper motor neuron lesion depend upon the site:

1. Lesion in pyramidal system causes hypertonia and spastic paralysis.

TABLE 82.5: Types of paralysis.

Paralysis	Parts of the body affected	Causes
Monoplegia	Paralysis of one limb	Isolated damage of central nervous system or peripheral nervous system
Diplegia	Paralysis of both the upper limbs or both the lower limbs	Isolated damage of brain
Hemiplegia	Paralysis of upper limb and lower limb on one side of the body	Lesion in motor cortex and corticospinal tracts in posterior limb of internal capsule on the side opposite to the paralysis
Paraplegia	Paralysis of lower half of the body	Injury to lower part of spinal cord
Quadriplegia or tetraplegia	Paralysis of all the four limbs	Injury to upper part of spinal cord (shoulder level or above, at which the motor nerves of upper limbs leave the spinal cord)

2. Lesion in basal ganglia produces hypertonia and rigidity involving both flexor and extensor muscles.
3. Lesion in cerebellum causes hypotonia, muscular weakness and incoordination of movements.

Paralysis

Paralysis is defined as the complete loss of strength and functions of muscle group or a limb.

Causes for paralysis

Common causes for paralysis are:

1. Trauma.
2. Tumor.
3. Stroke.
4. Cerebral palsy (condition caused by brain injury immediately after birth)
5. Neurodegenerative diseases.

Types of paralysis

Paralysis of the muscles in the body depends upon the type and location of motor neurons affected by lesion. Different types of paralysis are given in **Table 82.5**.

Chapter 83

Physiology of Pain

CHAPTER OUTLINE

- PAIN SENSATION
- BENEFITS OF PAIN SENSATION
- COMPONENTS OF PAIN SENSATION
- PATHWAYS OF PAIN SENSATION
- VISCERAL PAIN
- NEUROTRANSMITTERS INVOLVED IN PAIN SENSATION
- REFERRED PAIN
- ANALGESIA SYSTEM
- GATE CONTROL THEORY
- APPLIED PHYSIOLOGY

PAIN SENSATION

Pain sensation is defined as an unpleasant and emotional experience associated with or without actual tissue damage. Pain is described in many ways like sharp, pricking, electric, dull ache, shooting, cutting, stabbing, etc. Often it induces crying and fainting.

Pain is produced by real or potential injury to the body. Often it is expressed in terms of injury. For example, pain produced by fire is expressed as **burning sensation**. Pain produced by severe sustained contraction of skeletal muscles is expressed as **cramps**.

BENEFITS OF PAIN SENSATION

Pain is an important sensory symptom. Though it is an unpleasant sensation, it has protective or survival benefits.

Protective or survival benefits of pain.

1. Pain gives warning signal about the existence of a problem or threat. It also creates the awareness of injury.
2. Pain prevents further damage by causing reflex withdrawal of the body from the source of injury.
3. Pain urges the person to take required treatment to prevent major damage.

COMPONENTS OF PAIN SENSATION

Pain has two components:

1. Fast pain.
2. Slow pain.

Fast pain is the first sensation whenever a pain stimulus is applied. It is experienced as a bright, sharp and localized pain sensation. Fast pain is followed by the **slow pain** which is experienced as a dull, diffused and unpleasant pain.

PATHWAYS OF PAIN SENSATION

Pain sensation from various parts of body is carried to brain by different pathways which are:

1. Pathway from skin and the deeper structures.
2. Pathway from face.
3. Pathway from viscera.
4. Pathway from pelvic region.

1. PATHWAY OF PAIN SENSATION FROM SKIN AND DEEPER STRUCTURES

Receptors

Receptors for both the components of pain are the same i.e. free nerve endings which are distributed throughout the body.

First Order Neurons

First order neurons are the cells in the posterior nerve root ganglia which receive the impulses of pain sensation from the pain receptors through their dendrites. These impulses are transmitted to spinal cord through the axons of first order neurons.

Fast pain fibers

Fast pain sensation is carried by Aδ type afferent fibers which synapse with neurons of **marginal nucleus** in the posterior gray horn.

Slow pain fibers

Slow pain sensation is carried by C type afferent fibers which synapse with neurons of **substantia gelatinosa of Rolando** in the posterior gray horn **(Fig. 81.4)**.

Second Order Neurons

Neurons of marginal nucleus and substantia gelatinosa of Rolando form the second order neurons. Fibers from these neurons ascend in the form of the **lateral spinothalamic tract**.

Third Order Neurons

Third order neurons are **ventral posterolateral nucleus** of thalamus and **reticular formation**. Axons from these neurons reach the sensory area of **cerebral cortex**. Some fibers from reticular formation reach **hypothalamus**.

Center for Pain Sensation

Center for pain sensation is in the postcentral gyrus of **parietal cortex**. Fibers reaching **hypothalamus** are concerned with arousal mechanism due to pain stimulus.

2. PATHWAY OF PAIN SENSATION FROM FACE

Pain sensation from face is carried by **trigeminal nerve**. Refer Chapter 82 for details.

3. PATHWAY OF PAIN SENSATION FROM VISCERA

Pain sensation from thoracic and abdominal viscera is transmitted by **thoracolumbar** (sympathetic) **nerves**. Pain from esophagus, trachea and pharynx is carried by **vagus nerve** and **glossopharyngeal nerve**.

4. PATHWAY OF PAIN SENSATION FROM PELVIC REGION

Pain sensation from deeper structures of pelvic region is conveyed by **sacral parasympathetic nerves**.

VISCERAL PAIN

Pain from viscera is unpleasant. It is poorly localized.

CAUSES OF VISCERAL PAIN

1. Substances released during ischemic reactions such as bradykinin and proteolytic enzymes stimulate the pain receptors of viscera.
2. Chemical substances such as acidic gastric juice leaks from ruptured ulcers into peritoneal cavity and produce pain.
3. Spastic contraction of smooth muscles in gastrointestinal tract and other hollow organs of viscera cause pain by stimulating the free nerve endings.
4. Overdistention of hollow organs also causes pain.

NEUROTRANSMITTERS INVOLVED IN PAIN SENSATION

Glutamate and **substance P** are the neurotransmitters secreted by pain nerve endings. Glutamate is secreted by A afferent fibers, which transmit impulses of fast pain. Substance P is secreted by C type fibers, which transmit impulses of slow pain.

REFERRED PAIN

Referred pain is the pain that is perceived at a site adjacent to or away from the site of origin. The deep pain and some visceral pain are referred to other areas. But the superficial pain is not referred.

EXAMPLES OF REFERRED PAIN

1. Cardiac pain is felt at the inner part of left arm and left shoulder.
2. Pain in ovary is referred to umbilicus.
3. Pain from testis is felt in abdomen.
4. Pain in diaphragm is referred to right shoulder.
5. Pain in gallbladder is referred to epigastric region.
6. Renal pain is referred to loin **(Fig. 83.1)**.

MECHANISM OF REFERRED PAIN

Dermatomal Rule

According to dermatomal rule, pain is referred to a structure, which is developed from the same dermatome from which the pain producing structure is developed.

A **dermatome** includes the structures or parts of the body, which are innervated by afferent nerve fibers of one dorsal root. For example, the heart and inner aspect of left arm originate from the same dermatome. So, the pain in heart is referred to left arm.

ANALGESIA SYSTEM

Analgesia system means the **pain control system**. Body has its own analgesia system in brain which provides a short-term relief from pain. It is also called **endogenous analgesia system**.

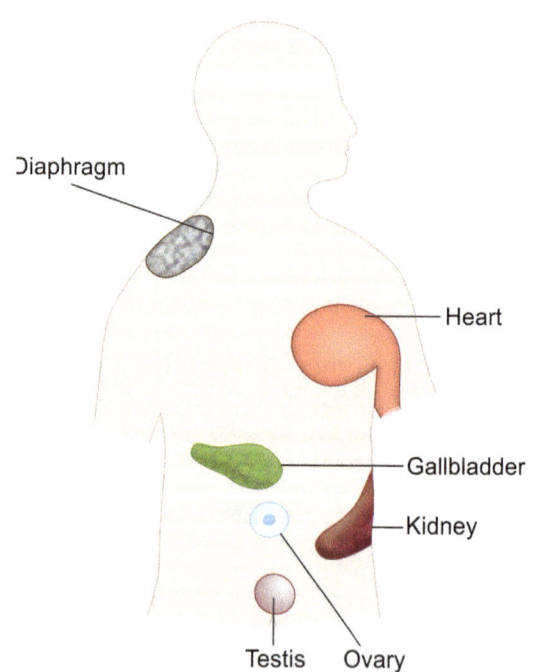

FIGURE 83.1: Sites of referred pain.

Analgesia system has got its own pathway through which it blocks the synaptic transmission of pain sensation in spinal cord and suppresses pain. In fact, analgesic drugs such as **opioids** act through this system and provide a controlled pain relief.

■ ANALGESIC PATHWAY

Analgesic pathway is considered as **descending pain pathway**, the ascending pain pathway being the afferent fibers that transmit pain sensation to the brain. Analgesic pathway commences from brainstem **(Fig. 83.2)**.

Nerve Fibers Forming Analgesic Pathway

1. Nerve fibers of analgesic pathway arise from two sources namely, periventricular nucleus and periaqueductal gray matter (PAG) situated in midbrain.
2. Nerve fibers from above areas terminate in two areas called nucleus raphe magnus and nucleus locus ceruleus situated in reticular formation of midbrain.
3. Fibers from the above nuclei descend through dorsal horn of spinal cord and synapse with interneurons.
4. Interneurons form synapses with the neurons of marginal nucleus and substantia gelatinosa of Rolando. Neurons of these nuclei form second order neurons of afferent (ascending) pathway for pain.

Mechanism of Analgesic Pathway in Inhibiting Pain Transmission

1. Whenever sensory cortex receives impulses of pain sensation via afferent pain pathway, it activates the periventricular nucleus and periaqueductal gray matter.

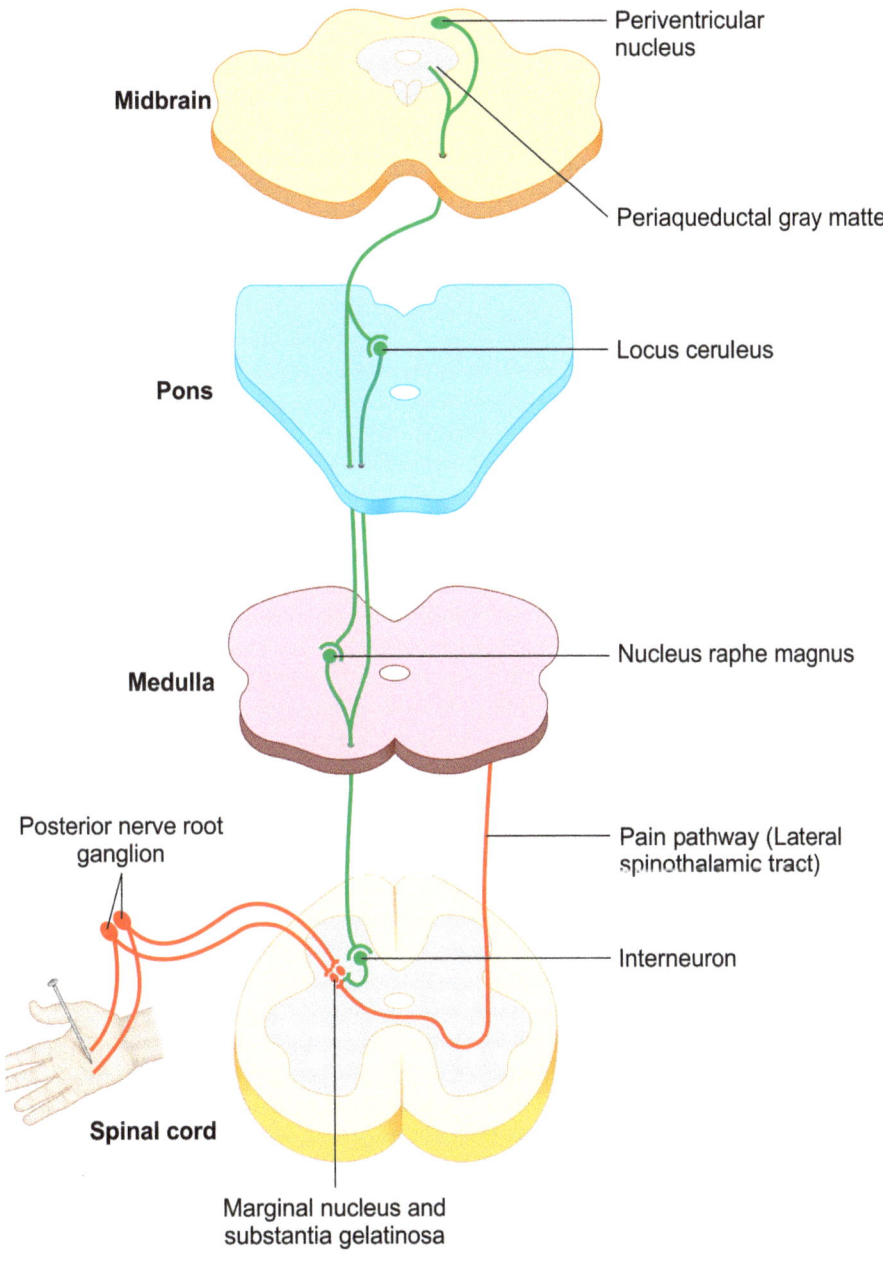

FIGURE 83.2: Analgesic pathway.

2. These two areas in turn activate nucleus raphe magnus and nucleus locus ceruleus of reticular formation.
3. Now, impulses from these two nuclei are transmitted to interneurons present in lateral horn of spinal cord.
4. Interneurons of spinal cord now, inhibit pain transmission at the synaptic level before being relayed to brain.

GATE CONTROL THEORY

Gate control theory explains the **pain suppression**. According to this theory, the pain stimuli transmitted by afferent pain fibers are blocked by gate mechanism located at the posterior gray horn of spinal cord. If the gate is opened, pain is felt. If the gate is closed, pain is suppressed. Brain also plays some important role in the gate control system of the spinal cord.

Significance of Gate Control

Thus, the gating of pain at spinal level is similar to **presynaptic inhibition**. It forms the basis for relief of pain through rubbing, massage techniques, application of ice packs, acupuncture and electrical analgesia. All these techniques relieve pain by stimulating the release of endogenous pain relievers such as **opioid peptides** which close the gate and block the pain signals.

APPLIED PHYSIOLOGY

1. Analgesia: Loss of pain sensation.
2. Hyperalgesia: Increased sensitivity to pain sensation.
3. Paralgesia: Abnormal pain sensation.

Chapter 84

Thalamus and Hypothalamus

CHAPTER OUTLINE

- **THALAMUS**
  - THALAMIC NUCLEI
  - FUNCTIONS OF THALAMUS
  - APPLIED PHYSIOLOGY
- **HYPOTHALAMUS**
  - HYPOTHALAMIC NUCLEI
  - FUNCTIONS OF HYPOTHALAMUS
  - APPLIED PHYSIOLOGY

THALAMUS

Thalamus is a large ovoid mass of gray matter, situated bilaterally in **diencephalon**. Both thalami form 80% of diencephalon.

THALAMIC NUCLEI

Thalamus on each side is divided into five main nuclear groups by means of 'Y' shaped internal medullary septum.

1. Midline Nuclei

It is a group of small nuclei, situated on the medial surface of thalamus **near midline**.

2. Intralaminar Nuclei

Intralaminar nuclei are smaller nuclei present in the **medullary septum** of the thalamus **(Fig. 84.1)**.

3. Medial Mass of Nuclei

Medial mass of nuclei is situated **medial to septum** and it comprises two nuclei:

1. Anterior nucleus.
2. Dorsomedial nucleus.

4. Lateral Mass of Nuclei

This group of nuclei is situated **lateral to septum**.

Lateral mass of nuclei is again divided into two subgroups:

a. Dorsal group of lateral mass with two nuclei:
   1. Dorsolateral nucleus.
   2. Posterolateral nucleus.
b. Ventral group of lateral mass with three nuclei:
   1. Ventral anterior nucleus.
   2. Ventral lateral nucleus.
   3. Posteroventral nucleus. It consists of two parts:
      i. Ventral posterolateral nucleus.
      ii. Ventral posteromedial nucleus.

5. Posterior Group of Nuclei

It is the continuation of lateral mass of nuclei. It has two subgroups:

a. Pulvinar.
b. Metathalamus which consists of two structures:
   1. Medial geniculate body.
   2. Lateral geniculate body.

Thalamic Reticular Nucleus

Thalamus also includes thalamic reticular nucleus, which is a thin layer of neurons covering the lateral aspect of thalamus.

FUNCTIONS OF THALAMUS

Thalamus is primarily concerned with somatic functions. Various functions of thalamus are given below.

1. Relay Center for Sensations

Thalamus forms the relay center for the sensations. Impulses of almost all the sensations reach the thalamic nuclei, particularly in the **ventral posterolateral nucleus**. After being processed in the thalamus, the impulses are carried to cerebral cortex.

2. Center for Processing of Sensory Information

Thalamus forms the major center for processing the sensory information. All the peripheral sensory impulses reaching thalamus are **integrated and modified** before being sent to specific areas of cerebral cortex.

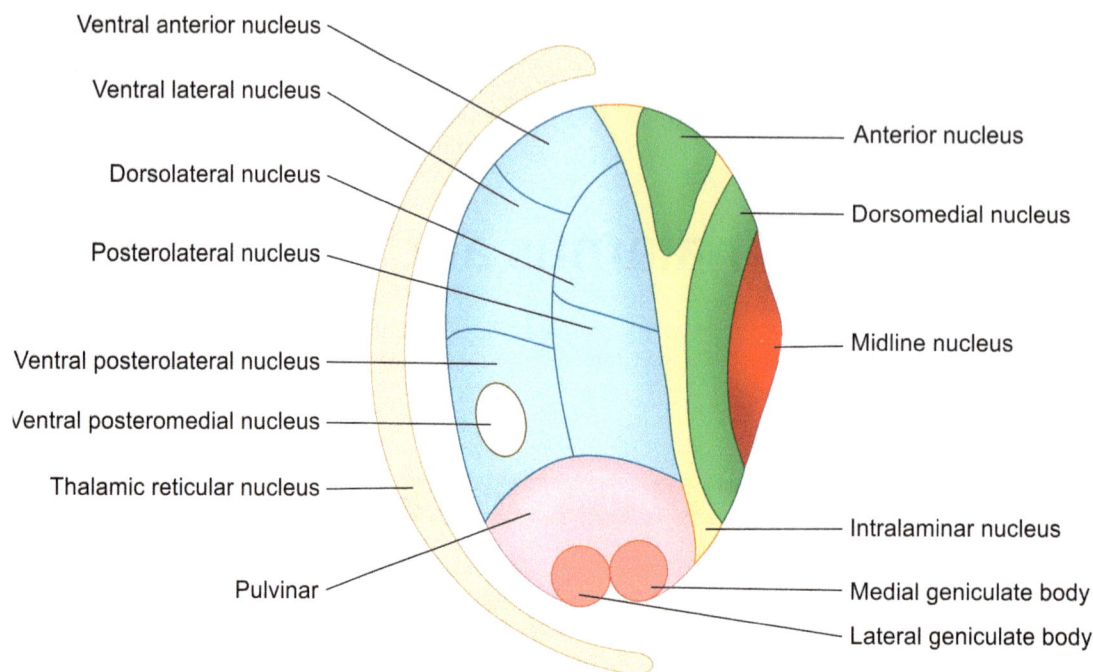

FIGURE 84.1: Thalamic nuclei.
Red = Midline nuclei, Yellow = Intralaminar nuclei, Green = Medial mass of nuclei, Blue = Lateral mass of nuclei, Pink = Posterior group of nuclei.

This function of thalamus is usually called the processing of sensory information.

Functional gateway for cerebral cortex

Almost all the sensations are processed in thalamus before reaching cerebral cortex. Very little information of somatosensory function is sent directly to cerebral cortex without being processed by the thalamic nuclei. Because of this function, thalamus is usually called a 'Functional gateway' for cerebral cortex.

3. Center for Determining Quality of Sensations

Thalamus is also the center for determining the quality of sensations, that is, to determine the affective nature of sensations.

Sensations have two qualities:

i. *Discriminative nature*: Ability to recognize the type, location and other details of the sensations. This is the function of cerebral cortex.
ii. *Affective nature*: Capacity to determine whether a sensation is pleasant or unpleasant and agreeable or disagreeable. This is the function of thalamus.

4. Center for Sexual Sensations

Thalamus forms the center for perception of sexual sensations.

5. Role in Arousal and Alertness Reactions

Because of its connections with nuclei of reticular formation, thalamus plays an important role in arousal and alertness reactions.

6. Center for Reflex Activity

Since the sensory fibers relay here, thalamus forms the center for many reflex activities.

7. Center for Integration of Motor Activity

Through the connections with cerebellum and basal ganglia, thalamus serves as a center for integration of motor functions.

■ APPLIED PHYSIOLOGY

Thalamic Lesion

Thalamic lesion occurs mainly because of blockage (due to thrombosis) in blood vessel supplying thalamus. Lesion of thalamus leads to thalamic syndrome.

Thalamic Syndrome

Thalamic syndrome is the neurological disease caused by lesion of thalamus. Lesion occurs because of blockage in the **thalamogeniculate branch** of posterior cerebral artery.

Symptoms of thalamic syndrome are given below.

1. Loss of sensations

Loss of all sensations (anesthesia) occurs as the sensory relay system in thalamus is affected.

2. Astereognosis

Astereognosis is the loss of ability to recognize a known object by touch with closed eyes. It is due to the loss of tactile and kinesthetic sensations in thalamic syndrome.

3. Ataxia

Ataxia is the incoordination of voluntary movements.

TABLE 84.1: Nuclei of hypothalamus.

Anterior or preoptic group	Middle or tuberal group	Posterior or mammillary group
1. Preoptic nucleus 2. Paraventricular nucleus 3. Anterior nucleus 4. Supraoptic nucleus 5. Suprachiasmatic nucleus	1. Dorsomedial nucleus 2. Ventromedial nucleus 3. Lateral nucleus 4. Arcuate (tuberal) nucleus	1. Posterior nucleus 2. Mammillary body

4. Thalamic phantom limb

Persons with amputated limb, sometimes feel sensations in the missing limb. This is called **phantom limb**. It is because of response by thalamus to inputs from cut ends of sensory nerves.

5. Amelognosia

It is the illusion felt by the patient that his limb is absent.

6. Pain sensation

Spontaneous pain occurs often. The pain may be so intense, that it even resists the action of powerful sedatives like morphine. Sometimes, the patient feels pain even in the absence of pain stimulus.

7. Involuntary movements

Thalamic syndrome is always associated with some involuntary motor movements:

  i. **Athetosis** (slow writhing and twisting movements).
 ii. **Chorea** (quick jerky involuntary movements).
iii. Intention tremor: **Tremor** is defined as rapid alternate rhythmic and involuntary movement of flexion and extension in the joints of fingers and wrist or elbow. **Intention tremor** is the tremor that develops while attempting to do any voluntary act. Intention tremor is the common feature of thalamic syndrome.

8. Thalamic hand or athetoid hand

It is the abnormal attitude of the hand in thalamic lesion. It is characterized by moderate flexion at wrist and hyperextension of all fingers.

■ **HYPOTHALAMUS**

Hypothalamus is a diencephalic structure. It is situated just below thalamus in the ventral part of **diencephalon**. It is formed by groups of nuclei scattered in the walls and floor of third ventricle. It extends from optic chiasma to mammillary body.

■ **NUCLEI OF HYPOTHALAMUS**

Nuclei of hypothalamus are divided into three groups:

1. Anterior or preoptic group.
2. Middle or tuberal group.
3. Posterior or mammillary group.

Nuclei of each group are listed in **Table 84.1** and represented diagrammatically in **Figure 84.2**.

■ **FUNCTIONS OF HYPOTHALAMUS**

Hypothalamus is the important part of the brain concerned with **homeostasis** of the body. It regulates many vital functions of the body such as endocrine functions, visceral

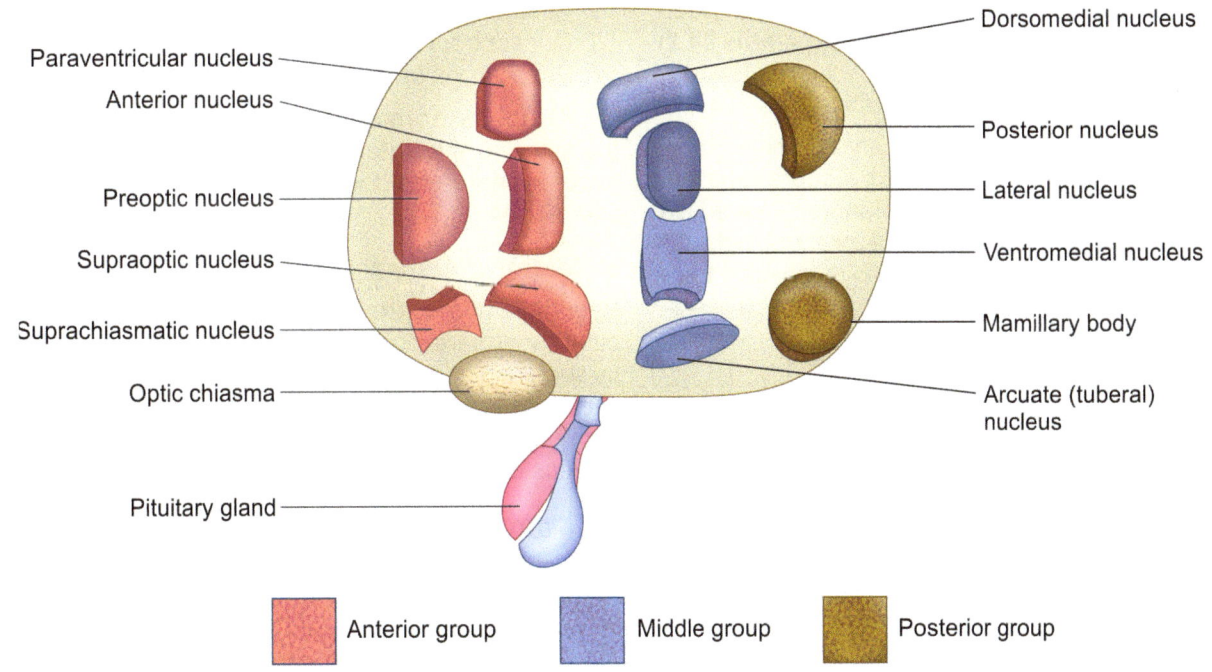

FIGURE 84.2: Nuclei of hypothalamus.

TABLE 84.2: Functions of hypothalamus.

Functions	Action/Center	Nuclei or parts involved
1. Control of anterior pituitary	By releasing hormones and inhibiting hormones	Discrete areas
2. Secretion of posterior pituitary hormones	Oxytocin Antidiuretic hormone (ADH)	Paraventricular nucleus Supraoptic nucleus
3. Control of adrenal cortex	By corticotropin-releasing hormone (CRH)	Paraventricular nucleus
4. Control of adrenal medulla	Catecholamines during emotion	Posterior nucleus Dorsomedial nucleus
5. Regulation of autonomic nervous system (ANS)	Sympathetic Parasympathetic	Posterior and lateral nuclei Anterior nucleus
6. Regulation of heart rate	Acceleration Inhibition	Posterior and lateral nuclei Preoptic and anterior nuclei
7. Regulation of blood pressure	Pressor effect Depressor effect	Posterior and lateral nuclei Preoptic area
8. Regulation of body temperature	Heat gain center Heat loss center	Posterior hypothalamus Anterior hypothalamus
9. Regulation of hunger and food intake	Feeding center Satiety center	Lateral nucleus Ventromedial nucleus
10. Regulation of water intake	Thirst center Water retention by ADH	Lateral nucleus Supraoptic nucleus
11. Regulation of sleep and wakefulness	Sleep Wakefulness	Anterior hypothalamus Mammillary body
12. Regulation of behavior and emotion	Reward center Punishment center	Ventromedial nucleus Posterior and lateral nuclei
13. Regulation of sexual function	Sexual cycle	Arcuate and posterior nuclei
14. Regulation of response to smell	Autonomic responses	Posterior hypothalamus
15. Role in circadian rhythm	Rhythmic changes	Suprachiasmatic nucleus

functions, metabolic activities, hunger, thirst, sleep, wakefulness, emotion, sexual functions, etc. **(Table 84.2)**.

1. Secretion of Posterior Pituitary Hormones

Posterior pituitary hormones namely, antidiuretic hormone (ADH) and oxytocin are secreted by supraoptic and paraventricular nuclei of hypothalamus. These two hormones are transported by means of axonic or axoplasmic flow through the fibers of hypothalamohypophyseal tracts to the posterior pituitary. Refer Chapter 44 for details.

2. Control of Anterior Pituitary

Hypothalamus controls the secretions of anterior pituitary gland by secreting releasing hormones and inhibitory hormones.

Hypothalamus secretes seven hormones:
  i. Growth hormone-releasing hormone (GHRH).
  ii. Growth hormone-releasing polypeptide (GHRP).
  iii. Growth hormone inhibitory hormone (GHIH) or somatostatin.
  iv. Thyrotropin-releasing hormone (TRH).
  v. Corticotropin-releasing hormone (CRH).
  vi. Gonadotropin-releasing hormone (GnRH).
  vii. Prolactin inhibitory hormone (PIH).

All these hormones are transported from hypothalamus to the anterior pituitary by the hypothalamo-hypophyseal portal blood vessels. Details are given in Chapter 44.

3. Control of Adrenal Cortex

Hypothalamus controls adrenal cortex through anterior pituitary. Anterior pituitary regulates the adrenal cortex by secreting adrenocorticotropic hormone (ACTH). ACTH secretion is in turn regulated by corticotropin-releasing hormone (CRH) which is secreted by the paraventricular nucleus of hypothalamus (Chapter 48).

4. Control of Adrenal Medulla

Dorsomedial and posterior hypothalamic nuclei are excited by emotional stimuli. These hypothalamic nuclei, in turn, send impulses to adrenal medulla through sympathetic fibers and cause release of catecholamines, which are essential to cope up with emotional stress.

5. Regulation of Autonomic Nervous System

Hypothalamus controls the autonomic nervous system (ANS). The sympathetic division of ANS is regulated by posterior and lateral nuclei of hypothalamus. The parasympathetic division of ANS is controlled by anterior group of nuclei. Cerebral cortex influences ANS through hypothalamus.

6. Regulation of Heart Rate

Hypothalamus regulates heart rate through vasomotor center in the medulla oblongata. Stimulation of posterior and lateral nuclei of hypothalamus increases the heart rate. Stimulation of preoptic and anterior nuclei decreases the heart rate (Chapter 62).

7. Regulation of Blood Pressure

Hypothalamus regulates the blood pressure by acting on the vasomotor center. Stimulation of posterior and lateral nuclei increases arterial blood pressure and stimulation of preoptic area decreases the blood pressure (Chapter 63).

8. Regulation of Body Temperature

Body temperature is regulated by hypothalamus which sets the normal range of body temperature. The **set point** under normal physiological conditions is 37°C.

Hypothalamus has two centers which regulate the body temperature:

i. Heat loss center that is present in preoptic nucleus of anterior hypothalamus.
ii. Heat gain center that is situated in posterior hypothalamic nucleus.

Regulation of body temperature is explained in Chapter 42.

9. Regulation of Hunger and Food Intake

Food intake is regulated by two centers present in hypothalamus:

i. Feeding center.
ii. Satiety center.

Feeding center

Feeding center is in the lateral hypothalamic nucleus. Normally feeding center is always active. That means it has the tendency to induce food intake always.

Satiety center

Satiety center is in the ventromedial nucleus of the hypothalamus. Satiety center regulates food intake by temporary inhibition of feeding center after food intake.

Mechanism of regulation of food intake

Under normal physiological conditions, appetite and food intake are well balanced and continues in a cyclic manner. Feeding center and satiety center of hypothalamus are responsible for regulation of appetite and food intake.

Hypothalamic centers are regulated by the following mechanisms:

a. Glucostatic mechanism.
b. Lipostatic mechanism.
c. Peptide mechanism.
d. Hormonal mechanism.
e. Thermostatic mechanism.

Glucostatic mechanism

Cells of the satiety center function as **glucostats** or **glucose receptors**. Glucostats are stimulated by increased blood glucose level during food intake. This develops the feeling of 'fullness'. The satiety center in turn, inhibits the feeding center, resulting in stoppage of food intake.

After few hours of food intake, the blood glucose level decreases and satiety center, becomes inactive. So, the feeding center is no longer inhibited. Now it becomes active and increases the appetite and induces food intake. After taking food, once again blood glucose level increases and the cycle is repeated (Fig. 84.3).

Lipostatic mechanism

Leptin is a peptide secreted by **adipocytes** (cells of adipose tissue). It plays an important role in controlling the food intake and adipose tissue volume. Details of leptin are given in Chapter 50.

When the volume of adipose tissues increases, adipocytes secrete and release a large quantity of leptin into the blood. While circulating through brain, leptin acts on hypothalamus and inhibits the feeding center resulting in loss of appetite and stoppage of food intake.

Peptide mechanism

Some peptides regulate the food intake either by stimulating or inhibiting the feeding center directly or indirectly.

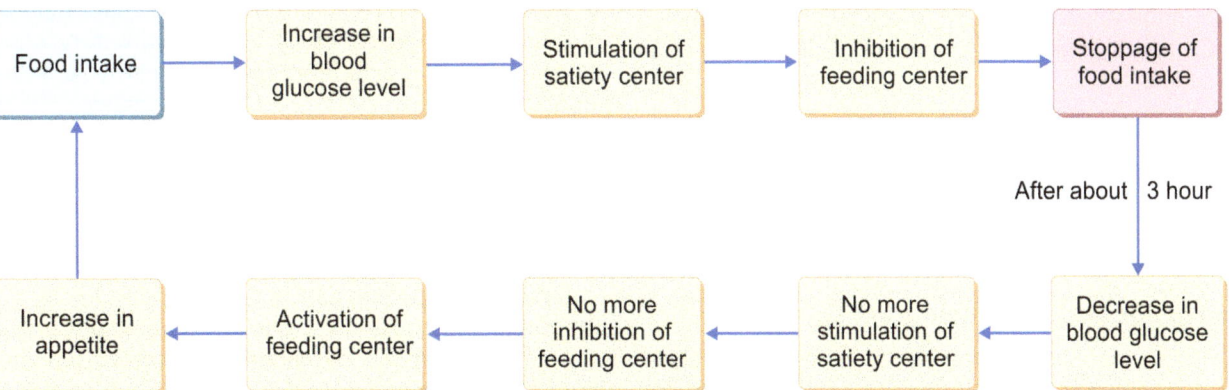

FIGURE 84.3: Glucostatic mechanism.

Peptides which increase the food intake are:
  i. Ghrelin.
  ii. Neuropeptide Y.

Peptides which decrease food intake are:
  i. Leptin.
  ii. Peptide YY.

Hormonal mechanism

Some of the endocrine hormones and GI hormones inhibit the food intake by acting through hypothalamus.

Hormones which inhibit food intake are:
  i. Somatostatin.
  ii. Oxytocin.
  iii. Glucagon.
  iv. Pancreatic polypeptide.
  v. Cholecystokinin.

Thermostatic mechanism

Food intake is inversely proportional to body temperature. So, in **fever**, the food intake is decreased due to the influence of preoptic **thermoreceptors** on feeding center.

10. Regulation of Water Balance

Hypothalamus regulates water content of the body by two mechanisms:
  i. Thirst mechanism.
  ii. ADH mechanism.

Thirst mechanism

Thirst center is in the lateral nucleus of hypothalamus. There are some **osmoreceptors** in the areas adjacent to thirst center. When the ECF volume decreases, the osmolality of ECF is increased and osmoreceptors are stimulated. Osmoreceptors in turn, activate the thirst center which induces water intake by causing thirst. Water intake increases ECF volume and decreases the osmolality.

ADH mechanism

When the volume of ECF decreases with increased osmolality, the supraoptic nucleus is stimulated and ADH is released. ADH causes retention of water by **facultative reabsorption** in the renal tubules. It increases the ECF volume and brings the osmolality back to the normal level.

On the contrary, when ECF volume is increased, the supraoptic nucleus is not stimulated and ADH is not secreted. In the absence of ADH, more amount of water is excreted through urine and the volume of ECF is brought back to normal.

11. Regulation of Sleep and Wakefulness

Mammillary body in the posterior hypothalamus acts as the **wakefulness center**. Stimulation of mammillary body causes wakefulness and its lesion leads to sleep. Stimulation of anterior hypothalamus also leads to sleep.

12. Role in Behavior and Emotional Changes

Behavior of animals and human beings is mostly affected by two responding systems in hypothalamus and other structures of limbic system. These two systems act opposite to one another. The responding systems are concerned with the affective nature of sensations, i.e. whether the sensations are pleasant or painful. These two qualities are called the **reward** (satisfaction) and **punishment** (aversion or avoidance).

Hypothalamus has two centers for behavior and emotional changes:
  i. Reward center.
  ii. Punishment center.

Almost all the activities of day to day life depend upon reward and punishment. While doing something, if the person is rewarded or feels satisfied, he or she continues to do so. If the person feels punished or unpleasant, he or she stops doing so. Thus, these two centers play an important role in the development of behavioral pattern of a person.

Rage

Rage is the violent and aggressive emotional expression with extreme anger. It is common in animals when punishment centers in hypothalamus are stimulated. Reactions of rage are expressed by developing a defense posture which includes:
  i. Extension of limbs with lifting of tail.
  ii. Hissing and spitting.
  iii. Piloerection.
  iv. Wide opening of eyeballs with pupillary dilatation.
  v. Severe savage attack even by mild provocation.

Sham rage

Sham rage means **false rage**. It is an extreme emotional condition that resembles rage and occurs in some pathological conditions in humans. Sham rage is due to release of hypothalamus from the inhibitory influence of cortical control.

13. Regulation of Sexual Function

Hypothalamus regulates sexual functions by secreting gonadotropin-releasing hormone. Arcuate and posterior hypothalamic nuclei are involved in the regulation of sexual functions.

14. Role in Response to Smell

Posterior hypothalamus and other structures such as hippocampus and brainstem nuclei are responsible for the autonomic responses of body to olfactory stimuli. The responses include feeding activities and emotional responses like fear, excitement and pleasure.

15. Role in Circadian Rhythm

Circadian rhythm is the regular recurrence of physiological processes or activities which occur in cycles of 24 hours. It is also called **diurnal rhythm**. Circadian rhythm occurs in response to recurring daylight and darkness. The cyclic changes taking place in various physiological processes are set by means of a hypothetical internal clock that is often called **biological clock**.

Suprachiasmatic nucleus of hypothalamus is responsible for setting the biological clock by its connection with retina via retinohypothalamic fibers. Through the efferent fibers, it sends circadian signals to different parts and maintains the circadian rhythm of sleep, hormonal secretion, thirst, hunger, appetite, etc.

Whenever body is exposed to a new pattern of daylight/darkness rhythm, the biological clock is reset, provided the new pattern is regular. Accordingly, the circadian rhythm also changes.

■ APPLIED PHYSIOLOGY: DISORDERS OF HYPOTHALAMUS

Following disorders develop in hypothalamic lesion that occurs due to tumors, encephalitis or ischemia.

■ 1. DIABETES INSIPIDUS

Diabetes insipidus is the condition characterized by excretion of large quantity of water through urine. Details are given in Chapter 44.

■ 2. DYSTROPHIA ADIPOSOGENITALIS

It is characterized by obesity and sexual infantilism, associated with dwarfism (if the condition occurs during growing period). It is also called **Frohlich's syndrome**. Details are given in Chapter 44.

■ 3. KALLMANN SYNDROME

Kallmann syndrome is a genetic disorder characterized by **hypogonadism**, associated with **anosmia** (loss of olfactory sensation) or **hyposmia** (decreased olfactory sensation). It is also called **hypogonadotropic hypogonadism**, since it occurs due to deficiency of gonadotropin-releasing hormone secreted by hypothalamus.

■ 4. LAURENCE-MOON-BIEDL SYNDROME

This disorder of hypothalamus is characterized by **moon face** (facial contours become round by hiding the bony structures), obesity, **polydactylism** (having one or more extra fingers or toes), mental retardation and hypogenitalism.

■ 5. NARCOLEPSY

Narcolepsy is a hypothalamic disorder with abnormal sleep pattern. There is sudden attack of uncontrollable desire for sleep and the person suddenly falls asleep. It occurs in the daytime.

■ 6. CATAPLEXY

It is the sudden uncontrolled outbursts of emotion associated with narcolepsy. Due to emotional outburst like anger, fear or excitement, the person becomes completely exhausted with muscular weakness. The attack is brief and last for few seconds to a few minutes. The consciousness is not lost.

Chapter 85

Cerebellum

CHAPTER OUTLINE

- PARTS
- DIVISIONS
- VESTIBULOCEREBELLUM
- SPINOCEREBELLUM
- CORTICOCEREBELLUM
- APPLIED PHYSIOLOGY: CEREBELLAR LESIONS

PARTS OF CEREBELLUM

Cerebellum is the largest part of hind brain. It consists of a narrow, worm like central body called **vermis** and two lateral lobes, the right and left **cerebellar hemispheres** (Fig. 85.1).

VERMIS

Part of vermis on the upper surface of cerebellum is known as **superior vermis** and the vermis on the under surface of cerebellum is called **inferior vermis**. Vermis of cerebellum is formed by nine parts which are listed in **Table 85.1**.

Nodulus has extension on either side called flocculus. Nodulus and flocculi are together called **flocculonodular lobe**. On either side of pyramid, there is another extension named **paraflocculus**.

CEREBELLAR HEMISPHERES

Cerebellar hemispheres are the extended portions on either side of the vermis.

Each hemisphere has two portions:

1. Lobulus ensiformis or ansiform lobe.
2. Lobulus paramedianus or paramedian lobe.

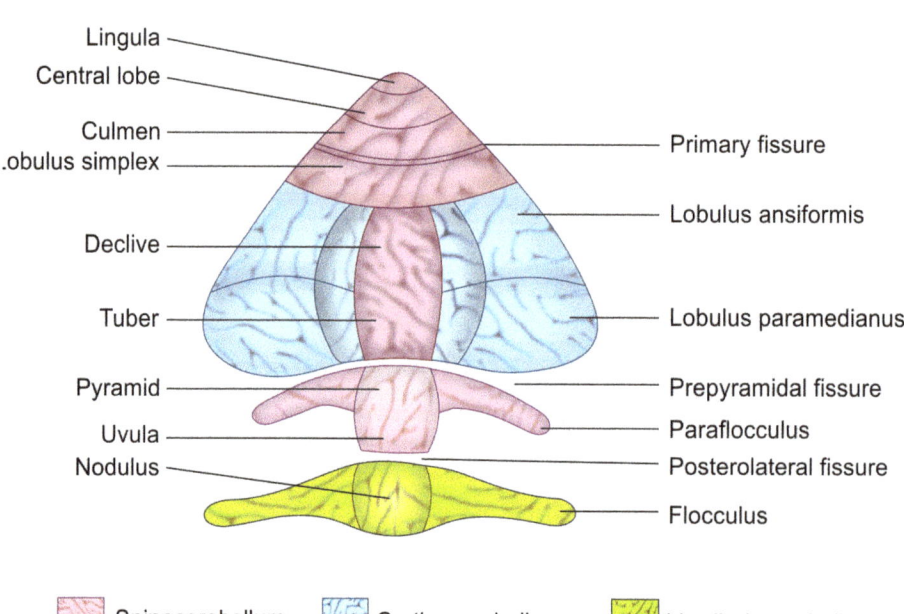

FIGURE 85.1: Parts and functional divisions of cerebellum.

TABLE 85.1: Parts of superior and inferior vermis.

Superior vermis	Inferior vermis
1. Lingula 2. Central lobe 3. Culmen 4. Lobulus simplex 5. Declive	6. Tuber 7. Pyramid 8. Uvula 9. Nodulus

■ DIVISIONS OF CEREBELLUM

Based on the functions, cerebellum is divided into three divisions:

1. Vestibulocerebellum.
2. Spinocerebellum.
3. Corticocerebellum.

■ VESTIBULOCEREBELLUM (ARCHICEREBELLUM)

This part of cerebellum is connected with the **vestibular apparatus** and so it is known as vestibulocerebellum. Since, vestibulocerebellum is the phylogenetically oldest part of cerebellum, it is also called archicerebellum.

■ COMPONENTS OF VESTIBULOCEREBELLUM

Vestibulocerebellum includes the **flocculonodular lobe** that is formed by the **nodulus** of vermis and its lateral extensions called **flocculi (Fig. 85.1** and **Table 85.2)**.

■ FUNCTIONS OF VESTIBULOCEREBELLUM

Vestibulocerebellum regulates **muscle tone, posture and equilibrium** by receiving impulses from vestibular apparatus regarding gravity and movements **(Table 85.3)**.

Mechanism of Action of Vestibulocerebellum

Normally, vestibular nuclei of brainstem facilitate the movements of trunk, neck and limbs. Medullary reticular formation inhibits the muscle tone.

After receiving information from vestibular apparatus, the vestibulocerebellum inhibits both vestibular nuclei and medullary reticular formation. As a result, the movements of neck, trunk and limbs are checked and the muscle tone increases. Because of these effects, any disturbance in posture and equilibrium is corrected.

Lesion of vestibulocerebellum, results in hypotonia (reduction of muscle tone) and failure to maintain posture and equilibrium.

■ SPINOCEREBELLUM (PALEOCEREBELLUM)

Spinocerebellum or paleocerebellum is connected with **spinal cord**. It forms the **major receiving area** of cerebellum for sensory inputs. Spinocerebellum is also phylogenetically older part of cerebellum.

■ COMPONENTS OF SPINOCEREBELLUM

Spinocerebellum consists of medial portions of cerebellar hemisphere, paraflocculi and the parts of vermis, viz. lingula, central lobe, culmen, lobulus simplex, declive, tuber, pyramid and uvula **(Fig. 85.1** and **Table 85.2)**.

■ FUNCTIONS OF SPINOCEREBELLUM

Spinocerebellum regulates **muscle tone, posture and equilibrium** by receiving sensory impulses form tactile receptors, proprioceptors, visual receptors and auditory receptors. It also receives the cortical impulses via pontine nuclei.

Spinocerebellum facilitates the discharge from gamma motor neurons. Increased discharge from gamma motor neurons increases the muscle tone.

The lesion in spinocerebellum causes stoppage of discharge from the gamma motor neurons resulting in hypotonia and disturbances in posture.

Spinocerebellum also receives impulses from optic and auditory pathway and helps in adjustment of posture and equilibrium in response to visual and auditory impulses.

■ CORTICOCEREBELLUM (NEOCEREBELLUM)

Corticocerebellum is largest part of cerebellum. Because of its connection with **cerebral cortex**, it is called corticocerebellum or **cerebrocerebellum**. It is phylogenetically newer part of cerebellum. So, it is also called **neocerebellum**. It is concerned with planning, programming and coordination.

■ COMPONENTS OF CORTICOCEREBELLUM

Corticocerebellum includes the lateral portions of cerebellar hemispheres **(Fig. 85.1** and **Table 85.2)**.

■ AFFERENT-EFFERENT CIRCUIT (CEREBRO-CEREBELLO-CEREBRAL CONNECTIONS)

It is a neuronal pathway through which corticocerebellum controls the voluntary movements.

Fibers from motor areas 4 and 6 in frontal lobe of cerebral cortex enter the pontine nuclei. These fibers are called **corticopontine fibers (Fig. 85.2)**. From pontine nuclei, the **pontocerebellar fibers** arise and pass through middle cerebellar peduncle of the opposite side and terminate in the cerebellar cortex.

TABLE 85.2: Components of divisions of cerebellum.

Division	Components
Vestibulocerebellum	Flocculonodular lobe (nodulus and flocculi)
Spinocerebellum	Lingula Central lobe Culmen Lobulus simplex Declive Tuber Pyramid Uvula Paraflocculi Medial portions of cerebral hemispheres
Corticocerebellum	Lateral portions of cerebral hemispheres

TABLE 85.3: Functions of cerebellum.

	Functions	Division of cerebellum involved
1. Regulation of tone, posture and equilibrium	By receiving impulses from vestibular apparatus	Vestibulocerebellum
	By receiving impulses from proprioceptors in muscles, tendons and joints, tactile receptors, visual receptors and auditory receptors	Spinocerebellum
2. Regulation of coordinated movements	i. Damping action ii. Control of ballistic movements iii. Timing and programming the movements iv. Servomechanism v. Comparator function	Corticocerebellum (neocerebellum)

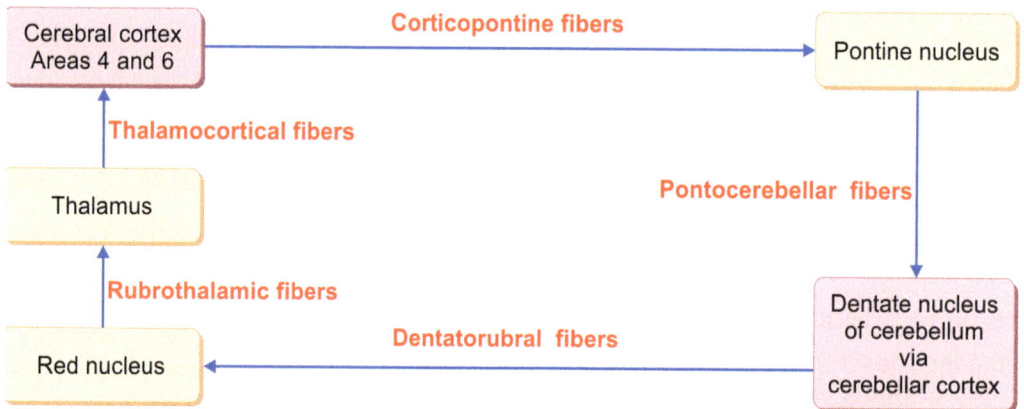

FIGURE 85.2: Schematic representation of cerebro-cerebello-cerebral circuit.

This pathway is called the **cerebropontocerebellar tract** or **corticopontocerebellar tract**.

Cerebellar cortex is, in turn, connected to the dentate nucleus. Fibers from the dentate nucleus pass via superior cerebellar peduncle and end in red nucleus of opposite side. These fibers are called **dentatorubral fibers**. From red nucleus, the **rubrothalamic fibers** go to thalamus. Thalamus is connected to areas 4 and 6 in motor cortex of cerebrum by **thalamocortical fibers**. This tract between dentate nucleus and cerebral cortex is called **dentatorubrothalamocortical tract**.

■ FUNCTIONS OF CORTICOCEREBELLUM

Corticocerebellum is concerned with the integration and regulation of **well-coordinated muscular activities** because of its connection with cerebral cortex through the cerebro-cerebello-cerebral circuit. Apart from its connections with cerebral cortex, cerebellum also receives feedback signals from the muscles through the nerve fibers of proprioceptors.

Mechanism of Action of Corticocerebellum

1. Damping action

Damping action refers to **prevention** of exaggerated muscular activity. This helps in making the voluntary movements **smooth and accurate**. All the voluntary muscular activities are initiated by motor areas of cerebral cortex. Simultaneously, corticocerebellum receives impulses from motor cortex as well as feedback signals from the muscles as soon as the muscular activity starts.

Corticocerebellum, in turn, sends information (impulses) to cerebral cortex to discharge only appropriate signals to the muscles and to cut off any extra impulses. Because of this damping action of corticocerebellum, the exaggeration of muscular activity is prevented and the movements become smooth and accurate. Literally, the word damping means any effect that decreases the amplitude of mechanical oscillation.

2. Control of ballistic movements

Ballistic movements are the **rapid alternate movements**, which take place in different parts of the body while doing any skilled or trained work like typing, cycling, dancing, etc. Corticocerebellum plays an important role in **preplanning** the ballistic movements during learning process.

3. Timing and programming the movements

Corticocerebellum plays an important role in timing and programming the movements particularly during **learning process**. While using a typewriter or while doing any other fast skilled work, a chain of movements occurs rapidly in a sequential manner. During the learning process of these skilled works, corticocerebellum plans the various sequential movements. It also plans schedule of time duration of each movement and the time interval between movements. All the information from corticocerebellum are communicated to **sensory motor area** of cerebral cortex and stored in the form of **memory**. So, after the learning process is over, these activities are executed easily and smoothly in sequential manner.

4. Servomechanism

Servomechanism is the **correction of any disturbance** or interference while performing skilled work. Once the skilled works are learnt, the sequential movements are executed without any interruption. Cerebellum lets the cerebral cortex to discharge the signals, which are already programmed and stored at sensory motor cortex, and, does not interfere much. However, if there is any disturbance or interference, the corticocerebellum immediately influences the cortex and corrects the movements.

5. Comparator function

Comparator function of the corticocerebellum is responsible for the integration and coordination of the various muscular activities. On one side, cerebellum receives the information from **cerebral cortex** regarding the cortical impulses which are sent to the muscles. On the other side, it receives the **feedback information** (proprioceptive impulses) from the **muscles** regarding their actions under the instruction of cerebral cortex.

By receiving the messages from both ends, corticocerebellum compares the cortical commands for muscular activity and the **actual movements** carried out by the muscles. If any correction is to be done, then, corticocerebellum sends instructions (impulses) to the motor cortex. Accordingly, the cerebral cortex corrects or modifies the signals to muscles, so that the movements become accurate, precise and smooth. This function of corticocerebellum is known as comparator function.

Simultaneously, it also receives the impulses from tactile receptors, eye and ear. Such additional information facilitates the comparator function of corticocerebellum.

■ APPLIED PHYSIOLOGY: CEREBELLAR LESIONS

Cerebellar lesions occur due to tumor, abscess, injury and excess alcohol intake. Cerebellar lesions cause disturbances in posture, equilibrium and the movements. In unilateral lesion, symptoms appear on the affected side because cerebellum controls the same (**ipsilateral**) side of the body.

■ DISTURBANCES IN TONE AND POSTURE

Atonia or Hypotonia

Atonia is the loss of tone and hypotonia is reduction in tone of the muscle. Atonia or hypotonia occurs because of the loss of facilitatory impulses from cerebellum to gamma motor neurons in the spinal cord.

Attitude

Attitude of the body changes in unilateral lesion of the cerebellum.

Changes in the attitude are:

1. Rotation of head towards the opposite side (unaffected side).
2. Lowering of shoulder on the same side.
3. Abduction of leg on the affected side. The leg is rotated outward.
4. Weight of the body is thrown on the leg of unaffected side. So, the trunk is bent with concavity towards the affected side.

Deviation Movement

It is the lateral deviation of arms when both the arms are stretched and held in front of the body with closed eyes. In bilateral lesion, both the arms deviate and in unilateral lesion arm of the affected side deviates.

Effect on Deep Reflexes

Pendular movements occur while eliciting a tendon jerk particularly the knee jerk (Chapter 80).

■ DISTURBANCES IN EQUILIBRIUM

While Standing

While standing, the legs are spread to provide a broad base. And, the body sways side-to-side with the oscillations of the head.

While Moving: Gait

Gait means the **manner of walking**. In cerebellar lesion, a **staggering, reeling and drunken like gait** is observed.

■ DISTURBANCES IN MOVEMENTS

Disturbances in movements during cerebellar lesions are explained in **Table 85.4**.

TABLE 85.4: Disturbances in movements during cerebellar lesions.

Disturbance	Explanation
1. Ataxia	Lack of coordination of movements
2. Asynergia	Lack of coordination between different groups of muscles
3. Asthenia	Weakness, easy fatigability and slowness of muscles
4. Dysmetria	Inability to check the exact strength and duration of muscular contractions required for any voluntary act. While reaching for an object, the arm may overshoot (hypermetria) or it may fall short (hypometria) of the object
5. Intention tremor	Tremor that occurs while attempting to do any voluntary act. Refer Chapter 84 for details of tremor
6. Astasia	Unsteady voluntary movements
7. Nystagmus	To and fro movement of eyeball. Refer Chapter 88 for details of nystagmus
8. Rebound phenomenon	While attempting to do a movement against a resistance, and if the resistance is suddenly removed, the limb moves forcibly in the direction in which the attempt was made
9. Dysarthriya	Disturbance in speech
10. Adiadochokinesis	Inability to do rapid alternate successive movements such as supination and pronation of arm

Chapter 86

Basal Ganglia

CHAPTER OUTLINE
- SITUATION
- COMPONENTS
- FUNCTIONS
- APPLIED PHYSIOLOGY: DISORDERS

■ SITUATION OF BASAL GANGLIA

Basal ganglia are the scattered **masses of gray matter** submerged in subcortical substance of cerebral hemisphere **(Fig. 86.1)**.

■ COMPONENTS OF BASAL GANGLIA

Basal ganglia include three primary components:
 I. Corpus striatum.
 II. Substantia nigra.
 III. Subthalamic nucleus of Luys.

I. Corpus Striatum

It is a mass of gray matter situated at the base of cerebral hemispheres in close relation to the thalamus **(Fig. 86.2)**.

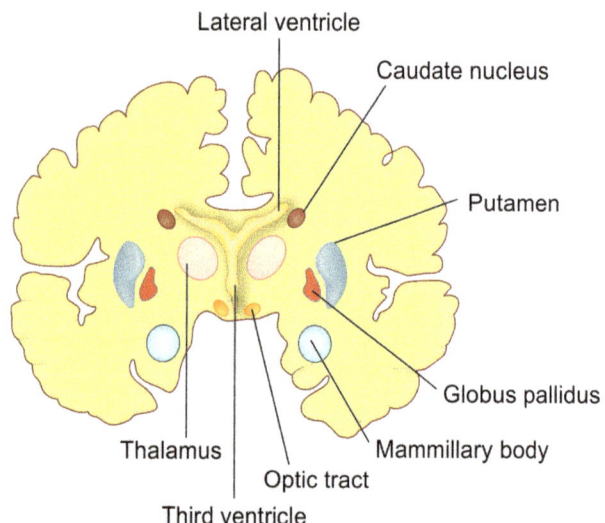

FIGURE 86.1: Basal ganglia.

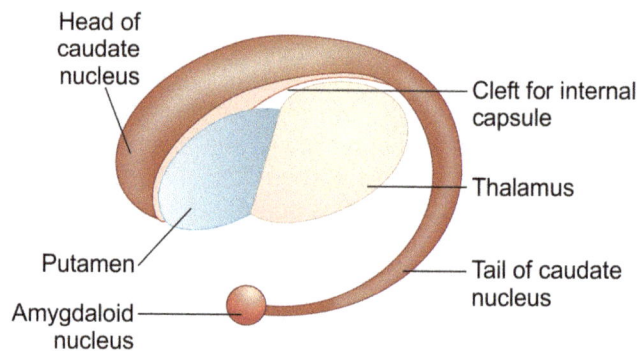

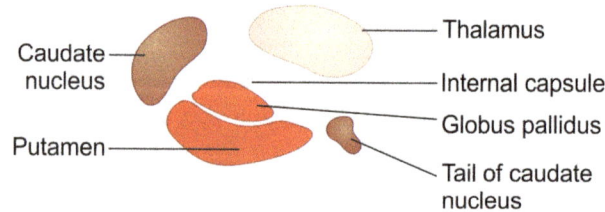

FIGURE 86.2: Corpus striatum.

Corpus striatum has two parts:
 1. Caudate nucleus.
 2. Lenticular nucleus which is divided into two portions:
    i. Putamen.
    ii. Globus pallidus.

II. Substantia Nigra

Substantia nigra is situated below red nucleus.

III. Subthalamic Nucleus of Luys

This nucleus is situated lateral to red nucleus and dorsal to substantia nigra.

FUNCTIONS OF BASAL GANGLIA

As a part of **extrapyramidal system**, basal ganglia are concerned with regulation of muscle tone and integration and the regulation of motor activities. The functions of basal ganglia are given below.

1. CONTROL OF MUSCLE TONE

Basal ganglia control the muscle tone. In fact, the **gamma motor neurons** of spinal cord are responsible for the tone of the muscles. Basal ganglia decrease muscle tone by inhibiting the gamma motor neurons through descending inhibitory reticular system in brainstem.

2. CONTROL OF MOTOR ACTIVITY

i. Regulation of Voluntary Movements

Voluntary motor activities initiated by cerebral cortex are controlled by basal ganglia. During lesions of basal ganglia, the control mechanism is lost and so the movements become inaccurate and awkward.

Basal ganglia control the motor activities because of the nervous (neuronal) circuits between basal ganglia and other parts of brain which are involved in motor activity.

ii. Regulation of Conscious Movements

Basal ganglia regulate the conscious movements. This function of basal ganglia is also known as the **cognitive control** of activity. For example, when a stray dog barks at a man, immediately the person understands the situation, turns away and starts running.

iii. Regulation of Subconscious Movements

Basal ganglia regulate the subconscious movements which take place during trained motor activities, i.e. skilled activities such as writing the learnt alphabet, paper cutting, nail hammering, etc.

3. CONTROL OF REFLEX MUSCULAR ACTIVITY

Some of the reflex muscular activities, particularly visual and labyrinthine reflexes, are important in the maintenance of posture. Basal ganglia are responsible for the coordination and integration of impulses for such reflex activities.

4. CONTROL OF AUTOMATIC ASSOCIATED MOVEMENTS

Automatic associated movements are the movements in the body, which take place along with some motor activities. Examples are the swing of the arms while walking, appropriate facial expressions while talking or doing any work. Basal ganglia are responsible for the automatic associated movements.

5. ROLE IN AROUSAL MECHANISM

Along with red nucleus, globus pallidus is involved in arousal mechanism because of their connections with reticular formation. Extensive lesion in globus pallidus causes drowsiness, leading to sleep.

APPLIED PHYSIOLOGY: DISORDERS OF BASAL GANGLIA

1. PARKINSON DISEASE

Parkinson disease is a slow progressive degenerative disease of nervous system associated with destruction of dopamine producing cells in brain. It is named after the discoverer **James Parkinson**. It is also called **parkinsonism** or **paralysis agitans**.

Causes of Parkinson Disease

Parkinson disease occurs due to **lack of dopamine** caused by damage of basal ganglia. It is mostly due to the destruction of substantia nigra and the nigrostriatal pathway, which has **dopaminergic fibers**. Basal ganglia are damaged during to viral infection of brain such as encephalitis and injury to basal ganglia.

This disease also occurs due to long-term treatment with drugs. Parkinsonism due to the drugs is known as **drug-induced parkinsonism**.

Signs and Symptoms of Parkinson Disease

Parkinson disease develops very slowly and the early signs and symptoms may be unnoticed for months or even for years. Often the symptoms start with a mild noticeable tremor in just one hand. When the tremor becomes remarkable, the disease causes slowing or freezing of movements followed by rigidity.

Common signs and symptoms of Parkinson disease are:

i. Tremor

Refer Chapter 84 for details of tremor. In Parkinson disease, static tremor or **resting tremor** occurs during rest. But it disappears while doing any work. It is also called **drum beating tremor**, as the movements are similar to beating a drum. The thumb moves rhythmically over the index and middle fingers. These movements are called **pill rolling movements**.

ii. Slowness of movements

Over the time, the movements start slowing down (**bradykinesia**) and it takes a long time even to perform a simple task. Gradually the patient becomes unable to initiate the voluntary activity (**akinesia**) or the voluntary movements are reduced (**hypokinesia**). It is because of hypertonicity of the muscles.

iii. Poverty of movements

Poverty of movements is the loss of all **automatic associated movements**. Because of absence of the automatic associate movements, the body becomes **statue like**. The face becomes **mask-like**, due to absence of appropriate expressions like blinking and smiling.

iv. Rigidity of limbs

Rigidity develops in limbs due to stiffness of muscles. **Muscular stiffness** occurs because of increased muscle tone which is due to the removal of inhibitory influence on gamma motor neurons. It affects both flexor and extensor muscles equally. So, the limbs become more **rigid like pillars**. The condition is called **lead pipe rigidity**. In later stages, the rigidity extends to neck and trunk.

v. Gait

Gait means **manner of walking**. Gait in Parkinson disease is called **festinant gait**. The patient walks quickly in short steps by bending forward, as if he is going to catch up the center of gravity.

vi. Speech problems

Many patients develop speech problems. They may speak very softly or sometimes rapidly. The words are repeated many times. Finally, speech becomes slurred and they hesitate to speak.

vii. Emotional changes

Persons affected by Parkinson disease are often upset emotionally.

viii. Dementia

In later stages, some patients develop dementia (Chapter 90).

2. WILSON'S DISEASE

Wilson's disease is an inherited disorder characterized by **excess of copper** in the body tissues. It is also known as **progressive hepatolenticular degeneration**. This disease develops due to damage of the lenticular nucleus.

In Wilson disease, copper is deposited in the liver, brain, kidneys and eyes. Copper deposits cause damage of tissues. And the affected organs stop functioning. In addition to symptoms of Parkinson disease, liver failure and damage of central nervous system are the most predominant effects of this disorder.

3. CHOREA

It is an abnormal involuntary movement. Chorea means **rapid jerky movements**. It mostly involves the limbs. It is due to lesion in caudate nucleus and putamen.

4. ATHETOSIS

It is another type of abnormal involuntary movement, which includes **slow rhythmic** and **twisting movements**. It is because of the lesion in caudate nucleus and putamen.

5. CHOREOATHETOSIS

It is the condition characterized by aimless involuntary muscular movements. It is due to combined effects of chorea and athetosis.

6. HUNTINGTON'S DISEASE

Huntington's disease is an inherited progressive neural disorder due to the degeneration of neurons secreting GABA in corpus striatum and substantia nigra. It is characterized by **chorea, hypotonia** and **dementia**.

7. HEMIBALLISMUS

It is a disorder characterized by **violent involuntary abnormal movements** on one side of the body involving mostly the arm. While walking, the arm swings widely. Hemiballismus occurs due to degeneration of subthalamic nucleus of Luys.

8. KERNICTERUS

Kernicterus is a form of brain damage in infants caused by **severe jaundice**. Basal ganglia are the mainly affected parts of brain. Refer Chapter 16 for details.

Chapter 87: Cerebral Cortex, Limbic System and Reticular Formation

CHAPTER OUTLINE

- CEREBRUM
- MORPHOLOGY OF CEREBRAL CORTEX
- NEOCORTEX AND ALLOCORTEX
- LOBES OF CEREBRAL CORTEX
- CEREBRAL DOMINANCE
- BRODMANN AREAS
- FRONTAL LOBE
- PARIETAL LOBE
- TEMPORAL LOBE
- OCCIPITAL LOBE
- LIMBIC SYSTEM
- RETICULAR FORMATION

■ CEREBRUM

Cerebrum is the largest part of brain. Cerebrum is responsible for perception of all sensations and initiation of various movements of the body.

Cerebrum is formed by two structures:

1. Outer layer of **gray matter** called **cerebral cortex** which includes nerve cell bodies.
2. Inner layer of **white matter** which includes of nerve fibers.

■ MORPHOLOGY CEREBRAL CORTEX

Cerebral cortex is formed by two **hemispheres** which are separated anteriorly and posteriorly by a deep **vertical fissure** (furrow or groove). But the middle portions are connected by **corpus callosum**.

Each hemisphere, has three surfaces namely, lateral, medial and inferior surfaces. Surface of the cerebral cortex is characterized by complicated pattern of **sulci** (singular = sulcus) and **gyri** (singular = gyrus). Sulcus is a slight depression or groove and gyrus is a raised ridge.

Cerebral cortex is formed by outer **gray matter** and inner **white matter**. It is formed by different types of nerve cells along with their processes and neuroglia which are arranged in **six layers**. It is not uniform throughout. It is thickest at the precentral gyrus, and thinnest at the frontal and occipital poles.

■ NEOCORTEX AND ALLOCORTEX

Part of the cerebral cortex that has **all six layers** of structures is called **neocortex**. It is also called **isocortex** or **neopallium**. It is the phylogenetically new structure of cerebral cortex. Neocortex forms the major portion of cerebral cortex.

Remaining part of the cerebral is called **allocortex**. It has **less than six layers** of structures. Allocortex includes **archicortex** and **paleocortex** which form the part of limbic system.

■ LOBES OF CEREBRAL CORTEX

Neocortex of each cerebral hemisphere consists of four lobes (Figs. 87.1 to 87.3):

1. Frontal lobe.
2. Parietal lobe.
3. Occipital lobe.
4. Temporal lobe.

Lobes of each hemisphere are demarked by four main fissures and sulci:

1. **Central sulcus** or Rolandic fissure between frontal and parietal lobes.
2. **Parieto-occipital sulcus** between parietal and occipital lobe.
3. **Sylvian fissure** or **lateral sulcus** between parietal and temporal lobes.
4. **Callosomarginal fissure** between temporal lobe and limbic area.

■ CEREBRAL DOMINANCE

Cerebral dominance is defined as the dominance of one cerebral hemisphere over the other in the control of cerebral functions. Cerebral dominance is related to handedness, i.e. preference of the individual to use right or left hand. More than 90% of people are **right-handed**.

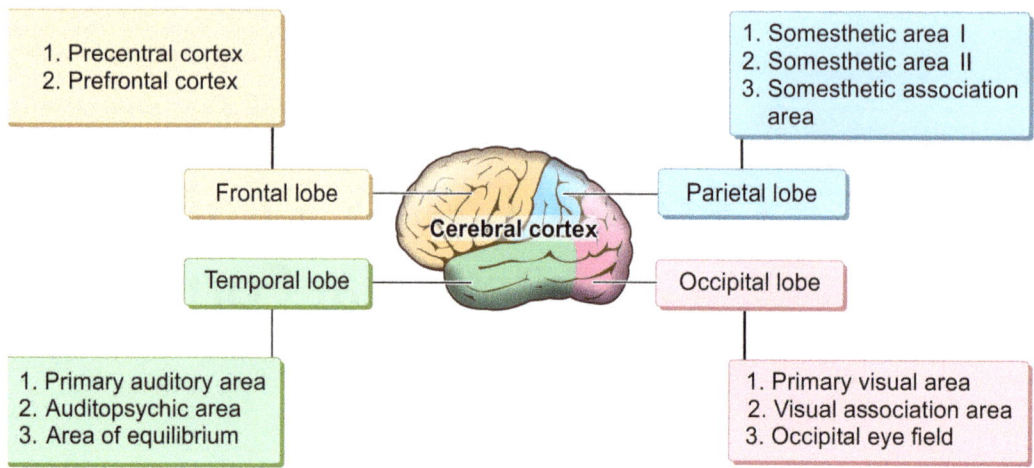

FIGURE 87.1: Parts of cerebral cortex.

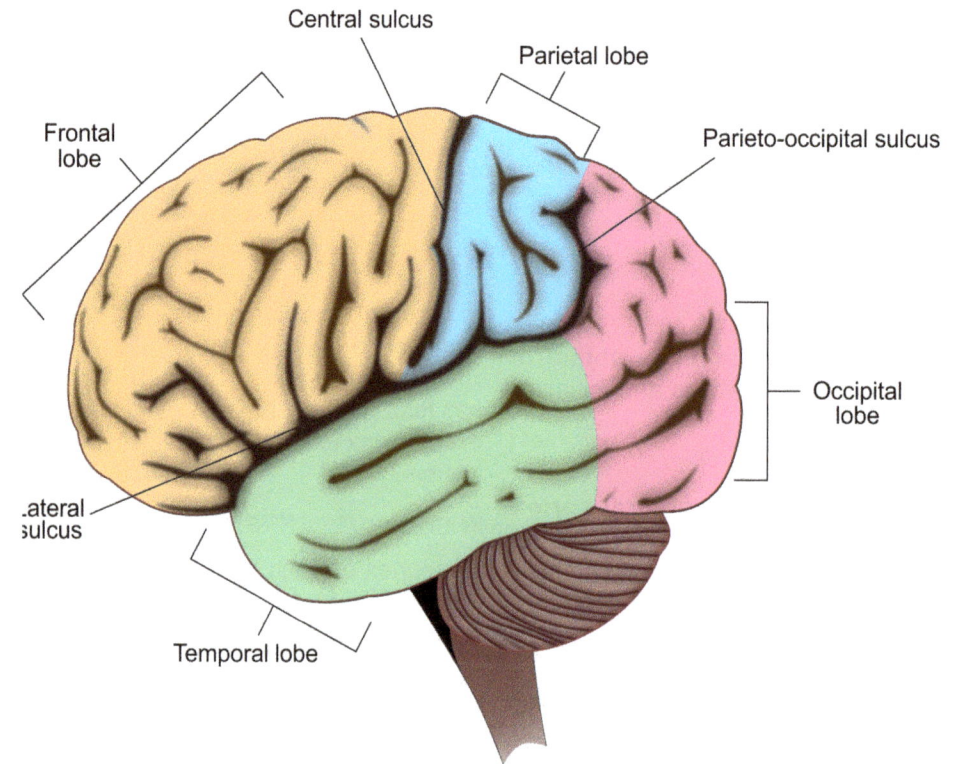

FIGURE 87.2: Lobes of cerebral cortex.

In these individuals, the **left hemisphere** is **dominant** and it controls the analytical process and language-related functions such as speech, reading and writing.

■ BRODMANN AREAS

Brodmann area is a region of cerebral cortex defined on the basis of organization of neurons. These areas were originally defined and numbered by **Korbinian Brodmann**. Some of these areas were given specific names based on their functions.

■ FRONTAL LOBE OF CEREBRAL CORTEX

Frontal lobe forms one-third of the cortical surface. It extends from frontal pole to the central sulcus and limited below by the lateral sulcus.

Frontal lobe of cerebral cortex is divided into two parts:
 I. Precentral cortex situated posteriorly.
 II. Prefrontal cortex situated anteriorly.

■ PRECENTRAL CORTEX

Precentral cortex includes the lip of central sulcus, whole of precentral gyrus and posterior portions of superior, middle and inferior frontal gyri. It also extends to the medial surface.

This part is also called **excitomotor cortex** or area, since the stimulation of different points in this area causes activity of discrete skeletal muscle. Precentral cortex is further divided into three functional areas **(Fig. 87.3)**:

Chapter 87: Cerebral Cortex, Limbic System and Reticular Formation   439

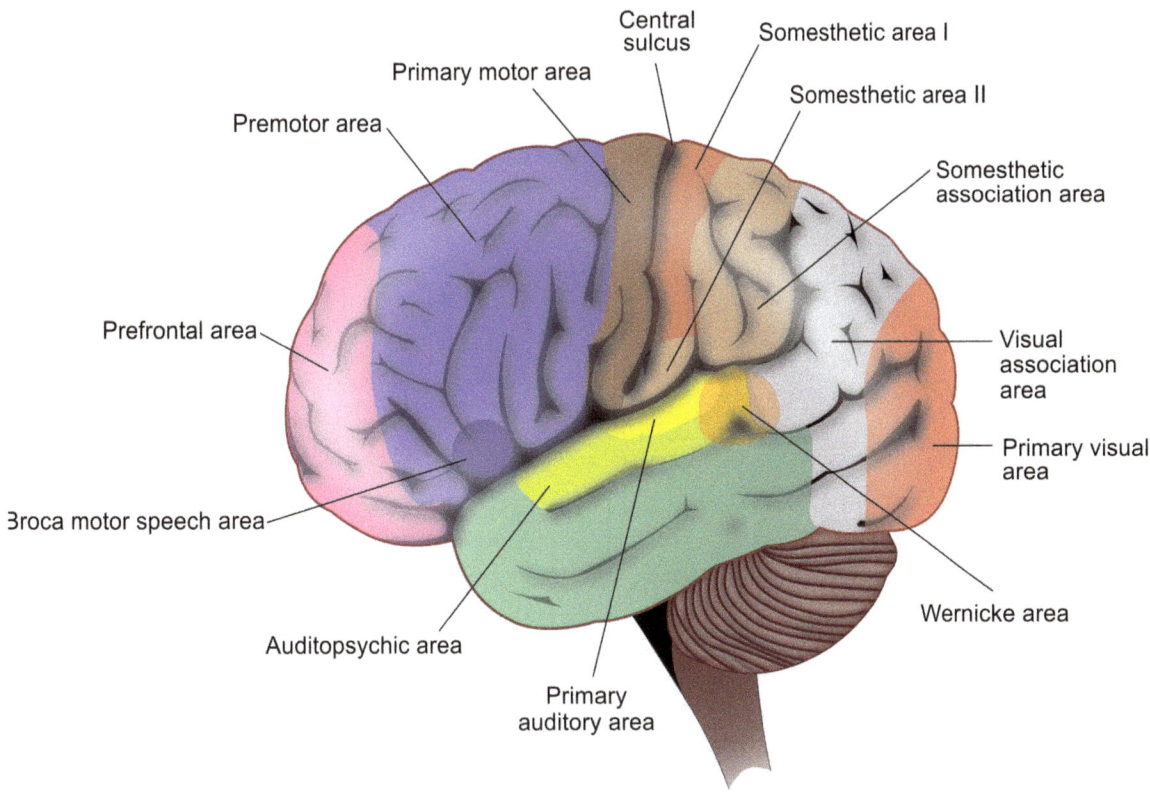

FIGURE 87.3: Functional regions on lateral surface of cerebral cortex.

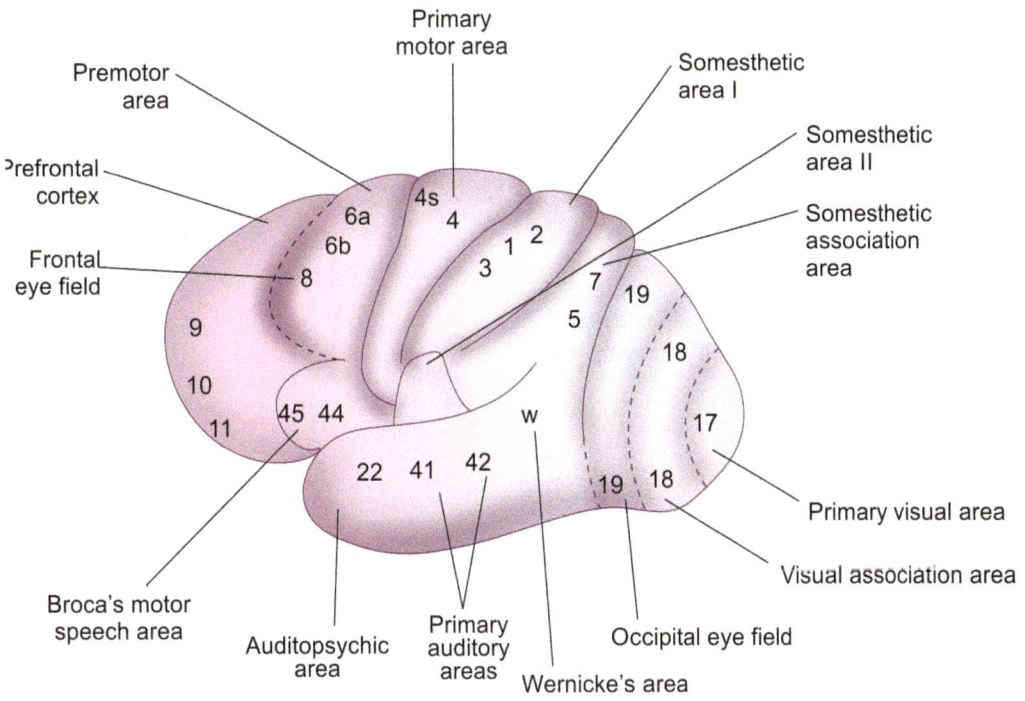

FIGURE 87.4: Lateral surface of cerebral cortex.

1. Primary motor area.
2. Premotor area.
3. Supplementary motor area.

1. Primary Motor Area

Primary motor area extends throughout the precentral gyrus and the adjoining lip of central sulcus. Areas 4 and 4S are present here **(Figs. 87.4** and **87.5)**.

Functions of primary motor area

Primary motor area is concerned with initiation of **voluntary movements** and speech.

Area 4

Area 4 is a tapering strip of area situated in precentral gyrus of frontal lobe **(Figs. 87.4** and **87.5)**.

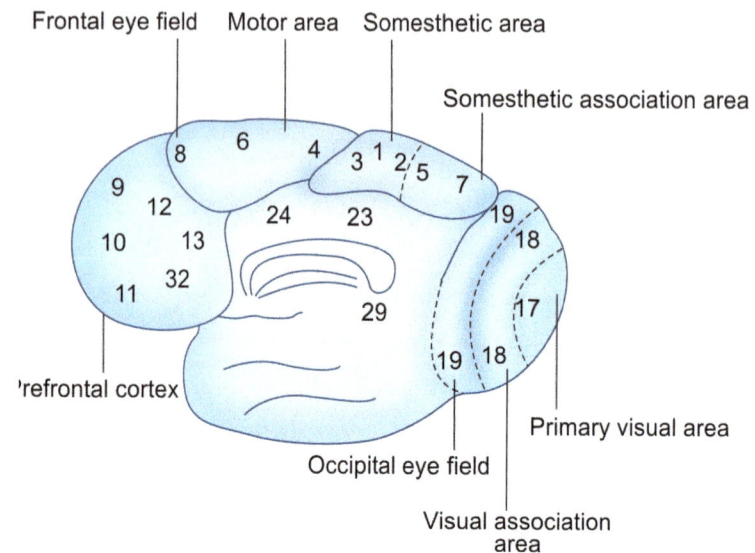

FIGURE 87.5: Medial surface of cerebral cortex.

It is the center for movement, as it sends all efferent (corticospinal) fibers of primary motor area. Through the fibers of corticospinal tracts, area 4 activates the **lower motor neurons** in the spinal cord. It activates both α-motor neurons and γ-motor neurons simultaneously by the process called **coactivation**.

Activation of α-motor neurons causes contraction of extrafusal fibers of the muscles. **Activation of γ-motor neurons** causes contraction of intrafusal fibers leading to increase in muscle tone.

Localization: Motor Homunculus

Muscles of various parts of the body are represented in area 4 in an inverted way from medial to lateral surface. Lower parts of body are represented in medial surface and upper parts of the body are represented in the lateral surface. Order of representation from medial to lateral surface is toes, ankle, knee, hip, trunk, shoulder, arm, elbow, wrist, hand fingers and face. However, parts of the face are not represented in inverted manner **(Fig. 87.6)**.

Area 4S

Area 4S is called **suppressor area**. It forms a narrow strip anterior to area 4. It scrutinizes and suppresses the extra impulses produced by area 4 and prevents **exaggeration of movements**.

2. Premotor Area

This has areas 6, 8, 44 and 45. Premotor area is anterior to primary motor area in the precentral cortex.

Functions of premotor area

Premotor area is concerned with control of **postural movements**.

Area 6

Area 6 is in the posterior portions of superior, middle and inferior frontal gyri. It is subdivided into 6a and 6b. It gives origin to some of the pyramidal tract fibers.

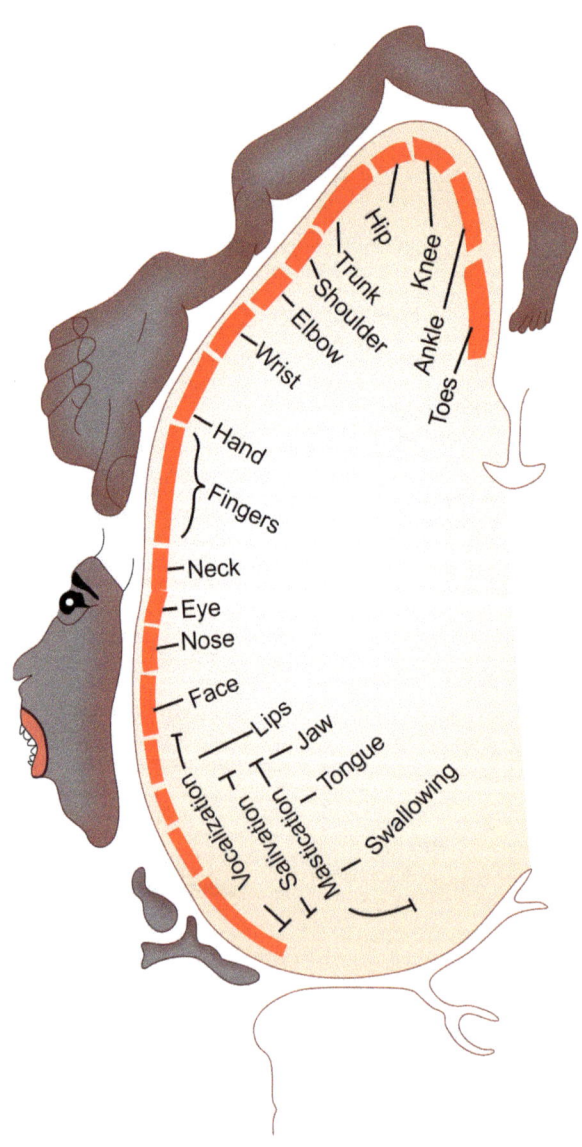

FIGURE 87.6: Topographical arrangement (homunculus) of motor areas in cerebral cortex.

Area 6 has two functions:

i. It is concerned with **coordination of movements** initiated by area 4. It helps to make the skilled movements more accurate and smoother.

ii. It is **cortical center** for extrapyramidal system.

Area 8

Area 8 is called **frontal eye field**. It lies anterior to area 6 in the precentral cortex. It is concerned with movements of eyeball.

Frontal eye field is concerned with **conjugate movement** of eyeballs.

Areas 44 and 45: Broca's area

Broca's area is the **motor area for speech**. It includes areas 44 and 45. Broca's area is present in left hemisphere (dominant hemisphere) of right-handed persons and in the right hemisphere of left-handed persons. It is a special region of premotor cortex situated in inferior frontal gyrus.

Broca's area is responsible for movements of tongue, lips and larynx, which are involved in speech.

3. Supplementary Motor Area

It is situated in medial surface of frontal lobe rostral to primary motor area.

Functions of supplementary motor area

This area is concerned with coordination of **skilled movements**.

■ PREFRONTAL CORTEX OR ORBITOFRONTAL CORTEX

Prefrontal or orbitofrontal cortex is the anterior part of frontal lobe of cerebral cortex, in front of areas 8 and 44. It occupies the medial, lateral and inferior surfaces, and includes orbital gyri, medial frontal gyrus and the anterior portions of superior, middle and inferior frontal gyri.

Areas present in prefrontal cortex are 9, 10, 11, 12, 13, 14, 23, 24, 29 and 32. Areas 12, 13, 14, 23, 24, 29 and 32 are in medial surface. Areas 9, 10 and 11 are in lateral surface.

Area 13 is concerned with **emotional reactions**.

Functions of Prefrontal Cortex

1. It forms the center for the **higher functions** like emotion, learning, memory and social behavior. Short term memories are registered here.
2. It is the center for **planned actions**.
3. It is the seat of intelligence. So, it is also called the **organ of mind**.
4. It is responsible for the **personality** of the individuals.
5. It is responsible for the various **autonomic changes** during emotional conditions, because of its connections with hypothalamus and brainstem.

■ APPLIED PHYSIOLOGY: FRONTAL LOBE SYNDROME

Frontal lobe syndrome is a disorder caused by injury or ablation of prefrontal cortex.

Features of frontal lobe syndrome are:

1. Emotional instability.
2. Lack of concentration and lack of fixing attention.
3. Lack of initiation and difficulty in planning any course of action.
4. Impairment of recent memory occurs. Memory of remote events is not lost.
5. Loss of moral and social sense is common, and there is loss of love for family and friends.
6. There is failure to realize the seriousness of the condition. Patient has the sense of well-being and also has flight of ideas.
7. Functional abnormalities:
    i. Hyperphagia (increased food intake).
    ii. Loss of control over sphincter of the urinary bladder or rectum.
    iii. Disturbances in orientation.
    iv. Slight tremor.

■ PARIETAL LOBE

Parietal lobe extends from **central sulcus** and merges with occipital lobe behind and temporal lobe below. This lobe is separated from occipital lobe by **parieto-occipital sulcus** and from temporal lobe by **Sylvian sulcus**.

Parietal lobe is divided into three functional areas:

A. Somesthetic area I.
B. Somesthetic area II.
C. Somesthetic association area.

In addition to these three areas, a part of **sensory motor area** is also situated in parietal lobe (see below).

■ SOMESTHETIC AREA I

It is also called **somatosensory area I** or primary somesthetic or **primary sensory area**. It is present in the posterior lip of central sulcus, in the postcentral gyrus and in the paracentral lobule.

Areas

Somesthetic area I has three areas which are called **areas 3, 1 and 2**. Anterior part of this forms area 3 and posterior part forms areas 1 and 2.

Localization: Sensory Homunculus

Different sensory areas of the body are represented in postcentral gyrus (**primary sensory area**) in an inverted manner as in the motor area. The toes are represented in lowest part of medial surface, legs at the upper border of hemispheres, then from above downwards knee, thigh, hip, trunk, upper limb, neck and face. The representation of face is not inverted. The representation of parts of face from above downwards is eyelids, nose, cheek, upper lip and lower lip **(Fig. 87.7)**.

Functions of Somesthetic Area I

1. Somesthetic area I is responsible for **perception and integration** of cutaneous and kinesthetic sensations.

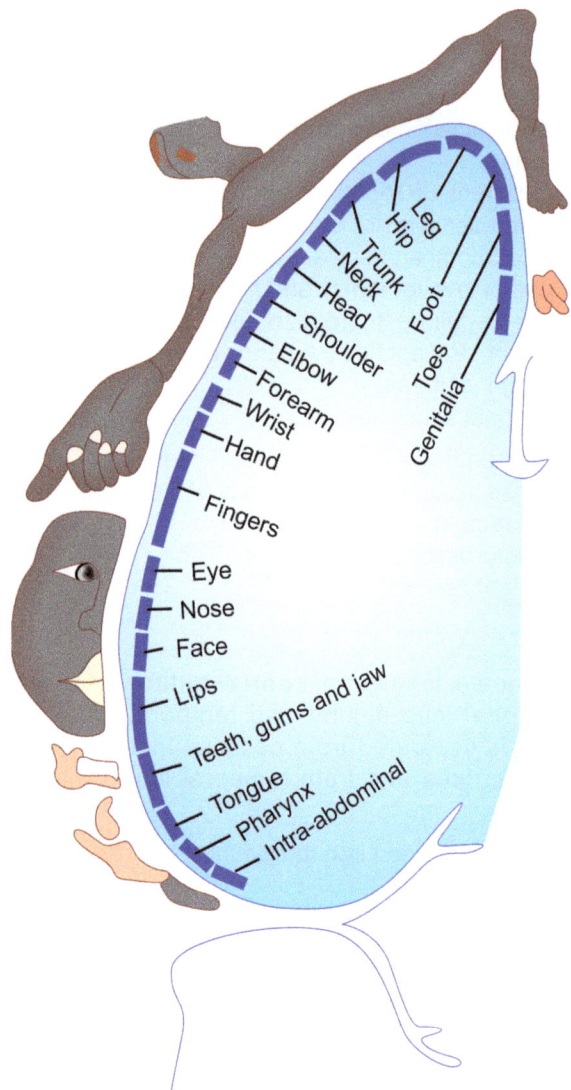

FIGURE 87.7: Topographical arrangement (homunculus) of sensory areas in cerebral cortex.

It receives sensory impulses from cutaneous receptors (touch, pressure, pain, temperature) and proprioceptors of opposite side through thalamic radiation. Area 1 is concerned with sensory perception. The areas 2 and 3 are involved in the integration of these sensations.

2. This area sends **sensory feedback** to the premotor area. It is also concerned with the movements of head and eyeballs.
3. **Discriminative functions**: In addition to perception of cutaneous and kinesthetic sensation, this area is also responsible for recognizing the discriminative features of sensations.

■ SOMESTHETIC AREA II

Otherwise called **somatosensory area II**, this area receives sensory impulses from somesthetic area I and from thalamus directly. This area is concerned with **perception of sensation**. Thus, the sensory parts of body have two representations, viz. in somesthetic area I and area II.

■ SOMESTHETIC ASSOCIATION AREA

This area is situated posterior to postcentral gyrus. It has two **areas, 5 and 7**. It is concerned with **synthesis of sensations** perceived by somesthetic area I.

Somesthetic association area is the center for combined sensations such as **stereognosis**.

Sensory Motor Area

Sensory motor area is the area of cerebral cortex in which the precentral gyrus of frontal lobe (where motor areas are located) and postcentral gyrus of parietal lobe (where sensory areas are located) are knit together by association nerve fibers.

Function of this area is to store the **timing and programing** of various sequential movements of complicated skilled movements which are planned by **neocerebellum** (Chapter 85).

■ APPLIED PHYSIOLOGY: EFFECTS OF LESION

Lesion or ablation of parietal lobe (sensory cortex) results in the following disturbances:

1. Contralateral disturbance in cutaneous sensations.
2. Disturbances in kinesthetic sensations.
3. Loss of tactile localization and discrimination.

■ TEMPORAL LOBE

Temporal lobe of cerebral cortex includes three functional areas:

A. Primary auditory area.
B. Secondary auditory.
C. Area for equilibrium.

■ PRIMARY AUDITORY AREA

Primary auditory area includes:

1. Area 41.
2. Area 42.
3. Wernicke's area.

Areas 41 and 42 are situated in anterior transverse gyrus and lateral surface of superior temporal gyrus. Wernicke's area is in upper part of superior temporal gyrus posterior to areas 41 and 42.

Functions of Primary Auditory Area

Primary auditory area is concerned with perception of auditory impulses, analysis of pitch and determination of intensity and source of sound.

Areas 41 and 42 are concerned only with the **perception** of auditory impulses **(Table 87.1). Wernicke's area** is responsible for the **interpretation of sound**. It carries out this function with the help of auditopsychic area (area 22).

■ SECONDARY AUDITORY AREA: AUDITOPSYCHIC AREA

Secondary auditory area is also called auditopsychic area or auditory association area. It is the **area 22** and it occupies

TABLE 87.1: Functions of cortical lobes.

Lobe			Functions
Frontal lobe	Precentral cortex	Primary motor area — Area 4	Initiates movements
		Primary motor area — Area 4S	Inhibits exaggeration of movements initiated by area 4
		Premotor area — Area 6	Coordinates movements initiated by area 4 Acts as higher center for extrapyramidal system
		Premotor area — Area 8	Frontal eye field Concerned with conjugate movements of eyeballs Concerned with voluntary movements of eyeballs
		Broca's area: Areas 44 and 45	Initiates movements involved in speech; motor speech area
		Supplementary motor area — –	Concerned with coordinated skilled movements
	Prefrontal cortex	Areas 9, 10, 11, 12, 13, 14, 23, 24, 29 and 32	Concerned with emotion, learning, memory and social behavior Act as the center for planned actions Form seat of intelligence Initiate autonomic changes during emotional conditions
Parietal lobe	Somesthetic area I	Area 1	Perceives cutaneous and kinesthetic sensations
		Areas 3 and 2	Integrate cutaneous and kinesthetic sensations
		Areas 3, 2 and 1	Send feedback to premotor area Concerned with movements of head and eyeballs Concerned with recognition of discriminative features of sensations
	Somesthetic area II	–	Perceives cutaneous and kinesthetic sensations
	Somesthetic association area	Areas 5 and 7	Synthesize sensations perceived by somesthetic area I (forms the center for combined sensations)
Temporal lobe	Primary auditory area	Areas 41 and 42	Perceives auditory sensation
		Wernicke's area	Interprets auditory sensation (along with area 22)
	Secondary auditory area	Area 22	Interprets auditory sensation (along with Wernicke's area)
	Area for equilibrium	–	Concerned with maintenance of equilibrium of body
Occipital lobe	Primary visual area	Area 17	Perceives visual sensation
	Secondary visual area	Area 18	Interprets visual sensation
	Occipital eye field	Area 19	Concerned with reflex movement of eyeballs Concerned with associated movements of eyeballs while following a moving object

the superior temporal gyrus. This area is concerned with **interpretation of sound** along with Wernicke's area.

■ AREA FOR EQUILIBRIUM

This area is in the posterior part of superior temporal gyrus. It is concerned with the maintenance of equilibrium of the body. Stimulation of this area causes dizziness, swaying, falling and feeling of rotation.

■ APPLIED PHYSIOLOGY: TEMPORAL LOBE SYNDROME

Temporal lobe syndrome is otherwise known as **Kluver-Bucy syndrome**. It is the disorder caused by bilateral lesion or bilateral ablation of temporal lobe along with amygdaloid and uncus.

Manifestations of this syndrome are:

1. Aphasia: Disturbance in speech.
2. Auditory disturbances: Such as frequent attacks of **tinnitus** (noise in ear), **auditory hallucinations** (feeling of a particular type of sensation without any stimulus) with sounds like buzzing, ringing or humming.
3. Disturbances in smell and taste sensations.
4. Dreamy states: Patient is not aware of his or her own activities, and has the feeling of unreality.
5. Visual hallucinations associated with hemianopia.

■ OCCIPITAL LOBE: VISUAL CORTEX

Occipital lobe is also called the visual cortex.

AREAS OF VISUAL CORTEX

Occipital lobe consists of three functional areas:

1. Primary visual area: Area 17.
2. Visual association area: Area 18.
3. Occipital eye field: Area 19.

Functions

1. Primary visual area: Area 17 is concerned with **perception of visual impulses**.
2. Visual association area: Area 18 is concerned with **interpretation of visual impulses**.
3. Occipital eye field: Area 19 is concerned with **movement of eyes**.

APPLIED PHYSIOLOGY: EFFECTS OF LESION

Lesion in the upper or lower part of visual cortex results in hemianopia. Bilateral lesion leads to total blindness.

LIMBIC SYSTEM OR LIMBIC LOBE

Limbic system or limbic lobe is a complex system of cortical and subcortical structures that form a ring around the hilus of cerebral hemisphere **(Figs. 87.8 and 87.9)**. Limbus means ring.

COMPONENTS OF LIMBIC SYSTEM

Structures of limbic system are classified into four groups:

1. Archicortical structures.
2. Paleocortical structures.
3. Juxtallocortical structures.
4. Subcortical structures

FUNCTIONS OF LIMBIC SYSTEM

1. Olfaction

Pyriform cortex and amygdaloid nucleus form the olfactory centers.

2. Regulation of Endocrine Glands

Hypothalamus plays an important role in regulation of endocrine secretion (Chapter 84).

3. Regulation of Autonomic Functions

Hypothalamus plays an important role in regulating the autonomic functions (Chapter 84) such as heart rate, blood pressure, water balance and body temperature.

4. Regulation of Food Intake

Along with amygdaloid complex, the feeding center and satiety center present in hypothalamus regulate food intake (Chapter 84).

5. Control of Circadian Rhythm

Hypothalamus is taking major role in the circadian fluctuations of various physiological activities.

6. Regulation of Sexual Functions

Hypothalamus is responsible for maintaining sexual functions.

7. Role in Emotional State

Emotional state of a person is maintained by hippocampus along with hypothalamus.

8. Role in Memory

Hippocampus plays an important role in memory (Chapter 90).

9. Role in Motivation

Reward and punishment centers present in hypothalamus and other structures of limbic system are responsible for motivation and the behavior pattern of human beings (Chapter 84).

Refer Chapter 84 for details of the hypothalamic functions.

RETICULAR FORMATION

Reticular formation is a diffused mass of neurons and nerve fibers forming an ill-defined meshwork of reticulum in the central portion of the brainstem. Reticular formation is situated in **brainstem**. It extends

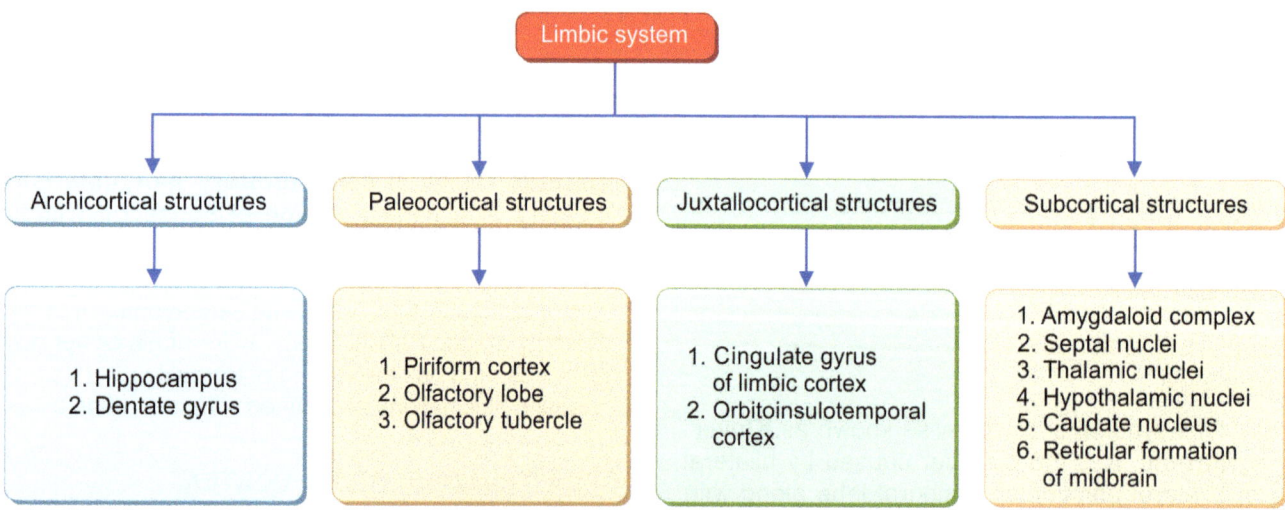

FIGURE 87.8: Components of limbic system.

Chapter 87: Cerebral Cortex, Limbic System and Reticular Formation · 445

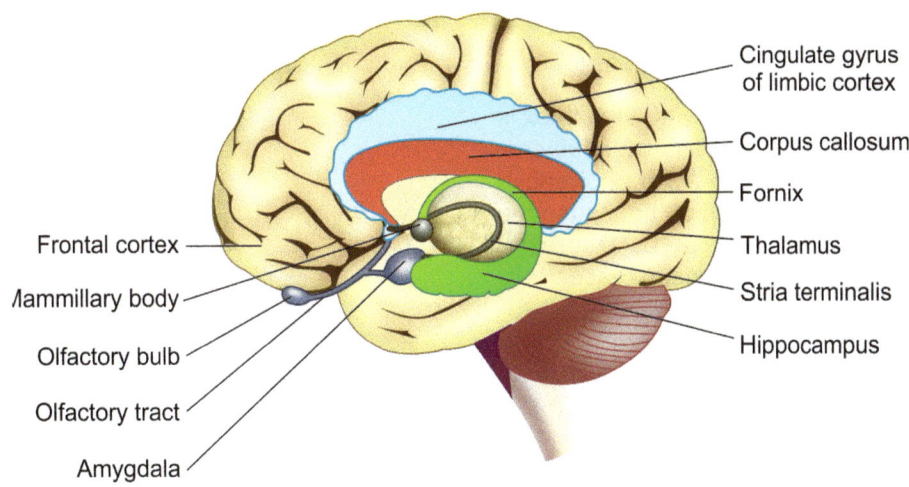

FIGURE 87.9: Limbic system.

downwards into spinal cord and upwards up to thalamus and subthalamus.

Reticular formation is divided into three divisions based on the location in brainstem:

1. Medullary reticular formation.
2. Pontine reticular formation.
3. Midbrain reticular formation.

Each division of reticular formation has its own collection of nuclei.

■ FUNCTIONS OF RETICULAR FORMATION

Based on functions, the reticular formation along with its connections is divided into two systems:

I. Ascending reticular activating system.
II. Descending reticular system.

Ascending Reticular Activating System (Aras)

Ascending reticular activating system (ARAS) begins in lower part of brainstem, extends upwards through pons, midbrain, thalamus and finally projects throughout the cerebral cortex.

ARAS receives fibers from the sensory pathways via long ascending spinal tracts **(Fig. 87.10)**.

Functions of ARAS

1. ARAS is concerned with arousal phenomenon, alertness, maintenance of attention and wakefulness. Hence the name ascending reticular activating system. Stimulation of midbrain reticular formation produces wakefulness.
2. ARAS also causes emotional reactions.
3. ARAS plays an important role in regulating the learning processes and the development of conditioned reflexes.

Mechanism of Action of ARAS

Impulses of all the sensations reach the cerebral cortex through two channels:
1. Classical or specific sensory pathways.

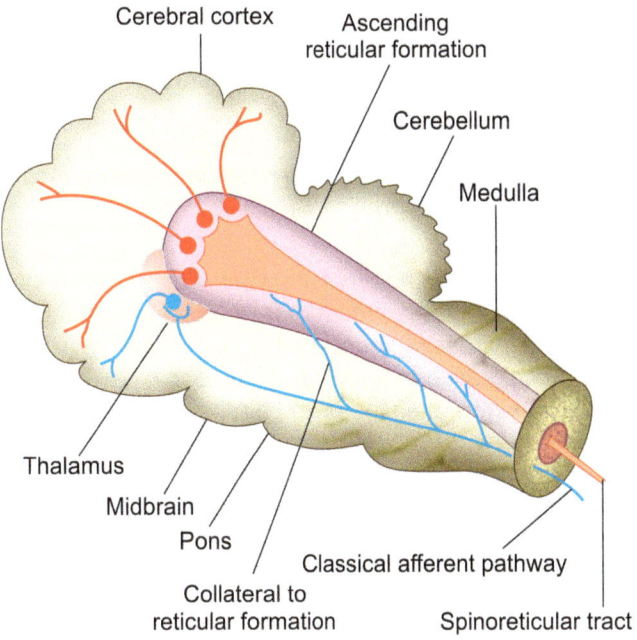

FIGURE 87.10: Ascending reticular formation.

2. Ascending reticular activating system or nonspecific specific pathway.

Classical or specific sensory pathways

Classical sensory pathways are the pathways which transmit the sensory impulses from receptors to cerebral cortex via thalamus. Some of the pathways carry impulses of a particular sensation only. For example, the auditory stimulus transmitted by the auditory pathway reaches the auditory cortex via thalamus and causes perception of sound. Such classical sensory pathways are called **specific sensory pathways**.

Ascending reticular activating system or nonspecific sensory pathway

All the sensory pathways send collaterals to diffused areas of ARAS. Spinal cord also sends sensory fibers directly to ARAS via **spinoreticular tract**. ARAS in turn sends the impulses to almost all the areas of cerebral cortex and other parts of brain. Hence, this pathway is called the **nonspecific sensory pathway**.

The nonspecific projection of ARAS into the cortex is responsible for the arousal, alertness and wakefulness. Impulses transmitted to cortex via ARAS do not cause the perception of any particular sensation but cause the generalized activation of almost all the areas of cerebral cortex and other parts of brain. This leads to reactions of arousal, alertness and wakefulness.

Descending Reticular System

Descending reticular system includes reticular formation in brainstem, the reticulospinal tract and reticular formation in spiral cord.

It modifies the activities of spinal motor neurons. Functionally, descending reticular system is divided into two subdivisions **(Fig. 87.11)**:

A. Descending facilitatory reticular system.
B. Descending inhibitory reticular system.

Descending Facilitatory Reticular System

Descending facilitatory reticular system is present in upper and lateral reticular formation.

Its functions are:
1. *Facilitation of somatomotor activities by:*
   i. Exciting the gamma motor neurons in spinal cord and increasing muscle tone.
   ii. Accelerating movements of the body.
   iii. Causing wakefulness and alertness.
2. *Facilitation of vegetative functions:* Descending facilitatory reticular system is the center for facilitation of the autonomic functions such as cardiac function, blood pressure, respiration, gastrointestinal function and body temperature.

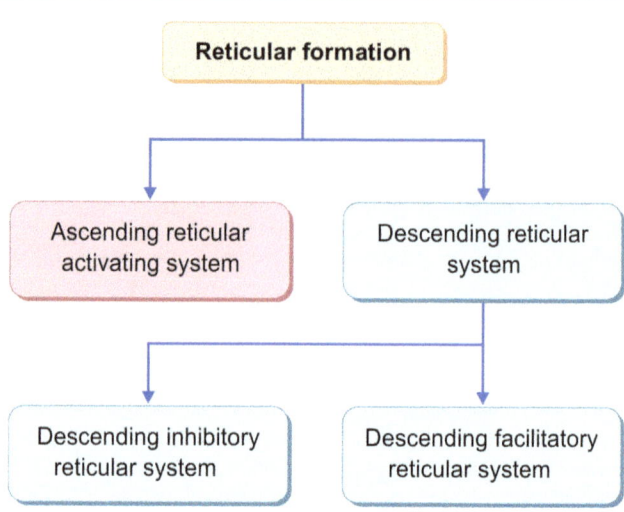

FIGURE 87.11: Functional divisions of reticular formation.

Descending Inhibitory Reticular System

Descending inhibitory reticular system is located in a small area in lower and medial reticular formation. Its functions are:
1. *Control of somatomotor activities by:*
   i. Inhibiting gamma motor neurons of spinal cord and decreasing muscle tone.
   ii. Inhibiting the α-motor neurons of spinal cord and producing smooth and accurate voluntary movements.
   iii. Controlling the reflex movements.
2. *Control of vegetative functions:* Descending inhibitory reticular system is the center for inhibition of several autonomic functions such as cardiac function, blood pressure, respiration, gastrointestinal function and body temperature.

Chapter 88: Proprioceptors, Posture, Equilibrium and Vestibular Apparatus

CHAPTER OUTLINE

- **PROPRIOCEPTORS**
  - MUSCLE SPINDLE
  - GOLGI TENDON ORGAN
  - PACINIAN CORPUSCLE
  - FREE NERVE ENDING
- **POSTURE**
  - BASIC PHENOMENA OF POSTURE
  - POSTURAL REFLEXES
  - STATIC REFLEXES
  - STATOKINETIC REFLEXES
- **VESTIBULAR APPARATUS**
  - LABYRINTH
  - FUNCTIONAL ANATOMY
  - RECEPTOR ORGAN
  - NERVE SUPPLY
  - FUNCTIONS
  - APPLIED PHYSIOLOGY

PROPRIOCEPTORS

Proprioceptors play a major role in the maintenance of posture and equilibrium. So, knowledge of proprioceptors is essential to understand maintenance of posture and equilibrium.

Proprioceptors or **kinesthetic receptors** are defined as the receptors, which give response to change in position of different parts of the body. Proprioceptors are situated in labyrinth, muscles, tendon of the muscles, joints, ligaments and fascia.

Different proprioceptors are:

1. Muscle spindle.
2. Golgi tendon organ.
3. Pacinian corpuscle.
4. Free nerve ending.
5. Proprioceptors in labyrinth.

MUSCLE SPINDLE

Muscle spindle is a spindle-shaped proprioceptor situated in the skeletal muscle. It is formed by modified skeletal muscle fibers called **intrafusal muscle fibers**.

Structure of Muscle Spindle

Muscle spindle has a central bulged portion and two tapering ends. Each muscle spindle is formed by 5 to 12 **intrafusal muscle fibers** which are enclosed by a connective tissue capsule. Intrafusal fibers are attached to the capsule on either end. The capsule is attached to either side of extrafusal fibers or the tendon of the muscle. Thus, the intrafusal fibers are placed parallel to the extrafusal fibers (Fig. 88.1).

Muscle spindle is formed by two types of intrafusal fibers.

1. Nuclear bag fiber.
2. Nuclear chain fiber.

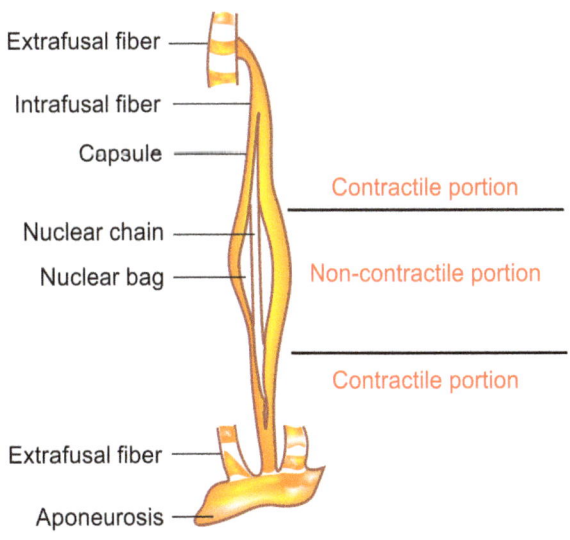

FIGURE 88.1: Muscle spindle.

Nerve Supply to Muscle Spindle

Muscle spindle is innervated by both sensory and motor nerves. It is the **only receptor** in the body, which has both sensory and motor nerve supply.

Sensory nerve supply

Each muscle spindle receives two types of sensory nerve fibers:

1. *Primary sensory (afferent) nerve fiber:* It belongs to type **Iα (Aα) nerve fiber**. Each sensory (afferent) nerve fiber has two branches. One branch supplies bag fiber **(Fig. 88.2)**. Another branch supplies nuclear chain fiber. The branches end in the form of **annul spiral endings** around central portion of the nuclear bag and nuclear chain fibers.
2. *Secondary sensory nerve fiber:* It is a type **IIβ (Aβ)** nerve fiber. It innervates only the nuclear chain fiber and ends in the form of **flower spray ending**.

Motor nerve supply

Motor nerve fiber supplying the muscle spindle belongs to gamma motor neuron **(Aγ) type**.

1. *Motor (efferent) nerve supply to nuclear bag fiber:* Gamma motor nerve fiber supplying nuclear bag fiber ends as motor **end plate**. Functionally this nerve is called dynamic gamma motor nerve.
2. *Motor nerve supply to nuclear chain fiber:* Gamma motor nerve fiber supplying the nuclear chain fiber divides into many branches, which form a network called **trail ending**. Sometimes, it gives a branch to nuclear bag fiber also. Functionally this nerve is called static gamma motor nerve.

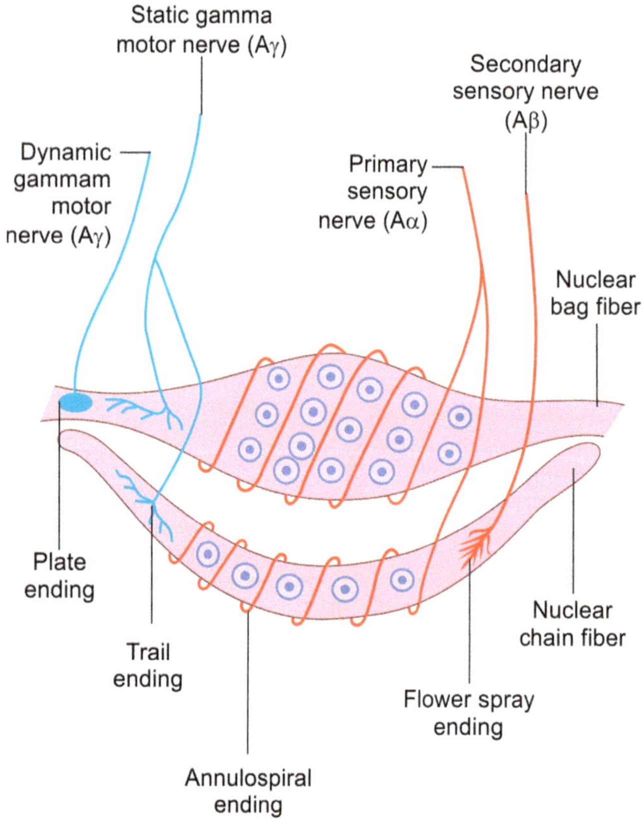

Functions of Muscle Spindle

Muscle spindle gives response to change in the **length of the muscle**. It detects how much the muscle is being stretched. By detecting the change in length of the muscle, the spindle plays an important role in **stretch reflex** and maintenance of **muscle tone** (see below).

■ GOLGI TENDON ORGAN

Golgi tendon organ is situated in the tendon of skeletal muscle. It is formed by a group of nerve endings covered by a connective tissue capsule **(Fig. 88.3)**.

Nerve Supply to Golgi Tendon Organ

Sensory nerve fiber supplying Golgi tendon organ belongs to **Ib type**.

Functions of Golgi Tendon Organ

Golgi tendon organ gives response to the change in the **force** or **tension** developed in the skeletal muscle during contraction.

■ PACINIAN CORPUSCLE

Pacinian corpuscle is a **mechanoreceptor** that senses pressure and vibration. It is situated in the deeper layers of skin, tendon, facia and joint capsule. Pacinian corpuscles situated in these tissues send information about **joint position** to central nervous system.

■ FREE NERVE ENDING

Free nerve ending is the receptor for pain sensation situated in skin, muscles, tendon, fascia and joints. It is stimulated during some specific joint positions. In turn, it sends information about **joint position** to central nervous system.

FIGURE 88.2: Nerve supply to muscle spindle.
Red = Sensory (afferent) nerve fibers,
Blue = Motor (efferent) nerve fibers,
Letters in parenthesis = Type of nerve fibers.

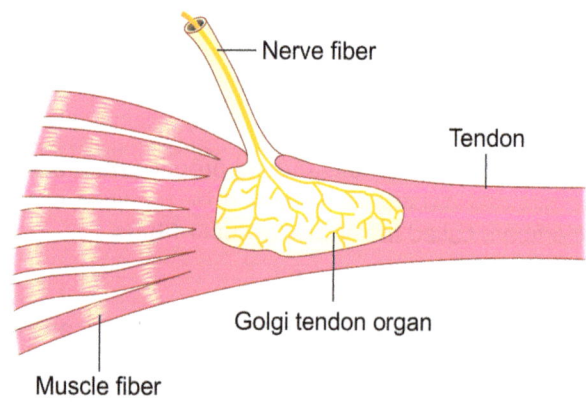

FIGURE 88.3: Golgi tendon apparatus.

Chapter 88: Proprioceptors, Posture, Equilibrium and Vestibular Apparatus

POSTURE

Posture is defined as the position or attitude of the body while standing or sitting.

Maintenance of posture is carried out by subconscious **adjustment of tone** in different muscles in relation to every movement of the body. Significance of maintenance of posture is to make the movement smooth and accurate and to keep the body in equilibrium with line of gravity.

BASIC PHENOMENA OF POSTURE

Basic phenomena for maintenance of posture are the muscle tone and stretch reflex.

Muscle Tone

Muscle tone or tonus is defined as the state of continuous and passive partial contraction of the muscle with certain vigor and tension. It is also defined as resistance offered by the muscle to stretch.

Muscle tone is responsible in maintenance of posture. Gamma motor neurons and muscle spindle are responsible for the development and maintenance of muscle tone **(Fig. 88.4)**.

Muscle tone is developed in the following sequence:

1. Impulses from the **gamma motor neurons** cause contraction of end portions of intrafusal fibers. This stretches and activates the central portion of the intrafusal fibers.
2. Impulses from the central portion of intrafusal fibers reach the spinal cord by passing through primary sensory nerve fibers and stimulate the **alpha motor neurons**.
3. Alpha motor neurons in turn, send impulses to extrafusal fibers of the muscle through spinal nerve fibers and produce **partial contraction** of the muscle fibers resulting in development of muscle tone.

Stretch Reflex

Stretch reflex or **myotatic reflex** is the reflex contraction of muscle when it is stretched. It is a **monosynaptic reflex** and the **quickest reflex**.

Stimulation of muscle spindle elicits the stretch reflex. Intrafusal muscle fibers are situated parallel to the extrafusal muscle fibers and are attached to the tendon of the muscle by means of capsule. So, stretching of the muscle causes stretching of the muscle spindle also. This stimulates the muscle spindle and it discharges the sensory impulses. These impulses are transmitted via the primary and secondary sensory (afferent) nerve fibers to the alpha motor neurons in spinal cord. Alpha motor neurons in turn send motor impulse to muscles through their fibers and cause contraction of extrafusal fibers.

Stretch reflex is the basic reflex involved in maintenance of posture.

POSTURAL REFLEXES

Postural reflexes are the reflexes which are responsible for the maintenance of posture.

Classification of Postural Reflexes

Postural reflexes are classified into two groups:

A. Static reflexes.
B. Statokinetic reflexes.

STATIC REFLEXES

Static reflexes are the postural reflexes that maintain posture at rest.

Static reflexes are of four types:

I. General static reflexes or righting reflexes.
II. Local static reflexes or supporting reflexes.
III. Segmental static reflexes.
IV. Statotonic or attitudinal reflexes.

I. General Static Reflexes or Righting Reflexes

General static or righting reflexes help to maintain an **upright position of the body**. Righting reflexes are of five types. First four reflexes are demonstrated on a **thalamic animal** or a **normal blindfolded animal**.

Sequential events of righting reflexes

1. *Labyrinthine righting reflexes acting upon the neck muscles*

When a thalamic animal (animal such as rabbit in which connections of the thalamus with cerebral cortex are

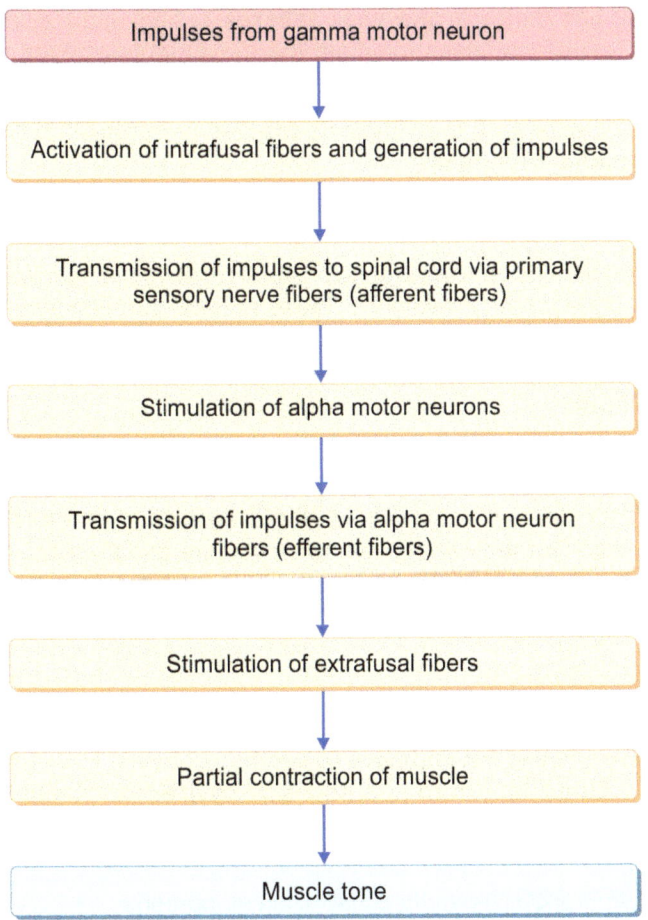

FIGURE 88.4: Schematic diagram showing development of muscle tone.

removed) is suspended by holding at the pelvic region, its head turns up, until it assumes its normal position. It is because of reflexes arising from labyrinth which act on neck muscles.

2. Neck righting reflexes acting upon the body

Now, the contraction of neck muscles produces proprioceptive impulses which act on the body and rotate the body in relation to position of head.

3. Body righting reflexes acting upon the head

If the animal is laid down upon its side on a table, pressure on that particular side of the body stimulates exteroceptors on the skin. Impulses thus generated by exteroceptors act on neck muscles and rotate the head.

4. Body righting reflexes acting upon the body

When the same animal is laid down on the table on its side with head held down to table, to eliminate labyrinthine and neck righting reflexes, the body attempts to right itself by raising the lower parts. It is because of the impulses from exteroceptors on that side of body acting on the body itself.

5. Optical righting reflexes

If the animal happens to be a **labyrinthectomized** one, then it makes an attempt to recover its upright position as a result of operation of the optical righting reaction. If the optical righting reflexes are abolished by covering the eyes, the righting ability is lost.

Optical righting reflexes are also demonstrated in 3 to 4 weeks old baby. When laid down on belly, i.e. prone position, the baby tries to raise the head to a vertical position.

Centers for righting reflexes

Centers for the first four righting reflexes are in the **red nucleus** situated in midbrain. The center for the optical righting reflexes is in the occipital lobe of **cerebral cortex**.

II. Local Static Reflexes or Supporting Reflexes

Local static reflexes or supporting reactions support the body in different positions against gravity and also protect the limbs against hyperextension or hyperflexion.

Supporting reactions are classified into two types:
1. Positive supporting reflexes.
2. Negative supporting reflexes.

1. Positive supporting reflexes

Positive supporting reflexes are the reactions, which help to **fix the joints** and make the limbs **rigid like pillars**, so that limbs can support weight of the body **against gravity**.

Positive supporting reflexes are developed **while standing**. Impulses for these reflexes arise from proprioceptors present in the muscles, joints and tendons and also the exteroceptors, particularly pressure (Pacinian corpuscles) receptors present in deeper layers of the skin of sole. This causes simultaneous reflex contractions of both extensor and flexor muscles and facilitate standing.

2. Negative supporting reflexes

Relaxation of the muscles and **unfixing of joints** enable the limbs to flex and move to a new position. It is brought about by raising the leg off the ground. When the leg is lifted off the ground, the exteroceptive impulses are stopped. It causes **unlocking of the limbs** and facilitates new movement.

Centers for the supporting reflexes are located in the **spinal cord**.

III. Segmental Static Reflexes

Segmental static reflexes are essential for walking. During walking, in one leg, the flexors are active and the extensors are inhibited. On the opposite leg, the flexors are inhibited and extensors are active. It is known as **crossed extensor reflex**. It is due to the **reciprocal inhibition** and the neural mechanism responsible for this reflex is called **reciprocal innervation**.

Centers for these reflexes are situated in the **spinal cord**.

IV. Statotonic or Attitudinal Reflexes

Statotonic or attitudinal reflexes are developed according to the attitude of the body and are of two types:
1. Tonic labyrinthine and neck reflexes acting on limbs: These reflexes maintain the movements of limbs in accordance to position of head.
2. Labyrinthine and neck reflexes acting upon eyes: These reflexes maintain the movements of eyes in accordance to position of head.

Centers for the statotonic reflexes are present in the **medulla oblongata**.

STATOKINETIC REFLEXES

Statokinetic reflexes are the postural reflexes that maintain posture during movement. These reflexes are concerned with both angular (rotatory), and linear (progressive) movements. **Vestibular apparatus** is responsible for these reflexes.

VESTIBULAR APPARATUS

Vestibular apparatus is the part of **labyrinth** or **inner ear**. It is concerned with maintenance posture and equilibrium through **statokinetic reflexes**. Other part of labyrinth is the cochlea, which is concerned with sensation of hearing.

LABYRINTH

Labyrinth (inner ear) consists of two structures, bony labyrinth and membranous labyrinth.

Bony labyrinth is a series of cavities or channels present in the petrous part of temporal bone. **Membranous labyrinth** is situated inside bony labyrinth (**Fig. 88.5**).

Membranous labyrinth consists of two portions:
1. **Cochlea** which is concerned with sensation of hearing (Chapter 97).

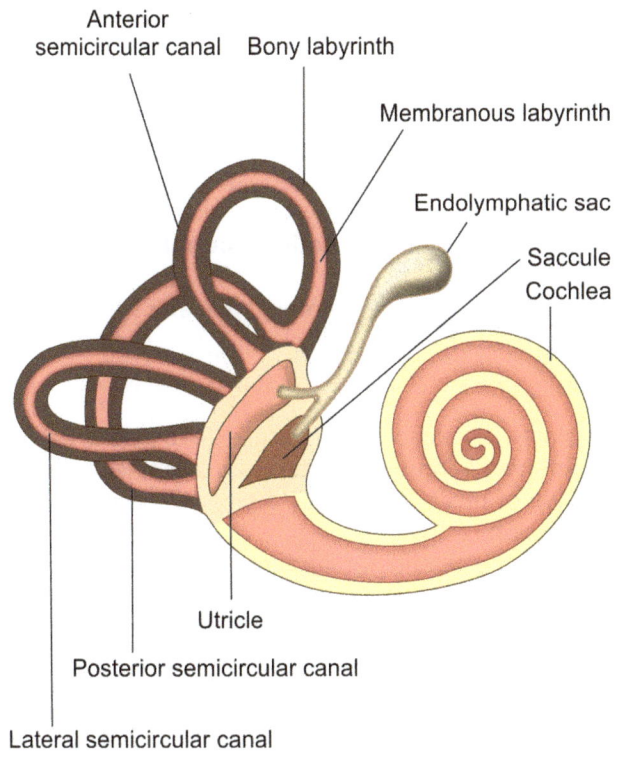

FIGURE 88.5: Labyrinth.

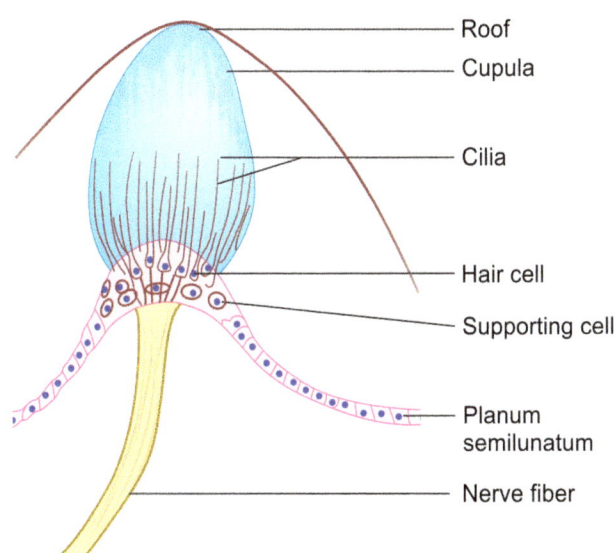

FIGURE 88.6: Crista ampullaris.

2. **Vestibular apparatus** which is concerned with posture and equilibrium.

FUNCTIONAL ANATOMY OF VESTIBULAR APPARATUS

Vestibular apparatus is formed by three semicircular canals and otolith organ or vestibule.

Semicircular Canals

Semicircular canals are:
1. Anterior or superior canal.
2. Posterior canal.
3. Lateral or horizontal or external canal.

Anterior and posterior canals are situated in vertical plane and the lateral canal is situated in horizontal plane.

Ampulla

Each semicircular canal has got two ends. One end is narrow and the other end is enlarged. The enlarged end is called ampulla. Ampulla contains the receptor organ of semicircular canals known as **crista ampullaris**. Ampulla of all the three canals and narrow end of horizontal canal open directly into the **utricle**. The narrow ends of anterior and posterior canals open into the utricle jointly, by forming the **common crus**. Thus, all the three semicircular canals open into the utricle by means of five openings. Utricle opens into **saccule**.

Otolith Organ or Vestibule

Otolith organ or vestibule is formed by **utricle** and **saccule**. Often utricle and saccule are together called **otoliths**. Utricle communicates with saccule through **utriculo-saccular duct**. Saccule communicates with cochlear duct through **ductus reuniens**. Another duct called **endolymphatic duct** arises from utriculo-saccular duct. It ends in a bag-like structure called **endolymphatic sac**.

RECEPTOR ORGAN IN VESTIBULAR APPARATUS

Receptor organ in semicircular canal is called **crista ampullaris** and that in otolith organ is called **macula**. These receptor organs contain the **proprioceptors**.

RECEPTOR ORGAN IN SEMICIRCULAR CANAL: CRISTA AMPULLARIS

Crista ampullaris is situated inside the ampulla of semicircular canals. It is formed by **receptor epithelium (neuroepithelium)** which consists of hair cells **(Fig. 88.6)**. It also has supporting cells and secreting epithelial cells which secrete the ground substance. These cells are arranged in **planum semilunatum** around hair cells.

Hair Cells

Hair cells are the **receptor cells** of crista ampullaris. There are two types of hair cells, type I and type II hair cells. Hair cells receive both afferent and efferent nerve terminals. Type I hair cells are flask shaped and Type II hair cells cylindrical. There are about 40 to 60 **cilia** called **stereocilia** arising from apex of hair cells. One of the cilia is very tall which is named as **kinocilium (Fig. 88.7)**.

From crista ampullaris, a dome shaped gelatinous structure extends up to the roof of the ampulla. It is known as cupula. The cupula encloses the cilia of hair cells. The cilia of hair cells are projected in the cupula.

RECEPTOR ORGAN IN OTOLITH ORGAN: MACULA

Receptor organ in otolith organ is called macula. Like crista ampullaris, the macula is also formed by **neuroepithelium** and supporting cells. Neuroepithelium

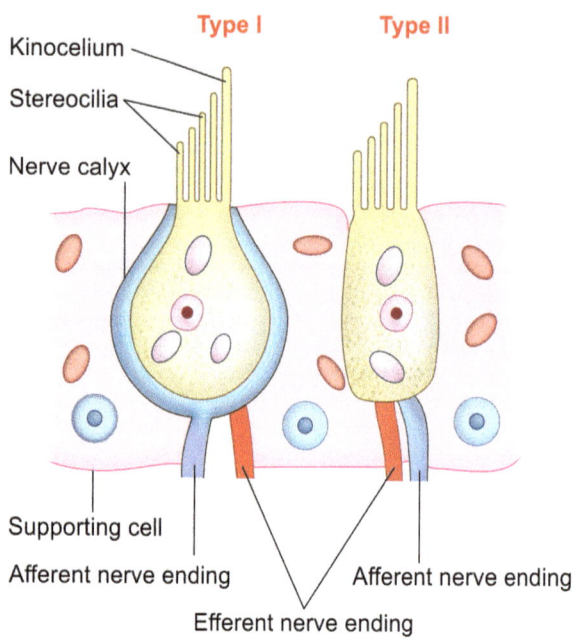

FIGURE 88.7: Hair cells of vestibular apparatus.

of macula also has two types of hair cells, the type I and type II hair cells **(Fig. 88.8)**.

Otolith Membrane

Like crista ampullaris, macula is also covered by a gelatinous membrane called **otolith membrane**. It is a flat structure and not dome shaped like cupula. **Stereocilia and kinocilium** of each hair cell are embedded in otolith membrane. Otolith membrane contains some crystals, which are called ear dust, **otoconia** or **statoconia**. The otoconia are mainly constituted by calcium carbonate.

Situation of Macula

In utricle the macula is situated in horizontal plane, so that the cilia from hair cells are in vertical direction. In saccule the macula is in vertical plane and the cilia are in horizontal direction.

■ NERVE SUPPLY TO VESTIBULAR APPARATUS

Impulses from the hair cells of crista ampullaris and maculae are transmitted to medulla oblongata and other parts of central nervous system through the fibers of **vestibular division** of **vestibulocochlear nerve** (VIII cranial nerve).

Hair cells also have efferent nerve fiber which controls the hair cells.

■ FUNCTIONS OF VESTIBULAR APPARATUS

Receptors of semicircular canals give response to **rotatory movements** or **angular acceleration** of the head. And, the receptors of utricle and saccule give response to **linear acceleration** of head.

Thus, the vestibular apparatus is responsible for detecting the position of head during different movements. It also causes the reflex adjustments in the position of eyeball, head and body during postural changes.

Functions of Semicircular Canals

Semicircular canals are concerned with **angular (rotatory) acceleration**. Semicircular canals sense the **rotational movement**. Each semicircular canal is sensitive to rotation in a particular plane.

Superior semicircular canal

Superior semicircular canal gives response to rotation in **anteroposterior plane** (transverse axis), i.e. front to back movements like nodding the head while saying '**yes – yes**'.

Horizontal semicircular canal

This semicircular canal gives response to rotation in **horizontal plane** (vertical axis), i.e. side to side movements (left to right or right to left) like shaking the head while saying '**no – no**'.

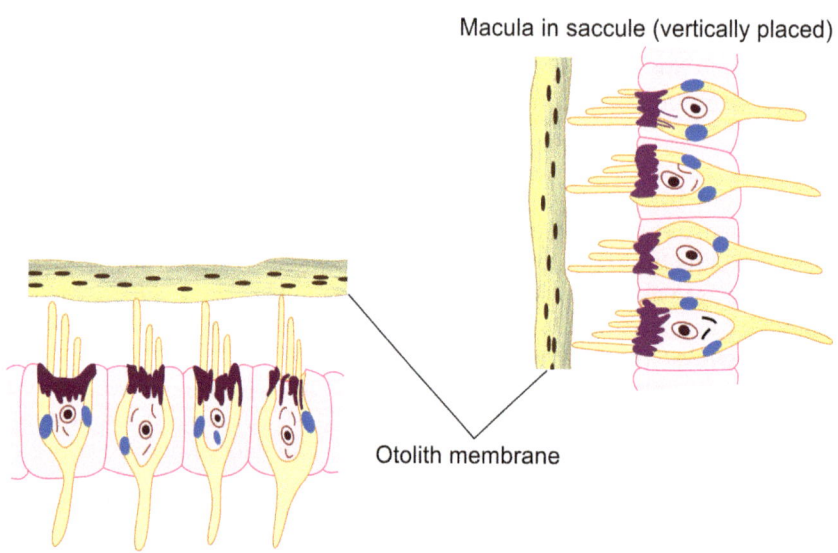

FIGURE 88.8: Macula in otolith organ.

Posterior semicircular canal

This semicircular canal gives response to rotation in the **vertical plane** (anteroposterior axis) by which head is rotated from **shoulder to shoulder**.

During rotation in anticlockwise direction

On the other hand, rotation in anticlockwise direction causes stimulation of hair cells in ampulla of horizontal canal in left ear only. Hair cells of horizontal canal in right ear are not stimulated. Stimulation of hair cells in left ear is followed by the process as in the case of clockwise rotation.

Electrical Potential in Hair Cells: Mechanotransduction

Mechanotransduction is a type of **sensory transduction** (Chapter 79) in the receptor cells (hair cells) of vestibular apparatus by which the mechanical energy (movement of cilia in hair cell) caused by stimulus is converted into **electrical energy** (action potentials) in the vestibular nerve fiber.

Resting membrane potential in hair cells is about – 60 mV. Movement of stereocilia of hair cells towards kinocilium causes development of **mild depolarization** in hair cells up to – 50 mV which is called **receptor potential**.

Receptor potential in hair cells causes generation of action potential in nerve fibers distributed to hair cells.

Movement of stereocilia in the opposite direction (away from kinocilium) causes **hyperpolarization** of hair cells which stops generation of action potential in the nerve fibers.

Nystagmus

Nystagmus is the rhythmic oscillatory involuntary movements of eyeball. It is common during rotation. It is due to the natural stimulatory effect of vestibular apparatus during rotational acceleration.

Nystagmus has two components of movement, which occur alternately:

1. *Slow component*: At the beginning of rotation, since eyes are fixed at a particular object (point), eyeballs rotate slowly in the direction opposite to that of rotation of the head. It is called slow component of nystagmus. It is due to vestibulo-ocular reflex.
2. *Quick component*: When the slow movement of eyeballs is limited, the eyeballs move to a new fixation point in the direction of rotation of head. This movement to a new fixation point occurs with a jerk. So, it is called the quick component. Quick component of nystagmus is due to the activation of some centers in brainstem.

Vestibulo-ocular reflex and nystagmus

Nystagmus is a reflex phenomenon that occurs in order to maintain the visual fixation. Since the movements of eyeballs occur in response to the stimulation of vestibular apparatus this reflex is called the vestibulo-ocular reflex.

Functions of Otolith Organ

Otolith organ is concerned with linear acceleration and detects acceleration in both horizontal and vertical planes. Utricle responds during **horizontal acceleration** and saccule responds during **vertical acceleration**.

■ APPLIED PHYSIOLOGY

Labyrinthectomy

Removal of labyrinthine apparatus on both sides leads to complete loss of equilibrium. The equilibrium could be maintained only by visual sensation. Postural reflexes are severely affected. There is loss of hearing sensation too.

Removal of labyrinthine apparatus on one side causes less effect on postural reflexes. However, severe autonomic symptoms such as nausea, vomiting and diarrhea occur.

Motion Sickness

Motion sickness is physiological response during movement (travel) to which the person is not adapted. It is characterized by nausea, vomiting, dizziness and other symptoms.

It can occur while traveling in any form of vehicle like automobile, ship, aircraft or spaceship. Motion sickness that occurs while traveling in a watercraft is called **seasickness**.

Cause

Motion sickness is due to excess and repeated stimulation of vestibular apparatus.

Symptoms

1. Nausea and vomiting.
2. Sweating.
3. Diarrhea.
4. Excess salivation.
5. Discomfort.
6. Headache.
7. Disorientation.

Responses of motion sickness can be prevented by avoiding greasy and bulky food before travel and by taking **antiemetic drugs** (drugs preventing nausea and vomiting).

Chapter 89

Electroencephalogram, Epilepsy and Sleep

CHAPTER OUTLINE

- **ELECTROENCEPHALOGRAM**
  - DEFINITIONS
  - SIGNIFICANCE OF EEG
  - METHOD OF RECORDING EEG
  - WAVES OF EEG
  - EEG DURING SLEEP
- **EPILEPSY**
  - DEFINITIONS
  - TYPES OF EPILEPSY
- **SLEEP**
  - DEFINITION
  - SLEEP REQUIREMENT
  - PHYSIOLOGICAL CHANGES DURING SLEEP
  - TYPES OF SLEEP
  - STAGES OF SLEEP AND EEG PATTERN
  - SLEEP CENTERS
  - APPLIED PHYSIOLOGY: SLEEP DISORDERS

ELECTROENCEPHALOGRAM

DEFINITIONS

Electroencephalography is the study of electrical activities of brain. **Electroencephalogram (EEG)** is the graphical recording of electrical activities of brain. German psychiatrist **Hans Berger** was the first one to analyze the EEG waves, hence the EEG waves are called as **Berger waves**.

Electroencephalograph is the instrument used to record EEG.

SIGNIFICANCE OF EEG

Electroencephalogram is useful in the diagnosis of neurological and sleep disorders.

EEG pattern is altered in the following neurological disorders:

1. **Epilepsy**, which occurs due to excessive discharge of impulses from cerebral cortex.
2. **Disorders of midbrain** which affect ascending reticular activating system.
3. **Subdural hematoma** during which there is collection of blood in subdural space over the cerebral cortex.

METHOD OF RECORDING EEG

For recording EEC, **scalp electrodes** from electroencephalographic instrument are placed over unopened skull or over the brain after opening the skull, or by piercing into the brain.

WAVES OF EEG

Electrical activity recorded by EEG may have synchronized or desynchronized waves. **Synchronized waves** are the regular and invariant waves, whereas **desynchronized waves** are irregular and variant.

Normally EEG has three frequency bands:

1. Alpha rhythm.
2. Beta rhythm.
3. Delta rhythm.

In children, in addition to these waves, theta rhythm appears.

1. *Alpha Rhythm*

Alpha waves are rhythmical waves, which appear at a frequency of 8 to 13 waves/second with the amplitude of 50 µV **(Table 89.1)**. Alpha waves are **synchronized waves** **(Fig. 89.1)**.

TABLE 89.1: Properties of EEG waves.

Rhythm	Frequency (per second)	Amplitude (µV)
Alpha	8 to 13	50
Beta	15 to 80	5 to 10
Delta	1 to 4	20 to 200
Theta	4 to 7	10

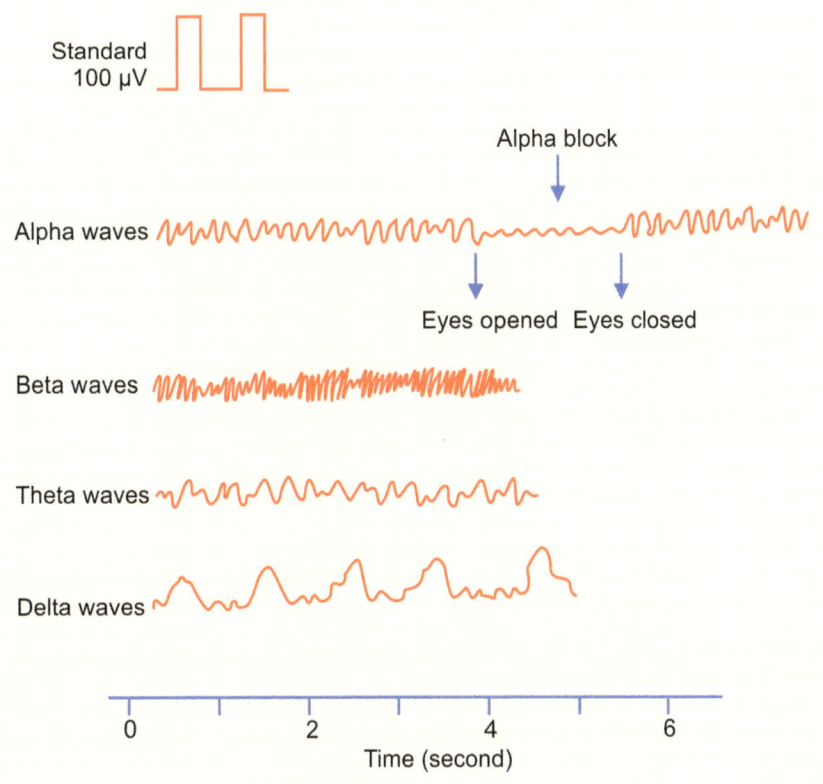

FIGURE 89.1: Waves of EEG.

Alpha waves are obtained in **inattentive brain** or **mind** as in drowsiness, light sleep or narcosis with closed eyes. These waves are abolished by any type of stimuli or mental effort and diminished when eyes are opened.

Alpha waves are most marked in parieto-occipital area.

Alpha block

Alpha block is the replacement of synchronized alpha waves in EEG by desynchronized and low voltage waves when the eyes are opened. Desynchronized waves do not have specific frequency. It occurs due to any form of sensory stimulation or mental concentration, such as solving arithmetic problems.

Desynchronization is the common term used for replacement of regular waves with irregular low voltage waves.

2. Beta Rhythm

Beta waves are high frequency waves of 15 to 80 per second. But their amplitude is low, i.e. 5 to 10 µV. Beta waves are **desynchronized waves** and are recorded during mental activity or mental tension or arousal state. These waves are not affected by opening the eyes.

3. Delta Rhythm

Delta waves are low frequency and high amplitude waves. Frequency of these waves is 1 to 4 per second and the amplitude is 20 to 200 µV. Delta waves are common in early childhood during waking hours. In adults, these waves appear mostly during deep sleep.

Presence of delta waves in adults during conditions other than sleep indicates the pathological process in brain such as tumor and epilepsy. These waves are not affected by opening the eyes.

Theta Rhythm

Theta waves are obtained generally in children below 5 years of age. These waves are of low frequency and low voltage waves. Frequency of theta waves is 4 to 7 per second and the amplitude is about 10 µV.

■ EEG DURING SLEEP

Changes in the EEG pattern during sleep are described later in this chapter.

■ EPILEPSY

■ DEFINITIONS

Epilepsy is a brain disorder characterized by convulsive seizures or loss of consciousness or both. **Convulsion** refers to uncontrolled involuntary muscular contractions. **Convulsive seizure** means sudden attack of uncontrolled involuntary muscular contractions. It occurs due to **paroxysmal** (sudden and usually recurring periodically) **uncontrolled discharge** of impulses from neurons of brain, particularly **cerebral cortex**.

Epileptic

Patient affected by epilepsy is called epileptic. The person with epilepsy remains normal in between seizures. Epileptic attack develops only when excitability of the neuron is increased, causing excessive neuronal discharge.

■ TYPES OF EPILEPSY

Epilepsy is divided into two categories:

1. Generalized epilepsy.
2. Localized epilepsy.

1. Generalized Epilepsy

Generalized epilepsy or **general onset seizure** or **general onset epilepsy** is the type of epilepsy that occurs due to excessive discharge of impulses from all parts of the brain.

Generalized epilepsy is subdivided into three types:

1. Grand mal.
2. Petit mal.
3. Psychomotor epilepsy.

Grand mal

Grand mal is characterized by sudden **loss of consciousness** followed by **convulsion**. Just before the onset of convulsions, the person feels the warning sensation in the form of some hallucination. It is called **epileptic aura**.

EEG recording shows fast waves with a frequency of 15 to 30 per second during initial stage. Later slow and large waves appear. In between seizures, the EEG shows delta waves in all types of epileptics.

Cause of grand mal epilepsy is the excess neural activity in all parts of the brain.

Petit mal

In this type of epilepsy, the person becomes **unconscious** suddenly without any warning. The unconsciousness lasts for a very short period of 3 to 30 seconds. Convulsions do not occur. However, the muscles of face show twitch like contractions and there is blinking of eyes. Afterwards, the person recovers automatically and becomes normal. The frequency of attack may be once in many months or many attacks may appear in rapid series. It usually occurs in late childhood and disappears completely at the age of 30 or above.

The EEG recording shows slow and large waves during the attack. Each wave is followed by a sharp spike. Delta waves appear in between the seizures.

Causes of petit mal are head injury, stroke, brain tumor and brain infection.

Psychomotor epilepsy

It is characterized by **emotional outbursts** such as abnormal rage, sudden anxiety, fear or discomfort. There is amnesia or a confused mental state for some period. Some persons have the tendency to attack others bodily or rub their own face vigorously. In most cases, the persons are not aware of their activities.

The EEG recordings show low frequency rectangular waves, ranging between 2 and 4 per second.

Causes of the psychomotor epilepsy are the abnormalities in temporal lobe and tumor in hypothalamus and other regions of limbic system such as amygdala and hippocampus.

2. Localized Epilepsy

Localized epilepsy or **Jacksonian epilepsy** is the epilepsy that occurs because of excess discharge of impulses from a **localized area of brain**.

Abnormality starts from a particular area and spreads to adjacent areas, developing slow-spreading muscular contractions. Contractions usually start in the mouth region and spread down towards the legs. Localized epilepsy is caused by brain tumor.

■ SLEEP

■ DEFINITION

Sleep is the natural state of rest for mind and body with closed eyes characterized by partial or complete **loss of consciousness**. Loss of consciousness leads to decreased response to external stimuli and decreased body movements.

Depth of sleep is not constant throughout the sleeping period and it varies in different stages of sleep.

■ SLEEP REQUIREMENT

Sleep requirement is not constant. Average sleep requirement per day at different age groups is:

Newborn infants	:	18 to 20 hours
Growing children	:	12 to 14 hours
Adults	:	7 to 9 hours
Old persons	:	5 to 7 hours

■ PHYSIOLOGICAL CHANGES DURING SLEEP

During sleep, most of the body functions are reduced to basal level. Important changes in the body during sleep are given below.

1. Plasma Volume

Plasma volume decreases by about 10% during sleep.

2. Cardiovascular System

Heart rate

During sleep, the heart rate reduces. It varies between 45 and 60 beats per minute.

Blood pressure

Systolic pressure falls to about 90 to 110 mm Hg. Lowest level is reached about 4th hour of sleep and remains at this level till a short time before waking up. Then, the pressure starts rising. If sleep is disturbed by exciting dreams, the pressure is elevated above 130 mm Hg.

3. Respiratory System

Rate and force of respiration are decreased. Respiration becomes irregular and **Cheyne-Stokes breathing** may develop.

4. Gastrointestinal Tract

Salivary secretion decreases during sleep. Gastric secretion is not altered or may be increased slightly. Contraction of empty stomach is more vigorous.

5. Excretory System

Formation of urine decreases and specific gravity of urine increases.

6. Sweat Secretion

Sweat secretion increases during sleep.

7. Lacrimal Secretion

Lacrimal secretion decreases during sleep.

8. Muscle Tone

Tone in all the muscles of body except ocular muscles decreases very much during sleep. It is called **sleep paralysis**.

9. Reflexes

Certain reflexes particularly knee jerk, are abolished. **Babinski sign** becomes positive during deep sleep. Threshold for most of the reflexes increases. Pupils are constricted. Light reflex is retained. Eyeballs move up and down.

10. Brain

Brain is not inactive during sleep. There is a characteristic cycle of brain wave activity during sleep with irregular intervals of dreams. Electrical activity in the brain varies with stages of sleep (see below).

■ TYPES OF SLEEP

Sleep is of two types:

1. Non-rapid eye movement sleep, NREM sleep or non-REM sleep.
2. Rapid eye movement sleep or REM sleep.

1. NREM Sleep

NREM sleep is the type of sleep without the movements of eyeballs. It is also called **slow wave sleep**. Dreams do not occur in this type of sleep and it occupies about 70 to 80% of total sleeping period. NREM sleep is followed by REM sleep.

2. REM Sleep

REM sleep is the type of sleep associated with **rapid conjugate movements** of the eyeballs which occurs frequently. Though the eyeballs move, the sleep is deep. So, it is also called **paradoxical sleep**. It occupies about 20 to 30% of sleeping period. Functionally, REM sleep is very important because, it plays an important role in consolidation of memory. Dreams occur during this period.

Differences between the two types of sleep are given in **Table 89.2**.

■ STAGES OF SLEEP AND EEG PATTERN

Generally, everybody passes through **five stages of sleep**, i.e. four stages of NREM sleep followed by REM sleep. All these stages occur periodically in cycles. One complete sleep cycle takes about 90 to 110 minutes. Usually, adults have 5 or 6 **sleep cycles** every night.

TABLE 89.2: REM sleep and NREM sleep.

Characteristics	REM sleep	Non-REM sleep
1. Rapid eye movement	Present	Absent
2. Dreams	Present	Absent
3. Muscle twitching	Present	Absent
4. Heart rate	Fluctuating	Stable
5. Blood pressure	Fluctuating	Stable
6. Respiration	Fluctuating	Stable
7. Body temperature	Fluctuating	Stable
8. Neurotransmitter	Noradrenaline	Serotonin

NREM Sleep

Stage 1: Stage of drowsiness

While feeling asleep and after going to bed, the person is in the **period of wakefulness**, i.e. while lying down, the eyes are closed and mind is relaxed. Then, the person proceeds to **drowsy state**. During drowsiness, the person can be awakened easily. Muscular activity slows down. Some persons may have feeling of falling followed by sudden muscular contractions. This period lasts for about 1 to 10 minutes.

EEC pattern in stage 1

During the stage of wakefulness, i.e. while lying down with closed eyes and relaxed mind, the **alpha waves** of EEG appear. Stage 1 of sleep is characterized by diminishing alpha waves and emerging **theta wave** activity in brain **(Fig. 89.2)**.

Stage 2: Stage of light sleep

When the person goes to **light sleep** from drowsiness, heart rate slows down and body temperature starts decreasing. Body prepares to go to deep sleep. This period lasts up to 20 minutes.

EEC pattern in stage 2

Theta wave continues in this stage also. In addition, theta waves are intermittently superimposed by **sleep spindles or spindle bursts** at a frequency of 14 per second. Sleep spindle is produced by electrical activity in thalamus and corticothalamic fibers.

During this stage of sleep, another type of wave called **K complex** also appears. It is a slow and large wave produced by the reaction to external stimuli while sleep.

Stage 3: Initial stage of deep sleep

Stage 3 is the **transitional period** between light sleep and deep sleep. Hence, it is considered as **initial stage of deep sleep**.

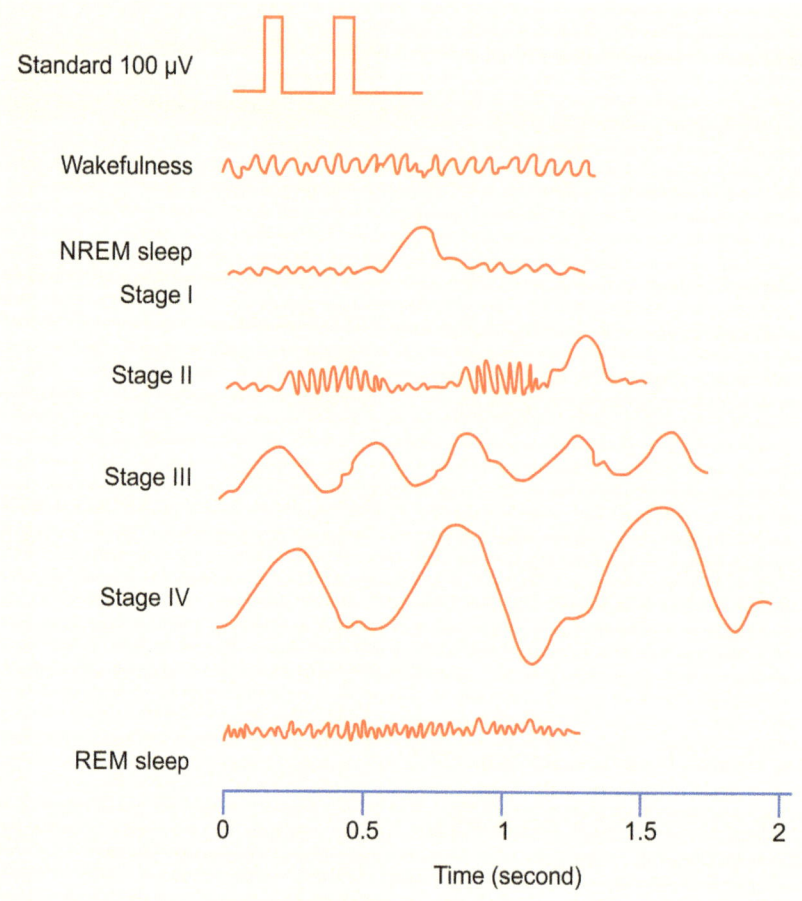

FIGURE 89.2: Electroencephalogram during wakefulness, different stages of NREM sleep and REM sleep.

EEC pattern in stage 3

During this stage, the spindle bursts and K complex disappear. Slow **delta waves** with high amplitude appear decreases to 1 or 2 per second and amplitude increases to about 100 µV.

Stage 4: Stage of deep sleep

Earlier, stages 3 and 4 were separated. But nowadays these two stages are combined together. When the person enters **deep sleep**, it is difficult to wake up. If someone wakes him or her up, there may be a feeling of disorientation for few minutes. In spite of having potential sleep disturbances such as noise, some persons may sleep without any reaction.

These stages of sleep help **rejuvenation of the body**. There is release of many vital hormones which induce growth and development. Immune system is boosted. Muscles and tissues are repaired. Body builds up energy for next day.

During this stage, children may have bedwetting, nightmares and sleepwalking. Even some adults may experience, nightmares and sleepwalking.

In most of the people, stages 3 and 4 together last for about 40 to 60 minutes.

EEC pattern in stage 4

During this stage, **delta waves** become more prominent with low frequency and high amplitude.

REM Sleep

Often, this is considered as **stage 5 of sleep**. During REM sleep, eyes move rapidly in all direction. Dreams occur. Muscles are relaxed or temporarily paralyzed. There is increase in heart rate and blood pressure. Respiration becomes rapid, shallow and irregular.

REM sleep during the first cycle of sleep lasts only for about 10 minutes. And the duration gradually increases in successive cycles and in final cycle it may last for about 1 hour.

EEC pattern in REM sleep

During REM sleep, electroencephalogram (EEG) shows irregular waves with high frequency and low amplitude. These waves are **desynchronized waves**.

■ SLEEP CENTERS

Sleep occurs due to the activity of some sleep inducing centers in brain. Complex pathways between the reticular formation of brainstem, diencephalon and cerebral cortex are involved in the onset and maintenance of sleep.

Brainstem has two centers which induce sleep:
1. Raphe nucleus.
2. Locus coeruleus

Inhibition of ascending reticular activating system also results in sleep.

1. Role of Raphe Nucleus

Raphe nucleus is situated in reticular formation of lower pons and medulla. Activation of this nucleus results in **NREM sleep**. It is due to release of **serotonin** by the nerve fibers arising from this nucleus. Serotonin induces NREM sleep.

2. Role of Locus Coeruleus

Locus coeruleus is situated in reticular formation of pons. Activation of this center produces **REM sleep**. **Noradrenaline** released by the nerve fibers arising from locus coeruleus induces REM sleep.

Inhibition of ascending reticular activating system

Ascending reticular activating system (ARAS) is responsible for **wakefulness** because of its afferent and efferent connections with cerebral cortex. Inhibition of ARAS induces sleep. Lesion of ARAS leads to coma.

■ APPLIED PHYSIOLOGY: COMMON SLEEP DISORDERS

1. Insomnia

Insomnia is the **inability to sleep** or abnormal wakefulness. It occurs due to systemic illness or mental conditions such as psychiatric problems, alcoholic addiction and drug addiction.

2. Hypersomnia

Hypersomnia is the **excess sleep** or excess need to sleep. It occurs because of lesion in floor of the third ventricle, brain tumors, encephalitis, chronic bronchitis and endocrine disorders such as myxedema and diabetes insipidus.

3. Somnambulism

Somnambulism or **sleep walking** is getting up from bed and walking in the state of sleep. The episode lasts for few minutes to half an hour.

4. Nocturnal Micturition

Nocturnal micturition or enuresis is the involuntary voiding of urine at bed. It is also called or **bedwetting**. It is common in children. Refer Chapter 40 for details.

Chapter 90: Higher Intellectual Functions

CHAPTER OUTLINE

- HIGHER INTELLECTUAL FUNCTIONS
- LEARNING
- MEMORY
- CONDITIONED REFLEXES
- SPEECH

HIGHER INTELLECTUAL FUNCTIONS

Higher intellectual functions are very essential to make up the human mind. Cerebral cortex is responsible for these functions. Important higher intellectual functions are learning, memory, conditioned reflexes and speech. Conditioned reflex forms the basis of all higher intellectual functions.

LEARNING

DEFINITION AND TYPES

Learning is defined as the process by which **new information** is acquired.

Learning is of two types:

1. Non-associative learning.
2. Associative learning.

1. Non-associative Learning

It involves response of a person to only one type of stimulus. It is based on two factors.

i. Habituation

Habituation means getting used to something to which a person is constantly exposed. When a person is exposed to a stimulus repeatedly, he starts ignoring the stimulus slowly. Finally, the person is habituated to the event and ignores it.

ii. Sensitization

Sensitization means a state in which the body becomes more sensitive to a stimulus. When a stimulus is applied repeatedly, habituation occurs. But if the same stimulus is combined with another type of stimulus, which may be pleasant or unpleasant, the person becomes more sensitive to the original stimulus.

For example, a woman gets habituated to different sounds around her and sleep is not disturbed by these sounds. However, she suddenly wakes up when her baby cries because she is sensitized to the crying sound of her baby.

2. Associative Learning

It involves learning about relations between two or more stimuli at a time. Classic example of associative learning is the conditioned reflex (see below).

MEMORY

DEFINITION AND TYPES

Memory is defined as the ability to recall the past experience. It is also defined as retention of learned materials.

Memory is classified by different methods:

Short-term Memories and Long-term Memories

Short-term or **recent memory** is the recalling of events that happened very recently, i.e. within hours or days. For example, telephone number that is known today may be remembered till tomorrow. If it is not recalled repeatedly, it may be forgotten on 3rd day.

Long-term or **remote memory** is the recalling of the events of weeks, months, years or sometimes lifetime. Examples are recalling 1st day of schooling, birthday celebration of previous year, picnic enjoyed last week, etc.

Explicit Memory and Implicit Memory

Explicit or **recognition memory** is defined as the memory that involves **conscious recollection** of past experience. It consists of memories regarding the events which occurred in the external world around us. The information stored may be about a particular event that happened at a particular time and place. Examples are recollection of a birthday party celebrated three days ago; the events taken place while taking breakfast, etc.

Explicit memory involves hippocampus and medial part of temporal lobe.

Implicit or **skilled memory** is defined as the memory in which past experience is utilized **without conscious awareness**. It helps to perform various skilled activities properly. For example, cycling, driving, playing tennis, dancing, typing, etc. are performed automatically without awareness.

Implicit memory involves the sensory and motor pathways.

■ PHYSIOLOGICAL BASIS OF MEMORY

Memory is stored in brain by the alteration of synaptic transmission between the neurons involved in memory. Storage of memory may be facilitated or habituated.

Facilitation

It is the process by which the memory storage is enhanced. It involves increase in synaptic transmission and increased postsynaptic activity.

Habituation

It is the process by which the memory storage is attenuated (attenuation means decrease in strength, effect or value). It involves reduction in synaptic transmission and slow stoppage of postsynaptic activity.

Basis for Short-term Memory

Basic mechanism of memory is the development of new neuronal circuits by the formation of new synapses and facilitation of synaptic transmission. Number of presynaptic terminals and the size of the terminals are also increased.

Basis for Long-term Memory

When the neuronal circuit is reinforced by constant activity, the memory is consolidated and encoded into different areas of the brain. This encoding makes memory a permanent or long-term memory.

Memory Encoding

Memory encoding occurs at synaptic level. Synapse for memory encoding is slightly different from other synapses. Two separate presynaptic terminals are present here. One of the terminal is **primary presynaptic terminal**, which ends on postsynaptic neuron as in conventional synapse. This terminal is called sensory terminal, because sensations are transmitted to the postsynaptic neuron through this terminal **(Fig. 90.1)**.

Another presynaptic terminal ends on the sensory terminal itself. This terminal is called **facilitator terminal**. When sensory terminal is stimulated alone without facilitator terminal, the firing from sensory terminal leads to habituation, i.e. the firing decreases slowly. On the other

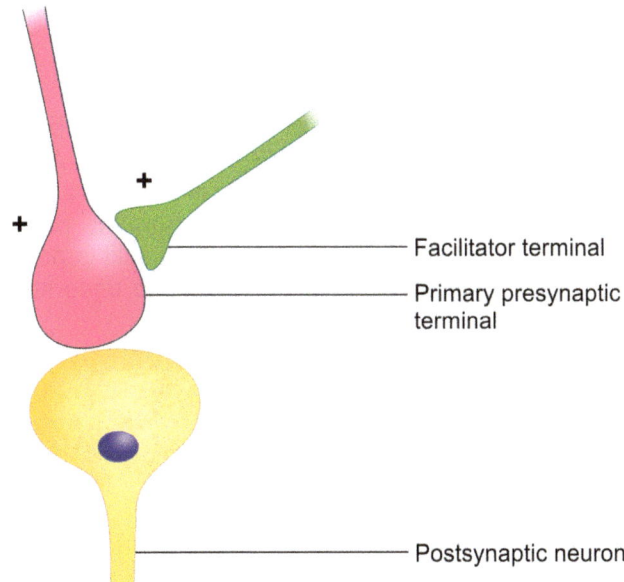

FIGURE 90.1: Synaptic terminal for memory encoding.

hand, if both the terminals are stimulated, facilitation occurs and the signals remain strong for long period, i.e. for few months to few years.

Sites of encoding

Hippocampus and the Papez circuit (the closed circuit between hippocampus, thalamus, hypothalamus and corpus striatum) are the main sites for **memory encoding**. Frontal and parietal areas are also involved in memory storage.

Consolidation of memory

Consolidation is the process by which a short-term memory is crystallized into a long-term memory.

■ APPLIED PHYSIOLOGY: ABNORMALITIES OF MEMORY

1. Amnesia

Amnesia is the loss of memory. It is classified into two types:

i. *Anterograde amnesia:* Failure to establish new memories after the onset of amnesia. It occurs because of lesion in hippocampus.

ii. *Retrograde amnesia:* Failure to recall past remote long-term memory. It occurs in temporal lobe syndrome.

2. Dementia

Dementia is the progressive deterioration of intellect, emotional control, social behavior and motivation associated with loss of memory. It is an age-related disorder that occurs above the age of 65 years. When it occurs before the age of 65, it is called **presenile dementia**.

Causes of dementia

Most common cause of dementia is **Alzheimer disease**. Other common causes of dementia are hydrocephalus, Parkinson disease, viral encephalitis, HIV infection, hypothyroidism, hypoparathyroidism, Cushing's syndrome, alcoholic intoxication, etc.

Features of dementia

Common features are loss of recent memory, lack of thinking and judgment and personality changes. As the disease progresses, psychiatric features begin to appear. Motor functions are also affected. Finally, the patient has to lead a vegetative life without any thinking power. The person is speechless and is unable to understand anything.

There is no effective treatment for this disorder. Physostigmine, which inhibits cholinesterase, causes moderate improvement.

3. Alzheimer Disease

Alzheimer disease is a progressive neurodegenerative disease. It is due to degeneration, loss of function and death of neurons in many parts of brain, particularly cerebral hemispheres, hippocampus and pons. There is reduction in the synthesis of most of the neurotransmitters.

CONDITIONED REFLEXES

DEFINITION AND TYPES

Conditioned reflex is the **acquired reflex** that requires learning, memory and recall of previous experience. It forms the basis of learning. Unconditioned reflex is the **inborn reflex** which does not require previous experience.

Conditioned reflexes are of two types:

A. Classical conditioned reflexes.
B. Instrumental conditioned reflexes.

Classical Conditioned Reflexes

Classical conditioned reflexes are those reflexes, which are established by a **conditioned stimulus** followed by an **unconditioned stimulus**.

Method of study: Pavlov's bell-dog experiments

Classical conditioned reflexes are demonstrated by the classical **bell-dog experiments** (salivary secretion experiments) done by **Ivan Pavlov** and his associates.

Types of classical conditioned reflexes

Classical conditioned reflexes are classified into two groups:

I. Positive or excitatory conditioned reflexes.
II. Negative conditioned reflexes.

I. Positive conditioned reflexes

Positive conditioned reflexes are of three types:

1. Primary conditioned reflex

It is the reflex developed with **one unconditioned stimulus** and **one conditioned stimulus**. The dog is fed with **food** (unconditioned stimulus). Simultaneously a **flash of light** (conditioned stimulus) is also shown. Both the stimuli are repeated for some days. After the development of reflex, the flash of light (conditioned stimulus) alone causes salivary secretion without food (unconditioned stimulus).

2. Secondary conditioned reflex

It is the reflex developed with **one unconditioned stimulus** and **two conditioned stimuli**. After establishment of a conditioned reflex with one conditioned stimulus, another conditioned stimulus is applied along with the first one. For example, the animal is fed with food (unconditioned reflex) and simultaneously a flash of light (first conditioned stimulus), and a **bell sound** (second conditioned stimulus) are applied. After the development of the reflex, the second conditioned stimulus, the bell sound alone can cause salivary secretion.

3. Tertiary conditioned reflex

In this reflex, a third conditioned stimulus is added and the reflex is established. But, the reflex with more than three conditioned stimuli is not possible.

II. Negative conditioned reflexes

In negative conditioned reflexes, the established conditioned reflexes are inhibited by some factors. For example, some disturbing factors such as sudden entrance of a stranger or sudden noise can abolish the conditioned reflex and inhibit salivary secretion.

Instrumental or Operant Conditioned Reflexes

Instrumental or operant conditioned reflexes are the reflexes in which the behavior of the person is instrumental. This type of reflexes is developed by the conditioned stimulus followed by a **reward** or **punishment**.

For example, if the animal is rewarded by a banana by pressing a bar, the animal repeatedly presses the bar. If the animal is given a tasty food along with electric shock, the animal starts avoiding that food.

Instrumental conditioned reflexes play an important role during the learning processes of a child. These conditioned reflexes are also responsible for **behavior pattern** of an individual.

SPEECH

DEFINITION

Speech is defined as the expression of thoughts by production of articulate sound, bearing a definite meaning. When a sound is produced verbally, it is called the **speech**. If it is expressed by visual symbols, it is known as **writing**.

MECHANISM OF SPEECH

Speech depends upon the coordinated activities of **central speech apparatus** and **peripheral speech apparatus**. The central speech apparatus consists of higher centers, i.e. the cortical and subcortical centers. The peripheral speech apparatus includes larynx or sound box, pharynx, mouth, nasal cavities, tongue and lips.

NERVOUS CONTROL OF SPEECH

Many parts of cortical and subcortical areas are involved in the mechanism of speech. Subcortical areas concerned with speech are controlled by cortical areas of dominant hemisphere.

Cortical areas concerned with speech:

I. Motor areas
II. Sensory areas
III. Wernicke's area

I. Motor Areas Concerned with Speech

1. Broca's area

Broca's area is also called **speech center**, motor speech area. It includes areas 44 and 45. These areas are situated in lower part of lateral surface of prefrontal cortex.

Broca's area controls the movements of structures (tongue, lips and larynx) involved in vocalization.

2. Upper frontal motor area

Upper frontal motor area is situated over the medial surface of cerebral hemisphere. It controls the coordinated movements involved in writing.

II. Sensory Areas Concerned with Speech

1. Secondary auditory area

Secondary auditory area or auditopsychic area includes area 22. It is situated in the superior temporal gyrus. It is concerned with the **interpretation of auditory sensation** and storage of memories of spoken words.

2. Secondary visual area

Secondary visual area or visuopsychic area includes area 18. It is present in angular gyrus of the parietal cortex. This area is concerned with the interpretation of visual sensation and storage of memories of the visual symbols.

III. Wernicke's Area

Wernicke's area is situated in the upper part of temporal lobe. This area is responsible for the **interpretation of auditory sensation.** It also plays an important role in speech. It is responsible for understanding the auditory information about any word and sending the information to Broca's area.

APPLIED PHYSIOLOGY: DISORDERS OF SPEECH

1. Aphasia

Aphasia is the loss or **impairment of speech**. It is due to damage of speech centers which occurs during stroke, head injury, cerebral tumors, brain infections and degenerative disease such as Parkinson disease.

Head's classification of aphasia

Henry Head has classified aphasia into four types:

i. *Verbal aphasia:* Disability in the formation of words.
ii. *Syntactical aphasia:* Inability to arrange words in proper sequence.
iii. *Semantic aphasia:* Inability to recognize the significance of words.
iv. *Nominal aphasia:* Difficulty in naming the object due to failure in recognizing the meaning of words.

2. Dysarthria or Anarthria

Dysarthria or anarthria is the difficulty or **inability to speak** because of paralysis of muscles involved in articulation. The spoken and written words are understood. It is caused by damage of brain areas or the nerves that control muscles involved in speech. It occurs in conditions like stroke, brain injury and degenerative disease.

3. Dysphonia

Dysphonia is a voice disorder characterized by **hoarseness** and a sore or **dry throat**. Hoarseness means the difficulty in producing sound while trying to speak or a change in the pitch or loudness of voice. It occurs due to diseases of vocal cords or larynx.

4. Stammering

Stammering or shuttering is a speech disorder in which the normal flow of speech is disturbed by repetitions or stoppage of sound and words. It is associated with some unusual facial and body movements. Stammering is due to genetic factors, brain damage, neurological disorders or anxiety.

Chapter 91: Cerebrospinal Fluid

CHAPTER OUTLINE

- DEFINITION
- PROPERTIES AND COMPOSITION
- FORMATION
- CIRCULATION
- ABSORPTION
- PRESSURE EXERTED BY CSF
- FUNCTIONS
- COLLECTION
- BLOOD-BRAIN BARRIER
- BLOOD-CEREBROSPINAL FLUID BARRIER
- APPLIED PHYSIOLOGY: HYDROCEPHALUS

DEFINITION

Cerebrospinal fluid (CSF) is the clear, colorless and transparent fluid that circulates through **ventricles of brain**, **subarachnoid space** and **central canal** of spinal cord. It is a **part of ECF**.

PROPERTIES AND COMPOSITION OF CSF

Properties

Volume : 150 mL
Rate of formation : 0.3 mL per minute
Specific gravity : 1.005
Reaction : Alkaline.

Composition

Composition of CSF is given in **Figure 91.1**. CSF is a part of ECF and contains more amount of sodium than potassium. It also contains some lymphocytes. CSF secreted by ventricle does not contain any cell. Lymphocytes are added when CSF flows in the spinal cord.

FORMATION OF CSF

CSF is secreted by **choroid plexuses** which are formed by tuft of capillaries in the ventricles of brain. Secretion of CSF involves active transport.

CIRCULATION OF CSF

Major quantity of CSF is formed in the **lateral ventricles** and passes through the **foramen of Monro** into the **third ventricle (Figs. 91.2 and 91.3)**. From here, it passes to the **fourth ventricle** through **aqueductus Sylvius**. From fourth ventricle, CSF enters into the cisterna magna and cisterna lateralis through **foramen of Magendie** (central opening) and **foramen of Luschka** (lateral opening).

From **cisterna magna** and **cisterna lateralis**, CSF circulates through **subarachnoid space** over spinal cord

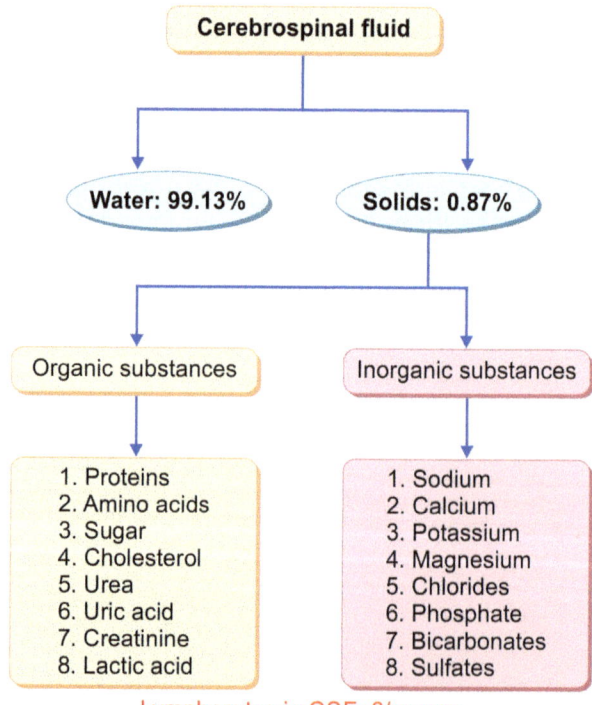

Lymphocytes in CSF: 6/cu mm

FIGURE 91.1: Composition of cerebrospinal fluid.

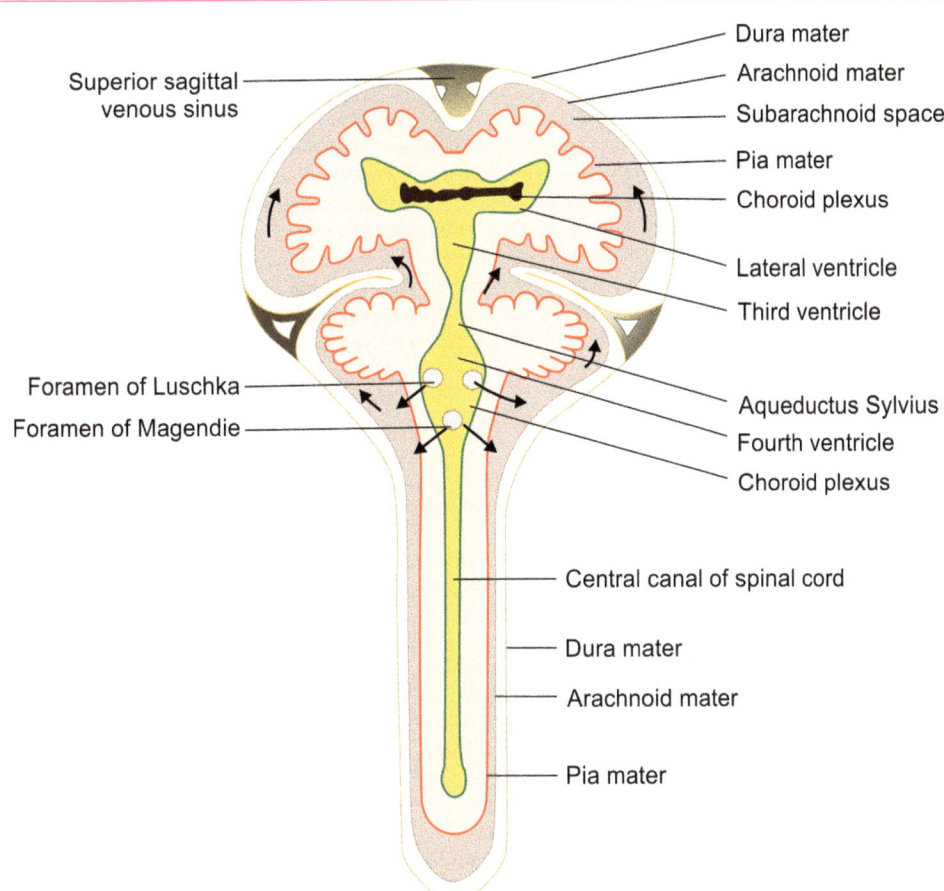

FIGURE 91.2: Circulation of cerebrospinal fluid.

and cerebral hemispheres. It also flows into **central canal** of spinal cord.

ABSORPTION OF CSF

CSF is absorbed by the **arachnoid villi** into **dural sinuses** and **spinal veins**. Small amount is absorbed into cervical lymphatics and perivascular spaces also. The mechanism of absorption is by **filtration**.

Normally, about 500 mL of CSF is formed every day and an equal amount is absorbed.

PRESSURE EXERTED BY CSF

Pressure exerted by CSF varies in different position, viz.:

Lateral recumbent position = 10 to 18 cm of H_2O
Lying position = 13 cm of H_2O
Sitting position = 30 cm of H_2O

Certain events like coughing, crying and compression of internal jugular vein increase the pressure.

FUNCTIONS OF CSF
PROTECTIVE FUNCTION

CSF acts as **fluid buffer** and protects the brain from **shock**. Since, the specific gravity of brain and CSF is more or less same, brain floats in CSF. When head receives a blow, CSF acts like a cushion and prevents the movement of brain against the skull bone and thereby prevents the damage of brain.

But severe blow affecting brain results in countercoup injury.

Contrecoup Injury

Contrecoup injury is the injury to brain, in which the damage is on the side opposite to the side on which head receives a severe blow.

When the head receives a severe blow, the brain moves forcefully and hits against the skull bone, leading to damage of brain tissues. Brain strikes against the skull bone at a point opposite to the point where the blow was applied. Hence the name contrecoup injury.

REGULATION OF CRANIAL CONTENT VOLUME

Regulation of cranial content volume is essential because, brain may be affected if the volume of cranial content increases. It happens in cerebral hemorrhage and brain tumors.

Increase in cranial content volume is prevented by greater absorption of CSF to give space for the increasing cranial contents.

MEDIUM OF EXCHANGE

CSF is the medium through which many substances, particularly the nutritive substances and waste materials are exchanged between blood and brain tissues.

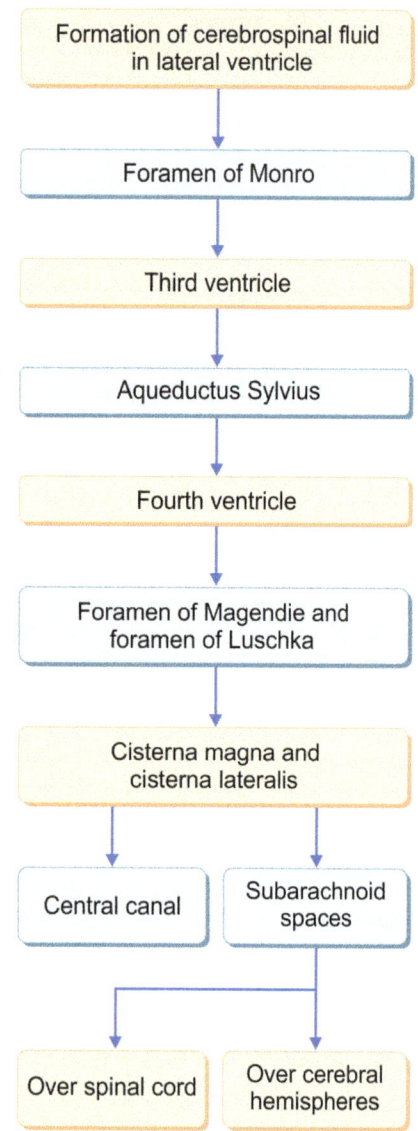

FIGURE 91.3: Schematic diagram of CSF circulation.

BOX 91.1: Substances which pass and substances which cannot pass through blood-brain barrier.

Substances which can pass through blood-brain barrier
1. Oxygen
2. Carbon dioxide
3. Water
4. Glucose
5. Amino acids
6. Electrolytes
7. Drugs such as L-dopa, 5-HT, sulfonamides, tetracycline and many lipid-soluble drugs
8. Lipid-soluble anesthetic gases such as ether and nitrous oxide
9. Other lipid-soluble substances
Substances which cannot pass through blood-brain barrier
1. Injurious chemical agents
2. Pathogens such as bacteria
3. Drugs such as penicillin and the catecholamines
4. Dopamine (so, parkinsonism is treated with L-dopa, instead of dopamine)
5. Bile pigments
However, since the barrier is not well developed in infants, the bile pigments enter the brain tissues. During jaundice due to erythroblastosis fetalis in infants, the bile pigments enter brain and causes damage of basal ganglia, leading to kernicterus (Chapter 16)

COLLECTION OF CSF

CSF is collected either by **cisternal puncture** or **lumbar puncture**. In cisternal puncture, the CSF is collected by passing a needle between the occipital bone and atlas, so that it enters the cisterna magna. In lumbar puncture, the lumbar puncture needle is introduced into the subarachnoid space in the lumbar region, between third and fourth lumbar spines.

BLOOD-BRAIN BARRIER

Blood-brain barrier (BBB) is a **neuroprotective structure** that prevents the entry of many substances and pathogens from blood into the brain tissues. Barrier exists in the capillary membrane of all parts of the brain except in some areas of hypothalamus.

BBB is formed by **tight junctions** in the endothelial cells of the brain capillaries. The cytoplasmic foot processes of **astrocytes** (neuroglial cells) develop around the capillaries and reinforce the barrier.

FUNCTIONS OF BLOOD-BRAIN BARRIER

1. BBB acts as a mechanical barrier and prevents harmful chemical substances from entering brain.
2. BBB provides a healthy environment for brain tissues by preventing injurious materials and organisms.
3. BBB permits metabolic and essential materials into the brain tissues.

Substances which can pass through blood-brain barrier and the substances which cannot pass through blood-brain barrier are listed in **Box 91.1**.

BLOOD-CEREBROSPINAL FLUID BARRIER

It is the barrier between the blood and cerebrospinal fluid that exists at the **choroid plexus**. The function of this barrier is similar to that of the BBB. It does not allow the movement of many substances from blood to cerebrospinal fluid. It allows the movement of only those substances, which are allowed by BBB.

APPLIED PHYSIOLOGY: HYDROCEPHALUS

Hydrocephalus is the **abnormal accumulation of CSF** in brain, associated with **enlargement of head**.

Types and Causes of Hydrocephalus

1. *Internal hydrocephalus or non-communicating hydrocephalus*

Internal hydrocephalus is the accumulation of CSF in **ventricles** of brain caused by **blockage of cerebral aqueduct**. It causes dilatation of ventricles resulting in enlargement of head and cortical atrophy.

2. External hydrocephalus or communicating hydrocephalus

External hydrocephalus is the accumulation of CSF in **subarachnoid space**. There is dilatation of ventricles and widening of subarachnoid space resulting in enlargement of head. It is due to **blockage of arachnoid villi**.

Features of Hydrocephalus

Hydrocephalus along with increased intracranial pressure causes headache and vomiting. In severe conditions, it leads to atrophy of brain, mental weakness and convulsions.

Chapter 92: Autonomic Nervous System

CHAPTER OUTLINE

- AUTONOMIC NERVOUS SYSTEM
- SYMPATHETIC DIVISION
- PARASYMPATHETIC DIVISION
- FUNCTIONS
- NEUROTRANSMITTERS
- SYMPATHOMIMETIC DRUGS
- SYMPATHETIC BLOCKERS
- PARASYMPATHOMIMETIC DRUGS
- PARASYMPATHETIC BLOCKERS
- GANGLIONIC BLOCKERS

AUTONOMIC NERVOUS SYSTEM

Autonomic nervous system (ANS) is a part of **peripheral nervous system** which is concerned with regulation of visceral or vegetative functions of the body. So, it is also called **vegetative** or **involuntary nervous system**.

DIVISIONS OF ANS

Autonomic nervous system is divided into two divisions:
1. Sympathetic division.
2. Parasympathetic division.

Differences between both the divisions of ANS are given in **Table 92.1**.

SYMPATHETIC DIVISION

It is otherwise called **thoracolumbar outflow** because, the **preganglionic neurons** are situated in lateral gray horns of 12 thoracic segments and first two lumbar segments of spinal cord. Fibers arising from here are called **preganglionic fibers**. Preganglionic fibers leave the spinal cord through anterior nerve root and white rami communicants, and terminate in the postganglionic neurons, which are situated in the **sympathetic ganglia**.

Sympathetic division supplies smooth muscle fibers of all the visceral organs such as blood vessels, heart, lungs, glands, gastrointestinal organs, etc.

SYMPATHETIC GANGLIA

Ganglia of sympathetic division are classified into three groups:
   I. Paravertebral or sympathetic chain ganglia.
   II. Prevertebral or collateral ganglia.
   III. Terminal or peripheral ganglia.

I. *Paravertebral or Sympathetic Chain Ganglia*

Paravertebral or sympathetic chain ganglia are present on either side of vertebral column. These ganglia are connected with each other by longitudinal fibers to form the sympathetic chains **(Fig. 92.1)**. Both the chains extend from skull to coccyx.

Ganglia of the sympathetic chain (trunk) on each side are divided into four groups.

1. Cervical ganglia : 8 in number
2. Thoracic ganglia : 12 in number
3. Lumbar ganglia : 5 in number
4. Sacral ganglia : 5 in number

II. *Prevertebral or Collateral Ganglia*

Prevertebral ganglia are situated in thorax, abdomen and pelvis in relation to aorta and its branches.

Prevertebral ganglia are:

1. Celiac ganglion.
2. Superior mesenteric ganglion.
3. Inferior mesenteric ganglion.

Prevertebral ganglia receive preganglionic fibers from T5 to L2 segments. The postganglionic fibers from these ganglia supply the visceral organs of thorax, abdomen and pelvis.

III. *Terminal or Peripheral Ganglia*

Terminal ganglia are situated within or close to structures innervated by them. Heart, bronchi, pancreas and urinary bladder are innervated by the terminal ganglia.

TABLE 92.1: Actions of sympathetic and parasympathetic divisions of ANS.

Effector organ		Sympathetic division	Parasympathetic division
1. Eye	Ciliary muscle	Relaxation	Contraction
	Pupil	Dilatation	Constriction
2. Lacrimal glands		Decrease in secretion	Increase in secretion
3. Salivary glands		Secretion of thick saliva and Vasoconstriction	Secretion of watery saliva and Vasodilatation
4. Gastrointestinal tract	Motility	Inhibition	Acceleration
	Secretion	Decrease	Increase
	Sphincters	Constriction	Relaxation
	Smooth muscles	Relaxation	Contraction
5. Gallbladder		Relaxation	Contraction
6. Urinary bladder	Detrusor muscle	Relaxation	Contraction
	Internal sphincter	Constriction	Relaxation
7. Sweat glands		Increase in secretion	–
8. Heart: Rate and force		Increase	Decrease
9. Blood vessels		Constriction of all blood vessels, except those in heart and skeletal muscle	Dilatation
10. Bronchioles		Dilatation	Constriction

Sympathoadrenergic System

Sympathoadrenergic system is a functional and phylogenetic unit that includes sympathetic division and adrenal medulla. Adrenal medulla is a modified sympathetic ganglion.

■ PARASYMPATHETIC DIVISION

Parasympathetic division of ANS is otherwise called **craniosacral outflow** because, the fibers of this division arise from brainstem and sacral segments of spinal cord. Cranial portion of parasympathetic division innervates the blood vessels of the head and neck, and many thoracoabdominal visceral organs.

Sacral portion of parasympathetic division innervates the smooth muscles forming the walls of viscera and the glands such as large intestine, liver, spleen, kidneys, bladder, genitalia, etc.

■ CRANIAL OUTFLOW

Cranial outflow or cranial portion of parasympathetic division arises from brainstem. It innervates the blood vessels of head and neck, and many thoracoabdominal visceral organs.

Cranial outflow includes the following cranial nerves:

1. Oculomotor nerve (III cranial nerve).
2. Facial nerve (VII cranial nerve).
3. Glossopharyngeal nerve (IX cranial nerve).
4. Vagus nerve (X cranial nerve).

Preganglionic fibers of these cranial nerves arise from neurons situated at two different levels:

1. Tectal or **midbrain outflow** (III cranial nerve).
2. Bulbar level or **bulbar outflow** (VII, IX and X cranial nerves).

Preganglionic fibers are longer and reach the postganglionic neurons, which are situated within the organs or close to the organs innervated by these nerves. Preganglionic fibers are myelinated, but the postganglionic fibers are nonmyelinated.

■ SACRAL OUTFLOW OR SACRAL PORTION OF PARASYMPATHETIC DIVISION

Sacral outflow or sacral portion of parasympathetic division arises from the sacral segments of spinal cord. It innervates smooth muscles forming the walls of viscera and the glands such as large intestine, liver, spleen, kidneys, bladder, genitalia, etc.

Preganglionic fibers arise from anterior gray horn cells of 2nd, 3rd and 4th sacral segments (from 1st also in some cases) of spinal cord and form the **pelvic nerve** (nervi erigens). Fibers end on postganglionic neurons, which are situated on or near the visceral organs. Fibers from postganglionic neurons supply descending colon, rectum, urinary bladder, internal sphincter, urethra and accessory sex organs.

Sacral parasympathetic fibers supply those visceral organs which are not supplied by **vagus**.

■ FUNCTIONS OF ANS

Autonomic nervous system is concerned with regulation of **vegetative functions**, which are beyond voluntary control. By controlling the various vegetative functions, ANS plays

470 Section 10: Nervous System

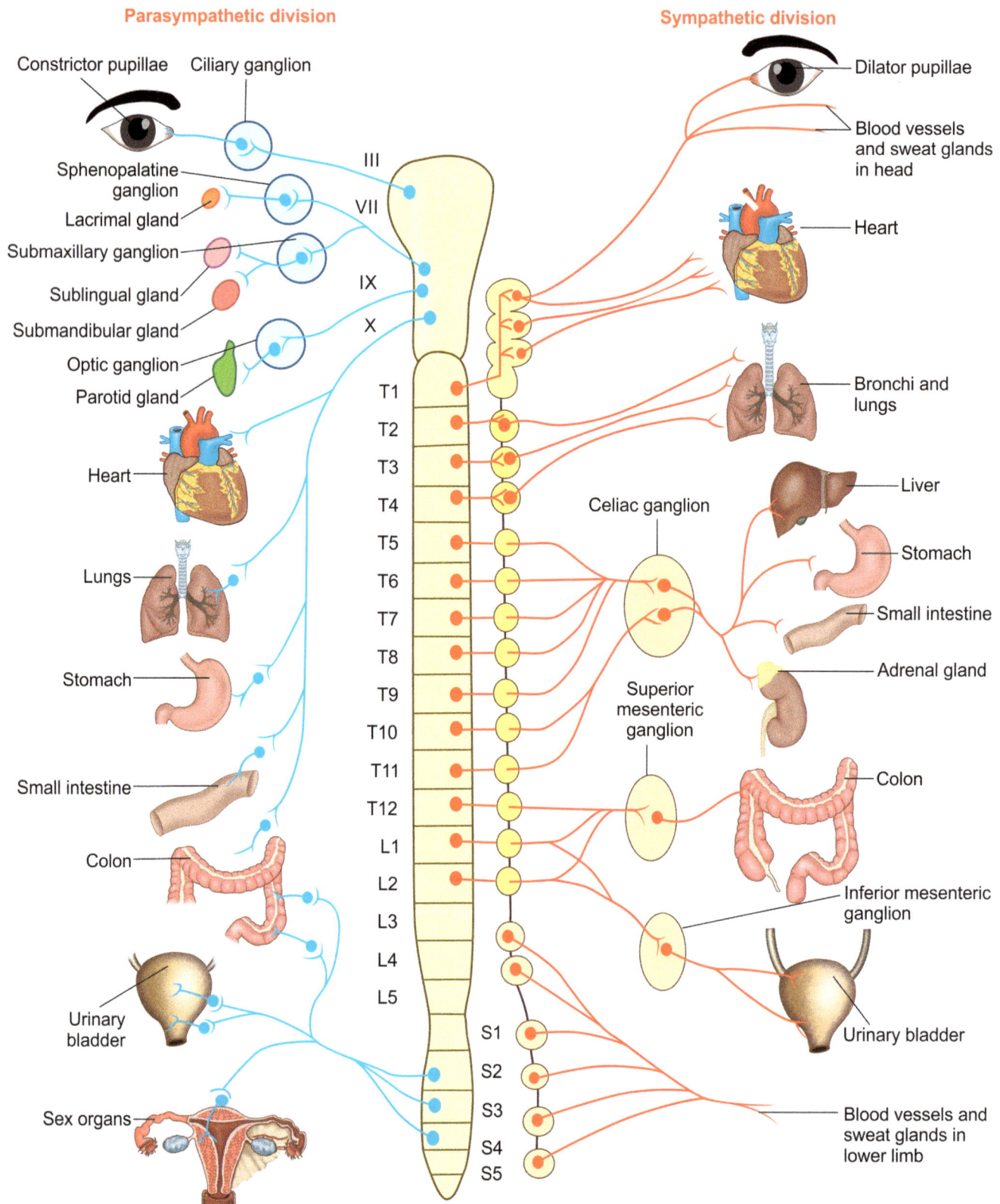

FIGURE 92.1: Autonomic nervous system.

an important role in maintaining homeostasis (constant internal environment).

Almost all the visceral organs are supplied by both sympathetic and parasympathetic divisions of ANS, and the two divisions produce antagonistic effects on each organ. When the fibers of one division supplying to an organ is sectioned or affected by lesion, the effects of fibers from other division on the organ become more prominent.

Actions of the sympathetic and parasympathetic fibers on various structures are given in **Table 92.1**.

Chapter 92: Autonomic Nervous System

■ NEUROTRANSMITTERS OF ANS

Different nerve fibers of ANS execute the functions by releasing some neurotransmitter substances.

■ SYMPATHETIC FIBERS

Neurotransmitters Released by Sympathetic Fibers:

1. Preganglionic fibers : Acetylcholine
2. Postganglionic sympathetic noradrenergic fibers : Noradrenaline.
3. Postganglionic sympathetic cholinergic fibers : Acetylcholine.

Postganglionic sympathetic cholinergic nerve fibers supply sweat glands and blood vessels in heart and skeletal muscle.

■ PARASYMPATHETIC FIBERS

Neurotransmitters Released by Parasympathetic Fibers:

1. Preganglionic fibers : Acetylcholine.
2. Postganglionic fibers : Acetylcholine.

■ SYMPATHOMIMETIC DRUGS

Sympathomimetic drugs or **adrenaline-like** drugs are the drugs, which produce the effects of sympathetic stimulation. Adrenaline and noradrenaline produced in the body act only for a short duration of about 1 to 2 minutes. Whereas, sympathomimetic drugs injected intravenously act for a longer period of about 30 minutes to 2 hours. Examples of sympathomimetic drugs phenylephrine, isoproterenol and albuterol.

■ SYMPATHETIC BLOCKERS

Sympathetic blockers are the drugs that prevent actions of sympathetic neurotransmitter. Sympathetic blockers act on all levels. Examples are reserpine and quanethidine.

■ PARASYMPATHOMIMETIC DRUGS

Parasympathomimetic drugs or acetylcholine (ACh) like drugs are drugs, which produce the effects of parasympathetic stimulation. ACh produced in the body acts only for a short period, whereas the injected ACh acts for a long time. Similarly, parasympathomimetic drugs also exhibit their actions for a longer time.

Parasympathomimetic drugs are as follows:

1. Drugs which Act on Muscarinic Receptors

Pilocarpine and methacholine produce their effects by acting on the muscarinic receptors.

2. Drugs which Prolong the Action of ACh

Action of ACh can be prolonged by preventing its destruction. Drugs like **neostigmine** and **physostigmine** inhibit the activity of acetylcholinesterase and so the ACh is not destroyed quickly.

■ PARASYMPATHETIC BLOCKERS

Parasympathetic blockers are drugs, which prevent the actions of parasympathetic neurotransmitter. Drugs **atropine**, **homatropine** and **scopolamine** inhibit the actions of ACh by blocking the muscarinic receptors.

■ GANGLIONIC BLOCKERS

Ganglionic blockers are the drugs that prevent the transmission of impulses from preganglionic neurons to postganglionic neurons. **Tetraethylammonium ion**, **hexamethonium ion** and **pentolinium** are some of the ganglionic blockers. These drugs block both sympathetic and parasympathetic ganglia. However, ganglionic blockers are commonly used to block sympathetic ganglia, rather than the parasympathetic ganglia because sympathetic blockade overshadows the parasympathetic blockade.

MODEL QUESTIONS IN NERVOUS SYSTEM

■ LONG QUESTIONS

1. What is neuron? Describe the structure of neuron and the properties of nerve fibers.
2. What are receptors? Classify them and explain their properties.
3. What is synapse? Explain the structure, functions and properties of synapse.
4. Define and classify reflex action. Explain reflex arc and the properties of reflexes.
5. Name the ascending tracts of the spinal cord and explain spinothalamic tracts.
6. What are the tracts of spinal cord? Describe the spinocerebellar tracts.
7. Give an account of tracts in the posterior white funiculus of spinal cord.
8. Enumerate the descending tracts of spinal cord. Describe in detail the pyramidal tracts. Write a note on the effects of upper and lower motor neuron lesions.
9. What are the thalamic nuclei? Describe the functions and effects of lesions of thalamus.
10. Name the hypothalamic nuclei. Explain the functions and effects of lesions of hypothalamus.
11. What are the different divisions of cerebellum? Explain the functions of each division. Add a note on cerebellar lesions.
12. What are the components of basal ganglia? Give an account of functions and disorders of basal ganglia.
13. Name lobes of cerebral cortex? Describe the functions of each lobe. Add a note on frontal lobe syndrome.
14. Describe the receptor organ in vestibular apparatus and explain role of vestibular apparatus in maintenance of equilibrium.
15. Explain divisions and functions of autonomic nervous system. Add a note on neurotransmitters of autonomic nervous system.

■ SHORT QUESTIONS

1. Structure of neuron.
2. Classification of nerve fibers.
3. Properties of nerve fibers.
4. Saltatory conduction.
5. Wallerian degeneration.
6. Neuroglia.
7. Cutaneous receptors.
8. Generator (receptor) potential.
9. Synaptic transmission.
10. Reflex arc.
11. Properties of reflexes.
12. Superficial reflexes.
13. Deep reflexes.
14. Upper/Lower motor neuron lesion.
15. Pathway for fine touch sensations.
16. Pathway for pressure sensation.
17. Pathway for temperature sensations.
18. Pathway for pain sensations.
19. Functions of thalamus.
20. Thalamic syndrome.
21. Regulation of food intake.
22. Disorders of hypothalamus.
23. Corticocerebellum (neocerebellum).
24. Spinocerebellum (paleocerebellum).
25. Vestibulocerebellum
26. Functions of basal ganglia.
27. Parkinsonism.
28. Frontal lobe of cerebral cortex.
29. Parietal lobe (or sensory areas) of cerebral cortex.
30. Functions of limbic system.
31. Muscle spindle.
32. Muscle tone
33. Righting reflexes.
34. Semicircular canal.
35. Otolith organ.
36. Motion sickness.
37. EEG.
38. EEG pattern during sleep.
39. Learning.
40. Memory.
41. Conditioned reflexes.
42. Speech.
43. CSF.
44. Functions of sympathetic division of ANS.
45. Functions of parasympathetic division of ANS.

■ VERY SHORT ANSWER QUESTIONS

1. Parts of brain.
2. Classification of neuron.
3. Myelin sheath.
4. Neurilemma and Schwann cells.
5. Myelinogenesis.
6. Nerve growth factor.
7. Action potential in nerve fiber.
8. Conduction through myelinated nerve fiber/saltatory conduction.
9. Degrees of injury to nerve fiber/Sunderland's classification.
10. Classify receptors on the basis of adaptation. Give examples.
11. Müller law.
12. Sensory transduction.
13. Classification of synapse.

14. Synaptic delay.
15. Functions of synapse.
16. Inhibitory postsynaptic potential.
17. Bell-Magendie law.
18. Reflex arc.
19. Babinski reflex.
20. Segments of spinal cord and spinal nerves.
21. Types of neuron present in gray matter of spinal cord.
22. Classify tracts of fibers in spinal cord.
23. Functions of ascending tracs situated in posterior white column of spinal cord.
24. Disk prolapse.
25. Types of somatic sensations.
26. Combined or synthetic sensations.
27. Paralysis.
28. Rage and sham rage.
29. Timing and programming the skilled movements.
30. Servomechanism.
31. Automatic associated movements.
32. Components of basal ganglia.
33. Crista ampullaris/macula.
34. Nystagmus/vestibulo-ocular reflex.
35. Labyrinthectomy.
36. Alpha block.
37. Differences between REM sleep and Non-REM sleep.
38. Definition of epilepsy, convulsion, convulsive seizures and epileptic.
39. Short-term and long-term memories/explicit and implicit memories/sensory, primary and secondary memories.
40. Amnesia and dementia.
41. Alzheimer's disease.
42. Head's classification of aphasia.
43. Blood-CSF barrier.
44. Hydrocephalus.
45. Neurotransmitters of ANS.
46. Sympathomimetic drugs.
47. Sympathetic blockers.
48. Parasympathomimetic drugs.
49. Parasympathetic blockers.
50. Ganglionic blockers.

SECTION 11 SPECIAL SENSES

CHAPTER 93

Eye

CHAPTER OUTLINE

- SPECIAL SENSES
- FUNCTIONAL ANATOMY OF THE EYEBALL
- WALL OF THE EYEBALL
- FUNDUS OCULI
- INTRAOCULAR FLUID
- INTRAOCULAR PRESSURE
- LENS
- OCULAR MUSCLES
- OCULAR MOVEMENTS
- APPLIED PHYSIOLOGY

SPECIAL SENSES

Special senses or **special sensations** are the complex sensations which involve **specialized sense organs**. Special sensations are different from somatic sensations that arise from skin, muscles, tendons and joints (Chapter 82).

Special senses are:

1. Sensation of vision.
2. Sensation of hearing.
3. Sensation of taste.
4. Sensation of smell.

FUNCTIONAL ANATOMY OF THE EYEBALL

MORPHOLOGY

Human **eyeball** (**bulbus oculi**) is made up of two segments, an anterior part and a posterior part.

Anterior part is small and forms one-sixth of the eyeball. Posterior part is larger and forms five-sixth of the eyeball. Posterior wall of this part is lined by the light-sensitive structure called **retina**.

Center of anterior curvature of the eyeball is called the **anterior pole**, and the center of posterior curvature is called the **posterior pole**. A line joining the two poles is called **optic axis**. And, another line joining a point in cornea little medial to anterior pole and the fovea centralis situated lateral to posterior pole is known as **visual axis**. Light rays pass through the visual axis of eyeball **(Fig. 93.1)**.

ORBITAL CAVITY

Except anterior one-sixth, the eyeball is situated in the bony **orbital cavity** or eye socket. A thick layer of areolar tissue is interposed between the bone and the eye. It serves as a cushion to protect the eyeball from external force. Eyeballs are attached to **orbital cavity** by **ocular muscles**.

EYELIDS

Eyelids protect the eyeball from foreign particles coming in contact with its surface and cutoff the light during sleep. Eyelids are opened and closed voluntarily as well as by reflex. Margins of eyelids have hairs called the **cilia**. Opening between the two eyelids is called **palpebral fissure**.

CONJUNCTIVA

It is a thin **mucous membrane**, which covers the exposed part of the eye. After covering the anterior surface, conjunctiva is reflected into the inner surfaces of eyelids. The part of conjunctiva covering the eyeball is called the **bulbar portion**. The part covering the eyelid is called the **palpebral portion**.

LACRIMAL GLAND AND TEAR

Lacrimal gland is situated in the shelter of bone, forming the upper and outer border of wall of the eye socket. From the lacrimal gland, **tear** flows over the surface of conjunctiva and drains into nose via lacrimal ducts, lacrimal sac and nasolacrimal duct.

Tear

Tear is a hypertonic fluid. Due to its continuous washing and lubrication, the conjunctiva is kept moist and is protected from infection. Tear also contains the enzyme

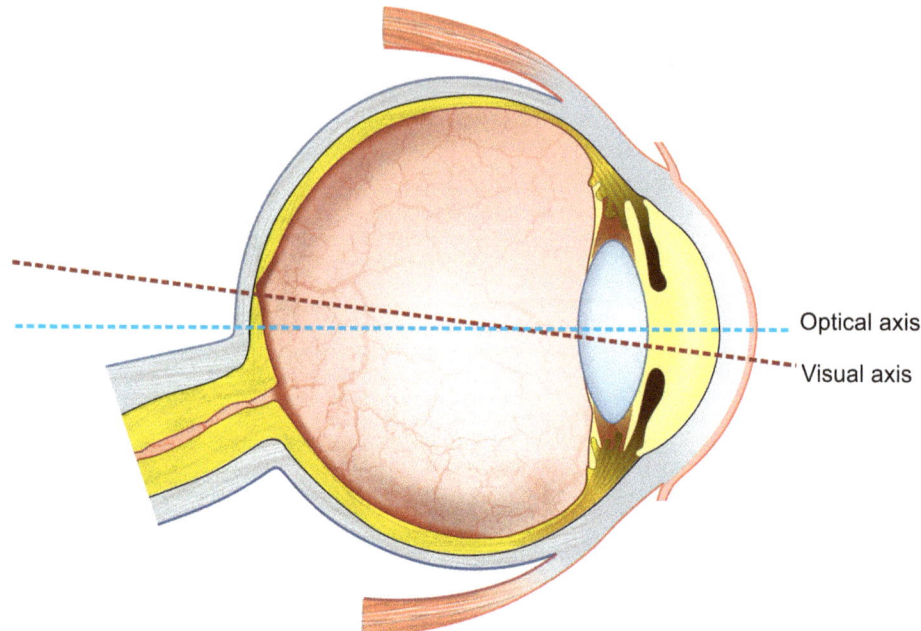

FIGURE 93.1: Optical and visual axis.

lysozyme that kills bacteria. Secretion of tears is controlled by the parasympathetic fibers of facial nerve.

WALL OF THE EYEBALL

Wall of the eyeball is composed of three layers:

I. Outer layer, which includes cornea and sclera.
II. Middle layer, which includes choroid, ciliary body and iris.
III. Inner layer, the retina.

OUTER LAYER OR TUNICA EXTERNA OR TUNICA FIBROSA

Anterior one-sixth of this layer is transparent and is known as **cornea**. It covers the **iris** and **pupil**. It is continuous with the sclera. Posterior five-sixth of this coat is tough, fibrous and opaque and it is called the **sclera**.

MIDDLE LAYER OR TUNICA MEDIA OR TUNICA VASCULOSA

This layer surrounds the eyeball completely except for a small opening in front known as the pupil.

Middle layer has three structures:

1. Choroid.
2. Ciliary body.
3. Iris.

1. Choroid

Choroid is the thin vascular layer of eyeball situated between sclera and retina. It forms posterior five-sixth of middle layer. Choroid is extended anteriorly up to the insertion of ciliary muscle (the level of **ora serrata**). Choroid is composed of a capillary plexus, numerous small arteries and veins.

2. Ciliary Body

Ciliary body is the thickened anterior part of middle layer of eye situated between choroid and iris. It is situated in front of ora serrata.

Ciliary body is in the form of a ring. Its outer surface is separated from the sclera by perichoroidal space. Inner surface of the ciliary body faces the vitreous body and lens. The **suspensory ligaments** from the lens are attached to ciliary body. Anterior surface of ciliary body faces towards the center of cornea. From this surface, the iris arises **(Fig. 93.2)**.

Ciliary body has three parts:

i. Orbiculus ciliaris.
ii. Ciliary body proper.
iii. Ciliary processes.

3. Iris

Iris is the thin curtain-like structure of eyeball. It forms the anterior most part of middle layer **(Fig. 93.3)**. It is like a thin **circular diaphragm**, placed in front of the lens. It has a circular opening in the center called **pupil**.

Iris is a muscular structure and has two muscles:

i. **Constrictor papillae** or sphincter pupillae: Contraction of this muscle causes constriction of pupil.
ii. **Dilator papillae** or pupillary dilator muscle: Contraction of this muscle causes dilatation of pupil.

Iris acts like the diaphragm of a camera. Iris separates the space between cornea and lens into two chambers namely, the anterior and posterior chambers. Both the chambers communicate with each other through **pupil**. The lateral border of anterior chamber is angular in shape. It is called **iris angle** or angle of anterior chamber.

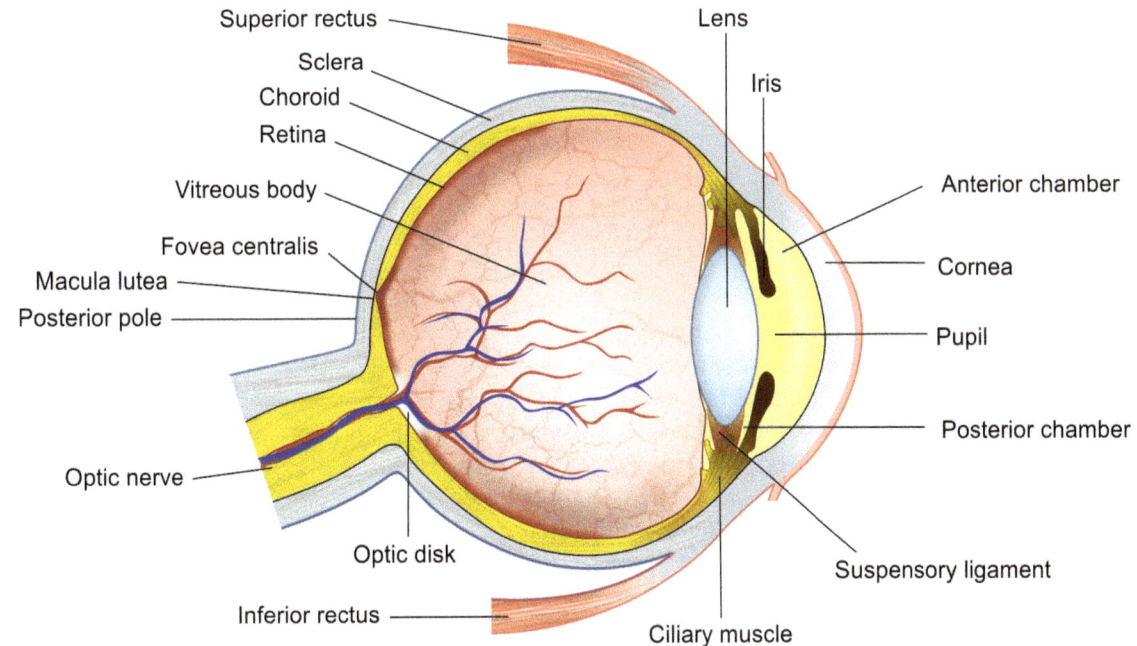

FIGURE 93.2: Structure of eyeball.

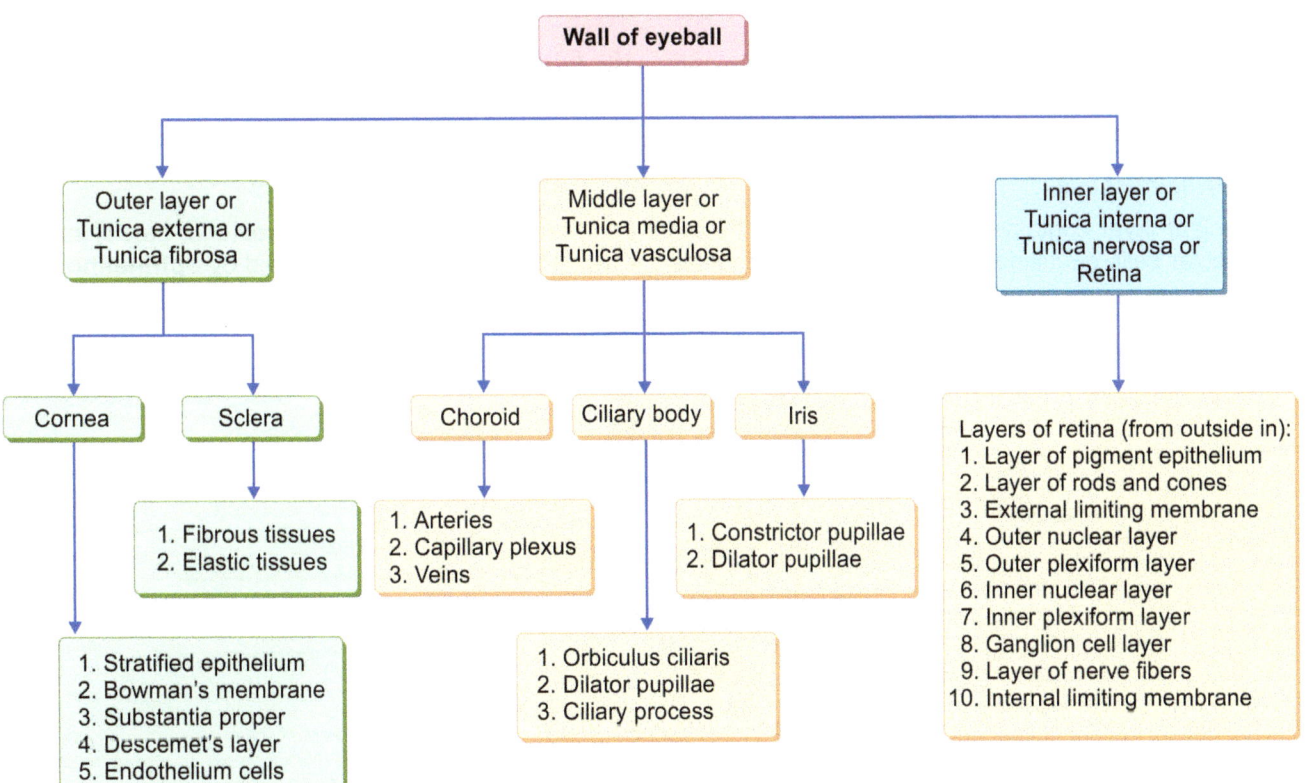

FIGURE 93.3: Wall of eyeball.

■ INNER LAYER OR TUNICA INTERNA OR TUNICA NERVOSA OR RETINA

Retina is the light-sensitive membrane that forms the innermost layer of eyeball. It extends from the margin of optic disk to just behind the ciliary body where, it ends abruptly as a dentated border known as **ora serrata**. Retina has the receptors of vision and it is made up of 10 layers of structures.

Layers of retina from outside in:

1. Layer of pigment epithelium.
2. Layer of rods and cones.
3. External limiting membrane.
4. Outer nuclear layer.
5. Outer plexiform layer.
6. Inner nuclear layer.
7. Inner plexiform layer.

8. Ganglion cell layer.
9. Layer of nerve fibers.
10. Internal limiting membrane.

1. Layer of Pigment Epithelium

Pigment epithelial layer is the outermost layer. It is a single layer of hexagonal epithelial cells which contain the pigment **melanin** (Fig. 93.4).

2. Layer of Rods and Cones

Rods and cones are the light-sensitive portions of the **visual receptor cells**, the rod cells and the cone cells.

Receptor cells are arranged in a parallel fashion and are perpendicular to the inner surface of the eyeball.

3. External Limiting Membrane

It is a thin layer, formed by the chief supporting elements of retina called **Müller's fibers**.

4. Outer Nuclear Layer

Fibers and granules of rods and cones are present in this layer. The granules of rods and cones contain nucleus.

5. Outer Plexiform Layer

This layer contains reticular meshwork formed by the terminal fibers of rods and cones and the dendrites from bipolar cells, situated in the inner nuclear layer.

6. Inner Nuclear Layer

Inner nuclear layer contains small **bipolar cells**. Axons of the bipolar cells go inside and synapse with dendrites of ganglionic cells in the inner plexiform layer. Dendrites synapse with fibers of rods and cones in the outer plexiform layer.

Inner nuclear layer also contains nuclei of Müller's supporting fibers. It also has some association neurons called **horizontal cells** and **amacrine cells**.

7. Inner Plexiform Layer

Inner plexiform layer of retina consists of synapses between dendrites of ganglionic cells and axons of bipolar cells.

8. Ganglion Cell Layer

Multipolar cells called ganglion cells are present in this layer. Axons from ganglion cells form the **optic nerve**. Dendrites of the ganglion cells synapse with axons of bipolar cells in the inner plexiform layer.

9. Layer of Nerve Fibers

This layer is formed by non-myelinated axons of ganglionic cells. After taking origin, the axons run horizontally to a short distance. Afterwards, the fibers converge towards the optic disk and form the **optic nerve**.

10. Internal Limiting Membrane

Inner limiting membrane forms the inner most layer of retina. It separates retina from the vitreous body.

■ FUNDUS OCULI OR FUNDUS

Fundus oculi or **fundus** is the posterior part of interior of eyeball (Fig. 93.5). It is examined by **ophthalmoscope**.

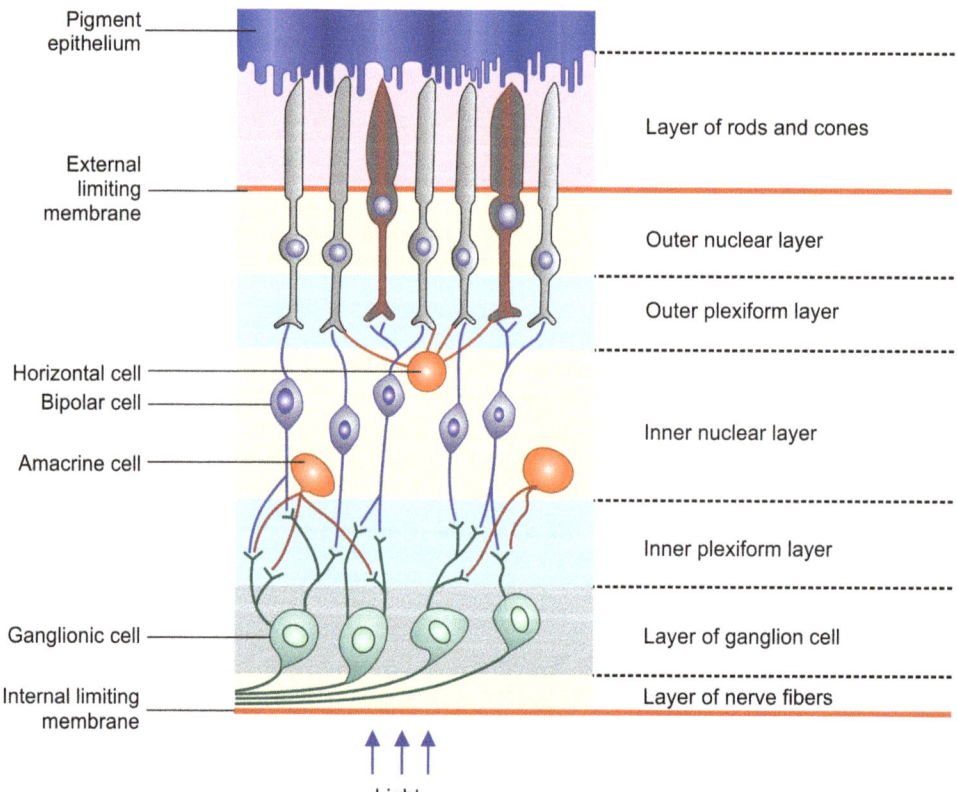

FIGURE 93.4: Layers of retina.

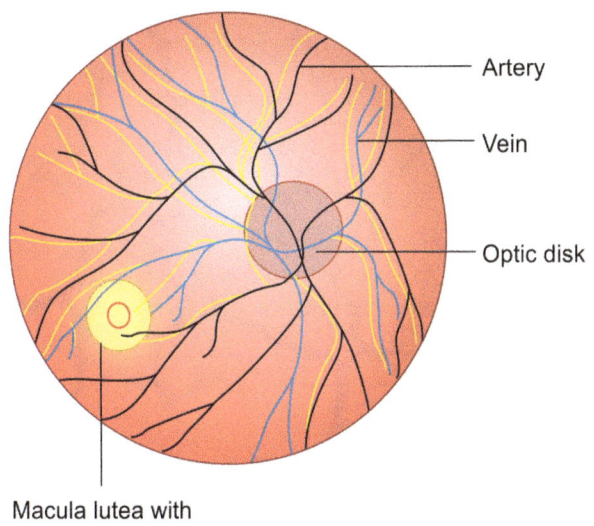

FIGURE 93.5: Fundus oculi.

Fundus has two important structures, optic disk and macula lutea with fovea centralis.

■ OPTIC DISK: BLIND SPOT

Optic disk or **optic papilla** is a disk-like structure situated near the center of posterior wall of eyeball. It is formed by the convergence of axons from ganglion cells, while forming the optic nerve.

Optic disk contains all the layers of retina except rods and cones. Therefore, it is insensitive to light. Hence, the optic disk is known as **blind spot**.

Blind Spot

Blind spot is a small portion of visual field of each eye that corresponds to the position of optic disk.

■ MACULA LUTEA

Macula lutea or yellow spot is a small yellowish area situated lateral to optic disk in retina. Yellow color of macula lutea is due to the presence of a **yellow pigment**. Macula lutea has fovea centralis in its center.

Fovea Centralis

Fovea centralis is a minute depression in the center of macula lutea and it is the region of acute vision because it contains only cones. When one looks at an object, if the image of that object falls on the fovea of each eye, the person can see the object very clearly. It is known as **foveal vision**.

Vision in other parts of retina is called peripheral or **extrafoveal vision**.

■ INTRAOCULAR FLUID

Intraocular fluid (fluid in eyeball) is responsible for the maintenance of shape of the eyeball. Intraocular fluid is of two types, vitreous humor and aqueous humor.

■ VITREOUS HUMOR OR VITREOUS BODY

Vitreous humor or vitreous body is present behind lens in the space between the lens and retina. It is a highly **viscous** and **gelatinous** substance. It is formed by a fine fibrillar network of **proteoglycan molecules**. Vitreous humor helps maintain the shape of the eyeball.

■ AQUEOUS HUMOR

Aqueous humor is a **thin fluid** present in front of lens. It fills the space between the lens and cornea. This space is divided into anterior and posterior chambers by iris. Both the chambers communicate with each other through pupil.

Aqueous humor is formed by **ciliary processes** by means of diffusion and ultrafiltration.

After formation, aqueous humor reaches the posterior chamber. From here it reaches the anterior chamber via pupil. From anterior chamber, the aqueous humor passes through the angle between cornea and iris, meshwork of **trabeculae** and **canal of Schlemm**, and reaches the venous system via anterior **ciliary vein**.

Functions of Aqueous Humor

1. Aqueous humor maintains shape of the eyeball.
2. It maintains the intraocular pressure.
3. It provides nutrients, oxygen and electrolytes to the avascular structures like lens and cornea.
4. Aqueous humor removes metabolic end products from lens and cornea.

■ INTRAOCULAR PRESSURE

Intraocular pressure is **fluid pressure** in the eye exerted by **aqueous humor**. Normal intraocular pressure varies from 12 to 20 mm Hg. It is measured by tonometer. When intraocular pressure increases above 60 mm Hg, **glaucoma** occurs (see below).

■ LENS

Lens of the eyeball is **crystalline** in nature. It is situated behind the pupil. It is a biconvex, transparent and elastic structure. Lens is avascular and receives its nutrition mainly from the aqueous humor.

Lens refracts light rays and helps to focus the image of the objects on retina. The focal length of human lens is 44 mm and its refractory power is 23 D.

Lens is supported by the **suspensory ligaments** (zonular fibers) which are attached with **ciliary bodies**.

■ STRUCTURE OF LENS

Lens is formed of three components:

1. *Capsule*

Capsule is an elastic membrane covering the lens.

2. *Anterior Epithelium*

Anterior epithelium is a single layer of cuboidal epithelial cells, situated beneath the capsule. Epithelial cells give rise to lens fibers present in the lens substance.

3. *Lens Substance*

Lens is formed by long lens fibers derived from anterior epithelium. Lens fibers are **prismatic** in nature and are arranged in concentric layers.

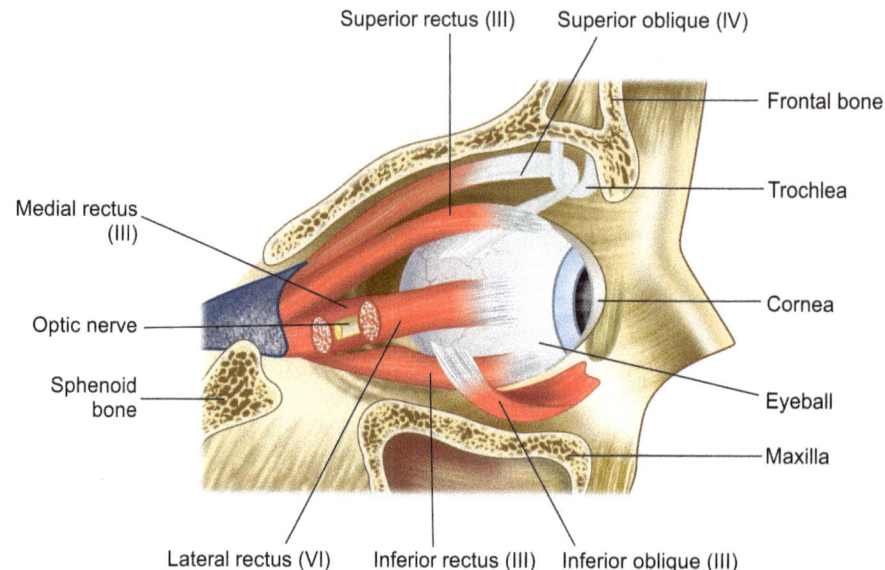

FIGURE 93.6: Extrinsic muscles of eyeball. Numbers in parenthesis indicate the cranial nerve supplying the muscle.

CHANGES IN THE LENS DURING OLD AGE

In old age, the elastic property of lens is decreased due to the physical changes in lens and its capsule. It causes **presbyopia**.

In old age, lens becomes opaque and this condition is called **cataract** (see below).

OCULAR MUSCLES

MUSCLES OF THE EYEBALL

Muscles of the eyeball are of two types, intrinsic muscles and extrinsic muscles.

I. Intrinsic Muscles

Intrinsic muscles are formed by **smooth muscle** fibers and are controlled by the **autonomic nerves**.

Intrinsic muscles of the eye are:

1. Constrictor pupillae.
2. Dilator pupillae.
3. Ciliary muscle.

2. Extrinsic Muscles

Extrinsic muscles are formed by **skeletal muscle** fibers and are controlled by the **somatic nerves**. The eyeball moves within the orbit by six extrinsic **(Fig. 93.6)**.

Extrinsic muscles of eye are:

1. Superior rectus.
2. Inferior rectus.
3. Medial or internal rectus.
4. Lateral or external rectus.
5. Superior oblique.
6. Inferior oblique.

INNERVATION OF OCULAR MUSCLES

Innervation of Intrinsic Muscles

Intrinsic muscles of eyeball are innervated by both sympathetic and parasympathetic divisions of autonomic nervous system.

Parasympathetic nerve fibers

Parasympathetic preganglionic fibers arise from **Edinger-Westphal nucleus** of III cranial nerve. After passing through III cranial nerve, these fibers synapse with postganglionic neurons in **ciliary ganglion**. Postganglionic fibers arising from here pass through **short ciliary nerves** and innervate the **ciliary muscle** and **constrictor pupillae**.

Stimulation of parasympathetic nerve fibers causes **contraction** of ciliary muscle and constrictor pupillae resulting in constriction of pupil.

Sympathetic nerve fibers

Sympathetic preganglionic nerve fibers arise from lateral horn of first thoracic segment of spinal cord, pass through **sympathetic chain** and synapse with neurons of superior cervical sympathetic ganglion. Postganglionic fibers arising from this ganglion run along with carotid artery and its branches, to reach the intrinsic muscles of the eyeball.

Stimulation of sympathetic nerve fibers causes **relaxation** of ciliary muscle and **contraction** of dilator pupillae resulting in dilatation of pupil.

Innervation of Extrinsic Muscles

Extrinsic muscles of the eyeball are innervated by somatic motor nerve fibers. Somatic nerve fibers arise from the cranial nerve nuclei in brainstem and reach the ocular muscles via three cranial nerves:

1. Oculomotor nerve (third cranial nerve) which supplies:
    i. Superior rectus.
    ii. Inferior rectus.
    iii. Medial rectus (internal rectus).
    iv. Inferior oblique.
2. Trochlear nerve (fourth cranial nerve) which supplies the superior oblique.
3. Abducens nerve (sixth) which supplies the lateral rectus (external rectus).

TABLE 93.1: Muscles taking part in ocular movements.

Movement	Primary muscle	Secondary muscle
1. Abduction	Lateral rectus	Superior oblique Inferior oblique
2. Adduction	Medial rectus	Superior rectus Inferior rectus
3. Elevation	Superior rectus	Inferior oblique
4. Depression	Inferior rectus	Superior oblique
5. Extorsion	Inferior oblique	Inferior rectus
6. Intorsion	Superior oblique	Superior rectus

OCULAR MOVEMENTS

Eyeball moves or rotates within the orbital socket in all the three primary axes, vertical, transverse and anteroposterior axis **(Table 93.1)**.

MOVEMENTS IN VERTICAL AXIS OR IN HORIZONTAL PLANE

1. *Abduction or Lateral Movement or Outward Movement*

Abduction of eyeball is due to the contraction of **lateral rectus** mainly. It is supported by the two **oblique muscles**.

2. *Adduction or Medial Movement or Inward Movement*

Adduction of the eyeball occurs because of the action of **medial or internal rectus,** along with action of **superior rectus** and **inferior rectus**.

MOVEMENTS IN TRANSVERSE AXIS OR IN SAGITTAL PLANE

1. *Elevation or Upward Movement*

Elevation of eyeball occurs because of the contraction of **superior rectus** and **inferior oblique muscles**.

2. *Depression or Downward Movement*

Depression of eyeball is brought out by **inferior rectus** and **superior oblique**.

MOVEMENTS IN ANTEROPOSTERIOR AXIS

Movements of eyeball in anteroposterior axis or in the frontal plane are called **torsion** or **wheel movements**. Torsion movements are two types, namely extorsion and intorsion.

1. *Extorsion*

During extorsion, the top of eyeball is rotated upward and outward direction away from nose. This movement is due to contraction of **inferior oblique** and **inferior rectus**.

2. *Intorsion*

During intorsion, the top of eyeball is rotated downward and inward direction towards nose. It is produced by the contraction of **superior oblique** and **superior rectus muscles**.

SIMULTANEOUS MOVEMENTS OF BOTH EYEBALLS

Simultaneous movements of both eyeballs are of four types.

1. *Conjugate Movement*

Conjugate movement is the movement of both eyeballs in the **same direction**. Visual axes of both eyes remain parallel. It is due to contraction of **medial rectus** of one eye and **lateral rectus** of the other eye.

2. *Disjugate Movement*

Disjugate movement is the movement of both eyeballs in **opposite direction**. There are two types of disjugate movement, namely convergence and divergence.

  i. *Convergence*: Convergence is the movement of both eyeballs towards nose. It is due to simultaneous contraction of **medial rectus** and simultaneous relaxation of lateral rectus of both eyes. Visual axes move close to each other. Convergence of eyeballs occurs during accommodation.
  ii. *Divergence*: Divergence is the movement of both eyeballs towards temporal side. It is due to the simultaneous contraction of **lateral rectus** and simultaneous relaxation of medial rectus of both eyes. Visual axes of the eyes move away from each other.

3. *Pursuit Movement*

Pursuit movement is the movement of eyeballs along with object, when eyeballs follow a moving object.

4. *Saccadic Movement*

Saccadic movement is the quick jerky movement of both eyeballs when the fixation of eyes (gaze) is shifted from one object to another object. It is also called **optokinetic movement**.

APPLIED PHYSIOLOGY

GLAUCOMA

Glaucoma is a disease characterized by increase in intraocular pressure above 60 mm Hg resulting in damage of optic nerve and blindness. Intraocular pressure increases due to the blockage in the drainage of aqueous humor.

CATARACT

Cataract is the **opacity** or **cloudiness** in the natural lens of the eye. It is the major cause of blindness worldwide. When the lens becomes cloudy, light rays cannot pass through it easily, and vision is blurred. Cataract develops in old age after 55 to 60 years.

Lens is situated within the sealed capsule. Old cells die and accumulate within the capsule. Over years, the accumulation of cells is associated with accumulation of fluid and denaturation of the proteins in the lens fibers causing cloudiness of lens and blurred image.

Cataract is treated by surgery. The cloudy lens is removed from the eye through a surgical incision. Natural lens is replaced with a permanent plastic **intraocular lens implant** (IOL implant).

Chapter 94

Visual Process and Field of Vision

CHAPTER OUTLINE

- **VISUAL PROCESS**
  - IMAGE FORMING MECHANISM
  - NEURAL BASIS OF VISUAL PROCESS
  - STRUCTURE OF VISUAL RECEPTORS
  - FUNCTIONS OF VISUAL RECEPTORS
  - CHEMICAL BASIS OF VISUAL PROCESS
  - ELECTRICAL BASIS OF VISUAL PROCESS
  - ACUITY OF VISION
- **FIELD OF VISION**
  - DEFINITION
  - BINOCULAR AND MONOCULAR VISION
  - DIVISIONS OF VISUAL FIELD
  - CORRESPONDING RETINAL POINTS
  - BLIND SPOT
  - VISUAL FIELD AND RETINA
  - MAPPING OF VISUAL FIELD

VISUAL PROCESS

Visual process is the series of actions that take place during **visual perception**. When the image of an object is focused on **retina**, the energy in visual spectrum is converted into **electrical potentials** (impulses) by rods and cones of retina through some chemical reactions. Impulses from **rods and cones** reach the **cerebral cortex** through **optic nerve**. And, the sensation of vision is produced in cerebral cortex.

Thus, process of visual sensation can be explained on the basis of image formation, and neural, chemical and electrical phenomena.

IMAGE FORMING MECHANISM

While looking at an object, the light rays from the object are refracted and brought to a focus upon retina. The image falls on the retina in an inverted position and reversed side to side. In spite of this, the object is seen in an upright position. It is because of the role of cerebral cortex.

Light rays are refracted by the lens and cornea. Refractory power is measured in diopter (D). A diopter is the reciprocal of focal length expressed in meters.

Focal length of cornea is 24 mm and refractory power is 42D. Focal length of lens is 44 mm and refractory power is 23D.

NEURAL BASIS OF VISUAL PROCESS

Retina has the **visual receptors** which are also called **photoreceptors**. The photoreceptors are rods and cones. There are about 6 million cones and 12 million rods in the human eye. Distribution of the photoreceptors varies in different areas of retina. Fovea has only cones and no rods. While proceeding from fovea towards the periphery of retina, the rods increase and the cones decrease in number. At the periphery of the retina, only rods are present and cones are absent.

STRUCTURE OF VISUAL RECEPTORS

Structure of Rod Cell

Rod cells are cylindrical structures with a length of about 40 to 60 µ and a diameter of about 2 µ. Each rod cell is formed by four structures.

1. *Outer segment*

Outer segment of rod cell is long, slender and gives the rod like appearance. It is in close contact with the pigmented epithelial cells. Outer segment of rod cell is formed by the modified cilia and it contains a pile of freely floating flat **membranous disks**. Disks in rod cells are closed structures and contain the photosensitive pigment, the **rhodopsin**.

2. *Inner segment*

Inner segment is connected to outer segment by means of a modified **connecting cilium**. Inner segment contains many types of organelles with large number of mitochondria.

3. *Cell body*

A rod fiber arises from inner segment of the rod cell and passes to outer nuclear layer through external limiting membrane. In outer nuclear layer, the enlarged portion of

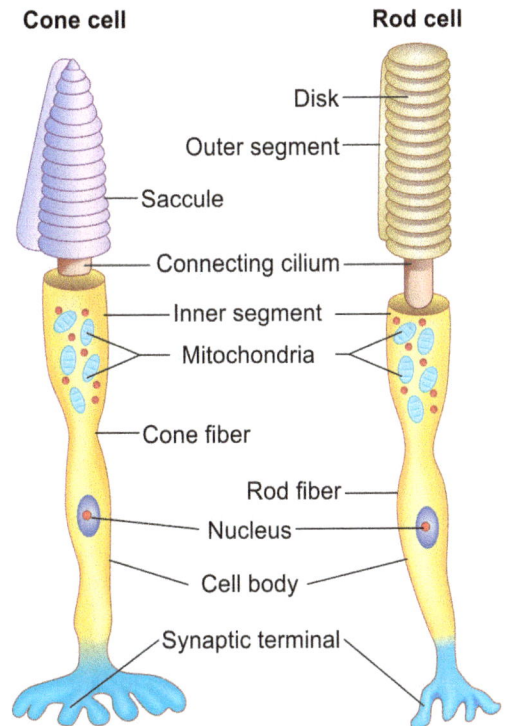

FIGURE 94.1: Structure of visual receptors.

this fiber forms the cell body or rod granule that contains the nucleus **(Fig. 94.1)**.

4. Synaptic terminal

A thick fiber arising from cell body passes to outer plexiform layer and ends in an enlarged synaptic terminal. Synaptic terminal synapses with dendrites of **bipolar cells** and **horizontal cells**. Synaptic vesicles present in the synaptic terminal contain neurotransmitter, **glutamate**.

Structure of Cone Cell

Cone cell is flask shaped. It has a length of 35 to 40 μ and a diameter of about 5 μ. Like rod cell, cone cell also has four parts.

1. Outer segment

Outer segment is small and conical without membranous disks. In cone, infoldings of cell membrane form **saccules,** which are the counterparts of rod disks. Photopigment of cone is synthesized in the inner segment and incorporated into the folding of surface membrane forming saccule.

2. Inner segment

In cones also, the inner segment is connected to outer segment by a connecting cilium as in the case of rods. This also contains various types of organelles including mitochondria.

3. Cell body

Cone fiber arising from inner segment is thick and it enters the inner nuclear layer. In the inner nuclear layer, cone fiber forms the cell body or cone granule that possesses nucleus.

4. Synaptic terminal

Fiber from cell body of cone enters outer plexiform layer and it ends in the form of synaptic terminal. Synaptic vesicle in the synaptic terminal of cone cell also possesses glutamate.

■ FUNCTIONS OF VISUAL RECEPTORS

Functions of Rods

Rods are very sensitive to light and have a **low threshold**. So, the rods are responsible for **dim light vision** or **night vision** or **scotopic vision**. But rods do not take part in visual acuity or color vision.

Functions of Cones

Cones have **high threshold** for light stimulus. So, the cones are sensitive only to bright light. Therefore, the cone cells are called receptors of **bright light vision** or **photopic vision** or **day light vision**. Cones are also responsible for **acuity of vision** and the **color vision**.

Differences between rods and cones are listed in **Table 94.1**.

TABLE 94.1: Rods vs cones.

Features	Rods	Cones
1. Number in each eye	12 million	6 million
2. Length	40 to 60 μ	35 to 40 μ
3. Diameter	2 μ	5 μ
4. Shape	Cylindrical	Flask shaped
5. Outer segment	Long and slender	Small and conical
6. Sensitivity to light	More sensitive	Sensitive only to bright light
7. Threshold	Low	High
8. Type of vision responsible for	Dim light vision or night vision or scotopic vision	Bright light vision or day light vision or photopic vision
9. Acuity of vision	Not responsible	Responsible
10. Color vision	Not responsible	Responsible
11. Photosensitive pigment	Rhodopsin	Porphyropsin or iodopsin or cyanopsin

CHEMICAL BASIS OF VISUAL PROCESS

Photosensitive pigments present in rods and cones form chemical basis of visual process. Chemical reactions of these pigments lead to the development of electrical activity in retina and generation of impulses (action potentials) in optic nerve. Photochemical changes in the visual receptors are called **Wald's visual cycle**.

Rhodopsin

Rhodopsin is the **photosensitive pigment** of rod cells. Rhodopsin is made up of a protein called **opsin** and a **chromophore**. Opsin present in rhodopsin is known as **scotopsin**. Chromophore is a substance that develops color in the cell. Chromophore present in the rod cells is called **retinal** which is the aldehyde of **retinol** or vitamin A.

Photochemical changes in rhodopsin

During exposure to light, rhodopsin is bleached and it is split into **retinine** and the protein called **opsin** through various intermediate photochemical reactions. The **metarhodopsin** produced during these reactions is the **activated rhodopsin**. It is responsible for development of receptor potential in rod cells.

Phototransduction: Visual Transduction

Phototransduction or **visual transduction** is the process in visual receptors by which **light energy** is converted into **electrical energy** (action potentials) in optic nerve fibers.

The resting membrane potential in other sensory receptor cells is usually between – 70 and – 90 mV. However, in the visual receptors in dark, the negativity is reduced and the resting membrane potential is about – 40 mV. When light falls on retina, the rhodopsin is converted into metarhodopsin which causes **mild hyperpolarization** which is called **receptor potential** in the rod cells.

Significance of hyperpolarization

Hyperpolarization in rod cells leads to the development of response in bipolar cells and ganglionic cells so that the action potentials are transmitted to cerebral cortex via optic pathway.

Photosensitive Pigment in Cone Cells

Photosensitive pigment in the cone cells are porphyropsin, iodopsin and cyanopsin. Only one of these pigments is present in each cone. Each type of cone pigment is sensitive to a particular light and the maximum response is shown at a particular light and wavelength.

The processes involved in phototransduction in cone cells are similar to those in the rod cells.

Dark Adaptation

Dark adaption is the process by which the person is able to see the objects in dim light. If a person enters a dim lighted room (darkroom) from a bright lighted area, he is blind for some time, i.e. he cannot see any object. After sometime his eyes get adapted and he starts seeing the objects slowly. Maximum duration for dark adaptation is about 20 minutes.

Causes for dark adaptation

1. *Resynthesis of rhodopsin:* Time required for dark adaptation is partly determined by the time to resynthesize rhodopsin. In bright light, much of the pigment is being bleached (broken down). But in dim light, it requires sometime for the regeneration of certain amount of rhodopsin, which is necessary for optimal rod function.
2. *Dilatation of pupil:* Dilatation of pupil during dark adaptation allows more and more light to enter the eye.

Light Adaptation

Light adaptation is the process in which eyes get adapted to bright light. When a person enters a bright lighted area from a dim lighted area, he feels discomfort due to the dazzling effect of bright light. After some time, when the eyes become adapted to light, he sees the objects around him without any discomfort. It is the mere disappearance of dark adaptation. The maximum period for light adaptation is about 5 minutes.

Causes for light adaptation

1. Reduced sensitivity of rods during light adaptation due to the breakdown of rhodopsin.
2. Constriction of pupil which reduces quantity of light rays entering the eye.

Night Blindness

Night blindness or **nyctalopia** is defined as the loss of vision in dim light.

Causes of night blindness

Night blindness is due to deficiency of vitamin A which is necessary for the functions of visual receptors.

Deficiency of vitamin A occurs because of:

1. Diet containing less amount of vitamin A.
2. Decreased absorption of vitamin A from the intestine.

Initially, vitamin A deficiency causes **defective rod function**. Prolonged deficiency leads to **anatomical changes** in rods and cones, and finally the **degeneration** of other retinal layers occurs. So, retinal function can be restored, only if treatment is given with vitamin A before the visual receptors start degenerating.

ELECTRICAL BASIS OF VISUAL PROCESS

Definition

Electroretinogram (ERG) is the record of electrical activity in retina. When light rays stimulate the retina, potential changes occur, which can be recorded in the form of ERG. Recording of ERG is a diagnostic procedure. It is useful in determining retinal disorders such as **cone dystrophy** (degeneration of cones) and **retinitis pigmentosa** (hyperactivity of the pigmented retinal epithelial cells, leading to damage of photoreceptors and blindness).

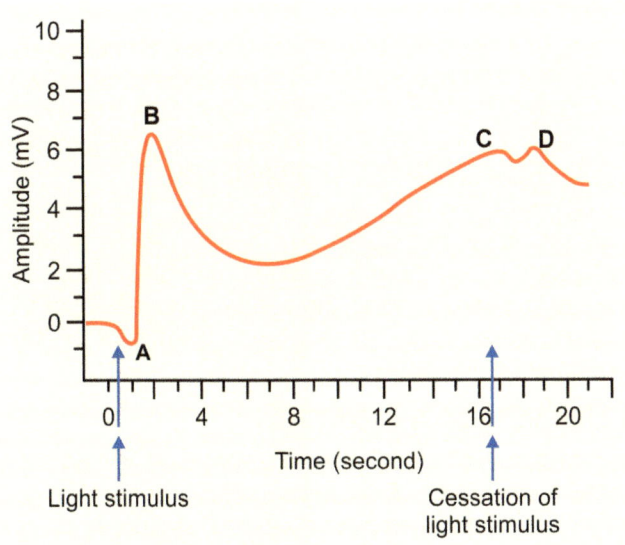

FIGURE 94.2: Electroretinogram.

Waves of ERG

Electroretinogram has 4 waves namely 'A', 'B', 'C' and 'D' **(Fig. 94.2)**. 'A' is the only negative wave and other three are positive waves. 'A', 'B' and 'C' waves occur when light stimulus falls on retina. 'D' wave occurs when light stimulus is stopped. 'A' and 'B' waves arise from rods and cones. 'C' wave arises from pigment epithelial layer and 'D' wave arises from inner nuclear layer.

■ ACUITY OF VISION

Definition

Acuity of vision is the ability of the eye to determine the precise shape and details of the object. It is also called **visual acuity**. **Cones** of the retina are responsible for acuity of vision. Visual acuity is highly exhibited in **fovea centralis**, which contains only cones. It is greatly reduced during the refractive errors.

Test for Acuity of Vision

Acuity of vision is tested for distant vision as well as near vision. If there is any difficulty in seeing the distant object or the near object, the defect is known as **refractive errors** (Chapter 96).

Distant vision is tested by using **Snellen's chart**. Near vision is tested by using **Jaeger's chart**.

■ FIELD OF VISION

■ DEFINITION

Part of the external world seen by one eye when it is fixed in one direction is called field of vision or **visual field** of that eye.

■ BINOCULAR AND MONOCULAR VISION

Binocular Vision

Binocular vision is the vision in which both the eyes are used together, so that a portion of external world is seen by the eyes together. In human and some animals, the eyeballs are placed in front of the head. So, the visual fields of both the eyes overlap. Because of this, a portion of the external world is seen by both the eyes.

Monocular Vision

It is the vision in which each eye is used separately. In some animals like dog, rabbit and horse, the eyeballs are present at the sides of head. So, the visual fields of both eyes overlap to a very small extent. Because of this, different portion of the external world is seen by each eye.

■ DIVISIONS OF VISUAL FIELD

Visual field of human eye has an angle of 160° in horizontal meridian and 135° in vertical meridian.

Visual field is divided into four parts:

1. Temporal field.
2. Nasal field.
3. Upper field.
4. Lower field.

Temporal and Nasal Fields

Visual field of each eye is divided into two unequal parts namely, outer or temporal field and the inner or nasal field by a vertical line passing through the fixation point **(Fig. 94.3)**. The **fixation point** is the meeting point of visual axis with the object.

Temporal part of visual field extends up to about 100°, but the nasal part extends only up to 60° because it is restricted by nose.

Temporal and nasal fields

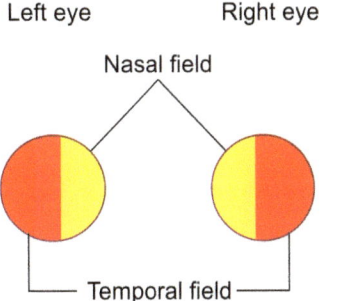

Upper and lower fields

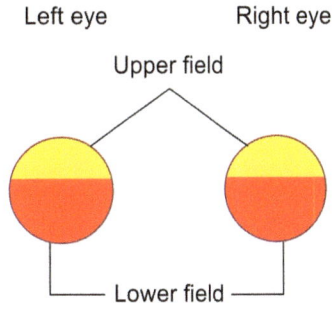

FIGURE 94.3: Divisions of visual field.

Upper and Lower Fields

Visual field of each eye is also divided into an upper field and a lower field by a horizontal line passing through the fixation point. The extent of the upper field is about 60° as it is restricted by upper eyelid and orbital margin. The extent of lower field is about 75°. It is restricted by cheek. Thus, the visual field is restricted in all the sides except in the temporal part.

■ CORRESPONDING RETINAL POINTS

Corresponding retinal points are the area in retina of both eyes on which the light rays from the object falls. It occurs in the binocular vision. Two images developed on retina of both eyes are fused into a single sensation. So, we see the objects with single image.

Diplopia

Diplopia means **double vision**. Normal single sensation is because of the ocular muscles, which direct the axes of the eyes in such a way, that the light rays from the object fall upon the corresponding points of both retinas. If the light rays do not fall on the corresponding retinal points, diplopia occurs.

■ BLIND SPOT

Blind spot is the small area of retina where visual receptors are absent. The **optic disk** in the retina does not have any visual receptors and, if the image of any object falls on the optic disk, the object cannot be seen. So, this part of the retina is blind hence the name **blind spot**.

Normally, the darkness in the visual field due to the blind spot does not cause any inconvenience because, the fixation of each eye is at different angles. Even when one eye is closed or blind, the person is not aware of blind spot. However, one can recognize blind spot by some experimental procedures.

■ VISUAL FIELD AND RETINA

Light rays from different halves of each visual field do not fall on the same halves of the retina. Light rays from temporal part of visual field of an eye fall on the nasal half of retina of that eye. Similarly, the light rays from nasal part of visual field fall on the temporal half of retina of the same side.

■ MAPPING OF VISUAL FIELD

Shape and extent of visual field is mapped out by means of an instrument called **perimeter**. The visual field is also determined by **Bjerrum screen** or by **confrontation test**.

Chapter 95: Visual Pathway

CHAPTER OUTLINE

- **VISUAL PATHWAY**
  - VISUAL RECEPTORS
  - FIRST ORDER NEURONS
  - SECOND ORDER NEURONS
  - THIRD ORDER NEURONS
- **COURSE OF VISUAL PATHWAY**
  - OPTIC NERVE
  - OPTIC CHIASMA
  - OPTIC TRACT
  - LATERAL GENICULATE BODY: SUBCORTICAL CENTER
  - OPTIC RADIATION
  - VISUAL CORTEX: CORTICAL CENTER
- **APPLIED PHYSIOLOGY: EFFECTS OF LESION IN VISUAL PATHWAY**

VISUAL PATHWAY

Visual pathway or **optic pathway** is the nervous pathway that carries the retinal impulses to cerebral cortex. In binocular vision, the light rays from temporal (outer) half of visual field (Chapter 94) fall upon the nasal part of corresponding retina. Light rays from nasal (inner) half of visual field fall upon the temporal part of retina.

VISUAL RECEPTORS

Rods and cones, which are present in the retina of eye, form the visual receptors. Fibers from the visual receptors synapse with dendrites of **bipolar cells** of inner nuclear layer of retina.

FIRST ORDER NEURONS

First order neurons are **bipolar cells** in the retina. Axons from the bipolar cells synapse with dendrites of ganglionic cells.

SECOND ORDER NEURONS

Second order neurons are the **ganglionic cells** in ganglionic cell layer of retina. Axons of the ganglionic cells form optic nerve. Optic nerve leaves the eye and terminates in lateral geniculate body.

THIRD ORDER NEURONS

Third order neurons are in the **lateral geniculate body**. Fibers arising from here reach the **visual cortex**.

COURSE OF VISUAL PATHWAY

Visual pathway consists of six components:

1. Optic nerve.
2. Optic chiasma.
3. Optic tract.
4. Lateral geniculate body.
5. Optic radiation.
6. Visual cortex.

1. OPTIC NERVE

Optic nerve is formed by the **axons of ganglionic cells (Fig. 95.1)**. Optic nerve leaves the eye through **optic disk**. Fibers from temporal part of retina are in lateral part of the nerve and carry the impulses from nasal half of visual field of same eye. Fibers from nasal part of retina are in medial part of the nerve and carry the impulses from temporal half of visual field of same eye.

2. OPTIC CHIASMA

Medial fibers of each optic nerve cross the midline and join the uncrossed lateral fibers of opposite side to form the optic tract **(Fig. 95.1)**. Area of crossing of the optic nerve fibers is called optic chiasma.

3. OPTIC TRACT

Optic tract is formed by uncrossed fibers of optic nerve on the same side and crossed fibers of optic nerve from the opposite side. All the fibers of optic tract run backward and outward, and terminate in the lateral geniculate body in thalamus. Few fibers just pass through medial geniculate

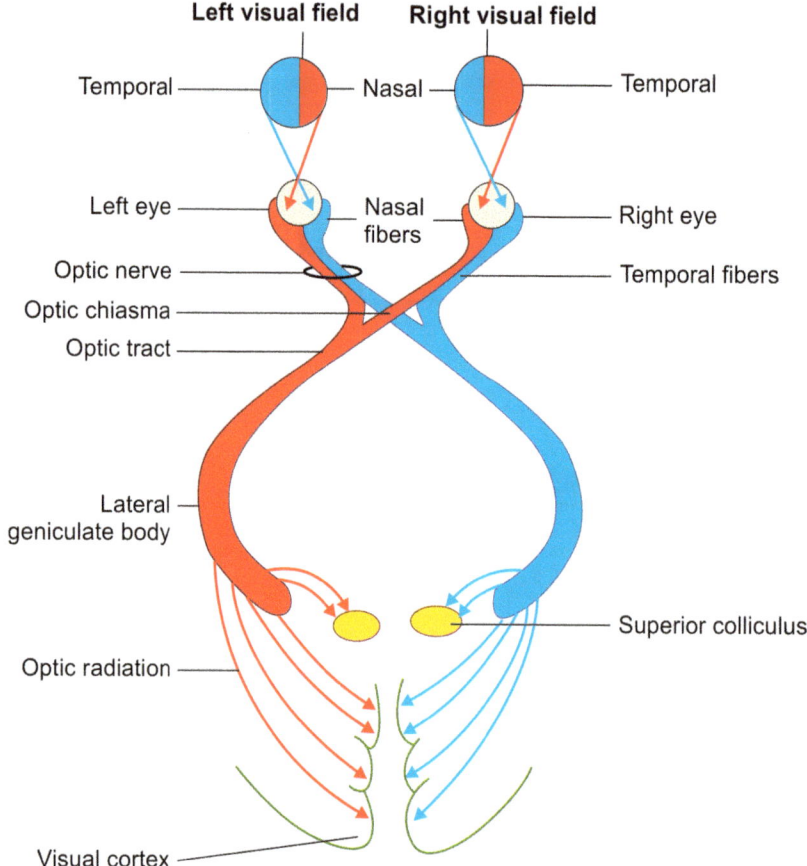

FIGURE 95.1: Visual pathway.

body and run towards superior colliculus in midbrain (see below).

Due to crossing of medial fibers in optic chiasma, the left optic tract carries impulses from temporal part of left retina and nasal part of right retina, i.e. it is responsible for vision in nasal half of left visual field and temporal half of right visual field. Right optic tract contains fibers from nasal half of left retina and temporal half of right retina. It is responsible for vision in temporal half of left visual field and nasal half of right visual field.

■ 4. LATERAL GENICULATE BODY: SUBCORTICAL CENTER

Majority of the fibers of optic tract terminate in lateral geniculate body, which forms the **subcortical center** for visual sensation. From here, the **geniculocalcarine tract** or **optic radiation** arises. This tract is the last relay of visual pathway.

Some of the fibers from optic tract do not synapse in lateral geniculate body, but pass through it and terminate in one of the following centers:

  i. **Superior colliculus** of midbrain which is concerned with **reflex movements of eyeballs** and head in response to optic stimulus.
 ii. **Pretectal nucleus** of midbrain which is concerned with **light reflexes**.
iii. **Supraoptic nucleus** of hypothalamus which is concerned with the retinal **control of pituitary**.

■ 5. OPTIC RADIATION

Fibers from lateral geniculate body pass through internal capsule and form optic radiation. Optic radiation ends in visual cortex **(Fig. 95.2)**.

■ 6. VISUAL CORTEX: CORTICAL CENTER

Cortical center for vision is called visual cortex that is located on the medial surface of **occipital lobe**. It forms the walls and lips of calcarine fissure in medial surface of occipital lobe.

Areas of Visual Cortex and Their Functions

1. **Primary visual area (area 17)** which is concerned with perception of visual impulses.
2. **Visual association area (area 18)** which is concerned with interpretation of visual impulses.
3. **Occipital eye field (area 19)** which is concerned with movement of eyes.

■ APPLIED PHYSIOLOGY

Injury to any part of optic pathway causes visual defect and the nature of defect depends upon the location and extent of injury.

■ ANOPIA

Anopia (blindness) is the loss of vision in one visual field.

■ HEMIANOPIA

Hemianopia is the loss of vision in one half of visual field **(Figs. 95.3 to 95.5)**. Hemianopia is classified into

Chapter 95: Visual Pathway

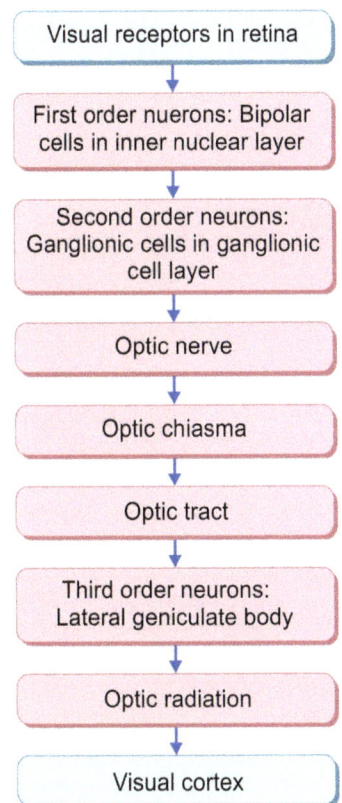

FIGURE 95.2: Schematic representation of visual pathway.

two types, homonymous hemianopia and heteronymous hemianopia.

1. Homonymous Hemianopia

Homonymous hemianopia means loss of vision in the **same halves** of both the visual fields. Loss of vision in right half of visual field of both eyes is known as **right homonymous hemianopia**. Similarly, **left homonymous hemianopia** means loss of vision in left half of visual field of both eyes.

2. Heteronymous Hemianopia

Heteronymous hemianopia means loss of vision in **opposite halves** of visual field. For example, **binasal heteronymous hemianopia** means loss of vision in right half of left visual field and left half of right visual field (nasal half of both visual fields).

Bitemporal heteronymous hemianopia is the loss of sight in left side of left visual field and right side of right visual field (temporal half of both visual fields).

■ EFFECTS OF LESION AT DIFFERENT LEVELS OF VISUAL PATHWAY

1. *Lesion of left optic nerve:* Total blindness (anopia) of left eye **(Fig. 95.5: A)**.
2. *Lesion of right optic nerve:* Total blindness (anopia) of right eye **(Fig. 95.5: B)**.
3. *Lesion of lateral fibers in left side of optic chiasma:* Left nasal hemianopia **(Fig. 95.5: C)**.
4. *Lesion of lateral fibers in right side of optic chiasma:* Right nasal hemianopia **(Fig. 95.5: D)**.
5. *Lesion of lateral fibers in both sides of optic chiasma:* Binasal hemianopia **(Fig. 95.5: C + D)**.
6. *Lesion of medial fibers in optic chiasma:* Bitemporal hemianopia **(Fig. 95.5: E)**.
7. *Lesion of left optic radiation:* Right homonymous hemianopia **(Fig. 95.5: F)**.
8. *Lesion of right optic radiation:* Left homonymous hemianopia **(Fig. 95.5: G)**.

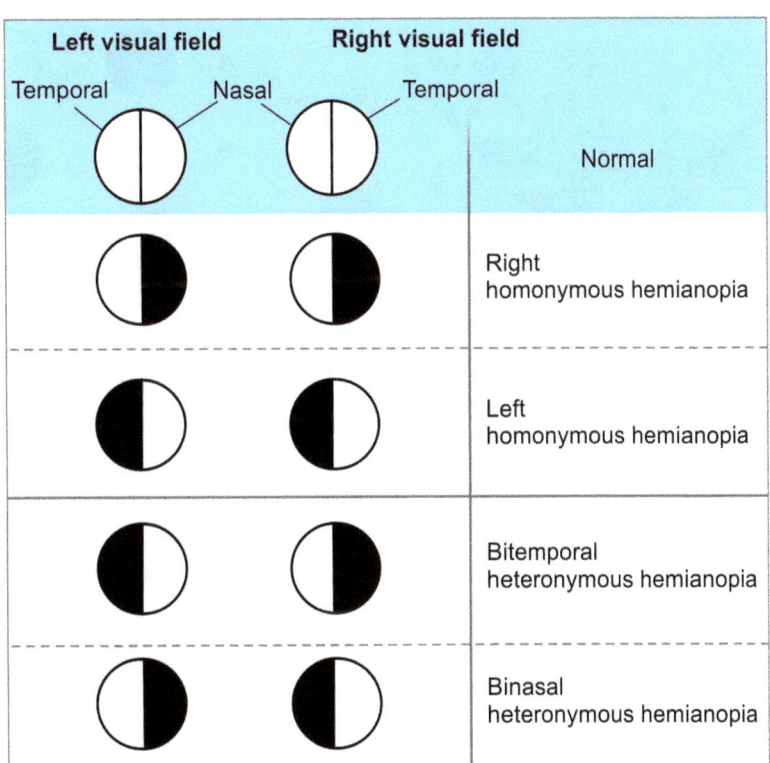

FIGURE 95.3: Types of hemianopia. Dark shade in circles indicates blindness.

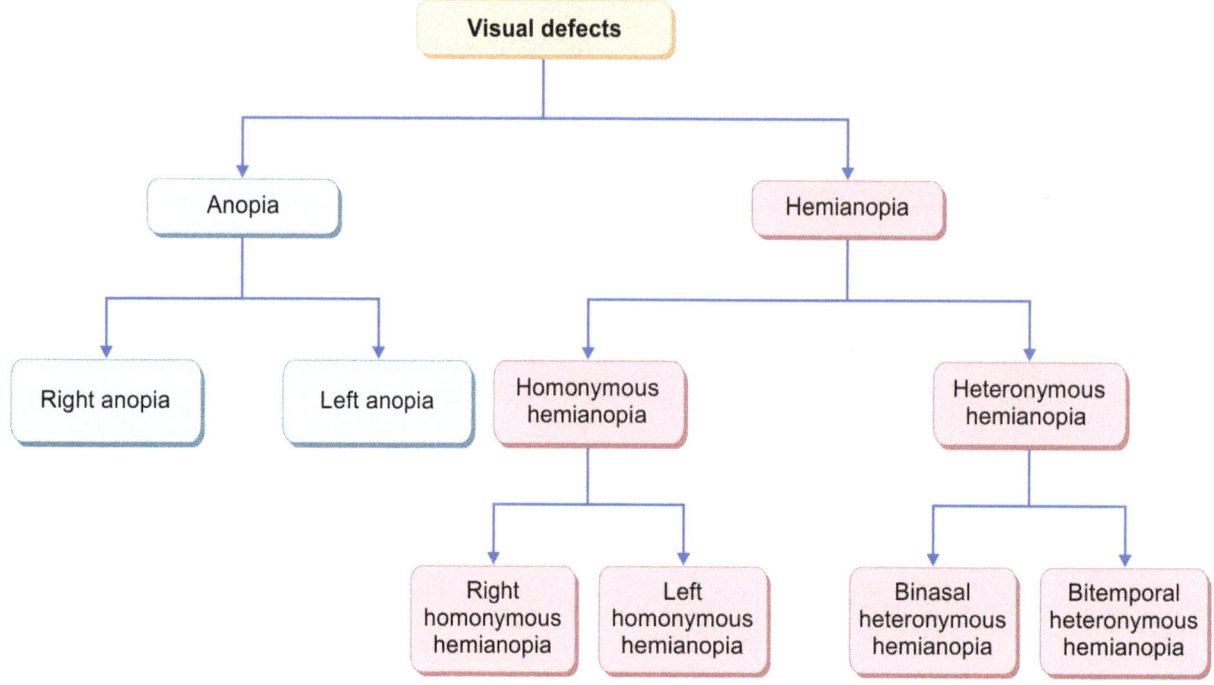

FIGURE 95.4: Visual defects.

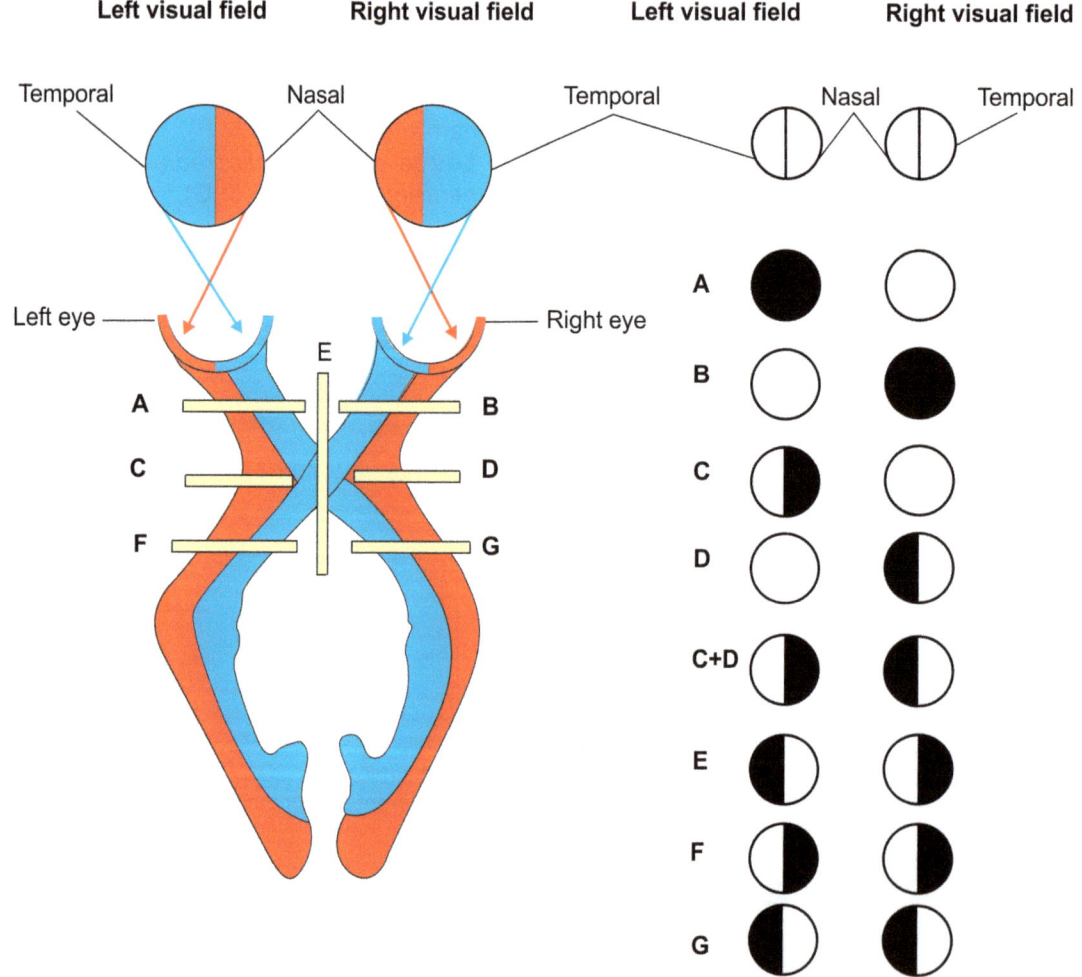

FIGURE 95.5: Effects of lesions of optic pathway. Dark shade in circles indicates blindness.

Chapter 96: Pupillary Reflexes, Refractive Errors and Color Vision

CHAPTER OUTLINE

- **PUPILLARY REFLEXES**
  - DEFINITION AND TYPES
  - LIGHT REFLEX
  - CILIOSPINAL REFLEX
  - ACCOMMODATION
  - APPLIED PHYSIOLOGY
- **REFRACTIVE ERRORS**
  - AMETROPIA
  - ANISOMETROPIA
- ASTIGMATISM
- PRESBYOPIA
- **COLOR VISION**
  - VISIBLE SPECTRUM
  - CONES AND COLOR VISION
  - COLOR SENSITIVE AREAS IN RETINA
  - APPLIED PHYSIOLOGY: COLOR BLINDNESS
  - TESTS FOR COLOR BLINDNESS

PUPILLARY REFLEXES

DEFINITION AND TYPES

Pupillary reflexes are the **visceral reflexes**, which alter the size of pupil. Pupillary reflexes are classified into three types:

1. Light reflex.
2. Ciliospinal reflex.
3. Accommodation reflex.

1. LIGHT REFLEX

It is the reflex in which the pupil constricts when light is flashed into the eyes.

Light reflex is of two types:

1. Direct light reflex in which there is constriction of pupil in an eye when light is thrown into that eye.
2. Indirect light reflex or consensual light reflex in which there is constriction of pupil in both eyes when light is thrown into one eye.

Pathway for Light Reflex

Afferent pathway

Pathway for light reflex is slightly deviated from visual pathway. When light falls on the eye, the visual receptors are stimulated. Afferent (sensory) impulses from the receptors pass through the optic nerve, optic chiasma and optic tract. At midbrain, some fibers get separated from optic tract and synapse with the neurons of pretectal nucleus.

Center

Pretectal nucleus of midbrain forms the center for light reflexes.

Efferent pathway

Efferent (motor) impulses from pretectal nucleus are carried by short fibers to **Edinger-Westphal** nucleus (parasympathetic nucleus) of **oculomotor nerve**. From this nucleus, preganglionic fibers pass through oculomotor nerve and reach the **ciliary ganglion**. Postganglionic fibers arising from ciliary ganglion pass through the **short ciliary nerves** and reach the eyeball. These fibers cause contraction of **constrictor pupillae** muscle of iris **(Fig. 96.1)** resulting in **constriction of pupil**.

2. CILIOSPINAL REFLEX

Ciliospinal reflex is the **dilatation of pupil** in eyes caused by painful stimulation of skin over neck. It is due to the contraction of **dilator pupillae** muscle. Sensory impulses pass through cutaneous afferent nerve. Center is in first thoracic spinal segment. Efferent impulses pass through sympathetic fibers and reach dilator pupillae.

3. ACCOMMODATION

Definition

Accommodation is the adjustment of the eye to see either near or distant objects clearly. It is the process, by which light rays from near objects or distant objects are brought to a focus on the sensitive part of retina.

Section 11: Special Senses

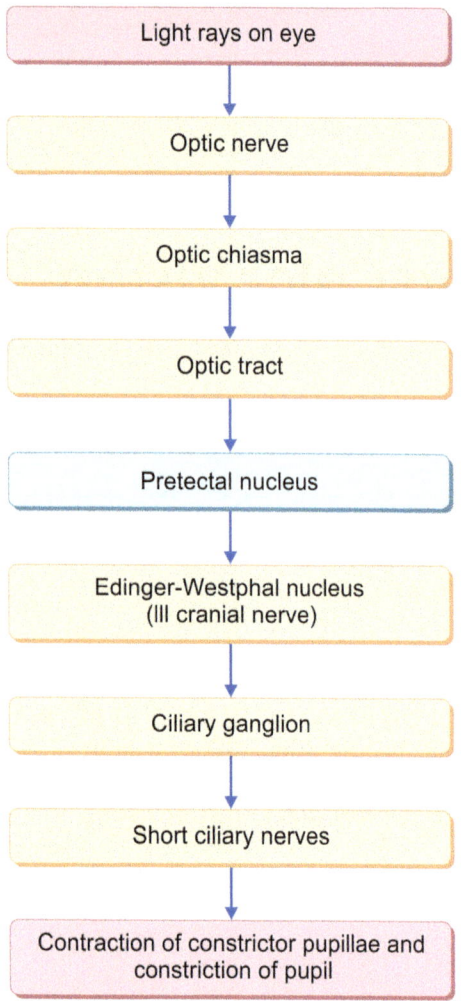

FIGURE 96.1: Pathway for light reflex.

Mechanism of Accommodation

Light rays from distant objects are approximately **parallel** and are less refracted while getting focused on retina. So, no adjustments are made in eye during distant vision.

But, the light rays from near objects are **divergent**. So, to be focused on retina, these light rays should be refracted (converged) to a greater extent. Some adjustments are made in eyes in order to converge the light rays from the objects.

Adjustments in eyeballs during accommodation

Accommodation in near vision occurs by means of three adjustments made in the eyeballs:

1. Increase in anterior curvature of lens, so that the refractory power of lens is increased.
2. Convergence of both eyeballs which brings the retinal images on to the corresponding points.
3. Constriction of pupil that causes:
   i. Increase in the visual acuity.
   ii. Reduction in the quantity of light entering eye.
   iii. Increase in the depth of focus through more central part of lens as its convexity is increased.

Young-Helmholtz theory

This theory describes how the curvature of lens increases and thereby, the refractive power of lens is enhanced. When the eyes are fixed on a distant object (distant vision), lens is flat due to the traction of **suspensory ligaments** which extend from the capsule of lens and are attached to the **ciliary processes**. The ciliary processes are attached to **choroid** through the **ciliary muscle** (Fig. 96.2).

When the vision is shifted from the distant object to a near object (near vision), ciliary muscle contracts and draws the choroid forward. Ciliary processes are brought closer to lens. Because of this, suspensory ligaments are slackened. Now, the tension on the lens is released. The **lens bulges** forward due to its elastic property. The anterior curvature (convexity) of lens increases greatly. A very little change occurs in posterior curvature.

In resting eye, the intraocular pressure sets up tension in choroids and pulls the ciliary processes backward and outward. Suspensory ligaments are tensed up and the lens becomes flat.

Accommodation Reflex

Accommodation is a reflex action. When a person looks at a near object after seeing a far object, three adjustments are made in the eyeballs:

1. Increase in the anterior curvature of the lens due to contraction of the ciliary muscle.

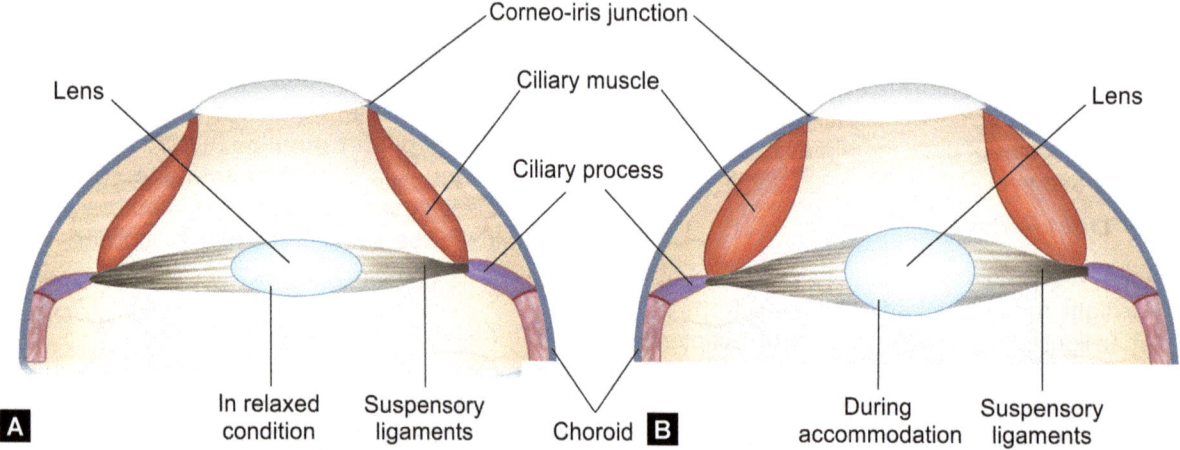

FIGURE 96.2: Accommodation. **A.** In relaxed condition; **B.** During accommodation.

2. Convergence of the eyeballs due to contraction of the medial recti.
3. Constriction of the pupil due to the contraction of constrictor pupillae of iris.

Thus, the accommodation reflex involves both skeletal muscle (medial recti) and smooth muscle (ciliary muscle and sphincter pupillae).

Pathway for Accommodation Reflex

Afferent pathway

Visual impulses from retina pass through the optic nerve, optic chiasma, optic tract, lateral geniculate body and optic radiation to visual cortex (area 17) of occipital lobe. From here, the association fibers carry the impulses to frontal lobe **(Fig. 96.3)**.

Center

Center for accommodation lies in **frontal eye field** (area 8) that is situated in the frontal lobe of cerebral cortex.

Efferent Pathway

1. *Efferent fibers to ciliary muscle and sphincter pupillae*

From area 8, the corticonuclear fibers pass via internal capsule to the **Edinger-Westphal nucleus** of III cranial nerve. From here, the preganglionic fibers pass through the III cranial nerve to the **ciliary ganglion**. Postganglionic fibers from ciliary ganglion pass via the **short ciliary nerves** and supply the ciliary muscle and the constrictor pupillae.

2. *Efferent fibers to medial rectus*

Some of the fibers from **frontal eye field** terminate in the somatic motor nucleus of oculomotor nerve. Fibers from this motor nucleus supply the medial rectus.

■ APPLIED PHYSIOLOGY

1. *Presbyopia*

Presbyopia is explained later in this chapter.

2. *Argyll Robertson Pupil*

Argyll Robertson pupil is a clinical condition in which the light reflex is lost but the accommodation reflex is present. It is due to lesion in pretectal nucleus or rostral portion of Edinger-Westphal nucleus. Argyll Robertson pupil is common in tertiary syphilis. It also occurs in diabetic and alcoholic neuropathy.

3. *Horner Syndrome*

Horner syndrome is an eye disorder caused by damage to cervical sympathetic nerve. Symptoms of Horner syndrome appear on the affected side.

Symptoms are:

i. **Ptosis** (drooping of upper eyelid).
ii. Swelling of lower eyelid.

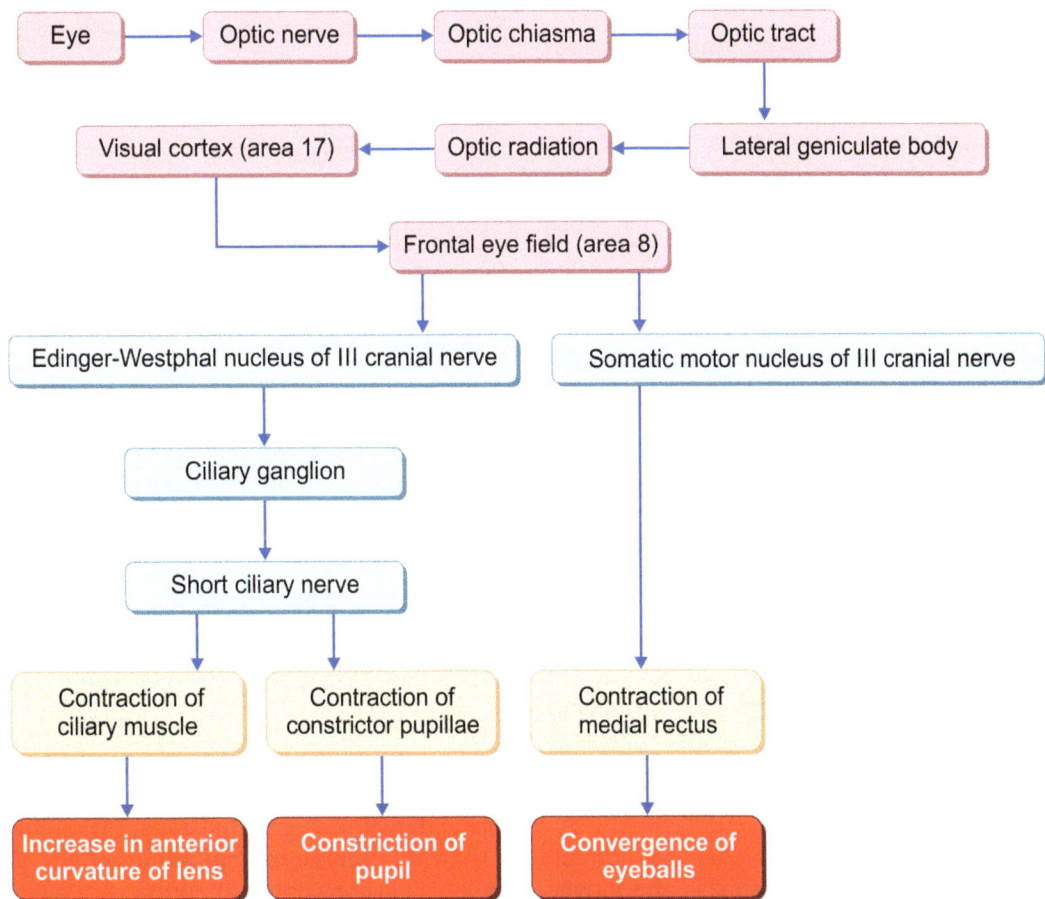

FIGURE 96.3: Pathway for accommodation reflex.

iii. **Miosis** or **myosis** (abnormal constriction of pupil).
iv. **Enophthalmos** (sinking of eyeball into its cavity).
v. Absence of sweating on affected side of the face.

■ REFRACTIVE ERRORS

Refractive error is defined as inability of the eye to focus the image of objects accurately on retina.

■ AMETROPIA

Emmetropia is the vision with lens having normal refractive power. And eye with normal refractive power is called **emmetropic eye**.

Any deviation in refractive power from normal condition resulting in inadequate focusing on retina is called **ametropia** and the eye is called **ametropic eye**. The defect is due to the change in shape of the eyeball.

Ametropia is of two types:
1. Hypermetropia.
2. Myopia.

1. Hypermetropia or Long Sightedness

Hypermetropia is the eye defect characterized by the inability to focus on near object. It is otherwise known as **long sightedness** because the person can see the distant objects clearly, but not the near objects. In this defect, the distant vision is normal, but the near vision is affected (metras = measure).

Causes of Hypermetropia

Hypermetropia is due to decreased anteroposterior diameter of the eyeball. So, even though the refractive power of the lens is normal, the light rays are not converged enough to form a clear image on retina, i.e. the light rays are brought to a focus **behind retina**. It causes a blurred image of near objects. Hypermetropia occurs in childhood, if the eyeballs fail to develop to the correct size. It is common in old age also.

Correction of Hypermetropia

Hypermetropia is corrected by using **biconvex lens**. Light rays are converged by convex lens before entering the eye **(Fig. 96.4)**.

2. Myopia or Short Sightedness

Myopia is the defect characterized by inability of the eye to focus on distant object. It is otherwise called **short sightedness**, because the person can see near objects clearly, but not the distant objects.

Normally, in emmetropia, the far point is infinite. In myopia, the near vision is normal, but the far point is not infinite, i.e. it is at definite distance **(Fig. 96.4 and Table 96.1)**. In extreme conditions, it may be only a few centimeters away from the eye (myo = half closed; ops = eye).

Causes of Myopia

In myopia, refractive power of the lens is usually normal. But, anteroposterior diameter of the eyeball is abnormally long. Therefore, the image is brought to a focus a little **in**

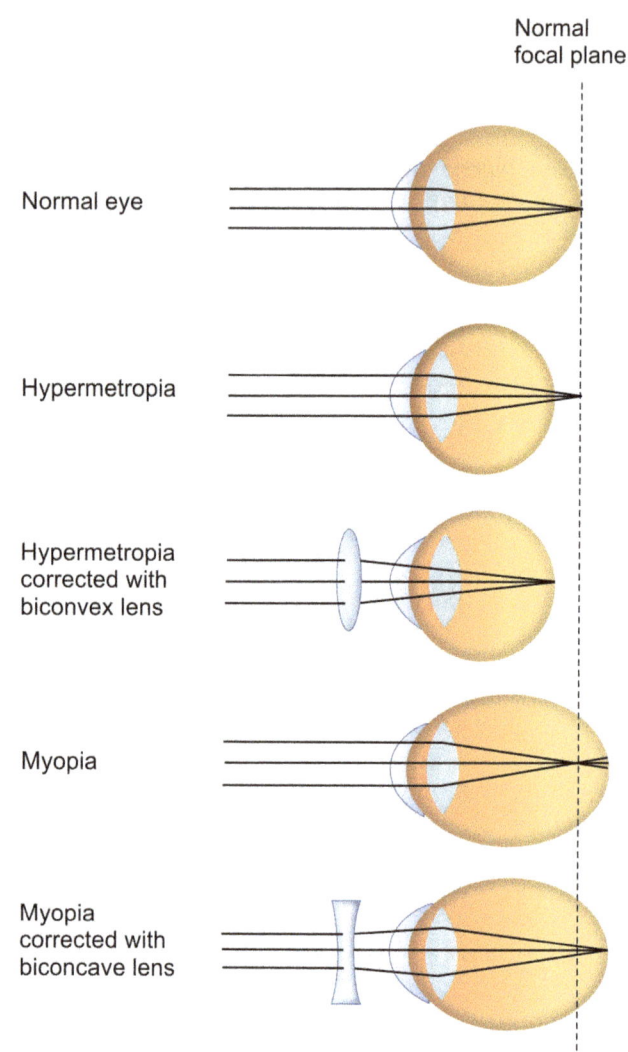

FIGURE 96.4: Refractive errors.

front of retina. In other words, refractory power of lens is too strong for the length of eyeball. The light rays, after coming to a focus, disperse again, so a blurred image is formed upon retina.

Correction of Myopia

In myopic eye, in order to form a clear image on the retina, light rays entering the eye must be divergent and not parallel. Thus, the myopic eye is corrected by using **biconcave lens**. Light rays are diverged by the concave lens before entering the eye **(Fig. 96.4)**.

■ ANISOMETROPIA

Anisometropia is the condition in which the two eyes have unequal **refractive power**. It is corrected by using different appropriate lens for each eye **(Table 96.1)**.

■ ASTIGMATISM

Astigmatism is the condition in which the light rays are not brought to a sharp point upon retina. It is the common optical defect present in all eyes. When it is moderate, it is known as **physiological astigmatism**. When it is well marked, it is considered abnormal. For example, the stars appear as small dots of light to a person with normal eye.

Chapter 96: Pupillary Reflexes, Refractive Errors and Color Vision

TABLE 96.1: Refractive errors.

Type of error	Cause	Correction
Hypermetropia	Decrease in anteroposterior diameter of the eyeball	Biconvex lens
Myopia	Increase in anteroposterior diameter of the eyeball	Biconcave lens
Anisometropia	Difference in refractive power of both eyes	Separate lens (biconcave or biconvex) for each eye as required
Astigmatism	Refractory power of lens is different in different meridians	
Regular astigmatism	Refractory power of lens is unequal in different meridians but uniform in one single meridian	Cylindrical lens
Irregular astigmatism	Refractory power of lens is unequal in different meridians as well as in different points in same meridian	
Presbyopia	Loss of elasticity in lens and weakness of ocular muscles due to old age	Biconvex lens

But in astigmatism, the stars appear as radiating short lines of light (a = not; stigma = point).

Cause of Astigmatism

Light rays pass through all meridians of a lens. In a normal eye, lens has approximately same curvature in all meridians. So, the light rays are refracted almost equally in all meridians and brought to a focus.

If the curvature is different in different meridians, vertical, horizontal and oblique, the refractive power is also different in different meridians. Meridian with greater curvature refracts the light rays more strongly than other meridians. So, these light rays are brought to a focus in front of the light rays, which pass through other meridians. Such irregularity of curvature of lens causes astigmatism.

Types of Astigmatism

1. **Regular Astigmatism**

In this type of astigmatism, the refractive power is unequal in different meridians because of alteration of curvature in one meridian. But it is uniform in all points throughout the affected meridian.

2. **Irregular Astigmatism**

Here, the refractive power is unequal not only in different meridians but it is also unequal in different points of same meridian.

Correction of Astigmatism

Astigmatism is corrected by using **cylindrical lens** having the convexity in the meridians corresponding to that of lens of eye having a lesser curvature, i.e. if the horizontal curvature of lens is less, the person should use cylindrical glass lens with the convexity in horizontal meridian.

PRESBYOPIA

Presbyopia is the condition characterized by progressive decrease in the ability of eyes to focus on near objects with age. It is due to the gradual reduction in the **amplitude of accommodation**. Presbyopia starts developing after middle age and progresses as the age advances (presbyos = old; ops = eye).

In presbyopia, the distant vision is unaffected. Only the near vision is affected. The near point is away from eye. In presbyopia, the anterior curvature of lens does not increase during near vision. So, the light rays from near objects are not brought to a focus on retina.

Causes of Presbyopia

1. Decreased elasticity of lens is because of the physical changes in lens and its capsule during old age. So, the anterior curvature is not increased during near vision.
2. Decreased convergence of eyeballs due to the concomitant weakness of ocular muscles in old age.

Correction of Presbyopia

Presbyopia is corrected by using **biconvex lens**.

COLOR VISION

VISIBLE SPECTRUM

Human eye can recognize about 150 different colors in the visible spectrum. Discrimination and appreciation of colors depend upon the ability of **cones** in retina.

Spectral Colors

When the sunlight or white light is passed through a glass **prism**, it is separated into series of colors called the **visible spectrum.** Colors which form the spectrum are called the **spectral colors**. Spectral colors are violet, indigo, blue, green, yellow, orange and red, (**VIBGYOR** or **ROYGBIV**).

In the spectrum, colors occupy the position according to their wavelengths. Wavelength is the distance between two identical points in the wave of light energy. Accordingly, violet has got the minimum wavelength of about 3,000 Å and red has got the maximum wavelength of about 8,000 Å.

Light rays shorter than violet are called the **ultraviolet rays**. And, light rays longer than red are called **infrared rays**. But, these two extraordinary types of rays do not evoke the sensation of vision.

Extra Spectral Colors

Extra spectral colors are the colors other than those present in visible spectrum. These colors are formed by the combination of two or more spectral colors. For example, purple is the combination of violet and red. Pink is the combination of red and white.

Primary Colors

Primary colors are those, which when combined together produce the white. Primary colors are **red**, **green** and **blue**. These three colors in equal proportion give white.

Complementary Colors

Complementary colors are the pair of two colors which produce white when mixed or combined in proper proportion. Examples of complementary colors are red and greenish blue; orange and cyan blue; yellow and indigo blue; violet and greenish yellow; and purple and green.

■ CONES AND COLOR VISION: YOUNG-HELMHOLTZ TRICHROMATIC THEORY

According to Young-Helmholtz theory, retina has three types of cones and each cone is supplied by a separate fiber of optic nerve. Each cone has its own photosensitive pigment and gives response to one of the primary colors namely, red, green and blue (Chapter 94).

Different color sensations are produced by the stimulation of various combinations of the three types of cones. White is perceived by equal stimulation of all three types of cones.

Color Sensitive Areas in Retina

Peripheral part of retina is devoid of cones. So, it is insensitive to color and gives sensation of white, black and gray only. Central portion of retina, fovea centralis has more cones so, it is more sensitive to color. In extrafoveal regions, cones are mingled with rods.

Retinal area sensitive to blue is largest and to green is smallest. Red comes next to blue and then comes yellow. All the color areas of retina are mapped out by using **perimeter**.

■ APPLIED PHYSIOLOGY: COLOR BLINDNESS

Color blindness is the failure to appreciate one or more colors. It is common in 8% of males and only in 0.4% of females, as mostly the color blindness is an inherited **sex-linked recessive character**. In addition to hereditary conditions, color blindness occurs due to acquired conditions also, such as ocular diseases or injury, or disease of retina.

Based on Young-Helmholtz trichromatic theory, color blindness is classified into three types:

1. Monochromatism.
2. Dichromatism.
3. Trichromatism.

1. Monochromatism

Monochromatism is the condition characterized by total inability to perceive color. It is also called **total color blindness** or **achromatopsia**. Monochromatism is very rare. Persons with monochromatism are called **monochromats**. The retina of monochromats is totally insensitive to color and they see the whole spectrum in only black, white and different shades of gray. So, their vision is similar to black and white photography.

2. Dichromatism

Dichromatism is the color blindness in which the subject can appreciate only two colors. Persons with this defect are called **dichromats**. They can match the entire spectrum of colors by only two primary colors because the receptors for third color are defective. Dichromatism is classified into three groups **(Fig. 96.5)**.

i. Protanopia

Protanopia is the type of dichromatism caused by the defect in the receptor of **first primary color**, i.e. **red**. So, the red color cannot be appreciated. The persons having protanopia are called **protanopes**. They use blue and green to match the colors. Thus, they confuse red with green.

ii. Deuteranopia

It is the dichromatism caused due to the defect in the receptor of the **second primary color**, i.e. **green**. **Deuteranopes** use blue and red colors and they cannot appreciate green color.

iii. Tritanopia

It is the dichromatism caused due to the defect in the receptor of **third primary color**, i.e. **blue**. **Tritanopes** use red and green colors and they cannot appreciate blue color.

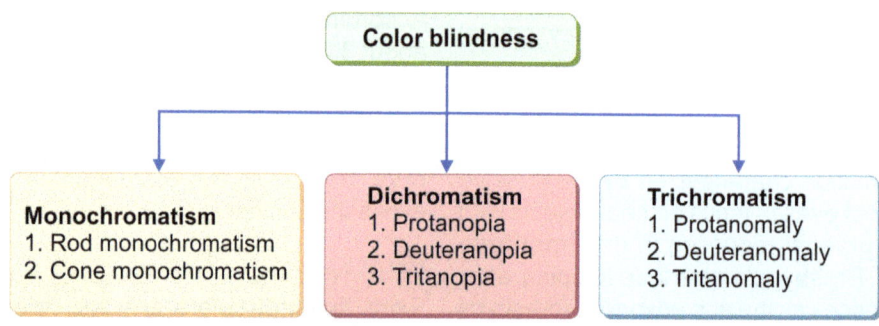

FIGURE 96.5: Color blindness.

3. Trichromatism

Trichromatism is the color blindness in which the intensity of one of the primary colors cannot be appreciated correctly though the affected persons are able to perceive all the three colors. Persons with this defect are called **trichromats**. Even the dark shades of one particular color look dull for them. Trichromatism is classified into three types.

i. Protanomaly

Protanomaly is the type of trichromatism in which the perception for **red** is weak. So, to appreciate the red color, the person requires more intensity of red than a normal person.

ii. Deuteranomaly

Deuteranomaly is the trichromatism in which the perception for **green** is weak.

iii. Tritanomaly

Tritanomaly the trichromatism with weak perception for **blue**.

■ TESTS FOR COLOR BLINDNESS

Color blindness is determined by using:

1. Ishihara's color charts.
2. Colored wool.
3. Edridge-Green lantern.

Chapter 97

Ear

CHAPTER OUTLINE

- EAR
- EXTERNAL EAR
  - AURICLE OR PINNA
  - EXTERNAL AUDITORY MEATUS
- MIDDLE EAR
  - AUDITORY OSSICLES
  - AUDITORY MUSCLES
  - EUSTACHIAN TUBE
- INTERNAL EAR
  - COCHLEA
  - COMPARTMENTS OF COCHLEA
  - ORGAN OF CORTI
  - AUDITORY RECEPTORS

■ EAR

Ear consists of cochlea, the sense organ for hearing and vestibular apparatus, the sense organ for equilibrium. Ear consists of three parts namely, external ear, middle ear and internal ear **(Fig. 97.1)**.

■ EXTERNAL EAR

External ear is formed by two parts:

1. Auricle or pinna.
2. External auditory meatus.

■ AURICLE OR PINNA

Auricle or pinna of the external ear consists of **fibrocartilaginous plate** covered by connective tissue and skin. This plate is characteristically folded and ridged. Skin covering this plate contains many fine hairs and sebaceous glands. On the posterior surface of auricles, many sweat glands are present. Depression of auricle, which forms the orifice of external auditory meatus, is called **concha**.

■ EXTERNAL AUDITORY MEATUS

External auditory meatus starts from the concha and extends inside as a slightly curved canal, with a length of about 55 mm.

External auditory meatus consists of two parts:

i. Outer Cartilaginous Part

Outer cartilaginous part is the initial part of external auditory meatus made up of cartilage. It is covered by

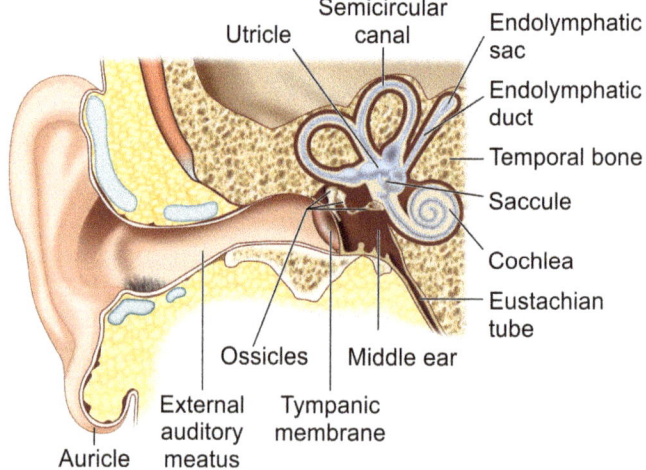

FIGURE 97.1: Diagram showing the structure of ear.

thick skin, which contains **stiff hairs**. These hairs prevent the entry of foreign particles. Large **sebaceous glands** and **ceruminous glands** are also present in the skin covering this portion. Secretions of sebaceous glands, ceruminous glands and desquamated epithelial cells form the **earwax**.

ii. Inner Bony Part

Inner part of the external auditory meatus is also covered by skin, which adheres closely to periosteum. Only sebaceous glands are present here. Skin covering this portion is continuous with cuticular layer of tympanic membrane.

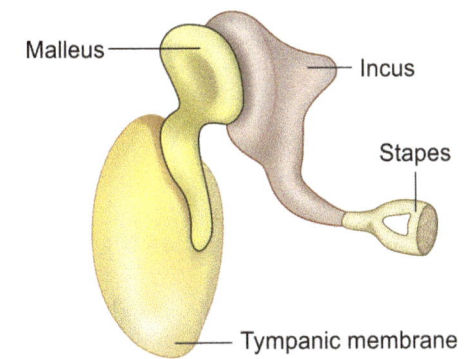

FIGURE 97.2: Tympanic membrane and auditory ossicles.

MIDDLE EAR

Middle ear or **tympanic cavity** is situated within the temporal bone. It is separated from external auditory meatus by a thin semitransparent membrane called **tympanic membrane (Fig. 97.2)**.

Middle ear consists of three structures:

1. Auditory ossicles.
2. Auditory muscles.
3. Eustachian tube.

AUDITORY OSSICLES

Auditory ossicles are the three **miniature bones**, which are arranged in the form of a chain extending across middle ear from **tympanic membrane** to **oval window**. Auditory ossicles are malleus, incus and stapes.

1. Malleus

Malleus or **hammer** has a handle, head and neck. Handle is otherwise known as **manubrium**. It is attached to the tympanic membrane. Head or capitulum articulates with the body of next bone incus.

2. Incus

Incus or **anvil** looks like a premolar tooth. It has a body, one long process and one short process. Anterior surface of the body articulates with head of malleus. The tip of the long process is like a knob, called **lenticular process** and it articulates with the next bone, stapes.

3. Stapes

Stapes or **stirrup**, is the **smallest bone** present in the body. It has a head, neck, anterior crus, posterior crus and a footplate. Head articulates with incus. **Footplate** fits into the oval window **(Fig. 99.1)**.

AUDITORY MUSCLES

Two skeletal muscles are attached to the ossicles:

1. Tensor Tympani

Tensor tympani muscle arises from cartilaginous portion of eustachian tube. Its tendon is inserted on manubrium of malleus which is in turn attached to tympanic membrane. It is supplied by mandibular division of **trigeminal nerve**.

Tensor tympani muscle pulls and keeps the tympanic membrane stretched constantly.

2. Stapedius

Stapedius is the **smallest skeletal muscle** in human body with a length of just over 1 mm. It arises from interior pyramid of tympanic cavity. Its tendon is inserted into the posterior surface of neck of stapes. It is supplied by branch of **facial nerve**.

Stapedius prevents excess movements of stapes. When it contracts, it pulls the neck of stapes backwards and reduces the movement of footplate against the fluid in cochlea.

Tympanic Reflex

Tympanic reflex is an **attenuation reflex** characterized by involuntary contraction of tensor tympani and stapedius muscles, in response to a **loud noise**.

When both the muscles contract, manubrium of malleus moves inward and stapes is pulled outward. These two actions result in stiffness of auditory ossicles, so that the transmission of sound is decreased.

Significance of tympanic reflex

i. Tympanic reflex protects the tympanic membrane from being ruptured by loud sound.
ii. It also prevents fixation of footplate of stapes, against oval window, during exposure to loud sound.
iii. Tympanic reflex helps to protect the cochlea from damaging effects of loud sounds. Contraction of tensor tympani and stapedius during exposure to loud sound develops stiffness of the auditory ossicles so that, the transmission of sound into cochlea is decreased.

EUSTACHIAN TUBE

Eustachian tube or the auditory tube connects the middle ear with posterior part of nose and forms the passage of air between middle ear and atmosphere. So, the pressure on both sides of tympanic membrane is equalized.

INTERNAL EAR

Internal ear or **labyrinth** is a membranous structure, enclosed by a **bony labyrinth** in petrous part of temporal bone. It consists of the sense organs of hearing and equilibrium. Sense organ for hearing is the **cochlea**. And, the sense organ for equilibrium is the **vestibular apparatus**. Vestibular apparatus is already explained in Chapter 88.

COCHLEA

Cochlea is a coiled structure like a snail's shell (cochlea = snail's shell).

Cochlea consists of two structures:

1. Central conical axis formed by spongy bone called **modiolus**.
2. Bony spiral canal, which winds around the modiolus.

Bony spiral canal makes two and a half turns, starting from the base of the cochlea and ends at the top (apex) of cochlea. End of the canal is called **cupula**. Base of modiolus forms the bottom of internal auditory meatus, through which cochlear nerve fibers pass and enter the modiolus. Thus, a section through the axis of cochlea reveals the central **bony pillar**, modiolus and **periotic or osseous canal**, which coils around the modiolus.

From modiolus, a bony ridge called **osseous spiral lamina** projects into the canal, winding around modiolus like the thread of a screw. Spiral lamina follows the spiral turns of cochlea and ends at the cupula in a hook-shaped process called **hamulus**.

■ COMPARTMENTS OF COCHLEA

Cochlea is divided into three compartments by two membranous partitions called **basilar membrane** and **vestibular membrane**.

Compartments of spiral canal of cochlea are:

1. Scala vestibuli.
2. Scala tympani.
3. Scala media.

All the three compartments are filled with fluid. Scala vestibuli and scala tympani contain **perilymph**. The scala media is filled with **endolymph**.

1. Scala Vestibuli

Scala vestibuli lies above the scala media. It arises from **oval window** which is closed by the **footplate of stapes**. It follows the osseous canal up to its apex. At the apex, it communicates with the scala tympani through a small canal called **helicotrema (Fig. 99.1)**.

2. Scala Tympani

It lies below the scala media. It is parallel to scala vestibuli and ends at the **round window**. The round window is closed by a strong thin membrane known as **secondary tympanic membrane**.

3. Scala Media

Scala media is otherwise called **cochlear duct**. It ends blindly at the apex and at the base of cochlea. The sensory part of cochlea called organ of Corti is situated on the upper surface of basilar membrane **(Fig. 97.3)**.

■ ORGAN OF CORTI

Organ of Corti is the receptor organ for hearing. It is the neuroepithelial structure in cochlea **(Fig. 97.4)**. It rests upon the lip of spiral lamina and the basilar membrane. It

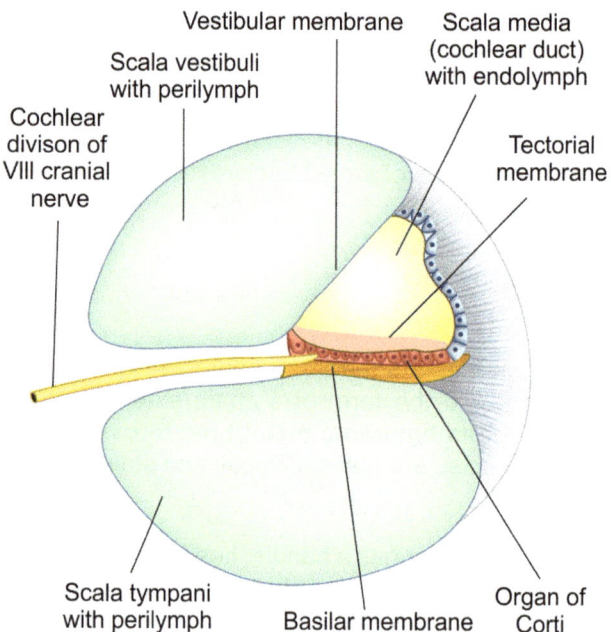

FIGURE 97.3: Cross-section of spiral canal of cochlea.

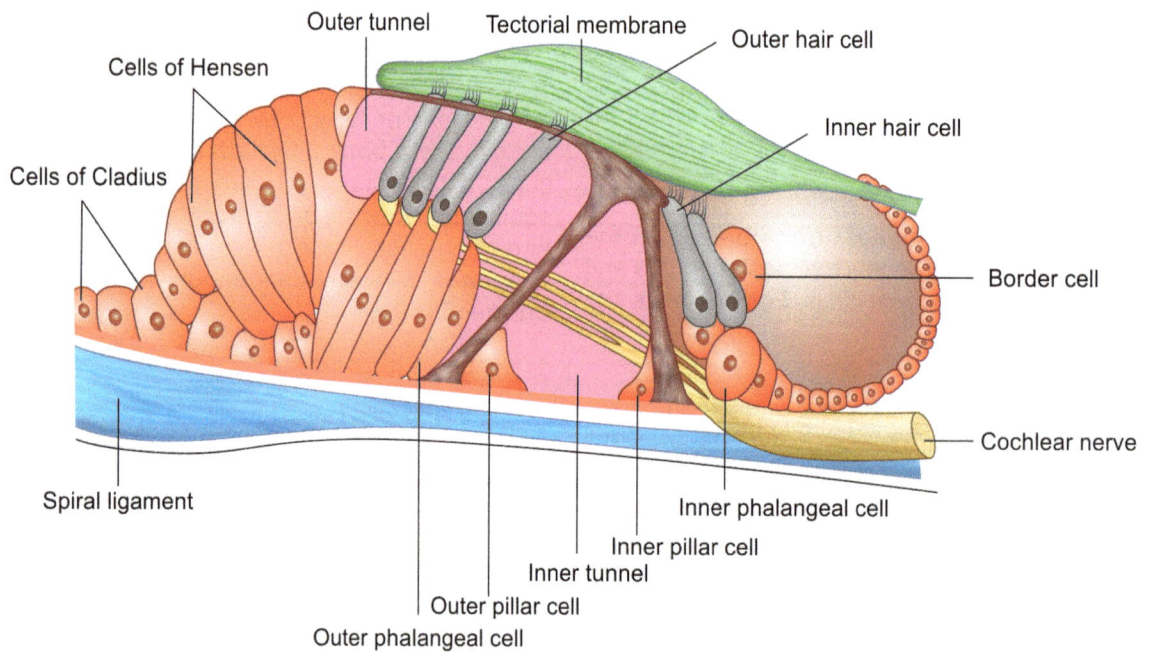

FIGURE 97.4: Organ of Corti.

extends throughout the cochlear duct, except for a short distance on either end. The roof of the organ of Corti is formed by gelatinous tectorial membrane.

Structure

Organ of Corti is made up of the auditory receptors called the **hair cells** and various **supporting cells**. All the cells of organ of Corti are arranged in order from center towards periphery of the cochlea.

Cells of organ of Corti:

1. Border cells.
2. Inner hair cells.
3. Inner phalangeal cells.
4. Inner pillar cells.
5. Outer pillar cells.
6. Outer phalangeal cells.
7. Outer hair cells.
8. Cells of Hensen.
9. Cells of Claudius.
10. Tectorial membrane and lamina reticularis.

■ AUDITORY RECEPTORS

Hair cells in organ of Corti are the receptors of the auditory sensation. The hair cells are of two types, outer hair cells and inner hair cells. Surface of the hair cell bears a **cuticular plate**. A number of short stiff hairs, called **stereocilia** arise from this cuticular plate. Each hair cell has about 100 stereocilia. One of the stereocilia is larger and it is called **kinocilium**. Stereocilia are in contact with the **tectorial membrane**. Sensory nerve fibers are distributed around the hair cells.

Chapter 98: Auditory Pathway

CHAPTER OUTLINE

- **AUDITORY PATHWAY**
  - RECEPTORS
  - FIRST ORDER NEURONS
  - SECOND ORDER NEURONS
- THIRD ORDER NEURONS
- SUBCORTICAL AUDITORY CENTERS
- CORTICAL AUDITORY CENTERS
- **APPLIED PHYSIOLOGY: EFFECT OF LESION**

■ AUDITORY PATHWAY

Fibers of auditory pathway pass through **cochlear division** of **vestibulocochlear nerve** (VIII cranial nerve). It is also known as **auditory nerve**.

■ RECEPTORS

Outer and inner **hair cells in organ of Corti** are the receptors of the auditory sensation (Chapter 97).

■ FIRST ORDER NEURONS

First order neurons of the auditory pathway are the **bipolar cells** of **spiral ganglion** situated in the modiolus of cochlea (Fig. 98.1).

Dendrites of the bipolar cells are distributed around the **hair cells** of organ of Corti. Their axons leave ear as cochlear nerve fibers and enter medulla oblongata. Immediately after entering the medulla oblongata, the fibers divide into two groups which end on ventral and dorsal **cochlear nuclei** of the same side in medulla oblongata.

■ SECOND ORDER NEURONS

Neurons of dorsal and ventral cochlear nuclei in the medulla oblongata form the second order neurons of auditory pathway.

Axons of the second order neurons run in four different directions:

1. First group of fibers cross the midline and run to the opposite side to form trapezoid body and go to the superior olivary nucleus.
2. Second group of the fibers terminate at the superior olivary nucleus of same side via trapezoid body of the same side.
3. Third group of fibers run in the lateral lemniscus of the same side and terminate in the nucleus of lateral lemniscus.
4. Fourth group of fibers cross the midline as intermediate trapezoid fibers and join the nucleus of lateral lemniscus of opposite side.

■ THIRD ORDER NEURONS

Third order neurons are in the **superior olivary nucleus** and **nucleus of lateral lemniscus**. Fibers from here end in medial geniculate body.

■ SUBCORTICAL AUDITORY CENTER

Medial geniculate body forms the subcortical auditory center. Fibers from medial geniculate body go to the temporal cortex, via internal capsule as **auditory radiation**.

Some fibers from medial geniculate body go to **inferior colliculus** of tectum in midbrain. These fibers are involved in reflex movement of head, in response to auditory stimuli.

■ CORTICAL AUDITORY CENTERS

Cortical auditory centers are in the **temporal lobe** of cerebral cortex (Chapter 87).

Auditory areas are:

1. **Primary auditory area**, which includes areas 41, and 42, and Wernicke's area.
2. **Secondary auditory area** or **auditopsychic area** or auditory association area, which includes area 22.

Functions of Cortical Auditory Centers

Cortical auditory centers are concerned with the perception of auditory impulses, analysis of pitch and intensity of sound and determination of source of sound.

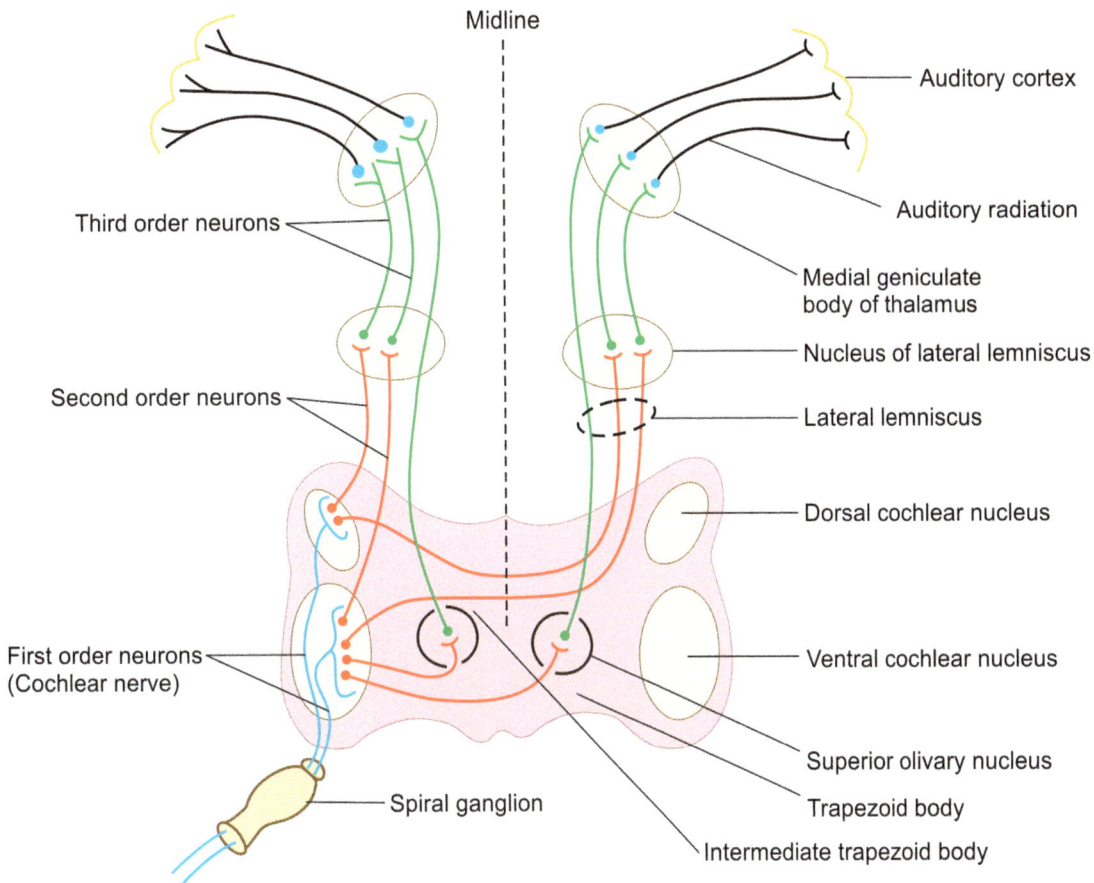

FIGURE 98.1: Auditory pathway.
Blue = First order neuron, Red = Second order neuron, Green = Third order neuron, Black = Auditory radiation.

Areas 41 and 42 are concerned with the perception of auditory impulses only. However, analysis and interpretation of sound are carried out by **Wernicke's area**, with the help of **area 22**.

APPLIED PHYSIOLOGY: EFFECT OF LESION

1. Lesion of cochlear nerve causes **deafness**.
2. Unilateral lesion of auditory pathway above the level of cochlear nuclei causes diminished hearing.
3. Degeneration of hair cells in organ of Corti leads to gradual loss of hearing. This is common in old age and the condition is called **presbycusis**.
4. Lesion in superior olivary nucleus results in poor localization of sound.

Mechanism of Hearing and Auditory Defects

CHAPTER OUTLINE

- PERCEPTION OF HEARING
- ROLE OF EXTERNAL EAR
- ROLE OF MIDDLE EAR
- ROLE OF INNER EAR
- ELECTRICAL EVENTS DURING PROCESS OF HEARING
- PROPERTIES OF SOUND
- APPRECIATION OF PITCH OF THE SOUND: THEORIES OF HEARING
- APPRECIATION OF LOUDNESS OF SOUND
- LOCALIZATION OF SOUND
- AUDITORY DEFECTS
- TESTS FOR HEARING

■ PERCEPTION OF HEARING

Sound waves travel through external auditory meatus and produce vibrations in the tympanic membrane. Vibrations from tympanic membrane travel through malleus and incus and reach the stapes resulting in the movement of stapes. Movements of stapes produce vibrations in the fluids of cochlea which stimulate the hair cells in the organ of Corti. This, in turn, causes the generation of action potential (auditory impulses) in the auditory nerve fibers. When the auditory impulses reach the cerebral cortex, perception of hearing occurs.

■ ROLE OF EXTERNAL EAR

External ear directs the sound waves towards the tympanic membrane. The sound waves produce pressure changes over the surface of **tympanic membrane**.

■ ROLE OF MIDDLE EAR

■ ROLE OF TYMPANIC MEMBRANE

Due to the pressure changes produced by sound waves, the tympanic membrane vibrates, i.e. it moves in and out of middle ear. Thus, the tympanic membrane acts as a **resonator** that produces the vibration of sound.

■ ROLE OF AUDITORY OSSICLES

Vibrations set up in tympanic membrane are transmitted through the malleus and incus and reach the stapes, causing to and fro movement of stapes against oval window and against the perilymph present in scala vestibuli of cochlea.

Impedance Matching

Impedance matching is the process, by which the tympanic membrane and auditory ossicles convert the sound energy into the mechanical vibrations in the fluid of internal ear with **minimum loss of energy** by matching the impedance offered by the fluid.

Impedance means obstruction or opposition to the passage of sound waves. When sound waves reach the inner ear, the fluid (perilymph) in cochlea offers impedance, i.e. the fluid resists the transmission of sound due to its own inertia. Tympanic membrane and the auditory ossicles effectively reduce the sound impedance which is called the impedance matching.

Significance of impedance matching

Impedance matching is the most important function of middle ear. Because of impedance matching the sound waves (stimuli) are transmitted to cochlea with minimum loss of intensity. Without impedance matching conductive deafness occurs.

Types of Conduction of Sound

Conduction of sound from external ear to internal ear through middle ear occurs by three routes:

1. Ossicular conduction.
2. Air conduction.
3. Bone conduction.

1. *Ossicular conduction*

Ossicular conduction is the conduction of sound waves through middle ear by auditory ossicles. This is the

Chapter 99: Mechanism of Hearing and Auditory Defects

normal way of conditions of the sound waves through middle ear.

2. Air conduction

Air conduction is the conduction of sound waves through air in middle ear. If the ossicular chain is broken, conduction occurs in an alternate route of air conduction. Air conduction is common in otosclerosis. **Otosclerosis** is the disease associated with fixation of stapes to oval window.

3. Bone conduction

It is the conduction of sound waves by **bones**. When middle ear is affected, bone conduction occurs. In this type of conduction, the sound waves are transmitted to cochlear fluid by the vibrations set up in the skull bones.

ROLE OF EUSTACHIAN TUBE

Eustachian tube is not concerned with hearing directly. However, it is responsible for **equalizing the pressure** on either side of tympanic membrane.

ROLE OF INNER EAR

TRAVELING WAVE

Movement of footplate of stapes against oval window causes movement of perilymph in scala vestibuli. This fluid does not move all the way from oval window toward round window through the helicotrema. It immediately hits the vestibular membrane near oval window and displaces the fluid in scala media **(Fig. 99.1)**. This causes bulging of basal portion of basilar membrane towards scala tympani.

Elastic tension developed in the bulged portion of basilar membrane initiates a wave called traveling wave. This wave travels along basilar membrane towards the helicotrema like arterial pulse wave.

Resonance Point

Resonance point is the part of **basilar membrane**, which is activated by traveling wave. In the beginning, each traveling wave is weak. While traveling through basilar membrane from base towards apex (helicotrema), the wave becomes stronger and at one point of basilar membrane, it becomes very strong and activates the basilar membrane. This part of basilar membrane which is activated by traveling wave is called resonance point. This resonance point of basilar membrane immediately vibrates back and forth. The traveling wave stops here and does not travel further.

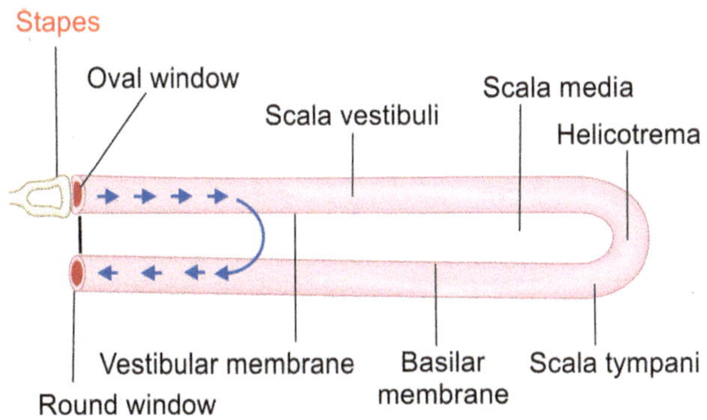

EXCITATION OF HAIR CELLS

Stereocilia of hair cells in organ of Corti are embedded in tectorial membrane (Chapter 97). Hair cells are tightly fixed by cuticular lamina reticularis and the pillar cells of Corti **(Fig. 97.4)**. When the traveling wave produces vibration of basilar membrane, all these structures move as a single unit. It causes movements of stereocilia leading to excitement of hair cells and generation of **receptor potential**.

ELECTRICAL EVENTS DURING PROCESS OF HEARING

SOUND TRANSDUCTION

Sound transduction or **auditory transduction** is a type of sensory transduction in the hair cell (receptor cells) in organ of Corti by which the **sound energy** is converted into **action potentials** in the auditory nerve fibers.

RECEPTOR POTENTIAL OR COCHLEAR MICROPHONIC POTENTIAL

Resting membrane potential in hair cells is about – 60 mV. Receptor potential or cochlear microphonic potential is the **mild depolarization** that is developed in the hair cells of cochlea when sound waves are transmitted to internal ear. Receptor potential in the hair cells causes generation of action potential in auditory nerve fibers.

PROPERTIES OF SOUND

Sound has two basic properties:

1. **Pitch** which depends upon the **frequency** of sound waves. Frequency of sound is expressed in hertz. The frequency of sound audible to human ear lies between 20 and 20,000 Hz or cycles/second. The range of greatest sensitivity lies between 2,000 and 3,000 Hz (cycles/second).
2. **Loudness** or **intensity** which depends upon the **amplitude** of sound waves. It is expressed in decibel (dB). The threshold intensity of sound wave is not constant. It varies in accordance to the frequency of the sound.

APPRECIATION OF PITCH OF THE SOUND: THEORIES OF HEARING

Though many theories are postulated to explain the mechanism by which the pitch of the sound is appreciated only few theories are accepted so far. Accepted theories are given below:

1. Place Theory

According to this theory, the nerve fibers from different portions (places) of organ of Corti on basilar membrane give response to sounds of different frequency. Accordingly, the corresponding nerve fiber from organ of Corti gives information to the brain regarding the portion of organ of Corti that is stimulated.

FIGURE 99.1: Diagrammatic representation of cochlea. Arrows show displacement of fluid.

2. Traveling Wave Theory

This theory explains how the traveling wave is generated in the basilar membrane. The generation, movement and disappearance of traveling wave are already described earlier in this chapter.

■ APPRECIATION OF LOUDNESS OF SOUND

Appreciation of loudness of sound depends upon the activities of auditory nerve fibers.

When the loudness of sound increases, it produces longer vibrations which spread over longer area of basilar membrane. This activates large number of hair cells and recruits many auditory nerve fibers. So, the frequency of action potential is also increased.

■ LOCALIZATION OF SOUND

Sound localization is the ability to detect the source from where the sound is produced or the direction through which the sound wave is traveling. It is important for survival and it helps to protect us from moving objects such as vehicles. Cerebral cortex and medial geniculate body are responsible for localization of sound.

■ AUDITORY DEFECTS

Auditory defects may be either partial or complete.

Auditory defects are of two types:

1. Conduction deafness.
2. Nerve deafness.

■ 1. CONDUCTION DEAFNESS

Conduction deafness occurs due to impairment in the transmission of sound waves in external ear or middle ear.

Causes of Conduction Deafness

i. Obstruction of external auditory meatus with dry wax or foreign bodies.
ii. Thickening of tympanic membrane due to infection.
iii. Perforation of tympanic membrane due to inequality of pressure on either side.
iv. **Otitis media** (inflammation of middle ear).
v. **Otosclerosis** (fixation of footplate of stapes against oval window).

■ 2. NERVE DEAFNESS

Nervous deafness is caused by damage of any structure in cochlea such as hair cell, organ of Corti, basilar membrane or cochlear duct or the lesion in auditory pathway.

Causes of Nerve Deafness

i. Degeneration of hair cells.
ii. Damage of cochlea by prolonged exposure to loud noise.
iii. Tumor affecting VIII cranial nerve.

■ TEST FOR HEARING

Various tests are available to assess the sensation of hearing. However, some simple tests called **bedside tests** are usually carried before doing routine (conventional) hearing tests.

■ BEDSIDE TESTS

Bedside tests are simple tests which are useful to know whether the hearing is normal or less.

Bedside tests are:

1. Whispering test.
2. Tickling of watch test.

1. Whispering Test

The examiner stands about 60 cm away from the subject at his side and whispers some words. If the subject is not able to hear the whisper, then hearing deficit is suspected.

2. Tickling of Watch Test

Wrist watch with tickling sound is kept near the ear of the subject. The subject suffering from hearing defects cannot hear the tickling sound of watch.

■ ROUTINE TESTS

Routine tests for hearing are of three types:

1. Rinne test.
2. Weber test.
3. Audiometry.

First two tests are done by using a tuning fork with high frequency. A tuning fork with 512 cycles per second is used. By turning fork tests, only the nature of auditory defect is determined. By audiometry, both nature and severity of auditory defects can be determined.

1. Rinne Test

Base of a vibrating tuning fork is placed on mastoid process, until the subject cannot feel the vibration and cannot hear the sound. When the subject does not hear the sound any more, the tuning fork is held in air in front of the ear of same side.

Normal person hears vibration in air even after the bone conduction ceases because, in normal conditions, air conduction via ossicles is better than bone conduction.

But in **conduction deafness**, the vibrations in air are not heard after cessation of bone conduction. Thus, in conduction deafness, the bone conduction is better than air conduction.

In **nerve deafness**, both air conduction and bone conduction are diminished or lost.

2. Weber Test

Base of a vibrating tuning fork is placed on the vertex of skull or the middle of forehead. Normal person hears the sound equally on both sides.

In unilateral **conduction deafness** (deafness in one ear), the sound is heard louder in diseased ear. In unaffected ear, there is a masking effect of environmental noise. So, the sound through bone conduction is not heard as clearly as on the affected side. In affected side, the sound is louder due to the absence of masking effect of environmental noise.

During unilateral **nerve deafness**, sound is heard louder in the normal ear.

3. Audiometry

Audiometry is the technique used to determine the nature and the severity of auditory defect. An electronic instrument called **audiometer** is used for this purpose. This instrument is capable of generating sound waves of different frequencies from lowest to highest. Intensity (loudness or volume) of sound also can be adjusted.

During the tests by audiometer, the subject's ability to hear the sounds with 8 to 10 different frequencies is observed and the hearing loss is determined for each frequency. By using these values, the audiogram is plotted.

Audiometer has an **electronic vibrator** also. It is used to test the bone conduction from mastoid process into the cochlea.

Chapter 100: Sensations of Taste and Smell

CHAPTER OUTLINE

- **TASTE SENSATION**
  - TASTE BUDS
  - PATHWAY FOR TASTE SENSATION
  - PRIMARY TASTE SENSATIONS
  - SUBSTANCES PRODUCING DIFFERENT TASTE SENSATIONS
  - TASTE TRANSDUCTION
  - FLAVOR
  - APPLIED PHYSIOLOGY: ABNORMALITIES OF TASTE SENSATION
- **OLFACTORY SENSATION**
  - OLFACTORY RECEPTORS
  - VOMERONASAL ORGAN
- OLFACTORY PATHWAY
- OLFACTORY TRANSDUCTION
- CLASSIFICATION OF ODOR
- THRESHOLD FOR OLFACTORY SENSATION
- ADAPTION
- ORTHONASAL OLFACTION AND RETRONASAL OLFACTION
- APPLIED PHYSIOLOGY: ABNORMALITIES OF OLFACTORY SENSATION

■ TASTE SENSATION

■ TASTE BUDS

Taste buds are the sense organs for **taste** or **gustatory sensation**. Taste buds are ovoid bodies with a diameter of 50 μ to 70 μ.

Situation of Taste Buds

Most of the taste buds are present on the **papillae of tongue**. Some taste buds are situated in the mucosa of epiglottis, palate, pharynx and proximal part of esophagus.

Types of papillae located on tongue:

1. Filiform papillae.
2. Fungiform papillae.
3. Circumvallate papillae.

1. Filiform papillae

Filiform papillae are small and conical shaped papillae situated over the **dorsum of tongue**. These papillae contain only few taste buds.

2. Fungiform papillae

Fungiform papillae are round in shape and are situated over the **anterior surface of tongue** near the tip. Numerous fungiform papillae are present. Number of taste buds in each is moderate (up to 10).

3. Circumvallate papillae

Circumvallate papillae are large structures arranged 'V' shape on the **posterior part of tongue** and are many in number. Each papilla contains many taste buds (up to 100).

Structure of Taste Bud

Taste bud is a bundle of taste receptor cells, with supporting cells embedded in the epithelial covering of the papillae **(Fig. 100.1)**. Each taste bud contains about 40 cells, which are the modified epithelial cells. The cells of taste bud are divided into four groups:

Types of cells in taste bud

1. Type I cells or sustentacular cells (supporting cells).
2. Type II cells (receptor cells).
3. Type III cells (receptor cells).
4. Type IV cells or basal cells (supporting cells).

Type I cells and type IV cells are supporting cells. Type II cells and type III cells are the **taste receptor** cells. Type I, II and III cells have projections called microvilli.

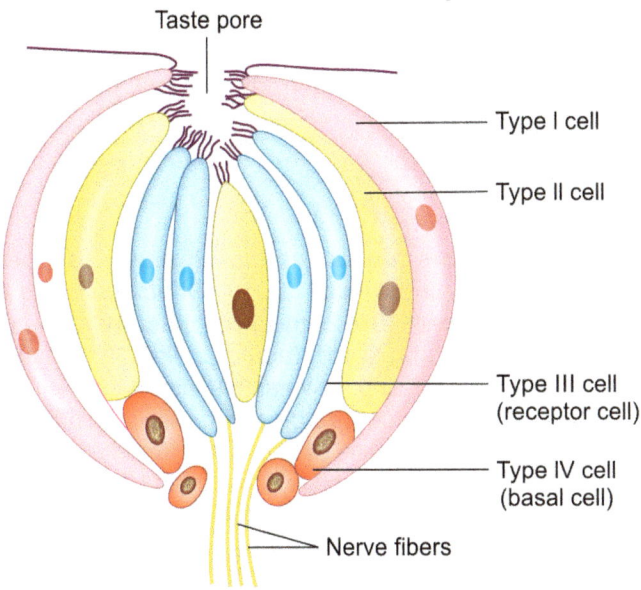

FIGURE 100.1: Taste bud.

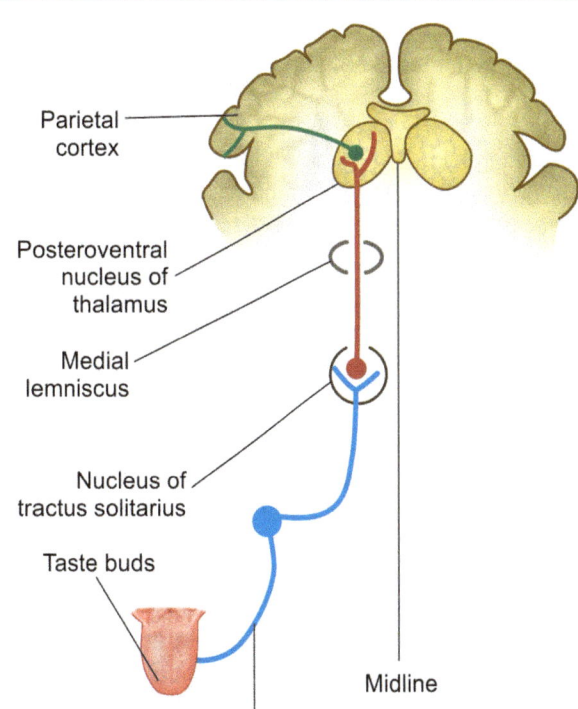

FIGURE 100.2: Pathway for taste sensation.

Microvilli project into an opening in the epithelium covering the tongue. The opening is called **taste pore**. All the cells of taste bud are surrounded by epithelial cells.

■ PATHWAY FOR TASTE SENSATION

Receptors

Receptors for taste sensation are the **type II and III cells** of taste buds. Each taste bud is innervated by about 50 sensory nerve fibers and each nerve fiber supplies at least 5 taste buds.

First Order Neuron

First order neurons of taste pathway are in the nuclei of three different cranial nerves, situated in medulla oblongata. Dendrites of the neurons are distributed to the taste buds. After arising from taste buds, the fibers reach the cranial nerve nuclei by running along the following nerves **(Fig. 100.2)**:

1. **Chorda tympani fibers** of facial nerve, which run from anterior two-third of tongue.
2. **Glossopharyngeal nerve fibers**, which run from posterior one-third of the tongue.
3. **Vagal fibers**, which run from taste buds in other regions.

Axons of the first order neurons run together in medulla oblongata and terminate in the nucleus of tractus solitarius.

Second Order Neuron

Second order neurons are in the **nucleus of tractus solitarius**. Axons of the second order neurons run through medial lemniscus and terminate in posteroventral nucleus of thalamus.

Third Order Neuron

Third order neurons are in the **posteroventral nucleus** of thalamus. Axons from the third order neurons project into cerebral cortex.

Taste Center

Center for taste sensation is in the **opercular insular cortex** (lower part of postcentral gyrus) in parietal lobe of cerebral cortex.

■ PRIMARY TASTE SENSATIONS

Primary or fundamental taste sensations are divided into five types:

1. Sweet.
2. Salt.
3. Sour.
4. Bitter.
5. Umami.

Man can perceive more than 100 different tastes. Other taste sensations are just the combination of two or more primary sensations.

Combination of Taste Sensation with Other Sensations

Sometimes, taste sensation combines with other sensations to give rise to a different sensation. For example, combination of taste, smell and touch senses, gives rise to **sensation of flavor**. Combination of taste with pain gives rise to **sensation of ginger**.

■ SUBSTANCES PRODUCING DIFFERENT TASTE SENSATIONS

1. Sweet Taste

Sweet taste is produced mainly by organic substances like monosaccharides, polysaccharides, glycerol, alcohol, aldehydes, ketones and chloroform. Inorganic substances producing sweet taste sensations are lead and beryllium.

2. Salt Taste

Salt taste is produced by chlorides of sodium, potassium and ammonium, nitrates of sodium and potassium. Some sulfates, bromides and iodides also produce salt taste.

3. Sour Taste

Sour taste is produced because of hydrogen ions in acids and acid salts.

4. Bitter Taste

Bitter taste is produced by organic substances like quinine, strychnine, morphine, glucosides, picric acid and bile salts, and inorganic substances like salts of calcium, magnesium and ammonium.

5. Umami

Umami is the recently recognized taste sensation. Umami is a Japanese word meaning 'delicious'. Receptors of this taste sensation respond to monosodium glutamate which is a common ingredient in Asian food.

Threshold for Taste Sensations

Sweet taste sugar	: 1 in 200 dilution
Salt taste sodium chloride	: 1 in 400 dilution
Sour taste hydrochloric acid	: 1 in 15,000 dilution
Bitter taste quinine	: 1 in 20,00,000 dilution

Bitter taste has very low threshold and sweet taste has a high threshold. Threshold for umami is not known.

TASTE TRANSDUCTION

Taste transduction is the process in taste receptors by which **chemical energy** is converted into **electrical energy** (action potentials) in the taste nerve fibers. Taste receptors **chemoreceptors**, which are stimulated by substances dissolved in mouth by saliva. The dissolved substances act on microvilli of taste receptors exposed in the taste pore. It causes development of receptor potential in the receptor cells. This in turn, is responsible for the generation of action potential in the sensory neurons.

FLAVOR

Flavor of food is the combination of two chemical sensations, namely taste and smell sensations.

Taste of the food is detected by the receptors in taste buds and the information is sent to brain. Smell of the food is detected by olfactory receptors in nose and the information is sent to brain. Ultimately, both taste and smell sensations combine and allow us to detect the flavors of food.

Retronasal olfaction is linked with flavor of the food (see below).

APPLIED PHYSIOLOGY: ABNORMALITIES OF TASTE SENSATION

1. *Ageusia:* Loss of taste sensation.
2. *Hypogeusia:* Decrease in the taste sensation.
3. *Taste blindness:* Inability to recognize substances by taste due to genetic disorder.
4. *Dysgeusia:* Disturbance in the taste sensation like hallucinations of taste.

OLFACTORY SENSATION

OLFACTORY RECEPTORS

Olfactory receptors are situated in **olfactory mucous membrane** that lines nasal cavity. Olfactory mucous membrane consists of 10 to 20 million of **olfactory receptor cells** supported by the **sustentacular cells**. Mucosa also contains mucus secreting Bowman glands.

Olfactory receptor cell is a **bipolar neuron**. Dendrite of this neuron is short. Expanded end of the dendrite is called **olfactory rod**. From the rod, about 10 to 12 cilia arise. **Cilia** are nonmyelinated with a length of 2 μ and a diameter of 0.1 μ. The cilia project to the surface of olfactory mucous membrane **(Fig. 100.3)**.

Mucus secreted by Bowman's glands continuously lines the olfactory mucosa. The mucus contains some proteins, which increase the actions of odoriferous substances on receptor cells.

VOMERONASAL ORGAN

Vomeronasal organ is an **accessory olfactory organ** found in many animals including mammals. It is enclosed in a cartilaginous capsule, which opens into the base of nasal cavity.

Olfactory receptors of this organ are sensitive to nonvolatile substances such as scents and **pheromones**. Vomeronasal organ helps the animals to detect even the trace quantities of chemicals. Impulses from this organ are sent to amygdala and hypothalamus via accessory olfactory bulb.

Vomeronasal Organ in Human Beings

In human beings, the vomeronasal organ was considered as vestigial or non-functional. Recently, it is claimed that vomeronasal organ is present in the form of **vomeronasal pits** on the anterior part of **nasal septum**. It is not known whether it is having olfactory function or not.

Receptors of vomeronasal pit detect human **pheromones** or **vomeropherins**, at a very low concentration in air. Refer Chapter 41 for details of pheromones. The subconscious detection of odorless chemical messengers in air is considered as the **sixth sense in human beings**.

OLFACTORY PATHWAY

Axons of the **bipolar olfactory receptors** pierce the **cribriform plate** of ethmoid bone and reach **the olfactory bulb**. Here, the axons synapse with dendrites of **mitral cells**. Different groups of these synapses form globular structures called **olfactory glomeruli**. Axons of mitral cells leave the olfactory bulb and form **olfactory tract**. Olfactory tract runs backwards and ends in **olfactory cortex**.

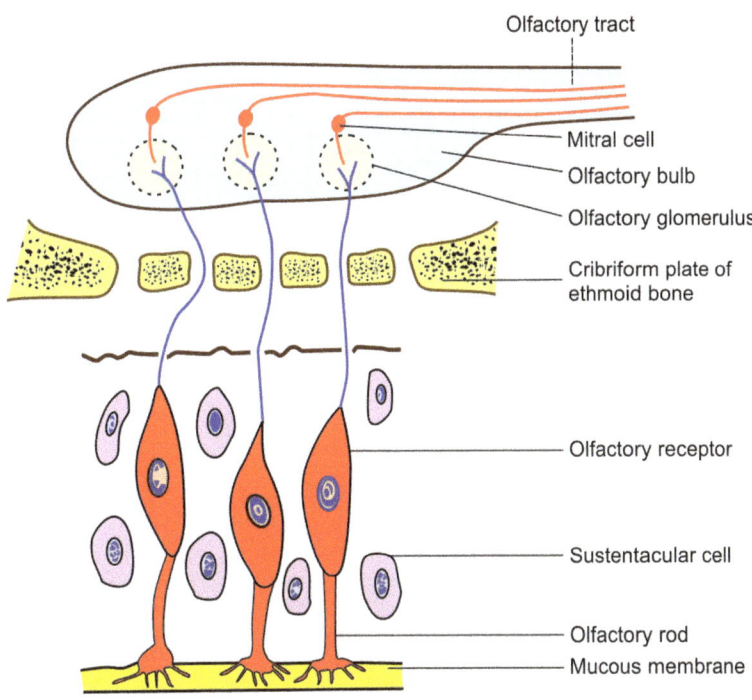

FIGURE 100.3: Olfactory mucous membrane and pathway for olfactory sensation.

Olfactory cortex includes the structures, which form a part of limbic system. These structures are anterior olfactory nucleus, prepyriform cortex, olfactory tubercle and amygdala.

■ OLFACTORY TRANSDUCTION

Olfactory transduction is the process in olfactory receptors by which **chemical energy** is converted into **electrical energy** (action potentials) in olfactory nerve fibers. Odoriferous substance stimulates the olfactory receptors, only if it dissolves in mucus, covering the olfactory mucus membrane. Molecules of dissolved substance, bind with receptor proteins in the cilia and form substance-receptor complex. Substance-receptor complex activates adenyl cyclase that causes the formation of cyclic AMP. Cyclic AMP in turn, causes opening of sodium channels, leading to influx of sodium and generation of receptor potential.

Receptor potential causes generation of action potential in the axon of bipolar neuron.

■ CLASSIFICATION OF ODOR

Odor is classified into various types. Each type is produced by different substance.

Substances Producing Different Types of Odor

1. *Aromatic or resinous odor:* Camphor, lavender, clove and bitter almonds.
2. *Ambrosial odor:* Musk.
3. *Burning odor:* Burning feathers, tobacco, roasted coffee and meat.
4. *Ethereal odor:* Fruits, ethers and beeswax.
5. *Fragrant or balsamic odor:* Flowers and perfumes.
6. *Garlic odor:* Garlic, onion and sulfur.
7. *Goat odor:* Caproic acid and sweet cheese.
8. *Nauseating odor:* Decayed vegetables and feces.
9. *Repulsive odor:* Bed bug.

■ THRESHOLD OLFACTION FOR OLFACTORY SENSATION

Ethyl ether	: 5.8 mg/L of air
Chloroform	: 3.3 mg/L of air
Peppermint oil	: 0.02 mg/L of air
Butyric acid	: 0.009 mg/L of air
Artificial musk	: 0.00004 mg/L of air
Methyl mercaptan	: 0.0000004 mg/L of air

Thus, the methyl mercaptan produces olfactory sensation even at a low concentration of 0.0000004 mg/L of air.

■ ADAPTATION

Olfactory receptors are phasic receptors and adapt very rapidly. Within one second, the adaptation occurs up to 50%.

■ ORTHONASAL OLFACTION AND RETRONASAL OLFACTION

Perception of smell occurs by two ways. One is via orthonasal olfaction and the other one is via retronasal olfaction.

Orthonasal Olfaction

Orthonasal olfaction is the **perception of smell** by means of sniffing into the **nose**. In this type of olfaction, the odor molecules pass through nostrils, reach the olfactory mucus membrane and stimulate the olfactory receptors.

Retronasal Olfaction

Retronasal olfaction is the **perception of odor** originating from **mouth** during eating or drinking. While chewing the food or while drinking, some of the odor molecules gently pass through the passage behind uvula, reach the nasal cavity and stimulate the olfactory receptors.

Retronasal olfaction is commonly linked with **flavor** of the food. Flavor is a combined sense which involves sensation of taste and sensation of smell.

■ APPLIED PHYSIOLOGY: ABNORMALITIES OF OLFACTORY SENSATION

1. *Anosmia:* Total loss of sensation of smell.
2. *Hyposmia:* Reduced ability to recognize and to detect any odor.
3. *Hyperosmia or olfactory hyperesthesia:* Increased or exaggerated olfactory sensation.

MODEL QUESTIONS IN SPECIAL SENSES

■ LONG QUESTIONS

1. Draw a diagram of visual pathway and explain it. Add note on hemianopia.
2. Explain the auditory pathway with suitable diagram. Add a note on auditory defects.
3. Explain the mechanism of hearing.

■ SHORT QUESTIONS

1. Retina.
2. Ocular muscles
3. Ocular movements.
4. Intraocular pressure.
5. Fundus oculi.
6. Lens of eye.
7. Visual receptors
8. Phototransduction.
9. Rhodopsin.
10. Dark adaptation.
11. Light adaptation.
12. Rhodopsin
13. Effects of lesion in optic pathway.
14. Light reflex and its pathway.
15. Accommodation reflex and its pathway.
16. Color blindness.
17. Refractive errors.
18. Auditory ossicles and auditory muscles.
19. Cochlea/Organ of Corti.
20. Role of middle ear in hearing (functions of middle ear).
21. Traveling wave.
22. Auditory defects.
23. Taste buds.
24. Taste pathway.
25. Olfactory pathway.

■ VERY SHORT ANSWER QUESTIONS

1. Lacrimal gland and tear.
2. Ciliary body.
3. Iris.
4. Blind spot.
5. Vitreous humor/aqueous humor
6. Cataract.
7. Photosensitive pigments in rod cells and cone cells.
8. Night blindness or nyctalopia.
9. ERG.
10. Acuity of vision and tests for acuity.
11. Divisions of visual field and mapping of visual field.
12. Corresponding retinal point and diplopia.
13. Subcortical and cortical centers for visual sensation.
14. Anopia and hemianopia.
15. Ciliospinal reflex.
16. Adjustments in eyeball during accommodation.
17. Young-Helmholtz theory.
18. Argyll Robertson pupil.
19. Horner syndrome.
20. Spectral colors, primary colors and complementary colors.
21. Monochromatism/dichromatism/trichromatism.
22. Myopia/hypermetropia/astigmatism.
23. Presbyopia.
24. Tympanic membrane.
25. Tympanic reflex.
26. Compartments and membranes of cochlea.
27. Subcortical and cortical centers for auditory sensation.
28. Effect of lesion of auditory pathway.
29. Types of conduction through middle ear.
30. Impedance matching.
31. Conduction deafness
32. Nerve deafness.
33. Primary taste sensations.
34. Abnormalities of taste sensation.
35. Flavor.
36. Substances producing different odor.
37. Orthonasal and retronasal olfaction.
38. Abnormalities of olfactory sensation.

Index

Page numbers followed by *b* refer to box, *f* refer to figure, and *t* refer to table.

A

Abdominal pain 123, 370
   severe 129
Abducens nerve 480
ABO group
   blood 69, 70*t*
   determination of 70
   incompatibility 71
   system 69
Abortion 271
Abrupt apnea, causes of 364
Absolute refractory period 92, 283, 383
Absorptive function 3, 133, 140, 141, 185
Accessory digestive organs 109, 110
Accessory olfactory 510
Accessory sex organs 239, 240, 249, 469
   development of 243
Acclimatization 367
Accommodation 383, 491, 492, 492*f*
Accommodation reflex 492
   pathway for 493, 493*f*
Acetoacetate 219
Acetone breath odor 222
Acetylcholine 97, 100, 101, 107, 115, 194, 236, 303, 307, 391, 471
   action of 101, 236
   depletion of 392
   destruction of 102, 236
   exhaustion of 91
   rapid destruction of 102
   receptor complex 101
   release of 101
   source of secretion of 236
   synthesis of 100
Achlorhydria 123
Achromatopsia 496
Acid
   hydroxylases 5
   neutralization of 140
Acid-base balance 170
   maintenance of 150
   regulation of 30, 32, 336
Acid-base status, disturbances of 171
Acidophilic cells 196
Acidosis 144, 171, 222
Acinar cells 125
Acini 114*f*
Acne 183
   development of 244
   vulgaris 183
Acquired immune deficiency syndrome 59
Acquired immunity 54
   types of 54
Acquired reflex 396, 462
Acromegalic face 202
Acromegalic gigantism 202
Acromegaly 201, 202*f*
   causes of 202
   signs of 202
   symptoms of 202

Acromicria 203
Acrosome 245
Actin
   filament 86
      part of 87*f*
   molecule 87
Activin 243
Actomyosin complex 96
   formation of 98
Acute heart failure 326
   signs of 327
   symptoms of 327
Adaptation 383, 389, 511
Addison's anemia 48
Addison's disease 229
Addisonian crisis 229
Adduction 481
Adenine 8, 9
Adenohypophysis 196
Adenosine 107, 162, 309
   diphosphate 17, 63, 97, 98
   triphosphate 87, 97, 98
Adherens junction 12
Adhesiveness 61
Adipocytes 427
Adipose tissue 237
   cell of 427
Adrenal cortex 156, 224, 250, 251, 264
   control of 426
   disorders of 228, 229*b*
   functional histology of 224
   hyperactivity of 228
   hypoactivity of 229
   layers of 225*t*
Adrenal crisis 229
Adrenal gland 224*f*
   functional anatomy of 224
Adrenal hyperplasia 230
Adrenal insufficiency 229
Adrenal medulla 224, 231
   control of 426
   functional histology of 231
Adrenal sex hormones 227
Adrenal virilism 229
Adrenaline 107, 221, 231, 309, 471
   actions of 231
   apnea 232
   secretion of 232
Adrenergic nerve fibers 382
Adrenergic receptors 231
Adrenocortical hormones 224
Adrenocorticotropic hormone 156, 193, 197, 199, 426
Adrenogenital syndrome 229
Adult hemoglobin 41
Adult respiratory distress syndrome 339
Aerobic exercise 328, 329
Aerobic metabolism 329
Afferent arteriole 151, 158
   constriction of 162
Afferent fibers 143
Afferent nerve 395
   fibers 381, 381*b*

Afferent neurons 379
Afferent pathway 357, 491, 493
Afferent-efferent circuit 431
Ageusia 510
Agglutination 58, 61, 70
Agglutinins 69
Aggregation 61
Agranular cells 155
   endoplasmic reticulum 3
Agranulocytes 49
Air 329
   conduction 505
   enters the spirometer 344*f*
   sickness 144
   volume of 342
   wasted 348
Akinesia 435
Alanine 171
   transaminase 135
Alcoholic intoxication 362, 462
Aldosterone 31, 163, 170, 225, 309
   antagonists 176
   escape 225
   inhibit action of 176
   secretion, regulation of 226*f*
Alkaline 259
   phosphatase 133, 135
   urine 362
Alkalosis 172
Allocortex 437
All-or-none law 283, 283*f*, 383
   causes for 283
Alpha motor neurons 414, 449
Alpha rhythm 454
Alpha-adrenergic receptors 231
Alpha-motor neurons, activation of 440
Alveolar air 349
Alveolar cells 335
Alveolar ducts 335
Alveolar macrophages 52
Alveolar sac 335
Alveolar ventilation 347
Alveoli 335
Alzheimer disease 461, 462
Amacrine cells 236, 470
Ambrosial odor 511
Ameboid movement 51
Amelognosia 425
Amenorrhea 48, 208
Ametropia 494
Amino acid 29, 163, 197, 392
   reabsorption of 165
   role of 220
   tyrosine 182, 231
Ammonia 171*f*
   mechanism 171
Ammonium, acetoacetate 171
Amnesia 461
Ampulla 451
   of Vater 125, 129, 131
Amylase test 129
Amylolytic enzyme 115, 127, 138
Anacrotic limb 313
Anacrotic pulse 315

Anaerobic exercise 328, 329
Anaerobic metabolism 329
Anal canal 140
Anal sphincter, internal 110, 146
Analgesia 422
   system 420
Analgesic pathway 421, 421*f*
   mechanism of 421
   nerve fibers of 421
Anaphylactic shock 51, 325
Anarthria 463
Anastomosis 278
Anchoring junction 11, 12
Androgen 243
   binding protein 240
Androstenedione 228
Anelectrotonic potentials 382
Anemia 31, 35, 44, 46-48, 326
   classification of 46
   etiological classification of 47*t*
   severe 72
   signs of 48
   symptoms of 48
Anemic hypoxia 361
Angina pectoris 318
Angiotensin 107, 156, 157, 162, 163, 308, 309
   actions of 156, 308
   converting enzyme 156, 308
   secretion of 336
Angiotensinases 156
Angiotensinogen 156, 237
Anisometropia 494
Ankle clonus 398
Anopia 488
Anorexia 123, 124
Anosmia 429, 512
Anovulatory cycle 261, 270
Ansiform lobe 430
Antagonistic muscles 399
Anterior gray
   commissure 401
   horn 401, 402
      cells 91
      nuclei in 401
Anterograde amnesia 461
Antibody 57, 70*t*
   actions of 58
   direct actions of 58
   functions, types of 58
   molecule, structure of 58*f*
   production of 57
   structure of 57
Anticoagulant 65
   function 336
Anticodon 9
Antidiuretic hormone 31, 107, 156, 163, 164, 166, 193, 199, 200, 218
   mechanism of action of 164
Antidromic vasodilator fibers 307
Antiemetic drugs 453
Antigen 56, 70*t*
   presentation of 56, 57
Antigenic materials 56

Antigen-presenting cell 56, 56f, 57, 335, 336
   role of 56, 57
Antigravity reflexes 396
Anti-inflammatory effects 227
Antiinsulin hormones 220
Antiperistalsis 144
Antiseptic action 133
Antiserum 70
Antrum 117
Anuria 169
Aortic area 291
Aortic baroreceptors 303
Aortic body 304
Aortic nerve 303, 304
Aortic pressure 288
Aortic regurgitation 315
Aphasia 463
   head's classification of 463
Aplastic anemia 46-48
Apnea 336, 360
Apneic period 363
Apocrine glands 184, 184t
   secretory activity of 184
Apoferritin 34
Apoptosis 6, 10
Appendicitis 141
Aptyalism 116
Aquaporins 164, 200
Aqueductus Sylvius 464
Aqueous humor 479
Arachidonic acid 235, 236
Arachnoid 465
   mater 400
   villi, blockage of 467
Archicerebellum 431
Archicortex 437
Archicortical structures 444
Arcuate artery 158
Arcuate fibers, internal 407
Areola 184
Argentaffin cells 137, 138
Argyll Robertson pupil 493
Aromatic odor 511
Arrhythmia 292, 295, 326
Arterial blood pressure 207, 305, 306, 306t, 307
   hormone regulating of 309
   mean 305
   measurement of 309
   regulation of 306-309
   variations of 305
Arterial blood, gases in 353t
Arterial pulse 313
   abnormal 315
   tracing 313
Arterial system 278
Arterioles 321
Arteriosclerosis 210, 306
Arteriovenous shunt 320
Artificial immunization, passive 59
Artificial respiration 371
   Holger-Nielsen method of 372f
   mouth-to-mouth method of 372f
Ascorbic acid 163
Aspartate aminotransferase 135
Asphyxia, effects of 363
Aspiration, vacuum 271
Asplenia 76
Astereognosis 408, 424
Asthenia 222
Asthma 345
Astigmatism 494
   causes of 495
   correction of 495
   types of 495
Astrocytes 385, 466
Astronauts 368

Ataxia 424
   posterior column 408
Atelectasis 365
Atherosclerosis 175, 210, 306, 318
Atherosclerotic plaque 318
Athetoid hand 425
Athetosis 425, 436
Atmospheric air 351
Atmospheric pressure 362
Atmospheric temperature 31
Atonia 433
Atonic bladder 181
Atretic follicles 248
Atrial complex 294
Atrial diastole 285
Atrial fibrillation 296, 297, 299, 315
Atrial flutter 296, 297
Atrial gallop 290
Atrial musculature 297
Atrial natriuretic
   factor 163
   peptide, actions of 235
Atrial reflex, right 304
Atrial systole 285, 290
Atrioventricular block 296
Atrioventricular node 297
Atrioventricular valves 277
   closure of 289
Atropine 471
Attenuation reflex 499
Attitude 433
Attitudinal reflexes 449, 450
Audiometer 507
Auditopsychic area 442, 502
Auditory area, secondary 442, 463, 502
Auditory defects 506
Auditory hallucinations 443
Auditory impulses 504
Auditory muscles 499
Auditory nerve 502
Auditory ossicles 499, 499f
   role of 504
Auditory pathway 502, 503f
Auditory radiation 502, 503f
Auditory receptors 501
Auditory sensation, interpretation of 463
Auditory transduction 505
Auerbach's plexus, functions of 110
Augmented limb leads 293
Auricle 498
Auscultation areas 290, 291f
Auscultatory method 310
Autoantibodies 59
Autoantigens 56, 59
Autocrine messengers 191
Autoimmune disease 31, 59, 221
Autoimmunity 59
Autologous blood transfusion 73
Automatic bladder 181
Automatic blood pressure instrument 310
Autonomic functions, regulation of 444
Autonomic nerve 480
   fibers 219, 381, 396
   role of 219
Autonomic nervous system 378, 427, 468, 470f
   divisions of 468
   regulation of 427
Autonomic reflexes 396
Autophagosome 3, 5
Autoregulation 159, 317, 319
Autosomes 7
Axilla 184
Axillary pulse 314

Axillary temperature 186
Axoaxonic synapse 390
Axodendritic synapse 390
Axolemma 380
Axon 378
   hillock 380
   internal structure of 380
   reflex 307
   terminal 100
Axonal flow 380
Axonotmesis 384
Axoplasm 380
Axosomatic synapse 390

B

B cell
   activation of 57
   immunity 57
   receptor 57
   transformation 57
B lymphocytes 52, 54, 55
   specificity of 58
   storage of 55
   types of 55
Babinski reflex 398
Babinski sign 398, 457
Back pressure arm lift method 372
Bacterial origin, substances of 36
Bactericidal agents, secretion of 75
Badminton 329
Bainbridge reflex 304
Ballistic movements 432
Ballistocardiography 300
Balsamic odor 511
Barometric pressure 366, 367t, 368, 368t
Baroreceptor 303, 359
   functions of 304, 307
   mechanism 307
   nerve supply to 303, 303f
   reflex 156
Basal body temperature 256
Basal ganglia 233, 417, 434, 434f
   disorders of 435
   functions of 435
Basal lamina 100, 391
Basal metabolic rate 207
   effect on 244
   measurement of 211
Basement membrane 160
Basilar artery 319
Basilar membrane 500
   part of 505
Basophilic cells 196
Basophilic erythroblast 38
Basophils 38, 50
   functions of 51
Bathmotropic action 277, 278
Bedwetting 181, 459
Belching 123
Bell sound 462
Bell's palsy 116
Bell-dog experiments 462
Bell-Magendie law 392
Berger waves 454
Beta-adrenergic receptors 231
Beta-cells, degeneration of 221
Beta-estradiol, potency of 250
Betz cells 91, 392, 408
Bezold-Jarisch reflex 304
Bicarbonate ions 125, 127, 163, 172
   reabsorption of 170, 171f
Biconcave lens 494
Biconvex lens 495
Bicuspid area 290
Bicuspid valve 275, 277

Bile
   alteration of pH of 134
   canaliculus 130
   composition of 132, 132f
   concentration of 134
   duct, tributary of 130
   functions of 133
   properties of 132
   secretion of 132, 134
   storage of 132, 134
Bile pigments 42, 132, 133
Bile salt 132, 174
   activated lipase 127, 128
   functions of 132
   stimulate 132
Biliary system 130, 131, 131f
   pressure in 134
Bilirubin 34, 42, 133, 174
   direct 133
   encephalopathy 72
   normal plasma levels of 133
   total 135
Biliverdin 42
Binasal heteronymous hemianopia 489
Binocular vision 485
Biological transducers 387
Biot's breathing 364
Biphasic action potential 96
Bipolar cells 478, 483, 487
Bipolar limb leads 293
Bipolar neuron 379, 510
Bipolar olfactory receptors 510
Birth control 268
Bitemporal heteronymous hemianopia 489
Bitter taste 510
Bjerrum screen 486
Bleeding disorders 67
Bleeding time 67
Blind spot 479, 486
Blood 28
   brain barrier 12, 466
   functions of 466
   buffering action in 34
   cancer, type of 51
   cerebrospinal fluid barrier 466
   coagulation of 21f, 62, 64
   composition of 28
   continuous circulation of 65
   effect on 207, 244
   examination of 174
   fluid 81
   free histiocytes of 75
   functions of 32
   in spleen, storage of 319
   in ventricles, significance of volume of 288
   indices 44, 46
   matching 70
   oncotic pressure in 30
   phosphate level 213, 215
   properties of 28
   reservoir for 319
   role in
      coagulation of 30
      viscosity of 30
   rushing of 290
   sinusoid, endothelium of 74
   substitutes 73
   sugar, high 319
   synthesized in 237
   testis barrier 240
   transfusion 69, 70, 72, 73
   viscosity of 306
   volume of 288
   wasted 337

Index

Blood calcium level 212, 214
   maintenance of 212
   regulation of 150, 215
Blood cells 28, 173
   destruction of 75
   formation of 75
   specific gravity of 28
Blood clot 64, 65
   role in 61
   stages of 64
Blood coagulation
   mechanism of 62
   process of 67
   stages of 66f
Blood flow 321, 323, 361
   normal 320, 321
   reversal of 323
   velocity of 306
Blood glucose level 220
   regulation of 220
   role of 219, 220
Blood group 69
   determination of 34, 70f
   systems 69
Blood loss
   anemia 47
   role in prevention of 61
Blood pressure 264, 305, 307, 330, 456
   action on 225, 232
   regulation of 150, 309f, 427
   systolic 207, 305
Blood sugar level
   hormones in maintenance of 221
   insulin in maintenance of 221
   normal 220
   regulation of 220
Blood typing 70
   principle of 70
   requisites for 70
Blood vessel 156, 207, 278, 321, 469
   action on 232, 236
   diameter of 306
   elasticity of 306
   ruptured 61
Blood volume 31, 306
   measurement of 25, 31
   normal 31
   reduced 329
   regulation of 31
   variations in 31
Body 117
   axial filament of 245
   built 306
   motor activities of 414
   normal cells 59
   parts of 100, 186t
   rejuvenation of 458
   surface area 298
Body fluid 23, 81, 329
   compartments of 23, 24f
   composition of 23
   concentration of 25
   distribution of 23
   volume 24
     measurement of 23
Body temperature 186-188
   normal 186
   regulation of 32, 185-187, 188f, 336, 427
   set point for 187
Body weight 31
   effect on 207
Bohr effect 354
Boiled starch 115
Bolus 142, 143

Bone 198
   action on 226
   conduction 505
   disease of 217
   effect on 212, 214, 251
   formation 217
   growth, effect on 244
   marrow 55
   physiology of 212, 216
   remodeling 217
   resorption 217
   structure of 216
Bony labyrinth 450, 499
Bony pillar 500
Bony spiral canal 499
Border cells 501
Botulinum toxin 102
Bowman's capsule 151, 153, 160-162, 168
Brachial pulse 314
Bradycardia 301, 304
Bradykinesia 435
Bradykinin 162
Bradypnea 360
Brain 156, 377
   attack 319
   damage 325
   derived neurotrophic growth factor 381
   localized area of 456
   natriuretic peptide 235
   parts of 377, 378f
   ventricles of 464
Brainstem nuclei 417
Braxton Hicks contractions 264
Breast
   enlargement of 247
   milk 267
     advantages of 267
Breath holding 360
   time 356
Breathing
   capacity, maximum 346
   difficulty in 318
   shortness of 326
   waxing of 363
   work of 341
Bright light vision 483
Broca's area 441, 463
Brodmann areas 438
Bromide 25
Bronchial artery 336, 337
Bronchial asthma 364
   causes of 364
Bronchial circulation 337
Bronchial veins 337
Bronchioles 334, 469
Bronchodilatation 236
Brown adipose tissue 187
Brown fat tissue 187
Brown-Séquard syndrome 410
Brucella 115
Brunner's glands 138
   secrete mucus 138
Buccinator muscle 142
Bucket handle movement 339
Buffer nerves 304, 308
Bulbar outflow 469
Bulbar portion 475
Bulbar reflexes 396
Bulk flow 15
   diffusion 350
Bulldog scalp 202
Bundle branches 282
Bundle of His 282
Bungarotoxin 102
Burn shock 325
Burning odor 511
Burning sensation 329, 419

C

C cells 205, 214
C wave 316
Calcitonin 205, 214
   role of 215, 216
   secretion, regulation of 215
Calcitriol 235
Calcium 163
   absorption of 213, 215
   calmodulin complex 106
   excretion of 215
   level, normal value of 215
   metabolism 215
   phosphate crystals, formation of 214
   pump 17
   receptor 215
   rigor 92
Calcium ion 107, 391
   role of 97
   influx of 281
   liberation of 99
   transport of 17
Callosomarginal fissure 437
Calmodulin 106
Calorigenic hormone 232
Canal of Schlemm 479
Canaliculi, presence of 118
Capillary blood
   flow, peculiarities of 321
   pressure 312, 312f
Capillary bulbs 77
Capillary circulation 317, 320
Capillary endothelium 161f
Capillary hemorrhage 324
Capillary hydrostatic pressure 312
Capillary loops 158, 321
Capillary membrane 162
Capillary plexus 336
Carbamino compounds 355
Carbamino proteins 355
Carbamylcholine 102
Carbhemoglobin 355
Carbohydrate 29
   digesting enzyme 115
   digestion of 127
   functions of 3
   metabolism 99, 198, 207, 218, 232
     action on 218, 219, 225
   starvation 144
Carbolic acid 36
Carbon dioxide 79, 172, 336, 350, 351t, 354
   diffusion of 351, 352f
   dissociation curve 355, 355f
   excess of 107, 360
   partial pressure of 360
   transport of 354, 354f, 355
Carbon monoxide 42
   effects of 364
   poisoning 364
   signs of 42
   symptoms of 42, 364
Carbon monoxyhemoglobin 42
Carbon particles, removal of 75
Carbonic acid 120, 171, 336, 354
Carbonic anhydrase 354
   inhibit activity of 176
   presence of 120
Carboxyhemoglobin 42
Carboxypeptidase 126, 128
   A 126
     actions of 127
   B 126
Carcinogens 4
Cardiac arrest 325
Cardiac bruit 291

Cardiac center 301
Cardiac chambers 337
Cardiac cycle 284, 286, 287, 287f, 287t, 288, 295
   atrial events of 285t
   ventricular events of 285, 285f, 285t
Cardiac diseases 326
Cardiac disorders 363
Cardiac failure 326
Cardiac glands 118
Cardiac index 298
Cardiac murmur 289, 291
Cardiac muscle 83, 84, 91, 280, 281, 283f
   action potential in 280
   disease 326
   fibers 276f
   properties of 280
   refractory period in 283
Cardiac output 264, 298, 299, 306, 329, 337
Cardiac pain 318
Cardiac region 117
Cardiac reserve 298
Cardiac shock 71
Cardiac sphincter 117
Cardiac syncytium 283
Cardiac tamponade 326
Cardioaccelerator 303
   center 302
   reflex 304
   tone 303
Cardiogenic shock 326
   types of 326
Cardiomyopathy 326
Cardiovascular accident 319
Cardiovascular hypertension 310
Cardiovascular system 48, 103, 207, 264, 275, 325, 329, 367, 456
   effects on 362
Carotid artery, internal 319
Carotid baroreceptors 303
Carotid body 304
Carotid pulse 314
Carotid sinus syncope 326
Carpopedal spasm 213, 214f
Carrier proteins 16, 16f
Carry sensory impulses 381
Caseinogens 126
Catacrotic limb 313
Catacrotic notch 314
Catacrotic waves 314
Catalase 42
Catamenia 257
Cataplexy 429
Cataract 480, 481
Catecholamines
   actions of 232
   hypersecretion of 301
   synthesis of 231
Cathelectrotonic potentials 382
Cathelicidins 335
Caudate nucleus 434
Celiac
   disease 129, 140
   ganglion 111, 468
   plexus 132
   sprue 140
Cell 1
   body 482, 483
   death 10
   drinking 18
   eating 18
   junctions 11, 12t
     types of 11f
   mediated immunity 54
     development of 56

murder 10
of Claudius 501
of Hensen 501
power house of 6
secretory function of 138*t*
shape and size of 3
signaling 191
structure of 1, 2*f*
suicide 10
to cell
    junction 12, 13
    signaling 191
to matrix junction 13
types of 137, 508
Cell membrane 1, 2*f*, 15*f*, 60, 193
    altering permeability of 193
    carbohydrate of 3
    composition of 1
    functions of 3, 3*b*
    lipids of 2, 2*f*
    permeability of 218
    protein layers of 2
    selective permeability of 94
    structure of 2
    transport through 14
Cellular immunity 54, 56
Cellular organelles 60
Cellulose 115
Central arterial pulse 313
Central canal 464, 465
Central chemoreceptors 359
Central nervous system 74, 208,
    377, 379, 385, 393, 448
    action on 226, 232
    development of 208
    effects on 362
    manifestations of 223
    normal function of 208
    parts of 377*f*
Central neuroglial cells 385
Central speech apparatus, activities
    of 462
Central sulcus 437, 441
Central venous pressure 311
Centrioles 6
Centrosome 3, 6, 378
Cephalic phase 121, 127
Cephalus 121
Cerebellar cortex 431
Cerebellar hemispheres 430
    lateral portions of 431
Cerebellar lesion 398, 433, 433*t*
Cerebellar reflexes 396
Cerebellum 417, 430, 431
    divisions of 431*t*
    functional divisions of 430*f*
    functions of 432*t*
    parts of 430
    vermis of 430
Cerebral aqueduct, blockage of 466
Cerebral blood
    flow, normal 319
    flow, regulation of 319
    vessels 319
Cerebral circulation 317, 319
Cerebral cortex 302, 303, 403, 417,
    431-433, 437, 440*f*, 442*f*,
    455, 482, 509
    frontal lobe of 438
    functional gateway for 424
    lateral surface of 439*f*
    lobes of 437, 438*f*
    medial surface of 440*f*
    morphology of 437
    occipital lobe of 450
    parts of 358, 438*f*
    sensory area of 420
    specific areas of 423

Cerebral dominance 437
Cerebral embolism 68
Cerebral palsy 418
Cerebri, epiphysis of 234
Cerebro-cerebello-cerebral
    circuit 432*f*
    connections 431
Cerebrocerebellum 431
Cerebropontocerebellar tract 432
Cerebrospinal fluid 377, 464
    abnormal accumulation of 466
    absorption of 465
    circulation of 464, 465*f*
    composition of 464*f*
Cerebrum 437
Ceruminous glands 498
Cervical
    cap 269
    enlargement 400
    ganglia 468
    mucus pattern 256
    sympathetic ganglia 303
    sympathetic nerves 303
Cervix 250
    effect on 252
Chemical barriers 269
Chemical energy 389, 510, 511
Chemical messengers 191, 192*f*
Chemical stimulus 89
Chemical substances 36, 191
Chemical synapse 12, 390, 390*f*
Chemical thermogenesis 189
Chemoattractants 51
Chemoreceptors 303*f*, 304, 359,
    387, 389, 510
    function of 304, 308
    types of 359
Chemosensitive area 359
Chemotaxis 51
Chest
    electrode 293
    leads
        position of 293
        unipolar 293
    pain 318, 327
Cheyne-Stokes breathing 361, 363,
    364, 456
Chicken chest 217
Chime, formation of 119
Chloride 25, 163
    shift 354, 355
Cholagogue 134
    action 133
Cholecalciferol 213, 235
Cholecystokinin 129, 219, 220, 428
Cholelithiasis 136
Choleretic action 132, 133
Cholestatic jaundice 135
Cholesterol 2
    ester hydrolase 127, 128
    high 319
Cholinergic nerve fibers 382
Cholinergic neurotransmitter 236
Cholinesterase inhibitors 102
Chorda tympani
    fibers 509
    syndrome 116
Chorea 425, 436
Choreoathetosis 436
Choroid 476
    plexus 464, 466
Christmas disease 68
Chromaffin cells 231
Chromatin 7
    network 38
Chromatolysis 385
Chromophil cells 196
    classification of 196

Chromophobe cells 196
Chromophore 484
Chromosomal disorders 9
Chromosomes 7
Chronaxie 90
Chronotropic action 277, 278
Chvostek's sign 214
Chyme 128, 144
Chymotrypsin 126, 128
Chymotrypsinogen 126
Cilia 451475
Ciliary body 476, 479
Ciliary ganglion 480, 491, 493
Ciliary muscle 480, 492
Ciliary neurotrophic factor 381
Ciliary processes 476, 479, 492
Ciliary vein 479
Ciliospinal reflex 491
Circadian rhythm 234
    control of 444
    role in 428
Circle of Willis 319
Circular diaphragm 476
Circulatory shock 222, 324
    types of 325, 325*f*
Circumvallate papillae 508
Cisterna 4
    lateralis 464
    magna 464
Cisternal puncture 466
Citrates 67
Clarke's nucleus 405
Classical pills, mechanism of action
    of 270
Clathrin 18
Clear cells 205, 214
Clonus 398
Clot
    fibrinolysin causes lysis of 257
    lysis of 241
    retraction 65
    role in 61
Clotting factors 64, 64*t*
Clotting mechanism, sequence
    of 64
Clotting time 67
Cloudiness 481
Cochlea 450, 499, 505*f*
    compartments of 500
    scala vestibuli of 504
Cochlear duct 500
Cochlear microphonic potential 505
Codons 9
Cold rigor 92
Cold temperature 92
Cold-blooded animals 187
Colipase 127, 128
Collagenase 127, 128
Collateral ganglia 468
Colliculus, inferior 502
Colloidal osmotic pressure 15, 161,
    162
Colloidal pressure 312
Colon
    ascending 140
    hypertrophy of 141
Colony-forming
    blastocytes 37, 53
    unit 37-39
Colony-stimulating factor 53, 58
    secretion of 75
Color blindness 496, 496*f*
    tests for 497
    total 496
Color index 46
Color sensitive areas 496
Color vision 483, 496
Colostrum 266

Columnar cells 138
Columns of Bertin 149
Coma 27
Combined pills 270
Combined sensations 413, 413*b*
Common autoimmune diseases 59
Common bile duct 125, 131
Common chromosomal disorders 9*b*
Common hepatic duct 131
Common sleep disorders 459
Complete heart block 296
Concha 498
Conduction 187
    block 384
Conduction deafness 506
    causes of 506
Conductive system 282, 282*f*, 282*t*
Conductivity 282
Cone 485, 487, 496
    dystrophy 484
    functions of 483
Cone cell 484
    structure of 483
Cone-shaped conus medullaris 400
Confrontation test 486
Congenital adrenal hyperplasia
    229, 230*f*
    causes of 229
    symptoms of 230
Congenital heart disease 301, 326
Congestive cardiac failure 31, 299
Congestive heart failure 326
Conjunctiva 475
Conn's syndrome 229
Connecting cilium 482
Connective tissue 1, 74, 75
    capsule 448
Connector neurons 395
Connexins 12
Conscious kinesthetic sensation
    407*f*, 408, 413
Conscious movements, regulation
    of 435
Consciousness, sudden loss of 456
Constipation 141, 147
    causes of 141
Constrictor papillae 476, 480, 491
Contact junction 107
Contain fixed cells 74
Contraceptive
    long-term 270
    methods 268, 271*t*
    pills 270
Contractile process 106
Contractile proteins 104
Contractility 90, 282
Contraction 480
    force of 299, 337
    period 91
    point of 90*f*
    time 91
Contrecoup injury 465
Convection 187
Convergence 392, 393*f*, 481
Convoluted tubules 149
Convulsion 213, 264, 455
Convulsive seizure 455
Copper intrauterine contraceptive
    device 269, 270
Copper T 269
Core temperature 186
Cornea 476
    radiata 255, 409
Coronary artery 317
    disease 292, 318, 326
Coronary blood flow 317, 318*f*
    normal 317
    regulation of 317

Index

Coronary blood vessels, distribution of 317
Coronary chemoreflex 304
Coronary circulation 317
Coronary collateral arteries 318
Coronary embolism 68
Coronary heart disease 318
Coronary occlusion 318
Coronary perfusion pressure 318
Coronary vasodilatation 318
Corpora cavernosa 241
Corpus 117
    albicans 256
    callosum 437
    hemorrhagicum 256
    spongiosum 241
    striatum 434, 434f
Corpus luteum 250, 251, 254f, 256, 256f, 257
    degeneration of 236
    development of 256
    fate of 256
    functions of 256
    graviditatis 257
    menstrualis 256
Corpuscular hemoglobin concentration, mean 46
Cortex 234, 248
Cortical auditory centers 502
Cortical center 441, 488
Cortical lobes, functions of 443t
Cortical nephrons 151
Cortical reflexes 396
Corticocerebellum 431
Corticomedullary junction 151
Corticopontine fibers 431
Corticopontocerebellar tract 432
Corticospinal tracts 408
Corticosteroid 224
Corticotrophs 197
Corticotropin releasing
    factor 227
    hormone 156, 197, 426
Cortisol 31, 220, 221
    secretion, regulation of 227f
Cough reflex 335
    causes of 336
Cough syncope 326
Coumarin derivatives 66
Countercurrent exchanger 167, 168f
Countercurrent flow 166
Countercurrent mechanism 166
Countercurrent multiplier 167, 167f
Countercurrent system 166
    divisions of 167
Coupling reactions 206
Covering sheath, formation of 254
Cracking voice 244
Cramps 419
Cranial content volume, regulation of 465
Cranial nerve 381
    nuclei 414, 417
Cranial outflow 469
Craniosacral outflow 469
Creatine phosphate 99, 374
Cretinism 210
Cricopharyngeal muscle 143
Crista ampullaris 451, 451f
Crohn's disease 140
Crude sensations 412
Crude touch
    impulses of 404
    sensation 403
Cryptorchidism 243
Crypts of Lieberkühn 137
Crystalline 479
Cumulus oophorus 254

Cushing's disease 202, 228
Cushing's syndrome 228, 228f, 462
Cutaneous blood vessels, architecture of 321
Cutaneous circulation 317, 321
Cutaneous receptors 387, 387f, 388t
Cutaneous reflexes 397t
Cutaneous vasoconstriction 370
Cuticular plate 501
Cyanocobalamin 40
Cyanosis 325, 363, 364
Cylindrical lens 495
Cystic duct 131
Cystic fibrosis 129
Cystometrogram 179, 180, 180t
Cystometry 179
Cytochrome 42
    oxidase 42
Cytokines 58
Cytoplasm 3, 60, 193
Cytoplasmic organelles 3b
    functions of 4t
Cytosine 8, 9
Cytoskeleton 3, 6, 7
    functions of 7
Cytotoxic T cells 54, 56, 59

■ D

D antigen 71
D cells 118, 129, 220
Dangerous hypertension 264
Dark adaptation 484
Dark band 85
Day light vision 483
Dead space 347
Decompression sickness 369
    causes of 369
    prevention of 369
    symptoms of 369
Deep inspiration 336, 343, 345
Deep reflexes 396, 398t
    effect on 433
Deep sea physiology 366, 368
Deep sensations 413
Deep sleep
    initial stage of 457
    stage of 458
Deeper reticular layer 182
Deeper structures 413
Deeper veins 321
Defecation 133, 146
Defecation reflex 146, 146f
    pathway for 147
Defective heart valves 326
Defective rod function 484
Defense mechanism, role in 30, 61
Defensins 138, 335
Defensive function 32
Deglutition 142
    apnea 143, 336
    reflex 143
Dehydration 26, 141, 204
    exhaustion 370
    mild 26
    moderate 26
    severe 26
    shock 325
    signs of 26
    symptoms of 26
    treatment of 26
Dehydrocholesterol 213
Dehydroepiandrosterone 228
Delirium 27
Delta rhythm 454, 455
Delta waves 458
Dementia 436, 461
    causes of 461

Demyelination 410
Dendrites 378
Dendritic cells 56, 336
Dengue
    fever 46
    shock syndrome 46
Densa 155
Dense bodies 104
Dense granules 60
Dentatorubral fibers 432
Dentatorubrothalamocortical tract 432
Deoxycholate 132
Deoxygenated blood 131, 336
Deoxyribonucleic acid 7, 8, 127
Depolarization 95, 96, 294, 382, 394
Depression 367, 481
Depressor area 302
Derebellum, divisions of 431
Dermatomal rule 420
Dermatome 420
Dermis 182
    capillaries of 182
Descending colon 140, 147
Descending facilitatory reticular system 446
Descending inhibitory reticular system 446
Desmosome 12, 13
Desquamated uterine tissues 257
Desynchronization 455
Desynchronized waves 454, 455, 458
Detoxification 4
    functions 134
Detrusor muscle 177
    contraction of 180
Deuteranopia 496
Dextrinase 138, 139
Diabetes 326
Diabetes insipidus 59, 202, 203, 221, 222, 319, 429
    causes of 203
    signs of 204
    symptoms of 204
Diabetes mellitus
    causes for 222
    classification of 221
    complications of 222
    diagnostic tests for 222
    non-insulin dependent 222
    signs of 222
    symptoms of 222
    type I 221, 221t
    type II 221t, 222
Diabetic nephropathy 222
Diabetic neuropathy 222
Diabetic retinopathy 222
Diabetogenic hormones 219
Dialysis 173, 175
Diapedesis 51
Diaphragm 338, 339
Diaphysis 216
Diarrhea 141
    causes of 141
Diastasis 286
Diastolic blood pressure 305
Diastolic murmur 291
Diastolic pressure 310
Dichromatism 496
Dichromats 496
Diencephalon 378
Dietary iron 42
Dietary source 215
Diffusion 14, 321
Digestion 109
Digestive enzymes 267
Digestive function 115, 119, 133, 138, 139
Digestive organs, primary 109

Digestive peristalsis 144
Digestive process 109
Digestive system 48, 103, 109, 264, 367
    changes in 264
    effects on 362
    functional anatomy of 109
Dihydroxycholecalciferol 150, 213, 215, 216, 235
Dihydroxyphenylalanine 182
Diiodotyrosine 206
Diisopropyl fluorophosphate 102
Dilator pupillae muscle 476, 480, 491
Dilute urine, formation of 166
Dim light vision 483
Diopter 482
Dipalmitoylphosphatidylcholine 339
Diplegia 411
Diploid cells 7
Diploid number 262
Diploid oogonia 248
Diplopia 486
Disk prolapse 411
    symptoms of 411
Distal convoluted tubule 152, 153, 169
Disulfide
    bonds 57
    bridges 218
Diuresis 169
Diuretics 173, 175, 176
    agents 175
    types of 175
    uses of 175
Diurnal rhythm 428
Diurnal variation 51, 234, 299, 306
Divergence 392, 393f, 481
Dizziness 370
Dopamine 233
    lack of 435
Dopaminergic fibers 435
Dopaminergic neurons 233
Doppler echocardiography 300
Dorsal cochlear nuclei 502
Dorsal spinocerebellar tract 405
Dorsalis pedis pulse 314
Dorsolateral nucleus 423
Dorsomedial nucleus 423
Double antigen-antibody reactions 265
Double vision 486
Douglas bag 345, 349
Down syndrome 9
Downhill movement 14
Downward movement 481
Drinker method 372
Dromotropic action 277, 278
Drowsiness, stage of 457
Drug-induced Parkinsonism 435
Drugs stimulating neuromuscular junction 102
Duct system 114f, 125
Ductless glands 192
Ducts cells 266
Ducts of Bellini 150, 154
Ductus arteriosus 322, 323
Ductus reuniens 451
Ductus venosus 322
Duke method 67
Dumbbell shape 60
Duodenal ulcer 123
Dura mater 377, 400
Dural sinuses 465
Dust particles, prevention of 335
Dwarfism 202, 204
    causes of 203
    signs of 203
    symptoms of 203
    types of 203b

Dye dilution
   method 300
   technique 25
Dynamic exercise 328
Dynamic gamma motor nerve 448
Dynamic lung function tests 342
Dysarthria 463
Dysgeusia 510
Dysphonia 463
Dyspnea 48, 360, 361, 363
   point 363
Dystrophia adiposogenitalis 204, 247, 429
   symptoms of 204

E

Ear 498
   structure of 498f
Early normoblast 38, 40
Earwax 498
Eccrine glands 184
   secretory activity of 184
Eccrine sweat glands 184t
Eclampsia 264
Ectopic arrhythmia 296
Ectopic foci 296
Ectoplasm, microfilament of 7
Edema 79
   generalized 79
   types of 79
Edinger-Westphal nucleus 480, 491, 493
Edridge-Green lantern 497
Efferent arteriole 151, 158
   constriction of 162
Efferent nerve 395
   fibers 381, 381b
Efferent neurons 379
Efferent pathway 357, 491, 493
Eicosanoids 235
Einthoven's triangle 293
Ejaculation 245
Ejaculatory duct 241
Ejection fraction 286, 298
Ejection period 286
Elastase 127, 128
Electrical activities, graphical registration of 292
Electrical energy 453, 484, 510, 511
Electrical potentials 280, 482
Electrical stimulus 89
Electrical synapse 390, 390f
Electrocardiogram 292
Electrocardiograph 292
Electrocardiographic grid 292
Electroencephalogram 454, 458, 458f
Electroencephalography 454
Electrolyte
   equilibrium 355
   imbalance 141
   loss 32
Electrolyte balance
   effect on 244, 251
   maintenance of 150
Electron-dense protein layers 2
Electronic vibrator 507
Electron-lucent lipid layer 2
Electroretinogram 484, 485f
Elevated jugular venous pulse 316
Embolism 68
Embolus 68, 318
Embryo 263
   development of 262
   implantation of 262
Emergency contraceptive pills 270
Emmenia 257
Emmetropia 494

Emmetropic eye 494
Emotion 31
Emotional changes 428, 436
Emotional conditions 35, 51, 299, 306
Emotional disturbances 319
Emotional fainting 326
Emotional reactions 441
Emotional state, role in 444
Emphysema 341, 345, 365
Empty stomach, contraction of 456
Emulsion 132
End knob
   anterior 245
   posterior 245
End stage renal disease 175
End-diastolic volume 286, 288
Endemic colloid goiter 211
Endocardium 277
Endocrine
   disorders 222
   function 125, 150, 263, 425
   glands 192, 208
   hormone 219
      role of 219
   hypertension 310
   messengers 191
   system 191, 264
Endocrinology 191
Endocytosis 17
   receptor-mediated 18
Endogenous analgesia system 420
Endolymphatic duct 451
Endolymphatic sac 451
Endometrial cells 259
Endometrium 85, 250, 259
Endoneurium 380, 384
Endopeptidase 126
Endoplasmic reticulum 3, 4f, 60
Endosmosis 15
Endosome 5, 18
Endosteum 216
Endothelin 107, 162, 309
Endothelium 350
   derived relaxing factor 107
Endplate potential, properties of 101
End-systolic volume 286, 288
Engulfed droplets 18
Enophthalmos 494
Enteric nervous system 110
Enterochromaffin cells 118, 137, 138
Enterocytes 137, 138
Enteroendocrine cells 118, 137, 138
Enterogastric reflex 123
Enterohepatic circulaiton 131, 131f, 132, 133
Enterokinase 126, 138
Enteropeptidase 126
Enuresis 181
Environmental temperature 299
Enzyme
   aromatase 240
   cascade theory 64
   secretion of 109
   transport of 32
Eosinophil 38, 50
   functions of 51
Epicritic sensations 412
Epidermis 182
Epididymis 240
Epilepsy 454, 455
   general onset 456
   localized 456
   types of 456
Epileptic aura 456
Epimysium 85
Epineurium 380
Epiphyseal cartilage 216

Epiphyseal fusion 198
Epiphyseal plate 216
Epiphysis 216, 234
   fusion of 201, 244, 251
Epithelial cells 173
Epithelial lining 110
Epithelial tissue 1
Epithelium 153t, 350
   anterior 479
Equalizing pressure 505
Equilibration 345
   area for 442, 443
Erb's sign 214
Erb-Westphal sign 214
Erlangergasser classification 382
Erythroblastosis fetalis 72
   complications of 72
Erythroblasts, presence of 72
Erythrocyte sedimentation rate 44
   normal values of 45t
   role in 30
Erythrocytes 33, 37, 52
Erythropoiesis 37-40, 40t
   process of 37
   site of 37
   stages of 38
Erythropoietic action 244
Erythropoietin 39, 150, 235, 329
Escape phenomenon 225
Esophageal Doppler transducer technique 300
Esophageal stage 142, 143
Esophagus 143
   disease of 116
Essential hypertension 310
Essential hypotension 311
Estrogen 243, 250, 258, 263
   forms of 250
   functions of 250
   secretion, regulation of 251, 251f
Estrogen-binding protein 240
Ethereal odor 511
Ethinyl estradiol 270
Ethmoid bone, cribriform plate of 510
Ethylenediaminetetra acetic acid 44, 67
Eukaryotes 7
Eunuchism 204, 246
Eupnea 360
Eustachian tube 499
   role of 505
Excess ketoacids, formation of 222
Excess sleep 459
Exchange transfusion 72, 73
Excitability curve 90
Excitation-contraction coupling 97, 106
Excitatory neurotransmitter 236, 237, 392
Excitatory postsynaptic potential 96, 391
Excitatory synapse 391
Excitomotor cortex 438
Excretory function 3, 32, 115, 119, 133, 134, 141, 185, 263
Excretory products 133
Excretory system 264, 457
Exercise
   effects of 374
   mild 329
   moderate 329
   severe 329
   types of 328
Exocrine function 125
Exocytosis 5, 17, 18, 101
   mechanism of 18
   process of 18f
Exopeptidases 127, 209

Exosmosis 15
Expansibility 340
Expiration 333, 343
   difficulty in 346
   normal 342, 343
Expiratory muscles 338, 357
Expiratory reserve volume 342, 344
Expired air 349
Explicit memory 460
Extensor muscles 399
Extensor reflexes 396
External anal sphincter 110, 146
External auditory meatus 498
External blood clot 65
External ear 498
   role of 504
External genitalia, development of 243
Exteroceptors 387, 388f
Extorsion 481
Extracellular fluid 1, 12, 15, 16, 17f, 20, 23, 24t, 31, 79, 101, 156, 175, 309, 391
   subunits of 24f
   volume
      action on 225
      measurement of 25
Extrafoveal vision 479
Extraglomerular mesangial cells 155, 157
Extrahepatic biliary apparatus 131
Extrahepatic jaundice 135
Extrapyramidal system 435
Extrapyramidal tracts 410
Extrasystole 296, 297
Extreme weakness 318
Extrinsic factor 40, 120
Extrinsic muscles 480
Eye 475
Eyeball 481
   conjugate movement of 441
   extrinsic muscles of 480f
   functional anatomy of 475
   muscles of 480
   reflex movements of 488
   structure of 477f
   wall of 476, 477f
Eyelids 475

F

F cells 220
Fabricius, bursa of 54
Facial nerve 111, 469
   branch of 499
Facial pulse 314
Facilitation 461
F-actin 87
   molecules 87
Fallopian tube 250
   effect on 250, 252
   recanalization of 272
False labor contractions 265
Family planning 268
Farrell and Ivy pouch 121
Fasciculus 380
   cuneatus 406
   dorsolateralis 406
   gracilis 406, 407
Fast muscles 91
Fast pain fibers 419
Fatigue 91, 367, 392, 399
   causes for 91
   first seat of 399
Fats
   absorption of 132
   addition of 78
   emulsification of 132

Index

metabolism 207, 232, 251
    action on 219, 226
    surface tension of 132
Fatty acids
    mobilization of 226
    synthesis of 219
Feces 146
    formation of 141
Feed-forward control 21
Feeding center 427
Female reproductive
    organs 248, 249f
    system 248, 249f
Female urethra 177
Feminization 229
Femoral pulse 314
Fencing function 12
Fenestra 151, 160
Ferrihemoglobin 42
Ferritin 34
Fertile period 268
Fertility control 268
Fertilization, prevention of 269
Festinant gait 436
Fetal circulation 321, 322f, 323
Fetal heart 321
Fetal hemoglobin 41
Fetal lungs 321, 322, 333
    nonfunctioning of 322
Fetal placenta 321
Fetal testes 263
Fetoplacental unit 263
Fetus
    delivery of 264
    expulsion of 200
Fever, causes of 189
Fibers
    thickest 382
    thinnest 382
    uncrossed 405
Fibrin monomer 65
Fibrinogen 29, 65, 245
    activated 65
    conversion of 64, 241
    presence of 80
Fibrinolysin 65, 245
Fibrinolysis 65
Fibroblast 182
    growth factor 381
Fibrocartilaginous plate 498
Fibrotic pleurisy 341
Fibrous band 323
Fick's principle 174, 300
Fifth degree injury 384
Filaments 60
Filiform papillae 508
Filtration membrane 160, 161f
Filtration pores 151, 160
Filum terminale 400
Fine tactile sensation 407
Fine touch sensation 407f
First breath 322, 333
First degree injury 383
First heart sound 286, 289
    causes of 289
    characteristics of 289
First order neurons 419, 487, 502, 503f, 509
First polar body 249, 262
First rapid filling period 286
Fissure 400
Fixation point 485
Fixed reticuloendothelial cells 74
Flaccid paralysis 93
Flaccidity 93
Flavor, sensation of 509
Flechsig's tract 405
Flexor muscles 399
Flexor reflex 396, 399

Flocculonodular lobe 430, 431
Fluid
    accumulation of 326
    buffer 465
    displacement of 505f
    loss 31, 32, 329
    osmolarity of 169t
    pressure 479
    retention 326
Fluid-filled cavities 410
Focal adhesions 12, 13
Folic acid 40
    deficiency 48
Follicle stimulating hormone 193, 197, 199, 240, 242, 251, 254, 258-260
Follicular cavity 205, 254
Follicular cells 205, 206
Follicular phase 253
Follicular sheath 254
Food intake, regulation of 444
Food substances, consumption of 109
Foramen magnum 377, 400
Foramen of Luschka 464
Foramen of Magendie 464
Foramen of Monro 464
Foramen ovale 322, 323
Forced expiratory volume 345
Forced inspiratory effort 311
Fourth degree injury 384
Fourth heart sound 285, 290
Fovea centralis 479, 485
Foveal vision 479
Fractional gastric analysis 123
Fractional test meal 123
Fragility 35, 511
Frank-Starling law 92, 299
Free bilirubin 133
Free fatty acid 183, 220
Frog-like husky voice 210
Fröhlich's syndrome 204, 247, 429
    type of 204
Frontal eye field 441, 493
Frontal lobe 437
    precentral gyrus of 439
    syndrome 441
Frostbite 367, 370
Fruity breath odor 222
Full-blown diabetes mellitus 198
Functional residual capacity 343, 344
    measurement of 345
Functional syncytium 104
Functional terminal artery 278
Fundic glands 118
Fundus 117, 478
    oculi 478, 479f
Fungiform papillae 508
Funiculi 402

G

G cells 118, 122, 138
G proteins 195
Gag reflex 143, 144
Galactopoiesis 266
Gallbladder 134, 469
    disorders of 135
    functions of 134
Gallstone 136
    features of 136
    formation
        causes for 136
        prevention of 133
Gamma globulins 30
Gamma glutamyl transferase 135
Gamma-aminobutyric acid 392, 393
Gamma-motor neurons 93, 416, 435, 449
    activation of 440

Ganglia, preverstebral 468
Ganglion cell layer 478
Ganglionic blockers 471
Ganglionic cells 487
    axons of 487
Gap junction 12, 104, 390
    functions of 12
    structure of 12
Garbage disposal system 5
Garlic odor 511
Gaseous exchange 348
Gases
    exchange of 3, 350
    expansion of 366
    transport of 352
Gastric acidity, measurement of 123
Gastric amylase 120
Gastric analysis 123
    method of 123
Gastric atrophy 123
Gastric cancer 123
Gastric disorders 123
Gastric function tests 123
Gastric gland 118, 118f
    cells in 118t
    parietal cell of 121f
    structure of 118
Gastric inhibitory peptide 122, 123, 219
Gastric juice
    collection of 123
    composition of 119, 119f
    digestive enzymes of 120t
    enzymes of 120
    functions of 119
    hyperacidity of 123
    properties of 119
    secretion of 120
Gastric lipase 120, 121, 127
Gastric pits 118
Gastric secretion 117
    phases of 121
    regulation of 120, 121, 122f
Gastric ulcer 123
Gastrin 122, 220
Gastritis 123
    common features of 123
Gastrocnemius-sciatic preparation 90
Gastrocolic reflex 147
Gastrointestinal hormones 123, 219, 237
    role of 219
Gastrointestinal mucosa 110
Gastrointestinal tract 78, 109, 109f, 133, 208, 456, 469
    effect on 213
    movements of 142
    nerve supply to 110
    somatostatin 220
    wall of 110
Gate control
    significance of 422
    theory 422
Gate function 12
Gelatinase 120
Gene 8
    expression 9
    control of 394
General vasoconstrictor 232
Genetic code
    transcription of 9
    translation of 9
Genetic disorders 9, 230
Geniculate body
    lateral 423, 487, 488
    medial 423, 502
Geniculocalcarine tract 488
Genital ridge 243
Genome 8

Germ
    cells 240
        primary 248
    hill 254
    hillock 255
Germinal epithelium 248
Gestation period 264
Gh-binding proteins 197
Ghrelin 428
    producing cells 118
Giant cells 408
Gigantism 201
    causes of 201
    signs of 201
    symptoms of 201
Glands of Littre 177, 241
Glandular cells 266
Glans penis 241
Glaucoma 479, 481
Glial cell 385
    line-derived neurotrophic factor 381
    morphology, control of 394
Globin 34, 41
Globus pallidus 434
Glomerular blood flow, regulation of 157
Glomerular capillary 151, 158
    membrane 160
    pressure 161, 162
Glomerular filtration 160
    process of 161
    rate 156, 157, 159, 161, 174, 176
        measurement of 174
Glomerular mesangial cells 155
    contraction of 162
Glomerulonephritis 175
Glomerulotubular balance 163
Glomerulus 151
Glossopharyngeal nerve 111, 420, 469
    fibers 509
Glucagon 219, 428
    actions of 219, 220
Glucocorticoids 215, 216, 224, 225
    functions of 225
    ketogenic effect of 226
    mode of action of 227
    permissive action of 226
    presence of 232
    role of 215, 216
    stimulate osteoclastic activity 226
Gluconeogenesis 219
Glucose 163, 174
    buffer system 221
    peripheral utilization of 218
    reabsorption of 164
    receptors 427
    reformation of 374
    renal threshold for 164
    storage of 218
    tolerance test 222
    transport maximum for 164
    tubular maximum for 164
Glucostatic mechanism 427, 427f
Glucostats 427
Glucosuria 222
Glutamate 420, 483
Glutamic acid 171
Glutamine 171
Gluten-sensitive enteropathy 140
Glycerol 509
Glycine 171
Glycocalyx 3
Glycogenesis 218
Glycogenolysis 219
Glycolipids 3
Glycoproteins 3
Goat odor 511

Goblet cells 137, 138
Goiter 210
Golgi apparatus 3, 4, 5f, 60, 380
    functions of 5
Golgi tendon apparatus 448f
Golgi tendon organ 447, 448
Gonadotrophs 197
Gonadotropic hormones 197
Gonadotropin 197
    releasing hormone 197, 244, 251, 252, 259, 426
Gong sound 310
Goormaghtigh cells 155
Gorilla face 202
Gower's tract 404
G-protein-coupled receptors 394
Graafian follicle 254, 255, 255f
    rupture of 255
Grand mal 456
Granular cells 155
Granular endoplasmic reticulum 3
Granules 60
    absence of 49
Granulocyte 37, 39, 49, 52, 53
Granulosa cells 248, 254, 262
Graves' disease 59, 209
Gravindex test 265
Gravitational force 368, 396
Gray horn
    lateral 401, 402
    posterior 401, 403
Gray matter submerged, masses of 434
Growth 207
    action on 219
Growth hormone 193, 197, 221, 242
    actions of 197
    inhibitory hormone 197-199, 220, 426
    releasing
        hormone 197-199, 426
        polypeptide 197-199, 426
    role of 215, 216
Guanosine nucleotide-binding proteins 195
Gustatory sensation 508
Guttural breathing 210
Gynecomastia 229, 247

H

Hair cells 451, 453, 501, 502
    excitation of 505
    inner 501
    stereocilia of 505
Hair distribution 251
    effect on 244
Hairpin bend 153
Haldane effect 355
    significance of 355
Haldane-Priestly tube 349
Hamburger phenomenon 354
Haploid cells 7, 255
Hashimoto's thyroiditis 59
Head, enlargement of 466
Headache 233, 367
Hearing
    and auditory defects, mechanism of 504
    perception of 504
    sensation of 475
    test for 506
    theories of 505
Heart 194, 207
    actions of 277, 278t
    attack 301, 318
    block 296, 299
    chambers, hypertrophy of 292
    conductive system of 282f, 282t
    contractile unit of 276
    disease 319
    left side of 275
    nerve supply to 302f
    regulation of actions of 277
    right side of 275
    section of 276f
    septa of 275
    shunt in 320
    valves of 277, 277f
Heart failure 324, 326, 336
    chronic 326
    signs of 326
    symptoms of 326
Heart rate 300, 301, 306, 329, 337
    acceleration of 307
    inhibition of 307
    normal 301
    regulation of 301, 427
Heart sound 289, 290, 290t
    abnormal 291
    classical 289
    different 289
    production of 289
Heart valve
    narrowing of 291
    stenosis of 291
    weakening of 291
Heartburn 124
Heat balance 186
Heat cramps 370
Heat exhaustion 370
Heat gain 186
    center 187
Heat loss 187
    center 187
    mechanism 336
    prevention of 188, 370
    promotion of 187
Heat production 134, 186, 369
    prevention of 188
    promotion of 188
Heat stroke 370
Heavy alcohol consumption 319
Heavy smoking 319
Helicobacter pylori 123
Helicotrema 500
Helium dilution technique 344, 345
Helper T cells 54, 56, 56f
    activation of 56
    role of 56, 57
Hematemesis 124
Hematocrit 28, 34
Hematopoietic function 150, 216
Hematopoietic growth factors 39, 53
Hematopoietic stem cells 37
Heme 41
Hemianopia 488
    types of 489f
Hemiballismus 436
Hemidesmosome 12, 13
Hemiplegia 417
Hemispheres 437
Hemoconcentration 329
Hemodialysis 175
Hemodilution 35
Hemodynamic events 315
Hemoglobin 38, 41, 353
    abnormal 41, 42
    content, normal 41
    derivative 42
    destruction of 42, 75
    formation 40
    functions of 41
    structure of 41
    synthesis of 42
    types of normal 41
Hemoglobinopathies 41
Hemolysins 36
Hemolysis 31, 35, 36, 47
Hemolytic anemia 46, 47
Hemolytic disease 72
Hemolytic jaundice 135
Hemolytic transfusion reaction 71
Hemophilia 67
    A 68
    B 68
    C 68
    causes for 67
    classic 68
    types of 67
Hemopoiesis 37
    stages of 39f
Hemopoietic function 119, 120, 134, 139, 140
Hemorrhage 299, 324
    accidental 324
    acute 324
    chronic 324
    effects of 324
    internal 324
    postpartum 324
Hemorrhagic anemia 46, 47
Hemorrhagic shock 325
Hemostasis 61, 62, 236
    stages of 62
    states of 63
Hemothorax 341, 345, 365
Henle's loop 167, 168, 169, 176
Henry head 463
Heparin 66, 237, 336
    actions of 237
    mechanism of action of 66
    uses of 66
Hepatic artery 131
    branch of 130
Hepatic blood vessels 320
Hepatic circulation 320
Hepatic ducts 131
Hepatic jaundice 135
Hepatic lobule 130, 131f
Hepatic plates 130
Hepatic portal vein 131
Hepatic stage 37
Hepatic vein 131
Hepatitis 135
Hepatocellular jaundice 135
Hepatocytes 130, 132
Hereditary unit 8
Hering's nerve 303, 304, 359
Hering-Breuer reflex 358
Hermaphroditism 239
Heterologous blood transfusion 73
Heteronymous hemianopia 489
Heterotopic arrhythmia 296
Hexamethonium ion 471
High barometric pressure 35
    effect of 369
High pressure bed 159, 312
Hilum 149
Hindbrain 378
Histamine 107, 237
    actions of 237
Histiocytes 182
Histocompatibility complex 56
Histone 7
Histotoxic hypoxia 361, 362
Holger-Nielsen method 371, 372, 372f
Homatropine 471
Homeostasis 20, 425
    role in 150
Homeostatic system
    components of 20, 20t
    mechanism of action of 20
Homeothermic animals 187
Homonymous hemianopia 489
Homotopic arrhythmia 296
Hormonal action, mechanism of 193
Hormonal contraceptives 270
Hormonal control 127, 128
Hormonal excretion 256
Hormonal function 139
Hormonal implants 270
Hormonal level, determination of 256
Hormonal mechanism 122, 307, 309, 427, 428
Hormonal receptors, situation of 193, 195f
Hormonal regulation 140
Hormonal substances, synthesis of 336
Hormone
    classical 191
    classification of 192, 194t
    inhibiting pancreatic secretion 129
    receptor 193
        complex 192
    replacement therapy 252
    role of 187, 266, 267f
    secretion of 256
    transport of 32
Horner syndrome 493
Human beings, sixth sense in 510
Human chorionic gonadotropin 194, 244, 263-265
Human chorionic somatomammotropin 263
Human eyeball 475
Human heart, parts of 281, 281t
Human immunodeficiency virus 59, 269
    infection 461
Human leukocyte antigen 56
Humoral immunity 54
    development of 57
Hunger contractions 144
Huntington's disease 436
Hyaline cartilage 216
Hyaluronidase 245, 262
Hydrocephalus 461, 466
    causes of 466
    types of 466
Hydrochloric acid 120
    functions of 120
    secretion of 120, 121f
Hydrocholeretic agents 134
Hydrogen
    excretion of 171f
    peroxide 75
    pump 17
Hydrogen ion
    concentration 107
        action on 225
    excretion of 171f
    removal of 170
    secretion of 170
    transport of 17
Hydrolytic enzymes 5
Hydrolytic function 140
Hydrolytic process 139
Hydroperoxyeicosatetraenoic acid 236
Hydrops fetalis 72
Hydrostatic pressure 79, 161, 162
Hydrothorax 341, 345, 365
Hydroxycholecalciferol 213
Hydroxyl ions 75
Hyperactive micturition reflex 181
Hyperactivity 222
Hyperaldosteronism 31, 229
    causes of 229
    primary 229
    secondary 229

signs of 229
symptoms of 229
types of 229
Hyperalgesia 422
Hyperbaric oxygen 362
Hyperbilirubinemia 133
Hypercalcemia 214
Hypercapnia 361, 362
Hypergonadism 247
　causes of 247
　symptoms of 247
Hyperhydration 27
Hyperinsulinism 222
Hypermetropia 494
Hyperosmia 512
Hyperosmolar coma 222
Hyperparathyroidism, causes of 214
Hyperphagia 441
Hyperplasia 214
Hyperpnea 360
　causes of 364
　stage of 363
Hyperpneic period 363
Hyperproteinemia 31
Hyperpyrexia 189, 213
Hypersalivation 116
Hypersensitivity reactions, acute 51
Hypersomnia 459
Hypersplenism 76
Hypertension 175, 222, 310, 319, 326
　primary 310
　secondary 310
　systolic 310
Hyperthermia 189
Hyperthyroidism 31, 209, 210, 299, 301, 326
Hypertonia 93
Hypertonic fluid 26
Hyperventilation 360, 374
Hypervolemia 31
Hypoactivity 221
Hypocalcemia 213
Hypocalcemic tetany 213
Hypocapnia 362
Hypochlorhydria 264
Hypogastric ganglion 178, 179
Hypogastric nerve 179
Hypogeusia 510
Hypoglycemia 223
Hypogonadism 247, 429
Hypogonadotropic hypogonadism 429
Hypokalemia 141
Hypokinesia 435
Hypokinetic hypoxia 361
Hypoparathyroidism 213, 462
Hypophyseal stalk 196, 199
Hypophysis 196
Hypoproteinemia 31
Hyposalivation 116
Hyposmia 429, 512
Hyposplenia 76
Hyposplenism 76
Hypotension 304, 311
　primary 311
　secondary 311
　types of 311
Hypothalamic eunuchism 204, 247
Hypothalamic hormone 259
Hypothalamic nucleus, posterior 187
Hypothalamic-pituitary-ovarian axis, hormone of 259
Hypothalamo-hypophyseal portal blood vessels 196
Hypothalamo-hypophyseal tract 200, 200f
　nerve fibers of 196

Hypothalamus 156, 188, 302, 303, 308, 420, 423, 425, 510
　anterior 187
　disorders of 429
　functions of 425, 426t
　nuclei of 425, 425f, 425t
　role of 187, 198, 209, 227
Hypothermia 189, 301
Hypothyroid goiter 210
Hypothyroidism 31, 209, 210, 299, 301, 462
　treatment for 211
Hypotonia 93, 418, 433, 436
Hypotonic fluid 26
Hypoventilation 360, 361
　causes of 361
　effects of 361, 361f
Hypovolemia 31
Hypovolemic shock 325
Hypoxia 39, 361
　causes of 361
　classification of 361
　development of 361
　effect of 362, 366
　treatment for 362
Hypoxic hypoxia 361

I

I cells 129, 138, 154
Icterus 135
Idiopathic nontoxic goiter 211
Idiopathic thrombocytopenic purpura 68
Idioventricular rhythm 296
Ileocecal junction 137
Ileocecal valve 137, 140
Immature ova 248
Immune
　deficiency diseases 59
　system 58
Immunity
　development of 55f
　specific 54
　types of 54
Immunization 58
　active 59
　passive 58
　type of 59
Immunoglobulins 30, 57, 267
Immunological test 265, 266f
Implicit memory 460
Impulse
　generation of 281
　spread of 281
　velocity of 382
Inborn reflex 396, 462
Incisura 314
Incus 499
Indigestion 264
Indole 234
Infantile sexual characters 246
Infarction 68
Infatigability 383
Inferior oblique muscles 480, 481
Inferior rectus 480, 481
Inferior vermis 430
　parts of 431f
Inflammatory bowel disease 140
Infrared rays 495
Inhibin 243
Inhibit osteoblastic activity 226
Inhibit pain transmission 422
Inhibitory impulses 303
Inhibitory neurotransmitter 237, 392, 393t
Inhibitory postsynaptic potential 96, 392

Inhibitory synapses 391
Inhibits cardiac function 236
Injury 367
　degrees of 383
Ink spot nucleus 38
Innate immunity 54
Inner ear 450
　role of 505
Inorganic phosphate 98, 215
Inorganic substances 23, 29b
Insensible perspiration 187
Insomnia 459
Inspiration 333, 343
　difficulty in 346
　normal 342
Inspiratory capacity 343, 344
Inspiratory impulses 358
Inspiratory muscles 338
Inspiratory neurons 357
Inspiratory ramp 358
Inspiratory reserve volume 342, 344
Inspired air 349
Insulin 218, 220
　action of 219
　actions of 218
　blood level of 218
　deficiency of 221
　dependent diabetes mellitus 221
　inhibits glycogenolysis 219
　receptors, deficiency of 222
　regulation of secretion of 219
Integral proteins 2
Intellectual functions, higher 460
Intention tremor 425
Interatrial septum 275
Intercalated cells 154
Intercalated disk 276
Intercellular communication 191
Intercellular junctions 11
Intercellular space 12
Interdigestive phase 121, 123
Interleukins, secretion of 75
Interlobular artery 158
Intermodal fibers 282
Internal ear 499
Internal sphincter 469
Internal urethra 241
　sphincter 177
Interneurons 395
Internuncial neurons 395
Interoceptors 387, 388, 389f
Interstitial cell
　of Leydig 240
　stimulating hormone 197, 199, 242, 244, 245
Interstitial fluid 20, 78
　volume, measurement of 25
Interventricular septum 275
Intervertebral disk, rupture of 411
Intestinal glands 137
Intestinal lipase 138, 139
Intestinal phase 121, 122, 127, 128
　initial stage of 122
　later stage of 123
Intestinal villi 137
Intestinal wall, structure of 110f
Intorsion 481
Intra-alveolar pressure 340, 341
　normal values of 340, 341t
　significance of 340
Intra-atrial pressure 286
Intracellular chemical mediators 191
Intracellular edema 79
Intracellular enzyme 194
Intracellular fluid 1, 15, 16, 17f, 23, 24f
　volume, measurement of 25
Intrafusal muscle fibers 416, 447

Intraglomerular mesangial cells 155
Intralaminar nuclei 423, 424f
Intralobular duct 125
Intraocular fluid 479
Intraocular lens implant 481
Intraocular pressure 479
Intrapleural fluid 334
　functions of 334
Intrapleural pressure 334, 339, 341
Intrapleural space 334
Intrapulmonary pressure 340
Intrarectal pressure 146
Intrathoracic pressure 339
Intrauterine contraceptive device 269
　disadvantages of 270
Intravascular blood clotting 68
Intraventricular pressure 287
Intravesical pressure 179
Intrinsic hemolytic anemia 47
Intrinsic muscles 480
Intrinsic nerve plexus 110f
Involuntary movements 425
Involuntary muscle 83, 103
Involuntary muscular activity 369
Involuntary nervous system 468
Iodide 206
　pump 206
　role of 209
　trapping 206
Iodinase 206
Iodination 206
Iodine 206
　deficiency goiter 211
Iodotyrosine residues 206
Iris 476
Iron
　absorption of 42
　daily loss of 43
　deficiency anemia 43, 47
　lung chamber 372
　metabolism 41, 42
　storage of 43
　transport of 43
Irregular astigmatism 495
Irregular heartbeat 295
Ischemia 68, 325
Ishihara's color charts 497
Islets of Langerhans 218, 218f
Isoagglutinin 70
Isocortex 437
Isoelectric period 294
Isometric contraction 90, 96, 328, 330
　period 285, 289
　significance of 286
Isometric relaxation
　period 286
　significance of 286
Isotonic contraction 90, 96, 328
Isotonic exercise 330
Isotonic fluid 26
Isotonic simple muscle curve 90f
Isovolumetric contraction 285
Isovolumetric relaxation 286
Isthmus 250
Ivan Pavlov 462

J

J point 295
Jacksonian epilepsy 456
Jaeger's chart 485
Jaundice 133, 135, 136b
　physiological 35
　severe 436
　types of 135, 135f
Jejunal mucosa 129
Jerky involuntary movements 425
Joints, unfixing of 450

Jugular venous pulse tracing 315
Juvenile diabetes 221
Juxtacapillary receptors 358
Juxtacrine messengers 191
Juxtaglomerular apparatus 155, 155f
    functions of 155
    structure of 155
Juxtaglomerular cells 155
Juxtallocortical structures 444
Juxtamedullary nephrons 151

K

K cells 138
K complex 457
Kallmann syndrome 429
Kernicterus 72, 436
Ketogenesis 220
Ketone 220
    bodies 163, 174
Ketosis 144, 198
Kidney 156, 235
    artificial 175
    different layers of 149
    effect on 213
    functional anatomy of 149
    functions of 150
    longitudinal section of 150f
    role of 170
    transplantation 175
    tubular structures of 150
Killer T cell 56
Kinesthetic receptors 447
Kinins 237
Kinocilium 451, 452, 501
Kluver-Bucy syndrome 443
Korbinian brodmann 438
Korotkoff sounds, phases of 310t
Kulchitsky cells 118
Kupffer cells 52, 74, 130, 134
Kussmaul's breathing 222
Kussmaul's sign 316
Kyphosis 202, 217, 341

L

Labor contractions commence 265
Labyrinth 451f
    part of 450
    proprioceptors in 447
Labyrinthectomy 453
Labyrinthine righting reflexes 449
Lacis cells 155
Lacrimal gland 469, 475
Lacrimal secretion 457
Lacrimal tear 475
Lactase 138, 139
Lactation, process of 267f
Lactic acid 91, 107, 374
Lactogenesis 266
    hormones in 266
Lactotrophs 197
Lambert-Eaton myasthenic
      syndrome 102
Lamina propria 110
Lamina reticularis 501
Landsteiner's law 69
Large intestinal juice 140
    composition of 140, 141f
    functions of 140
    parts of 140
Large intestine 137, 140
    disorders of 141
    functional 140, 141
    movements of 146
Large lymphocytes 50
Laryngeal stridor 214
Laryngospasm 214

Last menstrual period 264
Latchbridge mechanism 106
Late normoblast 38, 40
Latent tetany 214
Laurence-Moon-Biedl syndrome 429
Laxative action 133
Lead pipe rigidity 436
Left optic nerve, lesion of 489
Leishman's stain 50
Lemniscus, medial 407
Length-tension relationship 106
Lens 479
    bulges 492
Lenticular process 499
Leptin 237
Lesion, effects of 442, 444, 489, 503
Leukemia 51
Leukocyte 49, 259, 267, 335
    count 50
Leukocytosis 50, 51
Leukopenia 50, 51
Leukopoiesis 52, 52f, 53
Leukotrienes 236
Levonorgestrel 270
Leydig cells 244
Life-protecting hormone 225
Life-saving
    glands 224
    hormone 225
    procedure 72
Ligand-gated
    channels 15
    sodium channels 194
Light adaptation, causes for 484
Light energy 484
Light rays, effects of 367
Light reflex 488, 491
    pathway for 491, 492f
Light sleep, stage of 457
Limb
    ascending 153
    paralysis of 410
    rigidity of 435
Limbic lobe 444
Limbic system 437, 444, 445f
    regions of 456
Lipid derivatives 219
    role of 219
Lipid digesting enzyme 115
Lipid layer, functions of 2
Lipolytic activity 220
Lipolytic and ketogenic actions 219
Lipolytic enzyme 115, 120, 127,
    132, 138
Lipostatic mechanism 427
Lipoxins 236
Lippes loop 269
Lithium battery 297
Lithocholate 132
Liver 130
    cirrhosis of 31, 51, 135
    disorders of 135
    dual functions of 130
    dysfunction of 135
    fats 207
    function tests 134
    functions of 133
    nerve supply to 132
    posterior surface of 130f
Lobe, anterior 404
Lobules 234
Lobulus ensiformis 430
Local blood flow, regulation of 394
Local hormones 191, 194b, 235, 237
Local myenteric reflex 122
Local static reflexes 449, 450
Locke's solution 30
Locus coeruleus, role of 459

Long bone, parts of 216f
Long refractory period 283
Loop diuretics 176
Loop of Henle 152
Loose platelet plug 62
Lordosis 217
Loud noise 499
Low pressure bed 159, 312
Lower costal series 338, 339
Lower esophageal sphincter, role
    of 143
Lower eyelid, swelling of 493
Lower intensity 328
Lower motor neuron 409, 440, 417
    lesion 399, 417t
    nuclei of 401
Lower respiratory tracts 334
Lower right ventricle 275
Lower vaginal portion 250
L-tubules 88
Lubrication activity 140
Lubrication function 133
Lumbar enlargement 400
Lumbar ganglia 468
Lumbar puncture 466
Lung
    capacities 342
    collapse of 365
    collapsing tendency of 339
    compliance, variations in 341f
    covering of 333
    disorders 326
    expansion of 339
    function tests, types of 342
    movements of 339
    own defenses 335
    parenchyma 334
    tissues
        daily loss of 365
        inflammation of 365
    volumes 342, 343
Lusitropic action 277, 278
Luteal phase 256
Lutein cells 256
Luteinizing hormone 193, 197, 199,
    242, 244, 252, 254, 255,
    258, 259, 260
Luteolysis 236, 256
Lymph 78
    capillaries, meshwork of 77
    channels, system of 77
    composition of 78, 79f
    concentration of 78
    drainage 78f
    flow, rate of 78
    formation of 78
    functions of 78
    glands 77
    vessels join 77
Lymph node 77
    distribution of 77
    functions of 77
    lymphatic vessels to 77
    lymphoid tissues of 55
    structure of 77, 78f
    swelling of 78
Lymphatic duct, right 77
Lymphatic system 77
    drainage of 77
    organization of 77
Lymphatic tissue 77
Lymphatic vessels 78, 79
Lymphocyte 37, 38, 49, 50, 335
    activation of 54
    development of 54
    functions of 52
    processing of 54
    transport of 78

Lymphoid function 234
Lymphoid stem cells 37
Lysocephalin 127
Lysolecithin 127
Lysosomal enzymes, release of 217
Lysosome 3, 5
    functions of 5
    primary 5, 18
    secondary 5, 18
    types of 5
Lysozyme 184, 476

M

M cells 138
Macrocyte 46
Macrocytic hypochromic anemia 46
Macrocytic normochromic anemia 46
Macrogenitosomia praecox 230, 230f
Macromolecules 18
    degradation of 5
Macrophages 18, 56, 74, 75, 335
Macula densa 155, 162
    secretes thromboxane 157
Macula lutea 479
Magakaryocyte 52
Malabsorption syndrome 140
Male reproductive
    organs 239
    system 239, 239f
Male sex hormones 243
Male urethra 177
Malignant cells 335
Malleus 499
Malnutrition 129
Malpighian
    corpuscle 151
    pyramids 149
Maltase 115, 138, 139
Mammary glands 182, 200, 262, 265
    development of 265
    effect on 252
    growth of 266
Mammillary body 428
Manubrium 499
Marey's law 304
Marey's reflex 303, 304
Marginal nucleus 404, 419
Mass peristalsis 146
Masseter muscle 142
Mast cells 66, 335, 336
Mastication 142
    muscles and movements of 142
    significances of 142
Maturation
    factors 40
    stage of 242, 249
Measles 59
Mechanical energy 389
Mechanical stimulus 89
Mechanical trauma 36
Mechanotransduction 453
Mediastinum testis 240
Medulla 234, 248
    inner 149
    oblongata 378, 407, 450, 502
Medullary centers, role of 358
Medullary gradient 166
Medullary hyperosmolarity 166
Medullary pyramids 149
Medullary reflexes 396
Medullary reticular formation 431,
    445
Medullary septum 423
Megacolon 141
Megakaryocyte 38, 39, 61
Megaloblastic anemia 40, 48
Meissner's nerve plexus 110

Melanin 182, 478
    pigment, quantity of 244
Melanocyte 182
    stimulating hormone 227
Melatonin 234
Membrane junction 11
Membranous disks 482
Membranous labyrinth 450
Memory
    abnormalities of 461
    B cells, role of 57
    cells 55, 57
    consolidation of 461
    encoding 461
        synaptic terminal for 461f
    long-term 460, 461
    physiological basis of 461
    recognition 460
    role in 444
    short-term 460, 461
    T cells 54
        role of 57
Menarche 252, 253, 266
Meningocytes 74
Menopause 252, 253
Menorrhagia 48, 208
Menses 257
Menstrual bleeding 257
Menstrual cycle 253, 257f, 258t, 259, 260f
    abnormal 261t
    duration of 253
    phases of 259
    regulation of 259
    uterine changes during 257
Menstrual disorders 260
Menstrual phase 257
Menstrual symptoms 260
Menstruation 51, 257, 259
Mental retardation 207
Mercury, toxicity of 310
Mesencephalon 378
Mesenteric circulation 319
Mesenteric ganglia 111
Mesoblastic stage 37
Mesoepithelial cells 110
Meta-arterioles 320, 321
Metabolic acidosis 141, 170, 172
Metabolic activities 186
Metabolic alkalosis 172
Metabolic disorders 233, 363
Metabolic disturbances 172
Metabolic factors 318
Metabolic function 133, 216
Metabolic reactions 188
Metabolism 198
    actions on 232
    effect on 251
    general 232
Metabolites, accumulation of 91
Metaphysis 216
Metarhodopsin 484
Metencephalon 378
Methemoglobin 42
Micelles 132
Microcyte 46
Microcytic hypochromic anemia 46
Microglia 385
Micropills 270
Microtubule 6, 60
Micturition 177
    abnormalities of 181
    higher centers for 181
    reflex 180, 180f
    syncope 326
    urge for 180
    voluntary control of 180

Midbrain
    disorders of 454
    outflow 469
    reflexes 396
    reticular formation 445
Middle ear 499
    role of 504
Middle finger 314
Milieu interieur 20
Milk
    composition of 267
    curdling of 126
    digestion of 120, 126
    ejection reflex 200, 201f, 267
    fats 115
    let-down reflex 200
    secretion 266
Mineral metabolism, action on 226
Mineralocorticoids 224
    functions of 225
    mode of action of 225
Miniature bones 499
Minipills 270
Minor calyces 150, 154
Miosis 494
Mismatched blood transfusion, complications of 71f
Mitochondria 3, 60, 380, 391
Mitochondrion 6
Mitral cells, dendrites of 510
Mitral valve 275, 277
Mixed nerve 400
Modiolus 499
Mole 26
Monochromats 496
Monocular vision 485
Monocyte 37-38, 49, 50, 52, 53
    functions of 52
Monoiodotyrosine 206
Monoplegia 417
Monosaccharides 509
Monosynaptic reflex 396, 449
Morning sickness 264
Morula 263
Motion sickness 453
Motor activity, control of 435
Motor areas, topographical arrangement of 440f
Motor endplate 100
Motor homunculus 440
Motor impulses 379
Motor nerve
    fibers 381, 448f
    supply 448
Motor neuron 379, 409, 414
    lesion of 417
Motor pathways, classification of 417
Motor system, structure of 414
Mountain sickness 367
Mouth
    and salivary secretion 112
    functions of 113t
Movements, slowness of 435
Mucin, secretion of 134
Mucus 335
    function of 120
    layer 110
    membrane 110, 475
    neck cells 118
Muffled sound 310
Müller experiment 311
Müller maneuver 311, 312t
    uses of 312
Müllerian duct 243
Müllerian inhibiting substance 240
Müllerian regression factor 240, 243
Multiple sclerosis 410
Multipolar neurons 379

Multi-unit smooth muscle 106
    fibers 104, 104f
Mumps 59, 116
Murmur, classification of 291
Muscarinic receptors 471
Muscle
    action on 226
    cells, individual 85
    classification of 83
    composition of 88
    contractile elements of 87
    contraction of 414
    cramps, severe 370
    cross-section of 86f
    decreases, viscosity of 92
    excitability of 92
    fiber 85, 276, 277
        number of 102
    physiology 83
    pump 299
    relaxation of 98
    sustained contraction of 92
    tissue 1
    wastage 93
    wasting of 136
Muscle spindle 447, 447f, 448f
Muscle tone 93, 449, 457
    control of 435
    development of 449f
    maintenance of 93, 416, 448
Muscular activity 187, 432
Muscular contraction 94, 96, 98, 99, 321
    molecular basis of 97
    physical changes during 96
Muscular exercise 35
Muscular growth, effect on 244
Muscular stiffness 435
Muscular weakness 418
Muscularis mucosa 110
Myasthenia gravis 59, 102, 235, 311
Myelencephalon 378
Myelin sheath 380
    formation of 380
    functions of 381
Myelinated nerve fiber 380, 380f, 381, 383, 383f
Myelinogenesis 380, 381
Myeloid stage 37
Myenteric nerve 123
    plexus 110
Myocardial infarction 222, 318
Myocardial ischemia 292, 318
Myocarditis 326
Myocardium 276
    middle 276
    necrosis of 318
Myocytes 85
Myoepithelial cells 200
Myofibril 85, 104
    structure of 85
Myofibrillae 85
Myofilaments 104
Myometrium 250
Myopathy 217
Myopia 494
    causes of 494
    correction of 494
Myosin
    binding proteins 86
    filament 87, 87f
    head 87
    molecule 87, 87f
    occurs, phosphorylation of 106
Myosis 494
Myotatic reflex 449
Myotonia 93

Myxedema 209
    causes for 210
    signs of 210
    symptoms of 210

■ N

Narcolepsy 429
Narrow blood vessels 51
Nasal field 485
Nasal mucous membrane, receptors in 304
Nasal septum, anterior part of 510
Natriuretic peptide, B-type 235
Natural anticoagulant, presence of 65
Natural killer cell 37, 58, 335
Nausea 144, 370
Nauseating odor 511
Necrosis 10, 68, 257, 318
Necrotic endometrium 257
Neocerebellum 431, 442
Neocortex 437
Neopallium 437
Neoplasm 116
Neostigmine 102, 471
Nephrogenic diabetic insipidus 203
Nephron 151
    parts of 151, 153f, 169t
    structure of 152f
    tubular portion of 152
    types of 151, 152f
Nerve
    cell body 379, 384
    covering of 380
    cross-section of 380f
    growth factor 381
    impulse 382
    organization of 380
Nerve deafness 506, 507
Nerve fiber 379, 380, 382f, 382t, 383f, 448
    classification of 381
    degeneration of 383, 384f
    layer of 478
    properties of 382
    regeneration of 384f, 385
    types of 382t, 448f
Nervous disorders 364
Nervous erigens 179
Nervous factor 164, 107, 318, 319, 337
Nervous mechanism 122, 356
Nervous regulation 140
Nervous stimulation 277
Nervous system 264, 367, 377
    action on 236
    divisions of 377
    organization of 379f
Nervous tissue 1
Neural messengers 191
Neurilemma 380, 381
Neurocardiogenic syncope 326
Neurocrine 191
Neurodegenerative diseases 418
Neuroendocrine reflex 200, 201
Neuroepithelium 451
Neurofibrils 380
Neurogenic hypertension 310
Neurogenic shock 325
Neuroglia 377, 385
    functions of 386t
    types of 386t
Neuroglial cells 385f, 410
    classification of 385
    functions of 385
Neuroglycopenic symptoms 223
Neurohormone 192, 200
Neurohypophysis 196

Neuromodulators 394
Neuromuscular blockers 102
Neuromuscular junction 91, 97, 100, 100f, 101, 106, 193
   disorders of 102
   endplate potential in 96
   structure of 101f
Neuromuscular transmission 101, 101f
Neuron
   axon of 380
   classification of 378
   dendrites of 380
   dorsal respiratory group of 356, 357
   processes of 379
   situation, ventral respiratory group of 357
   structure of 379, 379f
   types of 379f
   ventral respiratory group of 356
Neuropeptide Y 428
Neuroplasm 379
Neuroprotective structure 466
Neurotmesis 384
Neurotransmitter 387, 392, 393t
   classification of 392
   receptor complex 391
   release of 391, 392
Neurotrophic factors 381
Neurotrophin 381
Neutrophil 38, 49, 50, 75, 267, 335
   functions of 51
Nexus 12
Nicotinic acetylcholine receptors 101
Night blindness 484
Night vision 483
Nissl bodies 380
Nissl granules 380
Nitric oxide 107, 309
Nitrobenzene 36
Nitrogen 345, 348
Nitrogen meter 348
Nitrogen narcosis 369
Nitrogen washout method 345, 348
Nocturnal micturition 181, 459
Node of Ranvier 380, 383
Nominal aphasia 463
Nonantibody proteins 58
Non-associative learning 460
Non-communicating hydrocephalus 466
Non-hemolytic transfusion reaction 71
Non-metabolizable saccharides 25
Non-myelinated nerve fiber 380, 380f, 381, 383f
Nonneural cells 385
Non-opioid neuromodulators 394
Non-pitting edema 80
Non-rapid eye movement 457
Non-respiratory functions 335
Nonsensory impulses 404
Non-specific immunity 54
Nonspecific sensory pathway 445, 446
Non-steroidal anti-inflammatory drugs 123
Non-striated muscle 83
Nontoxic goiter 210, 210f
Noradrenaline 107, 115, 162, 231, 303, 307, 309, 459, 471
   actions of 231
   secretion of 232
Normal color index 46
Normocyte 46
Normocytic normochromic anemia 46
Normotopic arrhythmia 296
Nose clip 343

Nuclear
   bag fiber 447
   chain fiber 447, 448
   layer, inner 477, 478
   membrane 7
Nuclei, lateral mass of 423, 424f
Nucleolus 7
Nucleoplasm 7
Nucleus 3, 7, 193, 379
   anterior 423
   cuneatus 407
   functions of 7, 7b
   gracilis 407
   medial mass of 423, 424f
   midline 423, 424f
   structure of 7
   ventral anterior 423
   ventral lateral 423
Numerical indicate osmolarity 167, 168f
Nutrients, lack of 91
Nutrition deficiency anemia 46, 47
Nutritional flow 320
Nutritive function 32, 263
Nyctalopia 484
Nystagmus 453

O

Obesity 204
Oblique muscles 481
Obstructive jaundice 301
Obstructive pulmonary disease, chronic 336, 348
Obstructive respiratory disease 346, 346t, 363, 365
Obstructive shock 326
Occipital eye field 488
Occipital lobe 437, 443, 488
Occluding junction 11
Ocular movements 481
   part in 481t
Ocular muscles 475, 480
   innervation of 480
Oculomotor nerve 469
   parasympathetic nucleus of 491
Odor
   classification of 511
   perception of 512
   types of 511
Olfaction 335
   type of 511
Olfactory
   bulb 510
   cortex 510
   glomeruli 510
   hyperesthesia 512
   mucous membrane 510, 511f
   pathway 510
   receptor cells 510
   rod 510
   sensation 335, 429, 510
      abnormalities of 512
      loss of 429
      pathway for 511f
      threshold olfaction for 511
   tract 510
   transduction 511
Oligodendrocytes 385
Oligomenorrhea 48, 208
Oliguria 169
Olivary nucleus, superior 502
Oocyte
   maturation inhibiting factor 254
   primary 248, 262
   secondary 249, 262
Oogenesis 248
Opacity 481
Opened glottis 336

Operant conditioned reflexes 462
Opercular insular cortex 509
Ophthalmoscope 478
Opioid neuromodulators 394
Opioid peptides 422
Opsin 484
Optic axis 475
Optic chiasma 487
   medial fibers in 489
   sides of 489
Optic disk 479, 486
Optic nerve 478, 482, 487
Optic papilla 479
Optic pathway 487
   lesions of 490f
Optic radiation 487, 488
Optic tract 487
Optical axis 476f
Optical righting reflexes 450
Optokinetic movement 481
Ora serrata 476, 477
Oral anticoagulants 67
Oral contraceptives 270
   disadvantages of 270
Oral rehydration
   solution 26
   therapy 26
Orbiculus ciliaris 476
Orbital cavity 475
Orbitofrontal cortex 441
Organ 1
Organ of Corti 500, 500f, 502
Organelles in cytoplasm 3
Organic acids 172
Organic substances 23, 29f
Orthochromatic erythroblast 38
Orthograde degeneration 384
Orthonasal olfaction 511
Orthostatic hypotension 311, 326
Orthostatic syncope 311
Oscillatory movements 398
Osmolality 25
Osmole 26
Osmoreceptors, role of 200
Osmosis 15, 16f
Osmotic diuresis 169, 175, 222
Osmotic equilibrium 36
Osmotic fragility 36
Osmotic pressure 15
Osseous canal 500
Osseous spiral lamina 500
Osseous tissue 216
Ossicular conduction 504
Osteoblastic activity 217, 251
Osteoblasts 216
   fate of 217
   functions of 216, 217
Osteoclastic activity 212, 217
Osteoclasts 212, 217
Osteocytes 217
Osteomalacia 217
Osteopontin 216
Osteoporosis 217, 251
Osteoprogenitor cells 216
Otitis media 506
Otoconia 452
Otolith membrane 452
Otolith organ 451
   functions of 453
   macula in 452f
Otoliths 451
Otosclerosis 505, 506
Ovarian changes 253
Ovarian follicles 253, 254f, 256f
   effect on 250
Ovarian hormones 250, 259

Ovary
   functional anatomy of 248
   functions of 248
   medulla of 248
Ovulation 255
Ovulation time, determination of 256
Ovulation
   process of 255f
   stages of 255
Ovum 254
   attains maximum size 255
   development of 262
   fertilization of 259, 262
   implantation of 259, 269, 270
Oxalate compounds 67
Oxidative enzymes 5
Oxygen 317, 329, 359
   carrying capacity 353, 361
   consumption of 374
   debt 374
   diffusion of 351, 352f
   extra amount of 374
   lack of 91, 107
   partial pressure of 359, 366, 367t
   poisoning 362
   pure 345
   rectifies lack of 359
   species, reactive 75
   therapy 362
   toxicity 362
   transport of 352, 353
   utilization of 362
Oxygenated blood 131, 336
Oxygen-hemoglobin dissociation curve 353, 353f
Oxyhemoglobin 353
Oxyntic cells 118
Oxyntic glands 118
Oxyphil cells 212
Oxytocin 107, 200, 428
   action of 200
   receptor 201

P

P cells 154
P wave 294
   causes of 294
Pacemaker 275, 277, 281
   abnormal 297
   artificial 297
   cells 277, 281
   current 281
   potential 281
   waves 105
Pacinian corpuscle 389, 447, 448
Packed cell volume 28, 34, 44, 45, 45f
Pain 303, 404
   control system 420
   fibers, slow 420
   impulses of 404, 406
   physiology of 419
   receptors 359
   referred 420
   sensation 419, 420, 425
      benefits of 419
      center for 420
      components of 419
      from face, pathway of 420
      from skin, pathway of 419
      from viscera, pathway of 420
   sites of referred 420f
   suppression 422
Painful stimuli 304
Pale muscles 91
Paleocerebellum 431
Paleocortex 437
Paleocortical structures 444

Index

Palpatory method 309
Palpebral fissure 475
Palpebral portion 475
Pancreas 125
    disorders of 129, 221
    dual functions of 125
    endocrine function of 218
    exocrine part of 125
    nerve supply to 125
Pancreatic amylase 127, 128
Pancreatic exocrine function
    tests 129
Pancreatic juice
    alkalinity of 125
    collection of 129
    composition of 125, 126f
    digestive enzymes of 128t
    digestive functions of 125
    neutralizing action of 127
    properties of 125
Pancreatic lipase 127, 128
    lack of 129
Pancreatic polypeptide 129, 220, 428
Pancreatic secretion, regulation of 127, 128f
Pancreatic somatostatin 123, 220
Pancreatic tumor 124
Pancreatitis 129
Paneth cells 138
Panhypopituitarism 203
Papilla 154, 508
Papillary ducts 154
Papillary muscle 277
    repolarization of 294
Para-aminohippuric acid 159, 174
Paracellular route 163
Paracrine messengers 191
Paradoxical sleep 457
Paraffin 183
Paraflocculus 430
Parafollicular cells 205, 214
Paralgesia 422
Paralysis 93, 370, 418
    agitans 435
    causes for 418
    types of 417t, 418
Paramedian lobe 430
Paramyxovirus 116
Paraplegia 417
Parasympathetic blockers 471
Parasympathetic division 378, 427, 469
Parasympathetic fibers 115, 471
Parasympathetic nerve 179, 337
    fibers 111, 125, 179, 302, 480
    functions of 179, 302
Parasympathetic tone 303
Parasympathetic vasodilator
    fibers 307
Parasympathomimetic drugs 471
Parathormone 163, 212
    actions of 212
    mode of action of 213
    receptor 213
    role of 215
    secretion, regulation of 213
Parathyroid function tests 214
Parathyroid gland 212, 212f, 214, 264
    disorders of 213
    functional histology of 212
    morphology of 212
Parathyroidectomy 213
Paratyphoid 51
Paraventricular nucleus 200
Parenchyma of testis 240
Parenchymal cells 234
Paresthesia 413
Parietal cells 118, 120
Parietal layer 151, 333

Parietal lobe 437, 441
Parieto-occipital sulcus 437, 441
Parkinson disease 435, 436, 461
Parkinsonism 435
Paroxysmal order 364
Paroxysmal tachycardia 296, 297
Pars distalis 196
Pars intermedia 196
Pars nervosa 199
Pars tuberalis 196
Particularly albumin 174
Parturition 51, 264
    stages of 265
Pasties 116
Patella clonus 398
Patent ductus arteriosus 291, 315, 323
Pathological reflexes 396, 398
Pavlov pouch 120, 121f
    use of 121
Pavlov's bell-dog experiments 462
Peak expiratory flow rate 346
Pectus carinatum 217
Pelvic
    bone, effect on 244
    colon 140
    nerve 111, 147, 179, 469
    outlet, narrowing of 244
    region, pathway of pain
        sensation 420
Pelvis
    funnel-like shape of 244
    lengthening of 244
    organs of 239f, 249f
Pendular movement 145, 398, 433
Pentolinium 471
Pepsin 119
Pepsinogen
    cells 118
    secretion of 120
Peptic activity, measurement of 123
Peptic ulcer 123
Peptidases 138, 139
Peptide mechanism 427
Peptide YY 129
Peptone shock 45
Periaqueductal gray matter 421
Pericardial 276
Pericardium 276
Perilymph 504
Perimenopause 261
Perimetrium 85, 250, 380
Periodic breathing 360, 363, 364f
Periosteum 216
Periotic canal 500
Peripheral arterial pulse 313
Peripheral chemoreceptors 304, 359
Peripheral ganglia 468
Peripheral membrane proteins 2
Peripheral nervous system 377, 378, 385, 400, 468
Peripheral neuroglial cells 385
Peripheral proteins 2
Peripheral speech apparatus 462
Peripheral venous pressure 311
Peristalsis 143
Peristalsis
    in fasting, significance of 146
    reverse 241
Peristaltic movement 145, 236
Peristaltic rush 145
Peristaltic waves 143, 179
Peritoneal dialysis 175
Peritoneum 117
Pernicious anemia 40, 48, 51, 120
Peroxidase 42
Peroxisome 3, 5
Peroxisomes, functions of 5
Petit mal 456

Phagocytic function 75
Phagocytosis 18, 51
    mechanism of 18
    process of 18f
Phagosomal contents 18
Phagosome 5, 18
Phalangeal cells 501
Phantom limb 425
Pharyngeal reflex 144
Pharyngeal stage 142, 143
Pharynx consists, wall of 110
Pheochrome cells 231
Pheochromocytoma 233
Pheromones 184, 510
Phlebogram 315, 316f
Phonocardiogram 287f
Phosphate 215
Phosphate buffer system 171
Phosphate ions 171f
Phosphate level
    normal value of 215
    regulation of 215
Phosphate mechanism 171, 215
Phosphates 163
Phosphaturic action 213
Phospholipids 2
Phosphoric acid 91
Phosphorus 215
Phosphorylcholine 127
Photopic vision 483
Photosensitive pigment 484
Physiology, high altitude 366
Physostigmine 102, 471
Pia mater 400
Pigeon chest 217
Pigment epithelium, layer of 477, 478
Pill method 270
Pill rolling movements 435
Pillar cells 501
Pillar cells, inner 501
Pineal gland 234
Pinna 498
Pinocytosis 18, 321
    mechanism of 18
    process of 18f
Pitting edema 80
Pituitary cachexia 203
Pituitary diabetes 201
Pituitary gland 196
    disorders of 201, 201t
    divisions of 196
    parts of 197f
    role of 208
Pituitary hormones
    anterior 197, 259
    regulation of secretion of 196
    secretion of posterior 426
Pituitary stalk 196
Pituitary tumors 201
Placenta 250, 251, 263, 265, 321, 333
    functions of 263
    premature detachment of 324
Placental estrogen, actions of 263
Placental progesterone, actions
    of 263
Plain muscle 83
Plantar reflex, abnormal 398
Planum semilunatum 451
Plasma 263, 207
Plasma cells 55, 57
    proliferation of 57
    role of 57
Plasma proteins 29, 80f, 161, 355
    functions of 30
    level 31
    molecular weight of 30t
    origin of 29
    properties of 30
Plasma transfusion 73

Plasma volume 456
    measurement of 25
Plasmapheresis 30
Plasmin 65
Plasminogen, inactive 65
Plastic tube 272
Platelet 38
    accelerate hemostasis 61
    activating factor 62, 63
    derived growth factor 61, 75
        secretion of 75
    development of 61
    disorders 61, 61b
    fate of 61
    functions of 61
    grouping of 61
    plug, formation of 62
    properties of 61
    secrete serotonin, activated 62
    shape of 60
    size of 60
    transfusion 72
    under electron microscope 60f
Plethysmograph 343-345
Pleural sac 333
Plexiform layer 477, 478
Pluripotent hematopoietic stem
    cells 37
Pneumocytes 335
Pneumonia 345, 365
Pneumotaxic center 357
Pneumothorax 341, 345, 365
Podocytes 161
Poikilothermic animals 187
Polar cushion 155
Polarized
    light 85
    state 94
Polkissen cells 155
Polychromatic erythroblast 38
Polycystic kidney disease 175
Polycythemia 35, 45
Polycythemia vera 35
    physiological 35
    primary 35
    secondary 35
Polydactylism 429
Polydipsia 204, 222
Polygraph 313
Polymenorrhea 208
Polymorphonuclear leukocytes 49
Polyphagia 222
Polypnea 360
Polysaccharides 509
Polysome 9
Polysynaptic reflexes 396
Polyuria 169, 204, 222
Pontine centers 357
    role of 358
Pontine reticular formation 445
Pontocerebellar fibers 431
Popliteal pulse 314
Porphyrin 34, 41
Portal system 158, 159
Portal vein, branch of 130
Postcatacrotic wave 314
Postcentral gyrus 441
Postcoital pills 270
Postganglionic
    fibers 111, 471
    neurons 469
    parasympathetic nerve 236
    sympathetic cholinergic nerves 236
    sympathetic noradrenergic fibers 471
Postmenopausal syndrome 252
Postprandial blood sugar level 220
Postsynaptic inhibition 392

Postsynaptic membrane 100, 391
Postsynaptic neuron 390, 391
Postural movements, control of 440
Postural reflexes 449
Postural syncope 326
Posture 31
  basic phenomena of 449
  maintenance of 449
Potassium 17, 163
  channels 392
  ion 392
    action on 225
    efflux of 281
    excess of 107
Potassium-retaining diuretics 176
Power stroke 98
Pre-Bötzinger complex 358
Precapillary sphincter 320
Precatacrotic wave 314
Precentral cortex 438
Pre-eclampsia 264
Pre-emulsified fats 115
Prefrontal cortex 441
Preganglionic fibers 468, 471
Preganglionic neurons 468
Pregnancy 262
  corpus luteum of 257
  hypertensive disorder of 264
  maintenance of 256
  medical termination of 271
  test strip 265
  toxemia of 264
Prehepatic jaundice 135
Preinspiratory position 338
Premenstrual syndrome 260
Premotor area, functions of 440
Preoptic nucleus 187
Presbycusis 503
Presbyopia 480, 493, 495
Presenile dementia 461
Pressure
  determining filtration 161
  diuresis 225, 308
  gradient 351
  natriuresis 308
  prolonged severe 384
  stimulus 389
  systolic 310
  ventilator 373
Presynaptic
  axon terminals 390
  inhibition 392, 422
  membrane 100, 390
  neuron 390
  terminal, primary 461
Presystolic gallop 290
Pretectal nucleus 488
Prevent blood clotting 67
Primordial follicle 248, 254
Procarboxypeptidases 127
Procoagulants agents 67
Procollagenase 127
Proelastase 127
Proerythroblast 38, 40
Profibrinolysin 245
Progestasert 270
Progesterone 251, 258, 263
  functions of 252
  influence of 259
  lack of 257
  mode of action of 252
  regulation of secretion of 252
Prognathism 202
Progressive hepatolenticular degeneration 436
Progressive inflammatory disease 410
Prokaryotes 7
Prolactin 199
  inhibitory hormone 197, 426

Proline-rich proteins 115
Propulsive movements 145, 146
Prosecretin, inactive 129
Prosencephalon 377, 378
Prostacyclin 236, 309
Prostaglandin 150, 162, 235, 236
  administration of 271
  types of 236
Prostate gland 241
Prostatic fluid 241
Protanopia 496
Protein
  addition of 78
  anabolism of 198
  channels 14
  conservation 219
  depletion 222
  digestion of 125, 126
  factories 6
  layers, functions of 2
  metabolism 207, 251
    action on 219, 226
  reserve 30
  role of 219
  sparing effect 219
  synthesis of 3
  total 135
Proteoglycan meshwork 80
Proteoglycan molecules 479
Proteolytic enzyme 119, 125, 126, 138, 245, 262
Prothrombin activator 61
  formation of 64, 65
Prothrombin time 67
Protodiastole 286
Protodiastolic period, end of 289
Protopathic sensations 412
Proximal convoluted tubule 152, 168
Psychological imbalance 264
Psychomotor epilepsy 456
Psychotherapy 252
Pterygoid muscles 142
Ptosis 493
Ptyalism 116
Pudendal nerve 147, 179, 181
Pulmonary arterial pressure 337
Pulmonary artery 275, 336
Pulmonary blood flow 337
Pulmonary blood pressure 337
Pulmonary blood vessels 336
Pulmonary capillary pressure 337
Pulmonary circulation 279, 317, 336, 337
Pulmonary congestion 345
Pulmonary edema 326, 365, 345
Pulmonary embolism 68
Pulmonary function tests 342
Pulmonary hypertension 368
Pulmonary surfactant 339
Pulmonary tuberculosis 345, 365
Pulmonary veins 275, 337
Pulmonary ventilation 347
Pulse
  abnormal 315
  examination of 314
  generator 297
  points 314, 314t
  pressure 305
  rate 315t
  transmission of 313
Pulses deficit 313, 315
Pulsus paradoxus 315
Pump handle movement 339
Pupil 476
  abnormal constriction of 494
  constriction of 491
  dilatation of 484, 491
Pupillary reflexes 491
Purkinje fibers 282, 294

Purpura 67, 68
Purpuric spots 68
Pursuit movement 481
Pus cells 51, 173, 329
Putamen 434
Pyelonephritis 175
Pyknosis 38
Pyloric canal 117
Pyloric glands 118
Pyloric region 117
Pyloric sphincter 117
Pyothorax 341, 345, 365
Pyramidal cells 408
Pyramidal decussation 409
Pyramidal lobules 240
Pyramidal tracts 408, 409f
Pyrexia 189
Pyrogens 189
Pyrrole rings 41

Q

QRS complex 294
Quadriplegia 417

R

Rabbit antiserum 265
Rachitic rosary 217
Radial pulse 309, 314
  examination of 314
  tracing 313
Radioactive sodium 25
Ramp fashion 358
Raphe nucleus 459
Raphe nucleus, role of 459
Rapid alternate movements 432
Rapid conjugate movements 457
Rapid eye movement sleep 457
Rapid hemolysis 71
Rapid jerky movements 436
Rare pituitary disorder 203
Ratchet theory 98
Reabsorption 163, 163f
Rebound phenomenon 399
Receptor cells 451
Receptor epithelium 451
Receptor organ 451
Receptor proteins 391
Reciprocal inhibition 399, 450
Reciprocal innervation 399, 450
Rectal temperature 186
Rectum 140, 469
Rectus 480
Red blood cells 28, 30, 33, 35, 38, 41, 44, 49t, 52, 265
  fate of 34, 34f
  functions of 34
  lifespan of 34
  morphology of 33
  properties of 34f
Red cell transfusion 72
Red muscles 91
Referred pain, mechanism of 420
Reflex 457
  action 127
  activity 395
    center for 424
    stage of 410
  arc 395
  classical conditioned 462
  classification of 395
  failure, stage of 410
  loss of 410
  muscular activity, control of 435
  positive conditioned 462
  positive supporting 450
  properties of 398
  protective 358, 396
  secondary conditioned 462

significance of 395
swallowing 336
unconditioned 115, 121, 127, 396
Refractive errors 485, 494, 494f, 495t
Refractive power 494
Relative refractory period 92, 283, 383
Relaxin 263
Releasing and inhibitory hormones 197
Remote memory 460
Renal artery 158
Renal autoregulation 159
Renal blood flow 158, 162, 174
  measurement of 159, 174
  regulation of 159
Renal blood vessels 158, 158f
Renal calculi 175
Renal capillaries 159f
Renal circulation 158, 317
  salient features of 159
Renal clearance 174
Renal columns 149
Renal corpuscle 151, 149, 152f, 161f
Renal failure 173-175
  acute 175, 325
  chronic 175
Renal function tests 173
Renal hypertension 310
Renal pelvis 149, 154
Renal plasma flow 174
Renal plasma flow, measurement of 174
Renal shutdown 71
Renal sinus 149
Renal system 103, 149
Renal tubule 163, 171f
  segments of 165
Renin 150, 162, 235
  actions of 235
  secretion of 155
Renin-angiotensin
  mechanism 308
  system 156, 156f
Renshaw cell 392
Renshaw cell inhibition 392
Reproduction system 48, 103, 239
Repulsive odor 511
Residual volume 342, 344
Resinous odor 511
Resistant vessels 300, 306
Respiration 333, 374
  action on 232
  altered patterns of 360
  disease of 360
  disorders of 360
  effect of 252, 311, 362
  external 333
  internal 333
  mechanics of 338
  muscles of 338
  nervous regulation of 356
  phases of 333
  rate of 347
  regulation of 356
Respiratory acid 172
Respiratory acidosis 172
Respiratory alkalosis 172
Respiratory bronchiole 334, 335
Respiratory centers 308, 356, 357t
  connections of 357
  integration of 358
Respiratory chain 6
Respiratory disorders 365
Respiratory distress syndrome 325
Respiratory disturbances 172
Respiratory exchange ratio 352
Respiratory function 32, 263
Respiratory gases
  exchange of 350, 351
  transport of 41, 350

Index

Respiratory membrane 335, 350
   layers of 350, 351*t*
   structure of 350*f*
   thickness of 351
Respiratory minute volume 346, 347
Respiratory movements 338
Respiratory muscle, paralysis of 345
Respiratory muscles 341
Respiratory pressures 339, 340*f*
Respiratory protective reflexes 336
Respiratory pump 299, 340
Respiratory quotient 352, 374
Respiratory rate 346
Respiratory sinus arrhythmia 296, 303
Respiratory system 48, 103, 264, 325, 333, 367, 456
   action on 236
Respiratory tract 334*f*, 335
   and pulmonary circulation 333
   functional anatomy of 333
Respiratory unit 334
   structure of 335, 335*f*
Respirometer 343, 345, 346
Resting membrane potential 94, 95, 104
Resting tremor 435
Restrictive respiratory disease 346
Resuscitation, manual methods of 371
Rete testis 240
Reticular activating system, ascending 406, 445, 459
Reticular cells 74
Reticular formation 302, 307, 420, 437, 444
   functional divisions of 446*f*
Reticular network 38
Reticulocyte 38, 40
Reticuloendothelial cells 74, 75
Reticuloendothelial system 74, 75
Reticulum 74
Retina 447, 475, 482, 486, 496
   amacrine cells of 236
   layers of 478
Retinine 484
Retinitis pigmentosa 484
Retinol 484
Retronasal olfaction 510-512
Rh
   incompatibility 72*f*
   negative blood 71
   system 69
Rheobase 90, 90*f*
Rhesus monkey 71
Rheumatoid arthritis 59
Rhodopsin 482, 484
   resynthesis of 484
Rhombencephalon 378
Rhythm 314
Rhythm method 268
Rhythmic discharge 358
Rhythmicity 281
Rib cage, effect on 244
Ribonucleic acid 7, 9, 127, 197
Ribosomes 3, 6
Rickets 217
Right optic nerve, lesion of 489
Right optic radiation, lesion of 489
Righting reflexes 449
   centers for 450
Rigor mortis 92
Ring finger 314
Rinne test 506
Rod cell, structure of 482
Rods 487
   and cones 482, 483*t*
   layer of 477, 478
   functions of 483
Rotatory acceleration 452

Rough endoplasmic reticulum 3
Rouleaux formation 30, 34, 34*f*
R-R interval, measurement of 295
Rubber tube 343
Rubrothalamic fibers 432
Ryle tube 123

S

S cells 129, 138
SA node 281
Saccadic movement 481
Saccules 483
Sacral ganglia 468
Sacral parasympathetic fibers 469
Sacral parasympathetic nerves 420
Saliva
   composition of 114
   enzyme lysozyme of 115
   functions of 114
   lack of 116
Salivary amylase 115
Salivary glands 114*f*, 125, 469
   major 113*f*
   nerve supply to 115
Salivary secretion
   disorders of 116
   reflex regulation of 115
   regulation of 115
Salt taste 510
Saltatory conduction 381, 383
Salt-retaining effect 225
Sarcolemma 85
Sarcomere 86, 98, 104
   parts of 88*f*
Sarcoplasm 85
   reticulum 87, 88
Sarcotubular system 87, 88*f*, 104
Satellite cells 385
Satiety center 427
Scala media 500
Scala tympani 500
Scala vestibuli 500
Scalp electrodes 454
Scars 410
Schwann cells 380, 381, 385
Sclera 476
Sclerosis 217, 341, 410
Scopolamine 471
Scotopic vision 483
Scotopsin 484
Sea sickness 144, 453
Sebaceous glands 183, 498
   secretory activity of 244
Sebum
   composition of 183
   functions of 183
Second heart sound 286, 289
Second order neuron 403, 407, 502, 503, 509
Second polar body 249
Secretes seminal fluid 240
Secretin 129, 219
Secretion, regulation of 200
Secretory function 5, 118*t*, 139, 141, 185, 196
Secretory lysosomes 5
Secretory vesicles 3, 5
Seddon neuropraxia 384
Segmental artery 158
Segmental static reflexes 449, 450
Seizures 27, 264
   general onset 456
Selective permeability 3
Self-antigens 59
Semantic aphasia 463
Semen 245
   clotting of 241
   composition of 245, 246*f*
   properties of 245

Semicircular canal 451
   functions of 452
   posterior 453
   superior 452
Semilunar valve 277, 315
   synchronous closure of 289
Seminal fluid 241
Seminal plasma 245
Seminal vesicles 240
Seminiferous tubules 240
Semipermeable membrane 1
Senile decay 203
Sensation 412
   abnormal 413, 413*b*
   classification of 413*f*
   complex 412
   loss of 410, 424
   perception of 442
   specific 389
   synthesis of 442
Sense organs, specialized 412, 475
Sensory 303
   adaptation 389
   area 302, 307
      functions of 302
      primary 441
      topographical arrangement of 442*f*
   ataxia 408
   fibers 381, 414
   function 184
   homunculus 441
   impulses 379
   information, processing of 423
   motor area 432, 442
      part of 441
   nerve 395
      fibers 448*f*
      supply 448
   neurons 379
   nucleus, chief 403
   pathways 413, 415*t*, 445
      disorders of 416*t*
   transduction 389
   type of 453
Septic shock 326
Septula testis 240
Sequential pills 270
Serosa 110
Serotonin 107, 236, 237, 309
Serous fluid 257
Serous layer 110
Serous membrane 110
Sertoli cells 240
   role of 242
Serum 28
   albumin 29
   globulin 29
   lipase test 129
   oozing of 65
Sex chromosomes 7, 262
Sex determination 262
Sex hormones 224
   role of 39
   secretion of 183
Sex-linked recessive character 496
Sex organs
   effect on 244
   primary 239
Sexual characters, effect on secondary 244, 251
Sexual function 208
   regulation of 428, 444
Sexual life in females 252
Sexual sensations, center for 424
Sexually transmitted infections 269
Sham feeding 121
Shivering 187, 188, 369
Shock 299, 326, 465

Short ciliary nerves 480, 493
Short sightedness 494
Shoulder, effect on 244
Shunt, physiological 317, 320, 337
SIADH 203
Sialolithiasis 116
Sialorrhea 116
Sickle cell anemia 45, 47
Sightedness, long 494
Sigmoid colon 140, 146, 147
Signaling cells 191
Silicon-coated container 67
Simmonds' disease 203
Simple diffusion 14
Simple muscle contraction 90
Simple muscle curve 90, 91
Simple muscle twitch 90
Simple reflex arc 395*f*
Single breath 343
Single-unit smooth muscle 104
   fibers 104*f*
   lies 106
Sinoaortic mechanism 304, 308
Sinoatrial block 296
Sinoatrial node 275, 282*f*
Sinus arrhythmia 296
Sinus bradycardia 296
Sinus tachycardia 296
Sjögren's syndrome 116
Skeletal muscle 83, 93, 95*f*, 177, 208, 236, 321, 330, 480
   action on 232
   activities of 414
   circulation 317, 321
   composition of 88*f*
   extra fusal fibers of 414
   fiber 110, 382*t*
   hyperexcitability of 214
   mass 86*f*
   properties of 89
   quick fatigue of 232
   structure of 85, 86*f*
   triad of 88
Skilled memory 461
Skin 182
   action on 232
   appendages of 182
   color of 182
   diffused bluish coloration of 364
   effect on 244
   functions of 184
   glands of 183
   pigmentation of 182
   structure of 182, 183*f*
Sleep 208, 454
   and wakefulness, regulation of 428
   apnea syndrome 312
   cycles 457
   paralysis 457
   physiological changes during 456
   stages of 457
   types of 457
Sliding mechanism 97
Slow ejection period 286
Slow-wave rhythm 104, 105
Small bile ducts 131
Small coenzyme 127
Small electronic device 297
Small intestine 137
   disorders of 140
   functional anatomy of 137
   functions of 139
   glands of 137, 138*t*
   movements of 145, 145*f*
   parts of 137
Small lymphocytes 50
Smallest bone 499
Smallpox 59

Smell
  perception of 511
  response to 428
  sensation of 475, 508
Smooth endoplasmic reticulum 3
Smooth muscle 83, 84, 93, 103, 105f, 106, 480
  action on 232
  activities, control of 107
  cells 155
  contraction of 107
    molecular basis of 106
  fibers 84t, 103, 104f, 110
    special structures of 104
    types of 104
  functions of 103
  relaxation of 107
  structure of 104
Sneezing reflex 335, 336
Snellen's chart 485
Soccer 329
Sodium 17, 18f, 163
Sodium acetoacetate 171
Sodium channels 391
Sodium chloride 168
  decreases infiltrate 162
Sodium citrate 44
Sodium cotransport 17
Sodium dependent glucose transporter 164
Sodium dihydrogen phosphate 171
Sodium hydrogen antiport pump 171
Sodium ions 281
  action on 225
Sodium potassium pump 94
Sodium, reabsorption of 164, 167
Solid tissue, free histiocytes of 75
Somatic autosomes 262
Somatic chromosomes 262
Somatic functions 378
Somatic nerve 179, 480
Somatic nerve fibers 381, 396
Somatic nerve supply 179
Somatic nervous system 378
Somatic reflexes 396
Somatic sensations 412
Somatomedin 198
Somatomotor, control of 446
Somatomotor, facilitation of 446
Somatomotor system 412, 414
Somatosensory area 441, 442
Somatosensory system 412
Somatosensory system, pathways 413
Somatostatin 129, 198, 220, 428
Somatotrophs 197
Somatotropic hormone 197
Somesthetic association area 441, 442
Somnambulism 459
Sound
  appreciation of loudness of 506
  appreciation of pitch of 505
  box 335
  disappearance of 310
  energy 505
  interpretation of 442, 443
  localization of 506
  murmuring 310
  properties of 505
  transduction 505
  types of conduction of 504
  waves, amplitude of 505
Sour taste 510
Spasm 213
Spastic paralysis 93
Spasticity 93
Spatial summation 392, 398
Special sensations 412, 475

Speech 439, 463
  apparatus 335
  center 463
  disorders of 51, 463
  impairment of 319, 463
  mechanism of 462
  motor area for 441
  nervous control of 463
  problems 436
  role in 115
Sperm 245
  count 245
  motility of 245
    maintenance of 241
  structure of 245
  survival time of 245
Spermatids 242
Spermatocyte
  primary 241
  secondary 242
Spermatogenesis 241, 242f
  hormones in 242, 243t
  stages of 241
Spermatogenic cells 240
Spermatogonia 240, 241
Spermatozoa 241
  precursor cells of 240
Spermiation 242
Spermicidal agent 269
Spermicide 269
Spermiogenesis 242
Sphincter of Oddi 131
Sphygmomanometer 309
Spike potential 96, 105
Spinal canal 401
Spinal cord 111f, 377, 400, 414, 431, 450
  ascending tracts of 402, 403, 403t
  coverings of 400
  descending tracts of 408, 408t, 410
  disease of 410
  enlargements of 400
  extent of 400
  features of 400
  gray horn of 402f, 402t
  gray matter of 401
  hemisection of 410
  incomplete transection of 410
  injury 381
  internal structure of 401
  interneurons of 422
  laminae of 401
  long tracts of 402
  nuclei in 401
  posterior white column of 407f
  sacral segments of 146f
  section of 401f
  segments of 400, 400t
  short tracts of 402
  symptoms of hemisection of 410
  tracts in 402, 404f
  transection of 410
  white matter of 402
Spinal disk 411
Spinal nerves 381, 400, 400t
Spinal reflexes 396
Spinal shock, stage of 410
Spinal veins 465
Spindle cells 254
Spinocerebellar tracts 406f
Spinocerebellum 431
Spino-olivary tract 406
Spinoreticular tract 406, 445
Spinotectal tract 406
Spinothalamic tract 405f
  anterior 403
  lateral 404, 405f, 420
Spinovestibular tract 406

Spinovisual reflex 406
Spiral filament 246
Spiral ganglion, bipolar cells of 502
Spirogram 343, 344f
Spirometer 343, 344f
Splanchnic circulation 317, 319
Splanchnic nerve 118, 125
Splanchnic region 300
Spleen 55, 74, 75
Splenic circulation 319
Splenic functions 76
Squalene 183
Stagnant hypoxia 361
Staircase phenomenon 283
Standard limb leads 293
Stapedius 499
Staphylococcus 36
Starling hypothesis 161
Starling's law 106
Static exercise 328
Static lung function tests 342
Static reflexes 449
Statoconia 452
Statokinetic reflexes 449, 450
Statotonic reflexes 449, 450
Steatorrhea 129, 140
Stem cell 37, 38f, 118, 267
  factor 39
Stercobilinogen 133
Stereocilia 451, 452, 501
Stereognosis 407f, 408, 413, 442
Sterilization 272
Steroid hormone 195
Sterols 183
Stiff hairs 498
Stigma 255
Stimulus 89, 143
  artifact 95
  number of 91
  point of 90f, 91
  qualities of 89
  response to 382
  rheobasic strength of 90
  strength of 91
  types of 89
  unconditioned 462
Stomach 117, 118
  emptying of 144
  filling of 144
  functions of 117, 119
  glands of 118
  movements of 144
  nerve supply to 118
  parts of 117, 117f
  wall, structure of 117
Stout collagen fibers 182
Strain 326
Stratum corneum 182
Stratum germinativum 182
Stratum granulosum 182
Stratum lucidum 182
Stratum spinosum 182
Streptococcus 36, 115
Stress 220
Stretch 303
  muscle 83
  receptors 110, 179, 180, 304
  reflex 396, 448, 449
Stridor 214
Stroke 319
  volume 298
Stunted skeletal growth 203
Stupor 369
Subarachnoid space 377, 464, 467
Subconscious kinesthetic sensation 404, 405, 406f, 413
Subconscious movements, regulation of 435
Subcortical area 403

Subcortical auditory center 502
Subcortical center 488
Subcortical structures 444
Subcutaneous tissue 74, 184
Subdural hematoma 454
Subliminal stimuli, summation of 283
Subliminal stimulus 383
Subliminal strength 382
Submaximal stimulus 89
Submucus layer 110
Submucus nerve plexus 110
Subneural clefts 101
Subpapillary venous plexus 321
Substantia gelatinosa, neurons of 420
Substantia nigra 434
Successive nodes 383
Succinylcholine 102
Succus entericus
  composition of 138
  digestive enzymes of 139t
  functions of 138, 139
  properties of 138
  regulation of secretion of 140
Sucrase 138, 139
Suicidal bags 5
Sulci 400
  complicated pattern of 437
Sulcus, lateral 437
Sulfates 163
Sulfhemoglobin 42
Summed electrical activity 292
Sunstroke 370
Superficial papillary layer 182
Superficial reflexes 396
  elicited from skin 397t
Superior colliculus 488
Superior vermis, parts of 431t
Superoxide 75
Supplementary motor area 439, 441
Supporting cell 240, 385
Supporting reflexes 449, 450
Suppressor area 440
Suppressor T cells 54, 56
Supramaximal stimulus 89
Supraoptic nucleus 200, 488
Suprarenal glands 224
Suspension stability 34, 44
  role in 30
Suspensory ligaments 476, 479
  traction of 492
Sustentacular cells 510
Swallowing apnea 143
Sweat glands 183, 184, 469
Sweat secretion 457
Sweet taste 509
Swinging 144
Swollen lymph nodes 78
Sylvian fissure 437
Sylvian sulcus 441
Sympathetic blockers 471
Sympathetic chain 480
  ganglia 468
Sympathetic cholinergic fibers 307
Sympathetic division 378, 468
Sympathetic fibers 115, 471
Sympathetic ganglia 468
Sympathetic nerve 179, 337
  fiber 111, 303, 480
  functions of 111, 179, 303
  mode of action of 303
Sympathetic postganglionic fibers 303
Sympathetic stimulation 162
Sympathetic tone 303, 307, 329
Sympathetic vasodilator fibers 307
Sympathomimetic drugs 471
Synapse 390
  functions of 391
  properties of 392
Synaptic cleft 100, 391

Index

Synaptic delay 392, 398
Synaptic inhibition, significance of 392
Synaptic transmission 391f
Synaptic vesicles 391
Synchronized alpha waves,
 replacement of 455
Synchronized waves 454
Syncope 326
Syncytium 276
Syntactical aphasia 463
Synthesis, regulation of 394
Synthetic estrogen 270
Synthetic function 133, 141, 185
Synthetic progesterone 270
Synthetic sensations 413
Syphilis 410
Syringomyelia 410
Systemic aorta 275
Systemic arterial pressure 162
Systemic circulation 279

T

T cell, 56
 specificity of 57
T lymphocytes 52, 54, 59, 235
 processing of 235
T wave 294
Tachycardia 233, 301
Tachypnea 360
Tactile discrimination 407, 407f, 412
Tactile localization 407, 407f, 412
Tank respirator 372
Tapping sound 310
Target cells 191
Taste 508
 appreciation of 114
 blindness 510
 bud 508, 509
 center 509
 pore 509
 receptor cells 508
 sensation 4756, 508-510
  pathway for 509, 509f
 transduction 510
Tear 475
Tectorial membrane 501
Telencephalon 378
Telereceptors 388
Temperature regulating
 capacity, loss of 370
 mechanism of 187
Temperature sensations 406
Temporal field 485
Temporal lobe 437, 442, 502
Temporal lobe syndrome 443, 461
Temporal muscle 142
Temporal pulse 314
Temporal summation 392, 300
Temporary endocrine gland 256
Tendon reflexes 396
Tensor tympani 499
Terminal bronchiole 334
Terminal cisternae 88
Terminal ganglia 468
Terminal portion 334
Tertiary bronchi 334
Tertiary conditioned reflex 462
Testes
 atrophy of 229
 coverings of 239
 descent of 243
 effects of extirpation of 246
 endocrine function of 243
 functions of 239, 241
 gametogenic functions of 241
 lobules of 240
 structure of 240f
 undescended 243

Testosterone 242
 functions of 243, 244
 mode of action of 244
 secretion 243
 regulation of 244, 245f
Tetanus bacillus 36
Tetany 213
Tetraethylammonium ion 471
Tetraiodothyronine 205
Tetraplegia 417
Thalamic animal 449
Thalamic hand 425
Thalamic lesion 424
Thalamic nuclei 423, 424f
Thalamic phantom limb 425
Thalamic reticular nucleus 423
Thalamic syndrome 424
Thalamocortical fibers 432
Thalamogeniculate branch 424
Thalamus 420, 423
Thalassemia 42, 47
Thebesian veins 337
Theca externa 254
Theca folliculi 254
Theca interna 250, 254
 cells 251
Thelarche 266
Therapeutic plasma exchange 30, 31
Thermal sensations 404
Thermal stimulus 89
Thermistors 300
Thermodilution technique 300
Thermogenic effect 252
Thermoreceptors 187, 359
Thermoregulatory disorders 189
Thermoregulatory system 329
Thermostatic mechanism 427, 428
Theta rhythm 455
Theta wave 457
Thiocyanate 211
Thioureylenes 211
Third degree injury 384
Third heart sound 286, 289, 290
Third order neuron 403, 420, 487,
 502, 503, 509
Thirst mechanism 428
Thoracic cage, movements of 338
Thoracic duct 77
Thoracic ganglia 468
Thoracic lid 338
Thoracic segment 402f
Thoracolumbar outflow 468
Thorax, abnormal 341
Thready pulse 315
Threshold stimulus 90
Threshold strength 90
Thrombasthenic purpura 68
Thrombocytes 60
Thrombocythemia 61
Thrombocytopenia 61, 68
Thrombocytopenic purpura 68
Thrombocytosis 61
Thrombophlebitis 321
Thrombopoietin 61, 134, 150, 235, 235
Thrombosis 68
Thrombosthenin 65
Thromboxane 236, 309
Thrombus 68, 318
Thymin 205
Thymopoietin 235
Thymosin 54, 235
Thymus 54, 234
 endocrine function of 235
 functions of 234
 hyperactivity of 235
 structure of 234
Thyroglobulin 205
 organification of 206
 synthesis 206

Thyroid
 adenoma 209
 disorders, treatment for 211
 follicles 205
 function tests 211
 peroxidase, presence of 206
Thyroid gland 205, 205f, 207, 264
 disorders of 209
 histology of 205f
 morphology of 205
 posterior surface of 212f
Thyroid hormone 195
 deficiency of 207
 functions of 207
 in blood, transport of 207
 mode of action of 208
 regulation of secretion of 208, 208f
 release of 207
 storage of 206
 synthesis of 206
Thyroid stimulating hormone 21,
 193, 197, 199, 208, 209
 receptor antibodies 209
Thyroidectomy 213
Thyrotoxicosis 209
Thyrotrophs 197
Thyrotropic hormone 197
Thyrotropin-releasing hormone 188,
 197, 209, 426
Thyroxine 39, 193, 194, 205, 221, 309
 binding
  globulin 207
  prealbumin 207
 hyposecretion of 208
 secretion of 21f
Tibialis pulse 314
Tidal volume 342, 344, 346
 product of 347
Tight collar dress 326, 398
Tight junction, functions of 11
Timed vital capacity 345
Tissue 1
 fluid 78
  formation of 79, 80f
  functions of 79
 macrophage 52, 74
 plasminogen activator 65
Tone, adjustment of 449
Tongue 508
 part of 508
Tonic contraction 106, 179
Tonic receptors 389
Tonicity 25, 26
Torsion 481
Total blood, specific gravity of 28
Total body water, measurement of 24
Total iron in body, regulation of 43
Total leukocyte count 50
Touch receptor 389
 plenty of 200
Toxemia 410
Toxic goiter 210
Toxic substances 184
Toxoids 59
Trabeculae 479
Tracheobronchial tree 334, 334f
Tractus solitarius, nucleus of 302, 509
Transcellular fluid 24f
Transcellular route 163
Transcytosis 17, 19
Transforming growth factor,
 secretion of 75
Transfusion reactions 71
Transmembrane proteins 2
Transneural degeneration 384
Transneuronal degeneration 385
Transport mechanism
 importance of 14
 role in 30

Transpulmonary pressure 340
Transverse colon 140
Transverse diameter 339
Traumatic shock 325
Traveling wave 505
 theory 506
Trehalase 138, 139
Trehalose glucohydrolase 138
Tremor 435
Trephone substances, production
 of 30
Tributyrin 120
Trichromatism 496, 497
Trichromats 497
Tricuspid area 290
Tricuspid valve 275, 277
Trigeminal ganglion 414
Trigeminal nerve 142
 divisions of 416t
 mandibular division of 499
 three divisions of 416f
Triglycerides 183, 219
Triiodothyronine 193, 194, 205
Triple heart sound 290
Tritanomaly 497
Tritanopia 496
Trochlear nerve 480
Tropic hormones 197
Tropical sprue 140
Tropomyosin 87
 role of 97
Troponin 87
 role of 97
Trousseau's sign 214
True capillaries 320
Trypsin 126, 128
 actions of 126
 autoactive action of 126
Trypsinogen 126
T-tubules 88
Tubectomy 272
 Tubercle bacilli 365
Tuberculosis 59, 175
Tubular necrosis 325
Tubular reabsorption 160, 163
Tubular secretion 160, 165
Tubules, U-shaped 166
Tubulin 60
Tubuloglomerular feedback 159, 162
Tumor necrosis factors, secretion 75
Tunica adventitia 278
Tunica albuginea 239, 248
Tunica externa 476
Tunica fibrosa 476
Tunica interna 477
Tunica intima, inner 278
Tunica media 476
 middle 278
Tunica nervosa 477
Tunica vaginalis 240
Tunica vasculosa 239, 476
Turner's syndrome 9
Twisting movements 436
Tympanic cavity 499
Tympanic membrane 499, 499f
 role of 504
 surface of 504
Tympanic reflex 499
Typhoid 51
Tyrosine 206

U

U wave 294
Ulcerative colitis 140
Ulnar pulse 314
Ultrafiltration 161
Ultrasonic Doppler transducer
 technique 300

Ultrasound scanning 256
Ultraviolet rays 367, 495
    protection from 184
Umbilical cord 263
Umbilical vein 322
Umbilical vessels 321
Umbilicus 184
Unipolar leads 293
Unipolar limb leads 293
Unipolar neurons 378
Universal donors 70
Universal recipients 70
Unnamed cells 118, 138
Uphill transport 16
Upper costal series 338
Upper esophageal sphincter 143
Upper frontal motor area 463
Upper motor neuron 409, 417
    lesion 398, 399
    effects of 417*t*
Upper respiratory tracts 334
Upper right atrium 275
Upper supravaginal portion 250
Uracil 9
Urea 168
    recirculation of 167, 168
Ureter 154, 177
    blockage of 175
    pelvis of 154
Urethra 177, 241, 469
    external 241
    functional anatomy of 177
    in female 178*f*
    in male 178*f*
Urethral constriction 175
Urethral sphincter 177, 179*t*
Uric acid 163
Urinary bladder 154, 177, 178*f*, 179*t*, 469
    and urethra, nerve supply to 178*f*
    filling of 179
    functional anatomy of 177
Urinary output 160
Urinary system 149*f*
Urine
    acidification of 170
    chemical analysis of 173
    color of 173
    composition of 173
    concentration 166, 168
    examination of 173, 174
    formation 160
    odor of 173
    osmolarity of 166
    passage of 154
    physical examination of 173
    properties of 173
Uriniferous tubules, parts of 150
Urobilinogen 133, 174
Uterine changes 253
Uterine vessels 321
Uterine wall, structure of 250
Uterus 200, 249
    contraction of 200
    divisions of 250
    effect on 250, 252
    section of 250*f*
Utriculo-saccular duct 451

■ V

V wave 316
Vacuoles 5
Vagal fibers 509
Vagal tone 303
Vagal trunks 118
Vagal withdrawal 329
Vagina 250
    epithelial cells of 259
Vaginal changes 253
Vaginal ring 271
Vaginal sponge 269
Vagovagal reflex 122
Vague pain 217
Vagus nerve 111, 125, 326, 420, 469
    dorsal nucleus of 302
    mode of action of 303
Valsalva experiment 311
Valsalva maneuver 311, 312*t*
Valvular diseases 291
Variable region 58
Varicose veins 321
Vas deferens 240
    ampulla of 241
    recanalization of 272
Vas efferens 240
Vasa recta 167
Vascular congestion 326
Vascular response, action on 226
Vascular spasm, severe 264
Vasectomy 272
Vasoactive intestinal
    peptide 122
    polypeptide 110, 123, 309
Vasoconstrictor area 302, 307
Vasoconstrictor center 307
Vasoconstrictor fibers 307
Vasodilatation 337
Vasodilator area 302, 307
Vasodilator fibers 307
Vasogenic shock 325
Vasomotor center 301, 307
Vasomotor system 307
Vasomotor tone 307
Vasopressin 309
Vasopressor action 200
Vasovagal syncope 326
Vegetative functions 469
    control of 446
Vena cava
    inferior 159, 275, 323
    superior 275, 323
Venous admixture 337
Venous blood pressure 311
    normal values of 311*b*
Venous drainage 317
Venous pressure 311
Venous pulse 313, 315
Venous return 299, 306, 337
Venous system 159, 279, 347
    vessels of 278
Ventilation
    method 372, 373
    volume, maximum 346
    wasted 348
Ventilation-perfusion ratio 348
Ventral posteromedial nucleus 423
Ventral root 400
Ventral spinocerebellar tract 404
Ventricular depolarization 294
Ventricular fibrillation 296, 297
Verbal aphasia 463
Vermis 430
Vertebral canal 400
Vesicular follicle 254
Vestibular apparatus
    functions of 451, 452
    hair cells of 452*f*
    nerve supply to 452
Vestibular membrane 500
Vestibulocerebellum 431
Vestibulocochlear nerve
    cochlear division of 502
    vestibular division of 452
Vestibulo-ocular reflex 453
Vibratory sensation 407*f*, 413
Villi 137
    movements of 146
Viral encephalitis 461
Viral infections 51
Virilism 230
Viropause 246
Visceral layer 151, 160, 333
Visceral muscle 84
Visceral organs 396
Visceral pain 420
Visceral pericardium, inner 276
Visceral reflexes 396
Visceral smooth muscle fibers 104
Visible spectrum 495
Vision
    acuity of 483, 485
    field of 482, 485
    sensation of 475
    test for acuity of 485
Visual acuity 485
Visual area
    primary 488
    secondary 463
Visual association area 488
Visual axis 475, 476*f*
Visual cortex 443, 487, 488
    areas of 444, 488
Visual defects 490*f*
Visual field 485, 486
Visual impulses
    interpretation of 444
    perception of 444
Visual pathway 487, 488*f*, 489
Visual perception 482
Visual process 482
    chemical basis of 484
    electrical basis of 484
    neural basis of 482
Visual receptor 482, 487
    cells 478
    functions of 483
    structure of 482, 483*f*
Visual transduction 484
Vital capacity 343-345
Vital organs 325
Vitamin 40
    A 484
    B_{12} 40
        deficiency 48
    D 40, 150
        activated 235
        metabolism 207
Vitreous body 479
Vitreous humor 479
Voice, effect on 244
Voltage-gated calcium channels 101, 391
Volume ventilator 373
Voluntary apnea 360
Voluntary breath holding 356
Voluntary hyperventilation 360
Voluntary movements
    initiation of 439
    regulation of 435
Voluntary muscle 83
Vomeronasal pits, form of 510
Vomeronasal receptors 184
Vomeropherins 184
Vomiting 144, 370
    reflex 145
von Willebrand disease 68
von Willebrand factor 62
    deficiency of 68

■ W

Waddling gait 217
Wakefulness
    center 428
    period of 457
Wald's visual cycle 484
Wall of heart, layers of 275
Wallerian degeneration 384
Wandering reticuloendothelial cells 74
Waning, causes for 363
Warm temperature 92
Warm-blooded animals 187
Waste
    disposal system 5
    materials diffuse 79
    products, excretion of 150
Watch test, tickling of 506
Water and electrolyte balance,
    regulation of 185
Water balance
    effect on 244
    maintenance of 26, 150, 336
    regulation of 32, 115, 428
Water diuresis 169
Water hammer pulse 315
Water intoxication 27
Water loss mechanism 336
Water metabolism, action on 226
Water pills 175
Waxing, causes for 363
Weber test 506
Weber-Fechner law 389
Wernicke's area 442, 443, 463, 503
Westergren method 44
Westergren tube 44, 45
Wheel movements 481
Wheezing 364
Whispering test 506
Whistling 364
White blood cells 28, 45, 49, 49*t*, 50*f*
    functions of 51
    lifespan of 50*t*, 51
    properties of 51
White commissure, anterior 402
White matter 377
    divisions of 402
White muscles 83
Whole blood transfusion 72
Wilson's disease 436
Wintrobe method 44
Wintrobe tube 44, 45
Wirsung's duct 125
Withdrawal reflex 396, 399
Wolffian duct 243
Worn-out organelles, degradation of 5
Wright's peak flowmeter 346

■ X

X wave 316
Xerostomia 116

■ Y

Y wave 316
Yellow body 256
Yellow fever 59
Yellow pigment 479
Young-Helmholtz trichromatic theory 492, 496

■ Z

Zollinger-Ellison syndrome 124
Zona fasciculata, glomerulosa, reticularis 224
    pellucida 254, 255
    vasculosa 248
Zygote 256, 262
Zymogen granules 120, 125

EU GSPR Authorised Reprsentative
Logos Europe, 9 rue Nicolas Poussin
1700, La Rochelle, France
Phone: +33 (0) 6 67 93 73 78
E-mail: contact@logoseurope.eu

www.ingramcontent.com/pod-product-compliance
Ingram Content Group UK Ltd.
Pitfield, Milton Keynes, MK11 3LW, UK
UKHW050430150426
5217IPUK00019B/1326